MEDICINE AND PHILOSOPHY
IN CLASSICAL ANTIQUITY

This work makes available for the first time in one dedicated volume Philip van der Eijk's selected papers on the close connections that existed between medicine and philosophy throughout antiquity. Medical authors such as the Hippocratic writers, Diocles, Galen, Soranus and Caelius Aurelianus elaborated on philosophical methods such as causal explanation, definition and division, applying concepts such as the notion of nature to their understanding of the human body. Similarly, philosophers such as Plato and Aristotle were highly valued for their contributions to medicine. This interaction was particularly striking in the study of the human soul in relation to the body, as illustrated by approaches to topics such as intellect, sleep and dreams, and diet and drugs. With a detailed introduction surveying the subject as a whole and a new chapter on Aristotle's treatment of sleep and dreams, this wide-ranging collection is essential reading for students and scholars of ancient philosophy and science.

PHILIP J. VAN DER EIJK is Professor of Greek at the University of Newcastle upon Tyne. He has published widely on ancient philosophy, medicine and science, comparative literature and patristics. He is the author of *Aristoteles. De insomniis. De divinatione per somnum* (Berlin: Akademie Verlag, 1994) and of *Diocles of Carystus. A Collection of the Fragments with Translation and Commentary* (2 vols., Leiden: Brill, 2000–1). He has edited and co-authored *Ancient Histories of Medicine. Essays in Medical Doxography and Historiography in Classical Antiquity* (Leiden: Brill, 1999) and co-edited *Ancient Medicine in its Socio-Cultural Context* (2 vols., Amsterdam and Atlanta: Rodopi, 1995).

MEDICINE AND PHILOSOPHY IN CLASSICAL ANTIQUITY

Doctors and Philosophers on Nature, Soul, Health and Disease

PHILIP J. VAN DER EIJK

Professor of Greek at the University of Newcastle upon Tyne

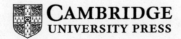

PUBLISHED BY THE PRESS SYNDICATE OF THE UNIVERSITY OF CAMBRIDGE
The Pitt Building, Trumpington Street, Cambridge, United Kingdom

CAMBRIDGE UNIVERSITY PRESS
The Edinburgh Building, Cambridge CB2 2RU, UK
40 West 20th Street, New York NY 10011-4211, USA
477 Williamstown Road, Port Melbourne, VIC 3207, Australia
Ruiz de Alarcón 13, 28014 Madrid, Spain
Dock House, The Waterfront, Cape Town 8001, South Africa

http://www.cambridge.org

© Philip van der Eijk 2005

This book is in copyright. Subject to statutory exception
and to the provisions of relevant collective licensing agreements,
no reproduction of any part may take place without
the written permission of Cambridge University Press.

First published 2005

Printed in the United Kingdom at the University Press, Cambridge

Typeface Adobe Garamond 11/12.5 pt.   *System* LATEX 2ε   [TB]

A catalogue record for this book is available from the British Library

Library of Congress Cataloguing in Publication data
Eijk, Ph. J. van der (Philip J.)
Medicine and philosophy in classical antiquity: doctors and philosophers
on nature, soul, health and disease / Philip J. van der Eijk.
p.   cm.
Includes bibliographical references and indexes.
ISBN 0 521 81800 1 (hardback)
1. Medicine, Greek and Roman.   2. Medicine, Ancient.
3. Medicine – Philosophy.   4. Soul.   5. Nature.   I. Title.
R135.E36 2005
610′.938 – dc22   2004056141

ISBN 0 521 818 001 hardback

For Arachne

Contents

Acknowledgements	*page* ix
Note on translations	xiii
Note on abbreviations	xiv
Introduction	1

I HIPPOCRATIC CORPUS AND DIOCLES OF CARYSTUS

1 The 'theology' of the Hippocratic treatise *On the Sacred Disease* — 45

2 Diocles and the Hippocratic writings on the method of dietetics and the limits of causal explanation — 74

3 To help, or to do no harm. Principles and practices of therapeutics in the Hippocratic Corpus and in the work of Diocles of Carystus — 101

4 The heart, the brain, the blood and the *pneuma*: Hippocrates, Diocles and Aristotle on the location of cognitive processes — 119

II ARISTOTLE AND HIS SCHOOL

5 Aristotle on melancholy — 139

6 Theoretical and empirical elements in Aristotle's treatment of sleep, dreams and divination in sleep — 169

7 The matter of mind: Aristotle on the biology of 'psychic' processes and the bodily aspects of thinking — 206

8	Divine movement and human nature in *Eudemian Ethics* 8.2	238
9	*On Sterility* ('*Hist. an.* 10'), a medical work by Aristotle?	259

III LATE ANTIQUITY

10	Galen's use of the concept of 'qualified experience' in his dietetic and pharmacological works	279
11	The Methodism of Caelius Aurelianus: some epistemological issues	299

Bibliography	328
Index of passages cited	379
General index	396

Acknowledgements

Since the original publication of these papers I have taken the opportunity to make some, mostly minor, revisions to some chapters, mainly on points of style and presentation, in order to enhance accessibility. Thus quotations from Greek and Latin are now accompanied by English translations or paraphrase, and in several cases words in Greek script have been transliterated. I have also in a number of cases taken account of publications that have come out since the paper was first published; there have, however, been no changes to the substance, and all revisions have been clearly marked by square brackets; in some cases I have presented them in the form of a postscript at the end of the relevant chapter, so as to facilitate reference to the original publication.

Chapter 1 was first published in *Apeiron* 23 (1990) 87–119, and is reprinted (with slight, mainly stylistic alterations) with the kind permission of Academic Printing and Publishing.

Chapter 2 was first published in R. Wittern and P. Pellegrin (eds.), *Hippokratische Medizin und antike Philosophie* (Medizin der Antike, Band 1), Hildesheim: Olms, 1996, 229–57, and is reprinted here with the kind permission of Olms Verlag; but the numeration of the Diocles fragments, and the translation of fr. 176 printed here have been modified in accordance with the relevant sections in my *Diocles of Carystus*, Leiden, 2000, which are reprinted here with the kind permission of Brill Academic Publishers.

Chapter 3 is a slightly expanded version of a paper published under the title 'The systematic status of therapy in the Hippocratic Corpus and in the work of Diocles of Carystus', in I. Garofalo, D. Lami, D. Manetti and A. Roselli (eds.), *Aspetti della terapia nel Corpus Hippocraticum*, Florence: Olschki, 1999, 389–404, reprinted with the kind permission of Olschki Editore; an abbreviated version in Dutch appeared under the title 'Helpen, of niet schaden. Enkele uitgangspunten van therapeutisch handelen in de klassieke Griekse geneeskunde' in *Hermeneus* 71 (1999) 66–71.

Chapter 4 was first published in Dutch under the title 'Hart en hersenen, bloed en pneuma. Hippocrates, Diocles en Aristoteles over de localisering van cognitieve processen' in *Gewina* 18 (1995) 214–29, and has been translated (and slightly adapted) for the present volume by Arachne van der Eijk-Spaan.

Chapter 5 was first published in German under the title 'Aristoteles über die Melancholie' in *Mnemosyne* 43 (1990) 33–72, and has been translated (and slightly adapted) for the present volume by Arachne van der Eijk-Spaan.

Chapter 6 is in its present form a new paper, although it is based on material published in my book *Aristoteles. De insomniis. De divinatione per somnum*, Berlin: Akademie Verlag, 1994, and in three articles: 'Theorie und Empirie in Aristoteles' Beschäftigung mit dem Traum und mit der Weissagung im Schlaf', in K. Döring and G. Wöhrle (eds.), *Antike Naturwissenschaft und ihre Rezeption*, vol. IV, Bamberg: Collibri Verlag, 1994, 31–46; 'Aristotle on "distinguished physicians" and on the medical significance of dreams', in P. J. van der Eijk, H. F. J. Horstmanshoff and P. H. Schrijvers (eds.), *Ancient Medicine in its Socio-Cultural Context* (Clio Medica/The Wellcome Institute Series in the History of Medicine 28–9), Amsterdam and Atlanta: Rodopi, 1995, vol. II, 447–59; and 'Aristotle on cognition in sleep', in T. Wiedemann and K. Dowden (eds.), *Sleep* (Nottingham Classical Literature Series / Midlands Classical Series 8), Bari: Levante Editori, 2003, 25–40.

Chapter 7 was first published in W. Kullmann and S. Föllinger (eds.), *Aristotelische Biologie. Intentionen, Methoden, Ergebnisse* (Philosophie der Antike, vol. VI), Stuttgart: Steiner Verlag, 1997, 221–58, and is reprinted with the kind permission of Steiner Verlag.

Chapter 8 was first published in *Hermes* 117 (1989) 24–42, and is reprinted (with alterations in presentation) with the kind permission of Steiner Verlag.

Chapter 9 was first published in *The Classical Quarterly* 49 (1999) 490–502, and is reprinted with the kind permission of Oxford University Press.

Chapter 10 was first published in A. Debru (ed.), *Galen on Pharmacology. Philosophy, History and Medicine* (Studies in Ancient Medicine 15), Leiden: Brill, 1997, 35–57, and is reprinted with the kind permission of Brill Academic Publishers.

Chapter 11 was first published in P. Mudry (ed.), *Le traité des Maladies aiguës et des Maladies chroniques de Caelius Aurelianus: nouvelles approches*, Nantes: Institut Universitaire de France, 1999, 47–83, and is reprinted with the kind permission of the Institut Universitaire de France.

Acknowledgements

I should further like to express my gratitude to the institutions, colleagues and friends who have provided financial, professional and personal support and encouragement during the many years in which the papers collected in this volume were produced. The earlier papers were written when I held a research assistantship, and subsequently a post-doctoral research fellowship, at the Classics Department of Leiden University. I am grateful to Leiden University for its institutional support, to the University Library for providing excellent resources, to the Leiden colleagues for their departmental support, and to the Netherlands Organisation for Scientific Research (NWO) for awarding the post-doctoral research fellowship.

The more recent papers date from my tenure of a Wellcome Trust University Award in the History of Classical Medicine at the University of Newcastle upon Tyne. I am grateful to the Governors of the Wellcome Trust for awarding me this fellowship, to Newcastle University for its institutional support in general – and for offering me a Personal Chair in Greek in particular – to the Newcastle University Arts and Humanities Research Fund for providing financial assistance towards the translation of chapters 4 and 5, to the Robinson Library for its support, and to my colleagues in the Newcastle Classics Department for providing a most congenial academic and social environment. I should further like to express my thanks to the Royal Netherlands Academy of Arts and Sciences (KNAW) for awarding me a fellowship at the Netherlands Institute for Advanced Study (NIAS) in 2000/1, which allowed me to pursue the study of ancient medicine in comparative context.

The papers collected here have greatly benefited from the comments made on oral presentations by audiences at a number of European and American universities, and from the many colleagues and friends who generously offered critical advice and encouragement on drafts. I should like to express a particular word of thanks to Jochen Althoff, Egbert Bakker, Lesley Dean-Jones, Armelle Debru, Jeanne Ducatillon, Sophia Elliott, Klaus-Dietrich Fischer, Hellmut Flashar, Sabine Föllinger, Elisabeth Foppen, Bill Fortenbaugh, Ivan Garofalo, Mark Geller, Hans Gottschalk, Mirko Grmek, Frans de Haas, Jim Hankinson, Donald Hill, Manfred Horstmanshoff, David Langslow, Charles van Leeuwen, Geoffrey Lloyd, James Longrigg, Daniela Manetti, Jaap Mansfeld, Phillippe Mudry, Vivian Nutton, Jan van Ophuijsen, Dobrinka Parusheva, Peter Pormann, Jonathan Powell, Marlein van Raalte, Amneris Roselli, Thomas Rütten, Trevor Saunders,

Mark Schiefsky, Piet Schrijvers, Chris Sicking, Wesley Smith, Richard Sorabji, Heinrich von Staden, Michael Stokes, Gisela Striker, Wim Verdenius, Henk Versnel, Jürgen Wiesner and Han Zuilhof.

I am grateful to Michael Sharp from Cambridge University Press for the interest he has taken in this volume and for his patience, to the anonymous referees for the Press for their comments on the proposal, and to the editorial staff at CUP for their care in bringing this publication to completion. I am also indebted to Sarah Francis (Newcastle) for her assistance with the technical preparation of the copy.

Finally, I owe a very special word of thanks to my wife Arachne, who translated two of the chapters for this volume and who has provided invaluable support and encouragement throughout all my academic work. I dedicate this volume to her with profound gratitude and affection.

Note on translations

All translations of Greek and Latin texts are my own, except in those cases where I have used the following:

the translations of the Hippocratic writings by W. H. S. Jones and P. Potter (quoted in the introduction and throughout part one), published by Harvard University Press in the Loeb Classical Library as *Hippocrates*, volumes 2/148 (1923), 4/150 (1931), 5/472 (1988) and 6/473 (1988);

the translation of Theophrastus' *On the Causes of Plants* by B. Einarson and G. K. K. Link (quoted in chapter 2), published by Harvard University Press in the Loeb Classical Library as Theophrastus, *De causis plantarum*, volumes 1/471 (1976) and 3/475 (1990);

the translation of Aristotle's *History of Animals*, Book 10, by D. M. Balme (quoted in chapter 9), published by Harvard University Press in the Loeb Classical Library as Aristotle, *History of Animals, Books VII-X*, volume II/439 (1991);

the translation of Theophrastus' fragments by W. W. Fortenbaugh et al. (quoted in chapter 2), published by Brill in 1992;

the translation of Theophrastus' *Metaphysics* by M. van Raalte (quoted in chapter 2), published by Brill in 1993;

the translation of Galen's *On Medical Experience* by R. Walzer (quoted in chapter 2), published by Oxford University Press in 1944 and reprinted by Hackett in 1985;

the translation of Caelius Aurelianus' *On Acute Affections* by I. Drabkin (quoted in chapter 4), published by the University of Chicago Press in 1950;

and the translation of Plato's *Republic* by G. Grube and D. Reeve (quoted in chapter 6), published by Hackett in 1997.

Note on abbreviations

Abbreviations of authors' names and works follow those used in the *Oxford Classical Dictionary*, ed. S. Hornblower and A. Spawforth (3rd edn, Oxford, 1999), apart from works of Galen, which follow G. Fichtner, *Corpus Galenicum* (Tübingen, 1990) and are explained in the text.

Hippocratic texts are normally cited by reference to the volume and page numbers of the Littré edition (L.): E. Littré, *Œuvres complètes d'Hippocrate* (10 vols., Paris, 1839–61). Thus 4.270 L. refers to vol. IV, p. 270, of Littré's edition.

Works of Galen are referred to according to the volume and page numbers of the edition by Kühn (K.): C. G. Kühn, *Claudii Galeni opera omnia*, 22 vols. (Leipzig, 1821–33, reprinted Hildesheim, 1964–5). Thus 5.244 K. refers to vol. V, p. 244, of Kühn's edition.

Introduction

Few areas in classical scholarship have seen such rapid growth as the study of ancient medicine. Over the last three decades, the subject has gained broad appeal, not only among scholars and students of Greek and Roman antiquity but also in other disciplines such as the history of medicine and science, the history of philosophy and ideas, (bio-)archaeology and environmental history, and the study of the linguistic, literary, rhetorical and cultural aspects of intellectual 'discourse'. The popularity of the subject even extends beyond the confines of academic communities, and ancient medicine has proved to be an effective tool in the promotion of the public understanding of medicine and its history.

The reasons for these changes are varied and complex, and to do justice to all would require a much fuller discussion than I can offer here.[1] In this introductory chapter, I will concentrate on what I perceive to be the most important developments and in so doing set out the rationale of the present collection of papers. Evidently, ancient medicine possesses remarkable flexibility in attracting interest from a large variety of people approaching the field from a broad range of disciplines, directions and backgrounds, for a number of different reasons and with a wide variety of expectations. The purpose of publishing these papers in the present form is to make them more easily accessible to this growing audience.

I FROM APPROPRIATION TO ALIENATION: DEVELOPMENTS IN THE STUDY OF ANCIENT MEDICINE

First, there has been a major shift in overall attitude and general perception with regard to the history and historiography of medicine in classical antiquity. Until about thirty years ago it was customary for Greek medicine to

---

[1] See also Nutton (2002).

be viewed as one aspect of what was sometimes referred to as *le miracle grec* or the 'Enlightenment' – the sudden, surprising rise of Greek civilisation, inexplicably emerging against the background of the primitive barbarism of earlier times. Like Greek literature, philosophy, art, architecture and democracy, ancient medicine was seen as one of those uniquely Greek contributions to the development of European culture and humanity. 'Rational' medicine, based on empirical observation and logical systematisation, and devoid of any superstitious beliefs in supernatural powers intervening in the human sphere, was believed to have been invented by the Greeks and to have developed teleologically into the impressive edifice of contemporary biomedical science and practice as we know it today.

This 'appropriating' claim was illustrated with such powerful examples as the sharp clinical observations recorded in the case histories of the Hippocratic *Epidemics*, the defiant rejection of supernatural explanations of disease by the author of *On the Sacred Disease*, the search for natural and empirically observable causes by the author of *On Ancient Medicine*, and of course the high ethical standards advocated by the Hippocratic *Oath*. These and other documents constituted the medical part of the Greek miracle, and they served very well as examples for classicists to cite when it came to promoting the study of Greek and Roman culture and demonstrating its relevance to the modern world. They also provided the cachet of a respectable historical tradition with which Western medicine believed it could identify and, perhaps legitimately, claim to stand in a special relationship of continuity, while at the same time taking pride in having emancipated itself from this tradition through the spectacular achievements of medical science in the nineteenth and twentieth centuries.

Yet, curiously, these examples and the underlying attitude and motivation for referring to them somehow also seem to have posed an obstacle to a closer study of the actual evidence. For while, in many other areas of classical studies, the belief in this 'Greek miracle' had long been eroded, if not abandoned, the perception of Greek and Roman *medicine* as the paradigm of rationality and the ancestor of contemporary biomedical science and practice was remarkably persistent.[2] One of the reasons for this was that, for a long time, the academic study of the field was a rather narrowly defined specialism, which very rarely had an impact beyond its own boundaries. It was mainly the territory of medical historians, often employed in (or retired from) medical faculties or other areas of the medical profession, and had

---

[2] Two exceptions that should be mentioned here are Kudlien (1967a), which is a relatively early examination of some of the more 'irrational' elements in Greek medicine, and of course Dodds (1951), although the latter does not deal specifically with medicine. On Ludwig Edelstein see below.

little appeal among classicists. Of course, there were exceptions on either side, and the names of such eminent historians of medicine as Karl Sudhoff, Henry Sigerist and Owsei Temkin, who devoted much attention to antiquity, could be paralleled by classicists such as Hermann Diels, Ludwig Edelstein, Karl Deichgräber and Hans Diller. But the reason why the latter are well known to most classical scholars is that they published also on mainstream, canonical classical subjects such as Aristophanes, Sophocles, the Presocratics, Plato, Aristotle and Posidonius. And at any rate (with the exception of Edelstein), their approach to ancient medicine had always been rather strictly philological, focusing on the texts of the great masters such as Hippocrates and Galen, but paying little attention to the social, cultural, economic, institutional, geographical and religious environment in which medical writing took place. For the rest, the subject was largely neglected: the majority of classicists considered it too medical and too technical, while the fact that the main texts were in Latin and Greek (and often in a quite technical, austere kind of Latin and Greek at that) did not help to secure the subject a prominent place in the attention of medical historians or members of the medical profession at large.

Nothing could be further from my intention than to dismiss the contribution of members of the medical profession to the study of ancient medicine – indeed, I myself have often benefited from the collaboration and dialogue with medically trained colleagues when studying ancient Greek medical texts. Still, it is fair to say that, especially in the first half of the twentieth century, the interest taken by medical people in Greek and Roman medicine was often motivated, apart from antiquarian intellectual curiosity, by what we could call a positivist, or presentist, attitude. There often was an underlying tendency to look for those respects in which Greek medicine was, as it were, 'on the right track', and to measure the extent to which the Greeks 'already knew' or 'did not yet know' certain things which contemporary biomedicine now knows, or claims to know, to be true.[3] This attitude led to a historiography of medicine (and science) which was predominantly conceived as a success story and which was preoccupied with great discoveries such as the nervous system or blood circulation, with heroic medical scientists such as Hippocrates, Galen, Harvey and Boerhaave, and with retrospective diagnosis of diseases in the past on the basis of great literary masterpieces such as Thucydides' account of the Athenian 'plague' or Daniel Defoe's *Journal of the Plague Year*. In other words, it was inspired by

---

[3] A striking example is the vigorous debate initiated by R. Kapferer in the 1930s on the question whether the Hippocratic writers were familiar with the process of blood circulation; for a review of this debate see Duminil (1998) 169–74.

a kind of teleological progressivism that pays particular attention to those aspects in which classical medicine still 'speaks' to us today.

But times have changed. Postmodernism, pluralism, cultural relativism and comparativism, as in so many other areas, have had their impact also on the study of Greek medicine and science. Questions have been asked about the uniqueness of Greek medical thought, and it has been suggested that its debt to earlier, Near Eastern and Egyptian thinking may have been much greater than was commonly assumed. Questions have also been raised about the rationality of Greek medical thought, about the assumption that Greek medicine developed 'from myth to reason',[4] and Greek medicine has been shown to have been much more open and receptive to superstition, folklore, religion and magic than was generally believed.

Furthermore, in the academic study of medical history – and to a certain extent also in the historiography of science – significant changes have occurred over the past decades, especially in the area of medical anthropology, the social, cultural and institutional history of medicine and science, the history of medical ethics, deontology and value systems, and the linguistic study and 'discourse analysis' of medical texts. There has been an increasing realisation of the social and cultural situatedness of medicine, healthcare and knowledge systems: individuals, groups of individuals and societies at large understand and respond differently to the perennial phenomena of sickness and suffering, health and disease, pain and death; and these reactions are reflected in different medical ideas, different 'healthcare systems', different value systems, each of which has its own social, economic and cultural ramifications. This appreciation of the variety of healthcare (and knowledge) systems – and indeed of the variety within one system – is no doubt related to the increasing acceptance of 'alternative' or 'complementary' medicine in the Western world and the corresponding changes in medical practice, doctor–patient relationship and the public perception of the medical profession. And the traditional assumption of a superiority of Western, scientific medicine over non-Western, 'primitive', 'folklore' or 'alternative' medicine has virtually reached the state of political incorrectness.

This shift in attitude has had rather paradoxical implications for the study of ancient medicine. In short, one could say that attention has widened from texts to contexts, and from 'intellectual history' to the history of 'discourses' – beliefs, attitudes, perceptions, expectations, practices and rituals, their underlying sets of norms and values, and their social and cultural ramifications. At the same time, the need to perceive continuity between

---

[4] For a more extended discussion of this development see the Introduction to Horstmanshoff and Stol (2004).

Greek medicine and our contemporary biomedical paradigm has given way to a more historicising approach that primarily seeks to understand medical ideas and practices as products of culture during a particular period in time and place. As a result, there has been a greater appreciation of the diversity of Greek medicine, even within what used to be perceived as 'Hippocratic medicine'. For example, when it comes to the alleged 'rationality' of Greek medicine and its attitude to the supernatural, there has first of all been a greater awareness of the fact that much more went on in Greece under the aegis of 'healing' than just the elite intellectualist writing of doctors such as Hippocrates, Diocles and Galen.[5] Moreover, it has been shown that although the Hippocratic writers did not positively encourage recourse to divine healing, they did not categorically reject it either. Thus, as I argue in chapter 1 of this volume, the author of *On the Sacred Disease*, in his criticism of magic, focuses on a rather narrowly defined group rather than on religious healing as such, and his insistence on what he regards as a truly pious way of approaching the gods suggests that he does not intend to do away with any divine intervention; and the author of the Hippocratic work *On Regimen* even positively advocates prayer to specific gods in combination with dietetic measures for the prevention of disease. Questions have further been asked about the historical context and representativeness of the Hippocratic *Oath* and about the extent to which Hippocratic deontology was driven by considerations of status and reputation rather than moral integrity. And the belief in the superiority of Greek medicine, its perceived greater relevance to modern medical science – not to mention its perceived greater efficacy – compared with other traditional healthcare systems such as Chinese or Indian medicine, has come under attack. As a result, at many history of medicine departments in universities in Europe and the United States, it is considered naïve and a relic of old-fashioned Hellenocentrism to start a course in the history of medicine with Hippocrates.

This change of attitude could, perhaps with some exaggeration, be described in terms of a move from 'appropriation' to 'alienation'. Greek, in particular Hippocratic medicine, is no longer the reassuring mirror in which we can recognise the principles of our own ideas and experiences of health and sickness and the body: it no longer provides the context with which we can identify ourselves. Nevertheless, this alienation has brought about a very interesting, healthy change in approach to Greek and Roman medicine, a change that has made the subject much more interesting and

---

[5] For an example see the case study into experiences of health and disease by 'ordinary people' in second- and third-century CE Lydia and Phrygia by Chaniotis (1995).

accessible to a wider group of scholars and students. An almost exclusive focus on medical ideas and theories has given way to a consideration of the relation between medical 'science' and its environment – be it social, political, economic, or cultural and religious. Indeed 'science' itself is now understood as just one of a variety of human cultural expressions, and the distinction between 'science' and 'pseudo-science' has been abandoned as historically unfruitful. And medicine – or 'healing', or 'attitudes and actions with regard to health and sickness', or whatever name one prefers in order to define the subject – is no longer regarded as the intellectual property of a small elite of Greek doctors and scientists. There is now a much wider definition of what 'ancient medicine' actually involves, partly inspired by the social and cultural history of medicine, the study of medical anthropology and the study of healthcare systems in a variety of cultures and societies. The focus of medical history is on the question of how a society and its individuals respond to pathological phenomena such as disease, pain, death, how it 'constructs' these phenomena and how it contextualises them, what it recognises as pathological in the first place, what it labels as a disease or aberration, as an epidemic disease, as mental illness, and so on. How do such responses translate in social, cultural and institutional terms: how is a 'healthcare system' organised? What status do the practitioners or 'providers' of treatment enjoy? How do they arrive at their views, theories and practices? How do they communicate these to their colleagues and wider audiences, and what rhetorical and argumentative techniques do they use in order to persuade their colleagues and their customers of the preferability of their own approach as opposed to that of their rivals? How is authority established and maintained, and how are claims to competence justified? The answers to these questions tell us something about the wider system of moral, social and cultural values of a society, and as such they are of interest also to those whose motivation to engage in the subject is not primarily medical. As the comparative history of medicine and science has shown, societies react to these phenomena in different ways, and it is interesting and illuminating to compare similarities and differences in these reactions, since they often reflect deeper differences in social and cultural values.[6]

From this perspective, the study of ancient medicine now starts from the basic observation that in the classical world, health and disease were matters of major concern which affected everyone and had a profound effect on the way people lived, what they ate and drank, how they organised their private

---

[6] See the work of G. E. R. Lloyd, especially his (1996a), (2002) and (2003).

and public hygiene and healthcare, and how they coped – physically as well as spiritually – with pain, illness and death. In this light, the emergence of Greek 'rational' medicine, as exemplified in the works of Hippocrates, Galen, Aristotle, Diocles, Herophilus, Erasistratus and others, was one among a variety of reactions and responses to disease. Of course, this is not to deny that the historical significance of this response has been tremendous, for it exercised great influence on Roman healthcare, on medieval and early modern medicine right through to the late nineteenth century, and it is arguably one of the most impressive contributions of classical antiquity to the development of Western medical and scientific thought and practice. But to understand how it arose, one has to relate it to the wider cultural environment of which it was part; and one has to consider to what extent it in turn influenced perceptions and reactions to disease in wider layers of society. The medical history of the ancient world comprises the role of disease and healing in the day-to-day life of ordinary people. It covers the relations between patients and doctors and their mutual expectations, the variety of health-suppliers in the 'medical marketplace', the social position of healers and their professional upbringing, and the ethical standards they were required to live up to.[7] And it also covers the material history of the ancient world, the study of diseases and palaeopathology; for in order to understand reactions to the pathological phenomena, and to explain differences between those reactions, it is obviously of vital importance to establish with as much certainty as possible the nosological reality of ancient Greece and the Eastern Mediterranean.[8]

As a result of these developments – and greatly helped by scholarly efforts to make the subject more accessible by means of modern translations of the original texts – increasing numbers of students of the Greek and Roman world have now embraced ancient medicine as a new area of research with very interesting implications for the wider study of classical antiquity. It is almost by definition an interdisciplinary field, involving linguists and literary scholars, ancient historians, archaeologists and environmental historians, philosophers and historians of science and ideas, but also historians of religion, medical anthropologists and social scientists. Thus, as we shall see in the next pages, medical ideas and medical texts have enjoyed a surge of interest from students in ancient philosophy and in the field of Greek and Latin linguistics. Likewise, the social and cultural history of ancient medicine, and the interface between medicine, magic

---

[7] See, e.g., Nutton (1992) and (1995).
[8] See Grmek (1983) and (1989); Sallares (1991) and (2003).

and religion has proved a remarkably fruitful area of research;[9] and similar observations can be made about areas such as women and gender studies and studies into 'the body'.[10]

2 PHILOSOPHY AND MEDICINE IN CONTEXT

A second, more specific impetus towards the contextualisation of ancient medicine has come from the study of ancient philosophy,[11] and this brings us closer to the title and rationale of this book. Indeed, my own interests in ancient medicine were first raised when I was studying Aristotle's *Parva naturalia* and came to realise that our understanding of his treatment of phenomena such as sleep, dreams, memory and respiration can be significantly enhanced when placing it against the background of medical literature of the fifth and fourth centuries. Fifteen years later the relevance of Greek medicine to the study of ancient philosophy is much more widely appreciated, not only by historians of science and medicine but also by students of philosophy in a more narrow sense.

Scholarship has, of course, long realised that developments in ancient medical thought cannot be properly understood in isolation from their wider intellectual, especially philosophical context.[12] But more recently there has been a greater appreciation of the fact that Greek medical writers did not just reflect a derivative awareness of developments in philosophy – something which led to the long-standing qualification of medicine as a 'sister' or 'daughter' of philosophy – but also actively contributed to the formation of philosophical thought more strictly defined, for example by developing concepts and methodologies for the acquisition of knowledge and understanding of the natural world. And even though this awareness has occasionally led to some philosophical cherry-picking, it has done much to put authors such as Galen, Diocles, Soranus and Caelius Aurelianus on the agenda of students of ancient thought.

Furthermore, the study of ancient medicine has benefited from a number of major developments within the study of ancient philosophy itself. First, as in the case of medicine, the notion of 'philosophy' too has been more explicitly contextualised and historicised, and there is now a much greater awareness of the difference between contemporary definitions of what constitutes philosophical inquiry and what Greek thinkers understood when

---

[9] See, e.g., section 3 in van der Eijk, Horstmanshoff and Schrijvers (1995).
[10] See especially the works by Gourevitch, H. King, Dean-Jones, A. E. Hanson, Flemming and Demand listed in the bibliography.
[11] See especially the titles by Hankinson, Frede, Barnes and Longrigg listed in the bibliography.
[12] See van der Eijk (2005c), sections from which have been adopted and adjusted to the present chapter.

Introduction 9

using the word – or if they did not, in what other terms they conceived their own activities.[13] Secondly, the activity of 'philosophers' in ancient Greece and Rome is now increasingly understood in social and cultural terms and with reference to their role in society, their practical activities and the ideas and values they shared with the communities in which they lived and worked.[14] Thirdly, and more specifically, scholars in ancient philosophy have come to realise that a number of 'philosophers' too had their own particular reasons for being interested in areas and themes that we commonly associate with medicine and for pursuing these interests in a variety of forms, theoretical as well as practical – and, in so doing, were interacting with medical writers in the setting of their agendas, the formation of their ideas, concepts and methodologies and in their practical activities.[15] And fourthly, students of ancient philosophy have drawn attention to the variety of modes and notions of 'rationality' in Greek thought;[16] important lessons can be learned from this for the claims about the 'rational' nature of Greek medical thought, and of 'rationality' as such.[17]

---

[13] For an example of this regarding the early classical Greek period see Laks and Louguet (2002).
[14] See, e.g., Griffin and Barnes (1989).
[15] For an older account see Schumacher (1940); for a more recent discussion see Frede (1986).
[16] See Frede and Striker (1996).
[17] The notion of 'rational' medicine has long been taken for granted, as it was felt that it was undeniable that there was such a thing as Greek rational medicine, which was perceived to lie in the examples of Hippocratic rationalism and empiricism as referred to above – aspects in which Greek medicine was perceived to be different from Egyptian or Babylonian medicine. As I have already indicated, this notion of rational medicine, together with the presuppositions underlying it, has come under attack more recently and is sometimes dismissed as an old-fashioned relic from a positivist way of thinking that is regarded as something that has long been superseded. Nevertheless one needs to be careful here and not give way too easily to relativism or deny to Greek medicine any distinctive character compared to what preceded it. The crucial question here, though, is how one defines 'rationality'. As far as medicine is concerned, it seems that the discussion would be clarified if an important distinction were made between two uses of the word 'rational'. First, there is the use of 'rational' as opposed to 'irrational' or 'supernatural', by which the characteristic element of Greek medicine is seen to lie in the absence of any appeal to gods or divine or supernatural powers. I have already discussed this above, when we saw that the view that Greek medicine was free from such appeals is too simplistic. In particular, one could ask what is so 'rational' about the claim made by the author of *On the Sacred Disease* that all diseases are divine and all are human (see ch. 1). Is this rational by his standards, or by ours? Or what is 'rational' about the assumption of the existence of four humours in the body, which the writer of *On the Nature of Man* simply posits, or about the role of the number seven in medicine, which the author of *On Fleshes* takes as a given? Examples like these could easily be multiplied. Yet a different use of the word 'rational' is in the sense in which ancient medical writers themselves used it, where 'rational' stands for 'rationalist', 'theoretical' (*logikos, rationalis*) as opposed to empirical/practical, thus denoting the speculative, theoretical nature of Greek medical thought and its close relation with natural philosophy, epistemology, etc. On this view, one can safely say – and comparisons with other ancient medical traditions have confirmed – that Greek medicine, with its emphasis on explanation, its search for causes, its desire for logical systematisation, its endeavour to provide an epistemic foundation for prognosis and treatment, and especially its argumentative nature and urge to give account (*logos, ratio*) of its ideas and practices in debate, does show a distinctive character.

The title of this volume still refers to 'medicine' and 'philosophy' as distinct disciplines, and to some extent this is appropriate, for there were important differences between the two areas. Yet the longer one studies this material, the more one realises that too rigid a use of these and similar labels is in serious danger of concealing the very substantial overlap that existed between the various areas of activity. In particular, it is in danger of misrepresenting the views which the main protagonists in Greek thought had about the disciplines or intellectual contexts in which they positioned themselves. Moreover, it would be quite misleading to present the relationship between 'doctors' and 'philosophers' in terms of interaction between 'science' and 'philosophy', the 'empirical' and the 'theoretical', the 'practical' and the 'systematical', the 'particular' and the 'general', or 'observation' and 'speculation'. To do this would be to ignore the 'philosophical', 'speculative', 'theoretical' and 'systematic' aspects of Greek science as well as the extent to which empirical research and observation were part of the activities of people who have gone down in the textbooks as 'philosophers'. Thus Empedocles, Democritus, Parmenides, Pythagoras, Philolaus, Plato, Aristotle, Theophrastus, Strato, but also later thinkers such as Sextus Empiricus, Alexander of Aphrodisias, Nemesius of Emesa and John Philoponus took an active interest in subjects we commonly associate with medicine, such as the anatomy and the physiology of the human body, mental illness, embryology and reproduction, youth and old age, respiration, pulses, fevers, the causes of disease and of the effects of food, drink and drugs on the body. As we shall see in chapter 3, according to one major, authoritative ancient source, the Roman author Celsus (first century CE), it was under the umbrella of 'philosophy' (*studium sapientiae*) that a theoretical, scientific interest in health and disease first started, and it was only when the physician Hippocrates 'separated' the art of healing from this theoretical study of nature that medicine was turned into a domain of its own for the first time – yet without fully abandoning the link with 'the study of the nature of things', as Celsus himself recognises when reflecting on developments in dietetics during the fourth century BCE.

This perception of the early development of medicine and its overlap with philosophy was more widely shared in antiquity, both by medical writers and by 'philosophers'. This is testified, for example, by ancient historiographical and doxographical accounts of the history of medicine and philosophy, which tend to provide an illuminating view of the 'self-perception' of ancient thinkers.[18] When reflecting on the past history

---

[18] See van der Eijk (1999a).

of their own subject, medical authors such as Galen – who wrote a treatise advocating the view that the best doctor is, or should be, at the same time a philosopher – and the so-called Anonymus Londiniensis (the first-century CE author of a medico-doxographical work preserved on papyrus) treated Plato's views on the human body and on the origins of diseases as expounded in the *Timaeus* on a par with the doctrines of major Greek medical writers; and Aristotle and Theophrastus continued to be regarded as authorities in medicine by medical writers of later antiquity such as Oribasius and Caelius Aurelianus. Conversely, as we shall see in chapter 6, a philosopher such as Aristotle commented favourably on the contributions by 'the more distinguished doctors' to the area of 'natural philosophy'. And in the doxographical tradition of 'Aëtius', in the context of 'physics' or 'natural philosophy', a number of medical writers such as Diocles, Herophilus, Erasistratus and Asclepiades are cited alongside 'philosophers' such as Plato, Aristotle and the Stoics for their views on such topics as change, the soul, the location of the ruling part of the soul (see chapter 4), dreams, respiration, monstrosities, fertility and sterility, twins and triplets, the status of the embryo, mules, seventh-month children, embryonic development, and the causes of old age, disease and fever.[19]

The subtitle of this volume, 'nature, soul, health and disease' indicates some of the more prominent areas in which such interaction between 'philosophers' and medical writers was most clearly visible. It is no coincidence that Aristotle's comments on the overlap between 'students of nature' and 'doctors' are made in his own *Parva naturalia,* a series of works on a range of psycho-physiological topics – sense-perception, memory, sleep, dreams, longevity, youth and old age, respiration, life and death, health and disease – that became the common ground of medical writers and philosophers alike. And, not surprisingly, Aristotle makes similar remarks in his zoological works concerning questions of anatomy, such as the parts of the body and structures like the vascular system, and embryology, especially the question of the origins of life, the mechanisms of reproduction and the ways in which inherited features are passed on from one generation to another, the question of the male and female contribution to the reproductive process, the origin of the semen, questions of fertility and infertility (see chapter 9), stages of embryonic development, the way the embryo is nourished, twins and triplets, and suchlike. This whole area was referred to in later antiquity as 'the nature of man', particularly man's physical make-up, ranging from the lowest, most basic level of 'principles'

[19] See Runia (1999).

(*archai*) or 'elements' (*stoicheia*) of organic substances through anatomical structures such as bones and the vascular system, fluids such as humours, qualities such as hot and cold, and physiological proportions and 'blendings' (*kraseis*) right through to the most sophisticated psycho-physical functions such as soul, sense-perception, thinking and reproduction. We perceive this 'agenda' in texts as early as the Hippocratic works *On Fleshes*, *On the Nature of Man* and *On Regimen*, or in such later works as Nemesius' *On the Nature of Man*, Vindicianus' *On the Nature of the Human Race* and in the treatise *On the Seed*, preserved in a Brussels manuscript and attributed to Vindicianus, and there are similar points of overlap in the doxographical tradition. Even a philosopher like Plato, who seems to have had very little reason to be interested in mundane matters like disease or bodily waste products, deals at surprising length and in very considerable detail with the human body and what may go wrong with it, using an elaborate classification of bodily fluids and types of disease (physical as well as mental) according to their physiological causes. Plato was of course not a doctor, but he was clearly aware of the medical doctrines of his time and took them sufficiently seriously to incorporate them into this account of the nature of the world and the human body as set out in the *Timaeus*.

Yet interaction was not confined to matters of content, but also took place in the field of methodology and epistemology. As early as the Hippocratic medical writers, one finds conceptualisations and terminological distinctions relating to such notions as 'nature' (*phusis*), 'cause' (*aitia, prophasis*), 'sign' (*sēmeion*), 'indication' (*tekmērion*), 'proof' (*pistis*), 'faculty' (*dunamis*), or theoretical reflection on epistemological issues such as causal explanation, observation, analogy and experimentation. This is continued in fourth-century medicine, with writers such as Diocles of Carystus and Mnesitheus of Athens, in whose works we find striking examples of the use of definition, explanation, division and classification according to genus and species relations, and theoretical reflection on the modalities and the appropriateness of these epistemological procedures, on the requirements that have to be fulfilled in order to make them work. In Hellenistic medicine, authors such as Herophilus and Erasistratus made important theoretical points about causation, teleological versus mechanical explanation, and *horror vacui*, and in the 'sectarian' debates between Empiricists, Dogmatists and Methodists major theoretical issues were raised about the nature of knowledge and science. Subsequently, in the Imperial period, we can observe the application and further development of logic and philosophy of science in writers such as Galen (chapter 10) and Caelius Aurelianus (chapter 11). And again, it is by no means the case that the medical writers were exclusively on the receiving end: theories about causation or inference from signs constitute good examples of areas in which major theoretical and conceptual distinctions were first formulated in medical discourse and subsequently incorporated in philosophical discussions.[20]

It would therefore be quite wrong to regard Aristotle's and Galen's perceptions of the overlap between medicine and philosophy as anachronistic distortions or projections of their own preoccupations, or to believe that, when 'philosophers' had medical interests, these were nothing more than eccentric curiosity. To the Greek thinkers, areas such as those mentioned above represented aspects of natural and human reality just as interesting and significant as the movements of the celestial bodies, the origins of earthquakes or the growth of plants and trees, and at least equally revealing of the underlying universal principles of stability and change. Nor were their interests in the medical area limited to theoretical study or the pursuit of knowledge for its own sake without extending to 'clinical' or 'therapeutic' practice. Some are known to have put their ideas into practice, such as Empedocles, who seems to have been engaged in considerable therapeutic activity, or Democritus, who is reported to have carried out anatomical research on a significant scale, or, to take a later example, Sextus Empiricus, who combined his authorship of philosophical writings on Scepticism with medical practice.

Such connections between theory and practical application, and such combinations of apparently separate activities, may still strike us as remarkable. Nevertheless we should bear in mind, first, that especially in the period up to about 400 BCE (the time in which most of the better-known Hippocratic writings are believed to have been produced), 'philosophy' was hardly ever pursued entirely for its own sake and was deemed of considerable practical relevance, be it in the field of ethics and politics, in the technical mastery of natural things and processes, or in the provision of health and healing. Secondly, the idea of a 'division of labour' which, sometimes implicitly, underlies such a sense of surprise is in fact anachronistic. We may rightly feel hesitant to call people such as Empedocles, Democritus, Pythagoras and Alcmaeon 'doctors', but this is largely because that term conjures up associations with a type of professional organisation and specialisation that developed only later, but which are inappropriate to the actual practice of the care for the human body in the archaic and classical period. The evidence for 'specialisation' in this period is scanty, for doctors

---

[20] See, e.g., Hankinson (1987) on the role of the Pneumatist physician Athenaeus of Attalia in the development of the notion of antecedent causation.

as well as mathematicians and other 'scientists', and there is good reason to believe that disciplinary boundaries, if they existed at all, were fluid and flexible. As we get to the Hellenistic and Imperial periods, the evidence of specialisation is stronger, but this still did not prevent more ambitious thinkers such as Galen or John Philoponus from crossing boundaries and being engaged in a number of distinct intellectual activities such as logic, linguistics and grammar, medicine and meteorology.

3 ARISTOTLE AND HIS SCHOOL

A case in point here is Aristotle, to whom the middle section of this volume is dedicated. It is no exaggeration to say that the history of ancient medicine would have been very different without the tremendous impact of Aristotelian science and philosophy of science throughout antiquity, the Middle Ages and the early modern period. Aristotle, and Aristotelianism, made and facilitated major discoveries in the field of comparative anatomy, physiology, embryology, pathology, therapeutics and pharmacology. They provided a comprehensive and consistent theoretical framework for research and understanding of the human body, its structure, workings and failings and its reactions to foods, drinks, drugs and the environment. They further provided fruitful methods and concepts by means of which medical knowledge could be acquired, interpreted, systematised and communicated to scientific communities and wider audiences. And through their development of historiographical and doxographical discourse, they placed medicine in a historical setting and thus made a major contribution to the understanding of how medicine and science originated and developed.

Aristotle himself was the son of a distinguished court physician and had a keen interest in medicine and biology, which was further developed by the members of his school. Aristotle and his followers were well aware of earlier and contemporary medical thought (Hippocratic Corpus, Diocles of Carystus) and readily acknowledged the extent to which doctors contributed to the study of nature. This attitude was reflected in the reception of medical ideas in their own research and in the interest they took in the historical development of medicine. It was further reflected in the extent to which developments in Hellenistic and Imperial medicine (especially the Alexandrian anatomists and Galen) were incorporated in the later history of Aristotelianism and in the interpretation of Aristotle's works in late antiquity. Aristotelianism in turn exercised a powerful influence on Hellenistic and Galenic medicine and its subsequent reception in the Middle Ages and early modern period.

Yet although all the above may seem uncontroversial, the relationship between Aristotelianism and medicine has long been a neglected area in scholarship on ancient medicine. The medical background of Aristotle's biological and physiological theories has long been underestimated by a majority of Aristotelian scholars – and if it was considered at all, it tended to be subject to gross simplification.[21] Likewise, on the medico-historical side, the contribution made by Aristotelianism to the development of medicine has long been largely ignored, especially as far as the later history of the Peripatetic school is concerned.[22] This seems to be due to a most unfortunate disciplinary dividing line between philosophers and historians of medicine: while the former used to regard the medical aspects of Aristotelian thought as philosophically less interesting, the latter usually did not engage in Aristotelianism because it was believed to be philosophy not medicine. These attitudes appear to have been based on what I regard as a misunderstanding of the Aristotelian view on the status of medicine as a science and its relationship to biology and physics, and on the erroneous belief that no independent medical research took place within the Aristotelian school. Aristotle's distinction between theoretical and practical sciences is sometimes believed to imply that, while doctors were primarily concerned with practical application, philosophers only took a theoretical interest in medical subjects.[23] As we have seen above, there are important exceptions to this rule; and Aristotle's own activities in the medical domain, too, have been more significant than has sometimes been appreciated. It is true that Aristotle was one of the first to spell out the differences between medicine and natural philosophy; but, as I argue in chapters 6 and 9, it is often ignored that the point of the passages in which he does so is to stress the substantial overlap that existed between the two areas. And Aristotle is making this point in the context of a theoretical, physicist account of psycho-physical functions, where he is wearing the hat of the *phusikos*, the 'student of nature'; but this seems not to have prevented him from dealing with more specialised medical topics in different, more 'practical' contexts. That such more practical, specialised treatments existed is suggested by the fact that in the indirect tradition Aristotle is credited with several writings on medical themes and with a number of doctrines on rather specialised medical topics. And as I argue in chapter 9, one of those medical works may well be identical to the text that survives in the form of book 10 of his *History of Animals*.

[21] For a discussion of an example of such simplification see ch. 9.
[22] Thus a recent medico-historical textbook like Conrad et al. (1995) devotes only two pages to Aristotle, and makes no reference at all to Theophrastus or the later Peripatos.
[23] For a fuller discussion see ch. 9.

Fortunately, there have recently been some encouraging signs of interest, such as the greater scholarly appreciation of Aristotle's awareness of, and receptivity to, Hippocratic and other medical literature (such as Diocles), the interest taken in early Peripatetic physiological ideas, the *opuscula* and fragments of Theophrastus, Strato, and the *Problems* (*Problemata physica*), and in the Anonymus Londiniensis.[24] Still, the subject of Aristotle's relationship to medicine is a vast area, and the study of the role of Aristotelianism in the development of ancient medicine is still in its infancy. Such a project would first of all have to cover the reception, transformation and further development of medical knowledge in the works of Aristotle and the early Peripatetic school. This would comprise a study of Aristotle's views on the status of medicine, his characterisation of medicine and medical practice, and his use and further development of medical knowledge in the areas of anatomy, physiology and embryology; and it would also have to comprise the (largely neglected) medical works of the early Peripatos, such as the medical sections of the *Problemata* and the treatise *On Breath*, as well as the works of Theophrastus and Strato on human physiology, pathology and embryology. It would further have to examine the development of medical thought in the Peripatetic school in the Hellenistic period and the reception of Aristotelian thought in the major Hellenistic medical systems of Praxagoras, Herophilus, Erasistratus and the Empiricists. Thirdly, it would have to cover the more striking aspects of Galen's Aristotelianism, such as the role of Aristotelian terminology, methodology, philosophy of science, and teleological explanation in Galen's work; and finally, it would have to consider the impact of developments in medicine after Aristotle – for example the Alexandrian discoveries of the nervous system and of the cognitive function of the brain, or the medical theories of Galen – on later Aristotelian thought and on the interpretation of Aristotle's biological, physiological and psychological writings in late antiquity by the ancient commentators, such as Alexander of Aphrodisias, Themistius, Simplicius and John Philoponus, or by authors such as Nemesius of Emesa and Meletius of Sardes. This is a very rich and challenging field, in which there still is an enormous amount of work to do, especially when artificial boundaries between medicine and philosophy are crossed and interaction between the two domains is considered afresh.

In the present volume, chapter 9 is a first step towards such a reassessment. It is concerned with what I claim to be an Aristotelian discussion

---

[24] In addition to older studies by Flashar (1962) and (1966) and Marenghi (1961), see the more recent titles by King, Manetti, Oser-Grote, Roselli, Fortenbaugh and Repici listed in the bibliography.

of the question of sterility, a good example of the common ground that connected 'doctors' and 'philosophers', in which thinkers like Anaxagoras, Empedocles, Democritus and Aristotle himself were pursuing very much the same questions as medical writers like the author of the Hippocratic embryological treatise *On Generation/On the Nature of the Child/On Diseases 4* or Diocles, and their methods and theoretical concepts were very similar.

But Aristotle's medical and physiological interests are also reflected in non-medical contexts, in particular in the fields of ethics and of psycho-physiological human functions such as perception, memory, thinking, imagination, dreaming and desire. Thus his concept of melancholy (ch. 5) presents a striking case study of an originally medical notion that is significantly transformed and applied to a completely new context, namely Aristotle's analysis of the physical causes of exceptional human success or hopeless failure, both in psychological and in ethical contexts. In the case of Aristotle's theory of sleep and dreams, too, there was a medical tradition preceding him, which he explicitly acknowledges; but as we will see in chapter 6, his willingness to accommodate the phenomena observed both by himself and by doctors and other thinkers before him brings him into difficulties with his own theoretical presuppositions. A similar picture is provided by the psychology and pathology of rational thinking (ch. 7), an area in which Aristotle recognises the role of bodily factors in the workings of the human intellect and where, again, an appreciation of the medical background of these ideas is helpful to our understanding of Aristotle's own position. And, moving to the domain of ethics, there is a very intriguing chapter in the *Eudemian Ethics*, in which Aristotle tries to give an explanation for the phenomenon of 'good fortune' (*eutuchia*), a kind of luck which makes specific types of people successful in areas in which they have no particular rational competence (ch. 8). Aristotle tackles here a phenomenon which, just like epilepsy in *On the Sacred Disease*, was sometimes attributed to divine intervention but which Aristotle tries to relate to the human soul and especially to that part of the soul that is in some sort of intuitive, instinctive way connected with the human *phusis* – the peculiar psycho-physical make-up of an individual. Thus we find a 'naturalisation' very similar to what we get in his discussion of *On Divination in Sleep* (see chapter 6). Yet at the same time, and again similar to what we find in *On the Sacred Disease*, the divine aspect of the phenomenon does not completely disappear: *eutuchia* is divine and natural at the same time. This is a remarkable move for Aristotle to make, and it can be better understood against the background of the arguments of the medical writers. Moreover, the phenomenon Aristotle describes has a somewhat peculiar, ambivalent status: *eutuchia* is natural yet not fully normal, and although it leads to success, it is not a desirable state to be in or to rely on – and as such it is comparable to the 'exceptional performances' (the *peritton*) of the melancholic discussed in chapter 5. We touch here on yet another major theme that has been fundamental to the development of European thought and in which ancient medicine has played a crucial role: the close link between genius and madness, which both find their origin in the darker, less controllable sides of human nature.

4 PHILOSOPHICAL INTERESTS OF MEDICAL WRITERS

As in the case of the pursuits of the 'philosophers' discussed above, it is, conversely, no exaggeration to say that what a number of Greek people whom we regard as medical thinkers were up to is very similar to, or at least coterminous with these. The fact that many of these writers and their works have, in the later tradition, been associated with Hippocrates and placed under the rubric of medicine, easily makes one forget that these thinkers may have had rather different conceptions of the disciplines or contexts in which they were working. Thus the authors of such Hippocratic works as *On the Nature of Man*, *On Fleshes*, *On the Nature of the Child*, *On Places in Man* and *On Regimen* as well as the Pythagorean writer Alcmaeon of Croton emphatically put their investigations of the human body in a physicist and cosmological framework. Some of them may have had very little 'clinical' or therapeutic interest, while for others the human body and its reactions to disease and treatment were just one of several areas of study. Thus it has repeatedly been claimed (though this view has been disputed) that the Hippocratic works *On the Art of Medicine* and *On Breaths* were not written by doctors or medical people at all, but by 'sophists' writing on *technai* ('disciplines', fields of systematic study with practical application) for whom medicine was just one of several intellectual pursuits. Be that as it may, the authors of *On Regimen* and *On Fleshes*, for instance, certainly display interests and methods that correspond very neatly to the agendas of people such as Anaxagoras and Heraclitus, and the difference is of degree rather than kind.

A further relevant point here is that what counted as medicine in the fifth and fourth centuries BCE was still a relatively fluid field, for which rival definitions were continuously being offered. And 'medicine' (*iatrikē*), like 'philosophy', was not a monolithic entity. There was very considerable diversity among Greek medical people, not only between the 'rational', philosophically inspired medicine that we find in the Hippocratic writings on the one hand and what is sometimes called the 'folk medicine' practised by drugsellers, rootcutters and suchlike on the other, but even among more intellectual, elite physicians themselves. One of the crucial points on which they were divided was precisely the 'philosophical' nature of medicine – the question of to what extent medicine should be built on the foundation of a comprehensive theory of nature, the world and the universe. It is interesting in this connection that one of the first attestations of the word *philosophia* in Greek literature occurs in a medical context – the Hippocratic work *On Ancient Medicine* – where it is suggested that this is not an area with which medicine should engage itself too much. It is clear from the context that what the author has in mind is approaches to medicine that take as their point of departure a general theory about 'nature' (*phusis*), more in particular theories that reduce all physical phenomena to unproven 'postulates' (*hupotheseis*), such as the elementary qualities hot, cold, dry and wet – theories which the author associates with the practice of Empedocles, who reduced natural phenomena to the interaction and combinations of the four elements earth, fire, water and air. The polemical tone of the treatise suggests that such 'philosophical' approaches to medicine were becoming rather popular, and this is borne out by the extant evidence such as that provided by the Hippocratic treatises mentioned above. There were a number of medical authors for whom what we call 'philosophy' would not have been an inappropriate term to describe their projects – regardless of whether or not they knew and used the term.

To this group certainly belongs the author of the treatise which is deservedly one of the most famous writings in the Hippocratic Corpus, *On the Sacred Disease*. As I alluded to above, this work has long been read as the paradigm of Greek fifth-century rationalism. And it is certainly true that this author, in claiming that epilepsy 'has a nature', is doing something very similar to what the Presocratics did in inquiring into the 'nature' (*phusis*) of things, namely their origin, source of growth and identifying structure – be they earthquakes and solar eclipses, or bodily processes and changes, illnesses, conditions, affections, symptoms, or substances like foods, drinks, drugs and poisons and the effects they produced on the bodies of human beings. And just like Ionian philosophers such as Anaximenes and Anaxagoras in their explanations of earthquakes, solar eclipses, thunderstorms and other marvellous phenomena, he produces a 'natural' explanation for a phenomenon – in his case 'the so-called sacred disease', epilepsy – that used to be seen as the manifestation of immediate divine agency. Epilepsy, the author argues, like all other diseases (and, one may add, like all other phenomena), has its own 'nature', its peculiar determined, normal, stable and self-contained identity. Knowledge of this identity, and of the regularity that results from this, will allow one to recognise and understand individual instances of the phenomenon, to predict its future occurrence and by medical intervention influence it or even prevent it from happening or spreading. And in making this claim, the author polemicises against people whom he calls 'magicians, quacks, charlatans', who regard the disease as a form of whimsical, unpredictable divine intervention or even demonic possession and whose therapeutic practice is determined by magical beliefs and procedures. He describes the development of the disease from its earliest, prenatal and indeed ancestral stages; he identifies the brain as the seat of consciousness (a theme I shall examine in greater depth in chapter 4) and as the primary organ affected by the disease; he discusses a whole range of additional factors, both internal and external, that set the disease in motion or influence its actual development; and he gives a vivid account of the various stages of an epileptic seizure, relating each of the symptoms to a particular underlying physiological cause.

Yet for all the emphasis on the naturalness and 'rationality' of his approach, we shall see in chapter 1 that the author rules out neither the divinity of the diseases nor the possibility of divine intervention as such. He is distinguishing between an appropriate appeal to the gods for purification from the 'pollution' (*miasma*) of moral transgressions (*hamartēmata*) that has disturbed the relationship between man and the gods, and an inappropriate appeal to the gods for the purification of the alleged pollution of the 'so-called sacred disease'. This is inappropriate, he says, for diseases are not sent by a god – to say so would be blasphemous, he insists – they are natural phenomena which can be cured by natural means, and they do not constitute a pollution in the religious sense. The text has often been read as if the author ruled out divine 'intervention' *as such*. But in fact, there is no evidence that he does – indeed, he does not even rule out that gods may cure diseases, if approached in the proper way and on the basis of appropriate premises.

Such negative readings of the text attributing to the author the ruling out of all forms of divine intervention have presumably been inspired by a wishful belief among interpreters to 'rationalise' or 'secularise' Hippocratic medicine – a belief possibly inspired by the desire to see Hippocratic medicine as the forerunner of modern biomedicine, and which can be paralleled with interpretative tendencies to 'demythologise' philosophers such as Parmenides, Pythagoras and Empedocles to make them fit our concept of 'philosophy' more comfortably. Yet recently, there has been a renewed appreciation of the 'mythical' or 'religious' aspects of early Greek thought, and a readiness to take documents such as the Dervenyi papyrus, the introduction of Parmenides' poem and the *Purifications* of Empedocles more seriously. Similar 'paradigm' shifts have taken place in the study of Hippocratic medicine, and there is now a much greater willingness among interpreters[25] to accept the religious and 'rational' elements as coexistent and – at least in their authors' conception – compatible. The question is not so much to disengage from their mythical context those elements which we, or some of us, regard as philosophically interesting from a contemporary perspective, but rather to try to see how those elements fit into that context. Within this approach, the author of *On the Sacred Disease* can be regarded as an exponent of a modified or 'purified' position on traditional religious beliefs without abandoning those beliefs altogether and, as such, he can be said to have contributed also to the development of Greek religious or theological thought; for his arguments closely resemble those found in Plato's 'outlines of theology' in the second book of the *Republic*, or, as I said above, Aristotle's arguments against the traditional belief that dreams are sent by the gods in his *On Divination in Sleep* (see also chapter 6).

One further, paradoxical aspect of *On the Sacred Disease* and its alleged 'rationality' is worth mentioning here. On the one hand, it is probably the best known of all the Hippocratic writings after the *Oath*, and its author (who is widely agreed to be also the author of *Airs, Waters, Places*) has often been regarded as one of the most plausible candidates for being identical with the historical Hippocrates. On the other hand, this is a fairly recent development, which stands in marked contrast to the rather marginal position the treatise occupied in ancient perceptions of Hippocrates. It hardly figures in ancient lists of Hippocratic writings, and it is particularly striking for its almost complete absence from Galen's references to the Hippocratic Corpus. This is all the more remarkable considering that it is by far the most suitable piece of evidence for Galen's claim that Hippocrates held an encephalocentric view of the mind (see chapter 4); there is even a suggestion that Galen may have regarded the treatise as spurious. This indicates the changeability of assessments of a treatise's importance and representativeness, and hence the danger of using ancient evaluations as evidence in the so-called 'Hippocratic question'.

5 MEDICINE BEYOND 'HIPPOCRATES'

I have already touched on the great diversity among the writings attributed to Hippocrates and, at some time long after they were written, assembled

---

[25] See, e.g., Jouanna (1998) and (2003); and Hankinson (1998c).

under the heading of 'Hippocratic Corpus'. As has been recognised ever since antiquity, these 'Hippocratic' writings are not the work of one author; rather, they constitute a heterogeneous group of over sixty treatises, which display great differences in content and style. None of these writings mention the name of their author, and none provide secure internal evidence as to date and geographical or intellectual provenance. Whether any of these works were written by the historical Hippocrates himself and, if so, which, has been the object of centuries of scholarly debate, but none of the proposed candidates have found widespread acceptance, and the question has proved unanswerable.[26] More recently, however, even the assumption that these works, regardless of the question of their authorship, all derive directly or indirectly from a Hippocratic medical 'school' or 'community' on the island of Cos has been exposed as the product of wishful thinking by scholars (and of anachronistic extrapolation of early twentieth-century models of medical institutional organisation) rather than something based on evidence.[27]

The upshot of all this is that there is no secure basis for regarding and studying the Hippocratic writings as a 'collection' and individual writings as part of such a collection, even though this has been the norm for many centuries. There is no intrinsic tie that connects these writings more closely with each other than with the works of other authors, medical and philosophical, of the same period that did not have the good fortune of having been preserved. It is true that some Hippocratic writings clearly refer or react to each other, or display such great similarities in doctrine and style that it is likely that they derive from a common background (and in some cases even from a common author). Yet similarly close connections can be perceived between some of these works and the fragments of some Presocratic philosophers (e.g. between the author of the Hippocratic *On Regimen* and philosophers such as Anaxagoras or Heraclitus), or of 'non-Hippocratic' medical writers such as Philistion of Locri or Alcmaeon of Croton. To suggest otherwise – a suggestion still implicitly present in most talk of 'Hippocratic medicine', 'Hippocratic thought' and so on – is in danger of making misleading use of traditional labels. In fact, it is almost certainly the case that none of these treatises were conceived and written with a view to the collection in which later tradition grouped them together (and there are good reasons to believe that the constitution of a Hippocratic 'Corpus' happened several centuries after they were written). The only thing the

---

[26] For a discussion see Lloyd (1991a) and Jouanna (1999).
[27] See Smith (1990a) for a discussion of the historical evidence.

'Hippocratic writings' have in common is that they are written in the Ionic dialect and that they were, at some stage of their tradition, attributed to, or associated with, Hippocrates – the latter on grounds we in most cases do not know, and which may have been different from one case to another. This fact of their being associated with Hippocrates may well have been the reason why they have been preserved, whereas the works of the many other medical and philosophical writers who are known to us by name only survive in fragments. Their attribution to Hippocrates may also have been the reason why the names of their original authors were suppressed – their anonymity, once stripped of their 'Hippocratic' label, standing in marked contrast to the confidence with which contemporaneous prose authors like Herodotus and Hecataeus put their names at the beginning of their works. Whatever the answer to these questions may be, there is no intrinsic reason to look for a unified doctrine in these works, and the fact that two treatises have been handed down as part of the Hippocratic collection does not provide any *a priori* indication regarding their intellectual affinity.

There is therefore every reason to study the Hippocratic writers in close connection with the many other medical thinkers that are known to have worked in the fifth and fourth centuries, such as Diocles of Carystus, Praxagoras of Cos, or the twenty-plus medical writers mentioned in the Anonymus Londiniensis. Again, the realisation of their importance is a very recent scholarly development, partly as a result of new discoveries or fresh examinations of existing evidence;[28] and although their works survive only in fragments, there is at least one respect in which these authors compare favourably to the Hippocratic Corpus. They provide an opportunity to form a picture of individual medical writers which we do not have in the case of the Hippocratic Corpus, where, because of the anonymity of the writings, it has become effectively impossible to appreciate the role of individual doctors in the formation of Greek medicine. By contrast, with people such as Diocles and Praxagoras, we have a considerable number of titles of works that they are reported to have authored as well as fragments reflecting a wide range of different areas of interest. And although for some of these works and areas our evidence is restricted to a few lines, it nevertheless gives us a good idea of the sheer scope and extent of their scientific interests and literary activity, which we simply cannot gain in the case of the writers of the Hippocratic Corpus.

One such 'non-Hippocratic' medical author was Diocles of Carystus, whose importance in antiquity was rated so highly that he was given the

---

[28] See van der Eijk (2000a) and (2001a); see also Manetti (1999a) and Orelli (1998).

title of 'younger Hippocrates' or deemed 'second in age and fame to Hippocrates'. He practised in the fourth century BCE, and although we know very little of his life, we can safely assume that he was one of the most prominent medical thinkers of antiquity.[29] His interests ranged widely, and he is reported to have written at least twenty works (some of them in at least four books) on a great variety of areas such as anatomy, physiology, digestion, fevers, prognostics, pathology, therapeutics, bandages, gynaecology, embryology, surgery, dietetics, hygiene and regimen in health, foods, wines, herbs, vegetables, olive oil, drugs, poisons, sexuality, and possibly also mineralogy and meteorology. He clearly had a keen interest in 'the phenomena' and in the practical aspects of medical care, and he rated the results of long-term medical experience very highly. Yet at the same time Diocles was known for his theoretical and philosophical outlook and for his tendency to build his medical views on a general theory of nature. There are good reasons to believe that he was well in touch with the medical and philosophical thinkers of his time, that he knew a number of the Hippocratic writings and that he was familiar with, and to, Aristotle and Theophrastus. Furthermore, he appears to have positioned himself prominently in the intellectual debates of the fourth century, and to have played a major role in the communication of medical views and precepts to wider audiences in Greek society by means of highly civilised literary writings in the Attic dialect. The basis for his fame may lie partly in the impressive range of subjects he dealt with, the almost encyclopaedic coverage of the subject of medicine and allied sciences such as botany, biology, and possibly mineralogy and meteorology, the considerable size of his literary production and the stylistic elegance his work displayed. But a further possible reason may have been Diocles' philosophical and theoretical orientation and his tendency to relate his medical views to more general theoretical views on nature (see frs. 61, 63, 64),[30] just like the 'Hippocrates' referred to by Socrates in the well-known passage in Plato's *Phaedrus* (270 c–d). For from the remains of his work Diocles emerges as a very self-conscious scientist with a keen awareness of questions of methodology, a fundamental belief that treatment of a particular part of the body cannot be effective without taking account of the body as a whole (fr. 61) and of the essence of disease (fr. 63), and a strong desire for systematisation of medical knowledge. Diocles' use of notions such as *pneuma*, humours and elementary qualities, his use of inference from signs

---

[29] For a collection and discussion of the evidence and an account of Diocles' views and historical importance see van der Eijk (2000a) and (2001a), from which the following paragraph is adapted.
[30] References to Diocles' fragments are according to the numeration in van der Eijk (2000a).

(cf. fr. 56), his references to obscure causes (fr. 177), his interest in cognition, sense-perception and locomotion, and even in the field of dietetics his endeavours to develop and systematise dietetics into a detailed regimen for health and hygiene aimed at disease prevention – all this confirms the 'theoretical', 'philosophical' nature of Diocles' medical outlook. It must have been these characteristics which prompted later Greek medical writers to reckon Diocles among the so-called Dogmatist or Rationalist physicians, who preferred to base medicine on a proper, theoretical and philosophical foundation, and who wanted to raise medicine from a craft to a systematic and explanatory intellectual discipline that obeyed the strict rules of logical coherence.

Nevertheless, as we have seen, there was also a tradition in antiquity that represented Hippocrates as being hostile to philosophy, indeed as the one who liberated medicine as an empirical, practical art aimed at treatment of diseases from the bondage of theoretical philosophical speculation (cf. fr. 2). And there is that side to Diocles as well; for, as we shall see in chapters 2 and 3, several fragments testify to Diocles' awareness that the use of theoretical concepts and explanatory principles constantly has to be checked against the empirical evidence, and that their appropriateness to individual circumstances has to be considered time and time again in each individual case. Diocles' reputation as the first to write a handbook on anatomy, in which he provided detailed descriptions of all the parts of the human body including the female reproductive organs, and his status as one of the leading authorities in the area of gynaecology, as well as the fame of some of his surgical instruments and bandages all suggest that we are dealing not only with a writer, communicator and thinker, but also with an experienced practitioner.

Yet whatever the title of 'younger Hippocrates' means, it certainly does not imply, and perhaps was not meant to suggest, that Diocles faithfully followed in the footsteps of the Father of medicine in all respects. For, as we will see in chapter 2, several fragments of his works bear out that, whatever the authority of Hippocrates may have been in Diocles' time, it did not prevent Diocles from taking issue with some ideas and practices that are similar to what is to be found in texts which we call Hippocratic. Diocles can therefore be regarded as an independent key figure in the interaction between medicine and natural philosophy (at least in its epistemological results) in one of the founding periods of Greek science who long exercised a powerful influence on later Greek medicine. Diocles provides an important connection between Hippocratic medicine and Aristotelian science, and he is a major contributor to the development of early Hellenistic medicine, especially because of his anatomical research and discoveries, his views on physiology, embryology and the role of *pneuma*, his views on gynaecology, and his development of a theory of regimen in health, food, and lifestyle, thus contributing to the increasing influence of doctors and medical writers on areas such as hygiene, cookery, gymnastics and sports.

Apart from Diocles' more specifically medical views, his relationship to the Hippocratic writers is also manifest in two issues that reflect the 'meta-medical' or philosophical nature of his approach to medicine. First, there are the principles of Dioclean therapeutics, which are at the heart of the question about the purposes of medical activity, and especially therapeutic intervention, in the light of more general considerations regarding the ethical aspects of medical practice and the question of the limits of doctors' competence with regard to areas not strictly concerned with the treatment of disease (ch. 3). The Hippocratic writings, and especially the famous *Oath*, first of all reflect on the duties and responsibilities the doctor has in relation to the patient, for example in articulating such famous principles as 'to do no harm', not to cause death, or in advocating confidentiality, self-restraint, discretion, gentleness, acting without fear or favour. Yet, interestingly, they also emphasise the need for moral and religious integrity of the practitioner and for correspondence between theory and practice. Furthermore, in the field of dietetics, the Hippocratics' development of the notions of moderation, 'the mean', and the right balance between opposites provided concepts and ways of thinking that found their way into ethical discussions as we find them in Plato and Aristotle; and, paradoxically, their tendency to 'naturalise' aspects of human lifestyle such as sexual behaviour, physical exercise, eating and drinking patterns by presenting these in terms of healthy or harmful provided useful arguments to those participants in ethical debates stressing the naturalness or unnaturalness of certain forms of human behaviour.

A further issue that occupied the interests of philosophers as well as medical writers like the Hippocratic writers and Diocles was the question of the location of the mind, or the question of the cognitive function of the heart, the blood and the brain (ch. 4). This was a question that later attracted great interest in Hellenistic philosophy, where medical evidence played a major (though by no means decisive) role in the discussion, but the way for this debate was already paved in the medical writings of the fifth century, though in a slightly different context, for in their discussions of disease, the Hippocratic writers frequently also discussed mental illness and other disturbances of the mental, cognitive, behavioural or motor functions of the body. What is striking here is that in many of these cases the authors do not make a categorical distinction between 'mind' and 'body': all mental affections are presented as being of a physical nature and having a physical cause. And even those authors who speak about 'soul' (*psuchē*) as distinct from the body, such as the author of *On Regimen*, still conceive of the soul as something physical, whose workings and failings can be described in material terms – for example a particular blend of fire and water – and influenced by dietary measures.

In this connection, a further major medical writer beyond the Hippocratic Corpus must be mentioned. Praxagoras of Cos is usually referred to in the handbooks of the history of medicine mainly for his 'discovery' of the difference between veins and arteries, his doctrine of the pulse and his assumption of the so-called 'vitreous' humour. A closer study of the extant material reveals interesting 'philosophical' features such as reflection on inference from signs, distinctions between various types of causes and symptoms; and of course Praxagoras presents a further intriguing example of a doctor connecting Hippocratic medical views (after all, he came from Cos), Alexandrian medicine (he was the teacher of Herophilus) and Chrysippus and the early Stoa.

Praxagoras thus marks the transition from the classical to what has come to be known as the 'Hellenistic' period. Here, again, interaction between the domains of philosophy, medicine and science was particularly lively. To do justice to all the relevant developments of that extremely significant period would require a separate volume; some brief remarks must suffice here, which are important for the understanding of what is at issue in chapters 10 and 11. As in the case of Diocles and Praxagoras, our knowledge of the actual views held by the main protagonists in Hellenistic medicine is obscured by the fact that all their works have been lost and the remaining evidence is fraught with difficulties as a result of fragmentation and distortion by the source-authors. Yet thanks in particular to some recent major scholarly contributions, both with regard to the ancient philosophical schools and their cultural context and to medicine and science, our view of the relevant stages has been significantly enhanced.[31]

First, as I have already mentioned, there is the very significant role of Aristotelianism in the development of medical research, as testified by the fragments of authors in the Peripatetic tradition itself such as Theophrastus and Strato, or by the compilation of medical ideas as found in the Pseudo-Aristotelian *Problemata physica*. But also later Peripatetics such as Clearchus and Dicaearchus display a keen interest in medical and physiological

---

[31] See especially von Staden (1989), Garofalo (1988) and Guardasole (1997).

questions; and moving on to the Imperial period, a particular mention must be made of Alexander of Aphrodisias, the second-century CE philosopher and commentator on Aristotle's works. Two works on medical topics (*Medical Problems, On Fevers*) are attributed to Alexander, and even though their authenticity is disputed, there is no question that Alexander had a great interest in medical issues (from a non-clinical, physiological point of view). And he is clearly taken seriously as an authority in these areas by his slightly later contemporary Galen. Furthermore, the two most striking representatives of early Hellenistic medicine, Herophilus and Erasistratus, are both reported to have held close connections with the Peripatetic school. This is most evident in the case of Erasistratus, whose ideas on mechanical versus teleological explanation mark a continuation of views expressed by Theoprastus and Strato and to some extent already by Aristotle himself. Likewise, Herophilus' famous, if enigmatic, aphorism that 'the phenomena should be stated first, even if they are not first', can be connected with Aristotelian philosophy.

Yet to suggest that Erasistratus and Herophilus were 'Aristotelians' would do grave injustice to their highly original ideas and the innovative aspects of their empirical research, such as Herophilus' discovery of the nervous system and Erasistratus' dissections of the brain and the valves of the heart. It also ignores their connections with developments in other sciences, notably mechanics, and with other philosophical movements, such as Scepticism (in particular regarding whether causes can be known) and Stoicism.

The Hellenistic period was also the time in which the medical 'sects' came into being: Empiricism, Dogmatism and Methodism. What separated these groups was in essence philosophical issues to do with the nature of medical knowledge, how it is arrived at and how it is justified. The precise chronological sequence of the various stages in this debate is difficult to reconstruct, but the theoretical issues that were raised had a major impact on subsequent medical thinking, especially on the great medical systems of late antiquity, namely Galen's and Methodism.

Galen is one of those authors who have been rediscovered by classicists and students of ancient philosophy alike, be it for his literary output, his mode of self-presentation and use of rhetoric, the picture he sketches of the intellectual, social and cultural milieus in which he works and of the traditions in which he puts himself, and the philosophical aspects of his thought – both his originality and his peculiar blends of Platonism, Hippocratism and Aristotelianism. Galen's work, voluminous in size as well as in substance, represents a great synthesis of earlier thinking and at the same time a systematicity of enormous intellectual power, breadth and versatility. In chapter 10, I shall consider Galen's theoretical considerations about pharmacology, and in particular his views on the relationship between reason and experience. Although in the field of dietetics and pharmacology he is particularly indebted to the Empiricists, his highly original notion of 'qualified experience' represents a most fortunate combination of reason and experience; and one of Galen's particular strengths is his flexibility in applying theoretical and experiential approaches to different domains within medical science and practice.

Among Galen's great rivals were the Methodists, a group of medical thinkers and practitioners that was founded in the first century BCE but came to particular fruition in the first and second centuries CE, especially under their great leader Soranus. Although their approach to medicine was emphatically practical, empirical and therapy-oriented, their views present interesting philosophical aspects, for example in epistemology and in the assumption of some kind of corpuscular theory applied to the human body. Regrettably, most works written by the Methodists survive only in fragments, and much of the evidence is biased by the hostile filter of Galen's perception and rhetorical presentation.[32] It is therefore most fortunate that we have a direct Methodist voice speaking in the work of Caelius Aurelianus, the (presumably) fifth-century CE author of several medical works, including two major treatises on acute and chronic diseases. Caelius has long been dismissed as an unoriginal author who simply translated the works of Soranus into Latin. However, recent scholarship has begun to appreciate Caelius' originality and to examine his particular version of Methodism.[33] My discussion (chapter 11) of a number of epistemological issues in Caelius' work such as causal explanation, definition, inference from signs, and reason and experience, ties in with this recent development.

6 THE TEXTUALITY AND INTERTEXTUALITY OF MEDICINE AND PHILOSOPHY

We have seen that ancient medicine and ancient philosophy, rather than being completely separate disciplines, interacted and overlapped in a number of ways. This overlap not only concerned the ideas, concepts and methodologies they entertained, but also the ways and forms in which they expressed and communicated these ideas, the modalities of dissemination and persuasion, and the settings in which they had to work and present

---

[32] For a collection of the fragments of the Methodists see now Tecusan (2004).
[33] See Mudry (1999).

their ideas. I touch here on a further aspect in which the study of ancient medicine – and philosophy – has recently been contextualised, and in this case the impetus has come from a third area of research we need to consider briefly because of its particular relevance to the papers collected in this volume, namely the field of textual studies or, to use a more recent and specific term, 'discourse analysis'.

One only needs to point to the twenty-two volumes of Kühn's edition of the works of Galen or the ten tomes of Littré's edition of the works of Hippocrates to realise that ancient medical literature has been remarkably well preserved, at least compared with many other areas of classical Greek and Latin literature. While much philological spade-work has been done to make these texts more accessible, especially in projects such as the *Corpus Medicorum Graecorum* or the *Collection des Universités de France*, many parts of this vast corpus of literature, to which newly discovered texts continue to be added, still await further investigation.

There still is, of course, a great basic demand for textual studies, editions, translations, commentaries and interpretative analyses – and in this respect, the triennial conferences on Greek and Latin medical texts have proved remarkably fruitful. Yet apart from this, there is an increasing interest being taken in medical, scientific and philosophical texts, not just because of their intellectual contents but also from the point of view of linguistics, literary studies, discourse analysis, narratology, ethnography of literature (orality and literacy), rhetoric and communication studies. This is related to a growing scholarly awareness of the communicative and competitive nature of Greek medicine and science. Greek doctors, philosophers, astronomers and mathematicians had to impress their audiences, to persuade them of their competence and authority, to attract customers and to reassure them that they were much better off with them than with their rivals. Medical, scientific and philosophical texts functioned in a specific setting, with a particular audience and purpose, and served as vehicles not only for the transmission of ideas but also for the assertion of power and authority.

These developments have given rise to a whole new field of studies and questions regarding the ways in which knowledge was expressed and communicated in the ancient world: the modes of verbal expression, technical idioms, stylistic registers and literary genres that were available to people who laid a claim to knowledge (healers, scientists, philosophers) in order to convey their views to their fellows, colleagues and their wider audiences; the rhetorical strategies they employed in order to make their ideas intelligible, acceptable, or even fashionable; the circumstances in which they had to present their ideas, and the audio-visual means (writing facilities, diagrams, opportunities for live demonstration) they had at their disposal; the interests and the expectations of their audiences, and the ways in which these influenced the actual form of their writings; and the respects in which 'scientific', or 'technical', or 'expert' language or 'discourse' differed from 'ordinary' and 'literary' language and 'discourse'.

After many years of considerable neglect, the last two decades have thus seen a significant increase in attention being given to the forms of ancient scientific writing, especially among students of the Hippocratic Corpus, but also, for example, on Latin medical literature, with some studies focusing on 'strictly' linguistic and textual characteristics, while others have attempted to relate such characteristics to the wider context in which the texts were produced.[34]

Again, it is important to view these developments in their wider context. First, general trends in the study of rhetoric and discourse analysis, in particular the study of 'non-literary' texts such as advertisements, legal proceedings, minutes of meetings, political pamphlets and medical reports, the study of rhetoric and persuasive strategies in apparently 'neutral' scientific writings, and the development of genre categories based on function rather than form have led to a growing awareness among classicists that even such seemingly 'unartistic', non-presumptuous prose writings as the extant works of Aristotle, the *Elements* of Euclid and the 'notebook-like' Hippocratic *Epidemics* do have a structure which deserves to be studied in its own right, if only because they have set certain standards for the emergence and the subsequent development of the genre of the scientific treatise ('tractatus') in Western literature. It is clear, for example, to any student of Aristotle that, however impersonal the tone of his works may be and however careless the structure of his argument may appear, his writings nonetheless contain a hidden but undeniable rhetoric aimed at making the reader agree with his conclusions, for example in the subtle balance between confident explanation and seemingly genuine uncertainty, resulting in a careful alternation of dogmatic statements and exploratory suggestions.

The study of these formal characteristics has further been enriched by a growing appreciation of the role of non-literal, or even non-verbal aspects of communication (and conversely, the non-communicative aspects of language). Aesthetics of reception, ethnography of literature and studies in orality and literacy have enhanced our awareness of the importance of

---

[34] For more detailed discussion and bibliographical references see van der Eijk (1997), from which the following paragraphs are excerpted.

the situation in which a text has, or is supposed to have, functioned, for example the audience for whom it is intended (as distinct from the audience by whom it has actually been received), the conditions in which it has been produced, 'published' and performed, the medium in which it has been transmitted, and so on. Here, again, discourse studies and ethnography of literature have provided useful instruments of research, for example D. Hymes' analysis of the 'speech event' into a number of components that can, not without some irony, be listed according to the initial letters of the word SPEAKING:

setting (time, place, and other circumstances),
scene (e.g. didactic, general or specialised audience, informal communication or festive occasion),
participants (speaker/writer, hearer/reader, addressee),
ends (objective of communication, e.g. conveying information, persuasion, entertainment),
act sequences (style, linguistic structure of the speech act),
keys (tone of communication, e.g. ironic, emotional),
instrumentalities (medium of communication: oral/written, letter/fax/ e-mail, illustrations, dialect, technical language),
norms (stylistic, social, scholarly),
genres.[35]

Though not all of these components are equally relevant in each particular case, models like this do provide a heuristic framework which may be helpful to the understanding of the actual linguistic form of *any* text, including scientific texts. A recent German collection of articles on 'Wissensvermittlung' ('transmission of knowledge') in the ancient world gives an impression of the kind of questions and answers envisaged from such an integrated approach.[36] Thus a number of syntactic peculiarities of texts like some of the 'case histories' of patients in the Hippocratic *Epidemics* might better be accounted for on the assumption that they represent private notes made by doctors for their own use; but further refinement of such an explanation comes within reach when stylistic variations *within* the *Epidemics* are related to a development in scientific writing towards greater audience-orientedness.

At this point, a most fortunate connection can be perceived between linguistically inspired approaches within classical philology and the recent surge of a 'contextual' approach in the history of science, whereby the text is seen as an instrument for scientists and practising doctors to use to define

---

[35] Hymes (1972) 58ff.   [36] Kullmann and Althoff (1993).

and assert themselves, to establish the position of their profession and to gain authority and power.[37] To be sure, the rhetorical nature of some of the Hippocratic writings has not been completely overlooked; but it used to be regarded with disdain and suspicion by scholars (such as Diels), apparently on the assumption that this was sheer stylistic, meaningless embellishment used in order to mask lack of substance, and consequently the authors of works such as *On the Art of Medicine* and *On Breaths* were deprecatingly labelled as 'iatrosophists'.[38] Historians of ancient science, however, have recently pointed to the competitive setting in which Greek scientists had to work and to the rhetorical devices doctors had to use to attract customers in what has appropriately been called the 'medical marketplace':[39] in a situation where no independently recognised qualifications and certificates were available and where everyone could call himself doctor, the Hippocratic physicians had to assert themselves not only against people they perceived as drugsellers, quacks, magicians and practitioners of temple-medicine, but also against intellectuals (such as Empedocles) who advocated healing on the basis of philosophical postulates. Again, the *variations* the Hippocratic Corpus displays with regard to the use of rhetoric (not only the well-known Gorgianic figures of speech but also argumentative techniques, analogies, metaphors, etc.) admit of greater appreciation and explanation if the social and cultural context (or, in Hymes' terminology, setting and scene) in which they were intended to function is taken into account.[40]

Finally, even within the traditional, content-oriented approach to ancient scientific writing, there has been a growing awareness of the relevance of the particular communicative situation of the text to its interpretation, such as the audience for whom the text was intended or the occasion for which it was produced. Such an awareness has led to greater caution in the establishment of doctrinal 'parallels' or 'inconsistencies' between different works of the same author, which would have been used as evidence of a development in doctrine or even as a basis for declaring a work genuine or spurious. (We will see interesting examples of this in chapters 8 and 9 below.) Indeed, it has prompted greater restraint in the establishment of the author's intention (in so far as it may be questioned whether it is appropriate to speak of an 'author' in cases such as the Hippocratic *Epidemics*). Such caution is inspired by a consideration of differences in genesis (single or multiple authorship), status (e.g. data collection, introductory work, rhetorical pamphlet, or

---

[37] See Barton (1994); Lloyd (1979); van der Eijk, Horstmanshoff and Schrijvers (1995).
[38] For a critical discussion of this concept see Jouanna (1988a) 48.
[39] Nutton (1992).
[40] On polemical writing in the Hippocratic Corpus see Ducatillon (1977).

comprehensive systematic account), intended audience (e.g. specialists or laymen), occasion (e.g. oral performance or written communication), and so on. Thus it has been attempted to relate varying degrees of philosophical sophistication in some of Plato's dialogues to differences between the audiences for whom they were intended (as indicated by the contribution of the interlocutors),[41] and something similar has been attempted with regard to differences in method – and to some extent also doctrine – between the three treatises on ethics preserved in the Aristotelian Corpus.[42] Likewise, in some cases apparent inconsistencies in one and the same Aristotelian work can better be accounted for on the assumption of a didactic strategy of the work and a 'progressive character of the exposition',[43] whereby the reader is psychagogically led to a number of new insights, which may be refinements or indeed modifications of views put forward in an earlier stage of the treatise.

Similar formal characteristics of medical and philosophical texts affecting the interpretation or evaluation of particular passages and their relation to other passages in the same work or in other works lie in the field of 'genre', where, again, the sheer variety in forms of expression is particularly striking. When, how and for what purposes prose came to be used for the transmission of knowledge in the late sixth century BCE and why some writers (such as Parmenides and Empedocles, or in later times Aratus and Nicander) preferred to write in verse when prose was available as an alternative, is not in all cases easy to say. Yet the Hippocratic Corpus provides opportunities to gain some idea of the process of text-production and genre-formation, and one can argue that medicine has played a decisive role in the formation of scientific literature.

The variety of forms of writing referred to above is manifest already within the Hippocratic Corpus itself. Some works (e.g. most of the gynaecological texts) show hardly any organisation and present themselves as seemingly unstructured catalogues of symptoms, prescriptions, recipes, and suchlike, though in some cases (e.g. *Epidemics* books 1 and 3) this lack of structure is only apparent. Other works, however (e.g. *Airs, Waters, Places; On the Sacred Disease; On the Nature of Man*), show a degree of care and elaboration on account of which they deserve a much more prominent place than they now occupy in chapters on prose in Greek literature.

The Corpus Aristotelicum presents different problems. Here we do have a large body of texts generally agreed to be by one author (although there

[41] Rowe (1992).
[42] For a summary of this discussion see Flashar (1983) 244; see also Lengen (2002).
[43] Kahn (1966) 56.

is disagreement about the authenticity of some of them). Yet any general account of Aristotle's philosophy is bound to begin with a discussion of the problems posed by the form and status of his writings. Do they represent the 'lecture notes' written by Aristotle himself on the basis of which he presented his oral teaching? Or are they to be taken as the 'minutes' or 'verbatims' of his oral teaching as written down by his pupils? Certainly, some characteristics of his works may be interpreted as evidence of oral presentation;[44] and with some (parts) of his works it is not easy to imagine how they might have been understood without additional oral elucidation – although this may be a case of our underestimating the abilities of his then audience and an extrapolation of our own difficulties in understanding his work. However, other parts of his work are certainly far too elaborate to assume such a procedure.[45] Some works display a careful structure of argumentation which may well be understood by reference to an audience which is supposed to go through a learning process; and certainly the 'dialectical' passages where he deals with the views of his predecessors reflect a very elaborate composition.[46] All in all, it is clear that not much is gained by premature generalisations and unreflective categorisations (such as 'lecture notes'),[47] and that we should allow for considerable variation in forms of expression and degree of linguistic and structural organisation between the various works in the Corpus Aristotelicum.

A further point that has attracted considerable attention is the relation between orality and literacy. Although the details and the precise significance of the process are disputed, the importance of the transition from orality to literacy for Greek culture and intellectual life can hardly be overstated. Since the majority of the Hippocratic writings were produced in the late fifth and early fourth centuries BCE, the Corpus testifies in a variety of ways to this transition. Thus it can safely be assumed that several treatises, especially the older gynaecological works *On Diseases of Women* and *On the Nature of the Woman*, which contain long catalogues of prescriptions and recipes, preserve traditional knowledge which has been transmitted orally over a number of generations. Moreover, several treatises explicitly refer to oral presentations of medical knowledge, such as the author of *On*

---

[44] For examples see Föllinger (1993) and van der Eijk (1994) 97; for direct references to the teaching situation see Bodéüs (1993) 83–96.
[45] E.g. *Metaphysics* 1.1 or *Nicomachean Ethics* (*Eth. Nic.*) 4.3; for other examples see Schütrumpf (1989) and Lengen (2002).
[46] E.g. *Generation of Animals* 1.17–18.
[47] On the problems inherent in this notion see Schütrumpf (1989) 178–80 with notes 12, 13, 17, 23 and 26.

Ancient Medicine[48] and the author of On Diseases 1, who seems to refer to a similar situation of public question and answer on medicine.[49] It is by no means inconceivable that some of the medical works preserved in the Hippocratic Corpus were actually delivered orally for a predominantly non-specialist audience, some possibly in the setting of a rhetorical contest; and it is quite possible that, for example, *On the Sacred Disease* was among this group too. Such a situation is almost certainly envisaged by the authors of the two rhetorically most elaborate works preserved in the Corpus, the already mentioned *On the Art of Medicine* and *On Breaths*, in which Gorgianic figures of speech and sound effects abound, such as parallelism, antithesis and anaphora.[50] As mentioned above, it has long been doubted whether these works were actually written by doctors; yet their style and character fit in very well with the competitive setting of ancient medicine referred to earlier, and they are apparently aimed at self-definition and self-assertion of a discipline whose scientific nature (*technē*) was not beyond dispute.

However, the oral transmission of medical knowledge not only served the purpose of self-presentation to a larger, non-specialised audience, but also had a didactic, educational justification: medicine being the practical art it naturally is, the importance of oral teaching and direct contact between the teacher and the pupil is repeatedly stressed. Thus both Aristotle and his medical contemporary Diocles of Carystus acknowledge the usefulness of written knowledge for the medical profession, but they emphasise that

---

[48] The author of *On Ancient Medicine* begins his work by referring to 'all who have attempted *to speak or to write* on medicine and who have assumed for themselves a postulate as a basis for their discussion' (1.1, 1.570 L.); and later on, in ch. 20 of the same work, he expresses his disdain for 'whatever has been *said or written down* by a sophist or a doctor about nature' (20.2, 1.622 L.). Likewise, the author of *On the Nature of Man* refers to an audience 'used to *listening to people who speak* about the nature of man beyond what is relevant for medicine' (ch. 1, 6.32 L.); and further on in the same chapter he describes how the people referred to are engaged in a rhetorical contest in which they try to gain the upper hand in front of an audience: 'The best way to realise this is to be present at their debates. Given the same debaters and the same audience, the same man never wins in the discussion three times in succession, but now one is victor, now another, now he who happens to have the most glib tongue in the face of the crowd. Yet it is right that a man who claims correct knowledge about the facts should maintain his own argument victorious always, if his knowledge be knowledge of reality and if he set it forth correctly. But in my opinion such men by their lack of understanding overthrow themselves in the words of their very discussions, and establish the theory of Melissus' (6.34 L., tr. Jones in Jones and Withington (1923–31) vol. IV, 5).

[49] 'Anyone who wishes to ask correctly about healing, and, on being asked, to reply and rebut correctly, must consider the following... When you have considered these questions, you must pay careful attention in discussions, and when someone makes an error in one of these points in his assertions, questions, or answers... then you must catch him there and attack him in your rebuttal', *On Diseases* 1.1 (6.140–2 L., tr. Potter (1988) vol. V, 99–101).

[50] A comprehensive account of these stylistic devices can be found in Jouanna's edition of the two works; Jouanna (1988a) 10–24 and 169–73.

this is not sufficient and of no use to those lacking the experience to put it into practice.[51] For what we know about the history of medical education in the ancient world, these remarks indeed reflect the standard situation.[52] The tradition of the *viva vox* as the preferred mode of teaching (not only in medicine) continued also in times in which literacy had established itself and in which medical literature was available on a very large scale; even Galen, the most learned physician of antiquity, who frequently recommends the use of the medical books written by the great authorities of the past, stresses the importance of learning from the master by direct oral teaching.[53]

All these references suggest that at least some of the medical works preserved in the Hippocratic Corpus were presented orally, and also that probably the majority of written texts were used in combination with oral teaching and transmission of knowledge. This means that they were not intended to stand on their own, and this fact may provide an explanation for some of the formal peculiarities they display and for some of the difficulties involved in their interpretation.[54]

At the same time, however, the Hippocratic writings refer on numerous occasions to 'written' information that is available and should be taken into account.[55] Thus at *Epidemics* 3.16 (3.100 L.) it is said that an important component of the medical art is the ability to form a correct judgement about 'what has been written down' (*ta gegrammena*), that is, the case histories of patients that have been put down in writing. Very similar instructions are found elsewhere in the Corpus, suggesting that this use of written information – probably in addition to oral information and the doctor's own observations – is by no means something self-evident, but needs to be encouraged and to be done correctly. It is further noted at several points

---

[51] In a comparison between legislation and medicine, Aristotle says: 'Neither do men appear to become expert physicians on the basis of medical books. Yet they try to discuss not only general means of treatment, but also how one might cure and how one should treat each individual patient, dividing them according to their various habits of body; these [discussions] appear to be of value for men who have had practical experience, but they are useless for those who have no knowledge about the subject' (*Eth. Nic.* 1181 b 2–6; cf. *Politics* 1287 a 35). And a report about Diocles' reply to someone who claimed to have purchased a medical book (*iatrikon biblion*) and therefore to be no longer in need of instruction makes the same point: 'Books are reminders for those who have received teaching, but they are gravestones to the uneducated' (fr. 6).

[52] See Kudlien (1970).

[53] Galen, *On the Powers of Foodstuffs* 1.1.47 (6.480 K.); *On the Mixtures and Powers of Simple Drugs* 6, proem (11.791 K.); *On the Composition of Drugs according to Places* 6.1 (12.894 K.).

[54] The brevity and obscurity of the Hippocratic writings were already noted and explained as a deliberate strategy by Galen; see the references mentioned by Langholf (1977) 11 n. 5, and the discussion by Sluiter (1995a).

[55] The evidence has been conveniently assembled by K. Usener (1990).

that a particular observation is 'worth writing down' (*axion graphēs*);[56] and an interesting passage in *On Regimen in Acute Diseases* refers to initial codification (*sungraphein*) of the 'Cnidian sentences' and subsequent revision (*epidiaskeuazesthai*) by a later generation in the light of further discoveries and growing experience (2.224–8 L.). Another remarkable reference to the use of written records is to be found at *Epidemics* 6.8.7 (5.346 L.), where a section of text is introduced by the words '(data) derived from the small writing-tablet' (*ta ek tou smikrou pinakidiou*), suggesting that the author is drawing on an existing collection (an archive or 'database') of information.[57] As Langholf has suggested, the fact that many 'chapters' or 'sections' in the Hippocratic *Epidemics* are of approximately the same length, may be explained by reference to the material conditions in which information was stored, such as the size of writing-tablets.[58]

These passages indicate that the Hippocratic writers gradually realised the importance of written documents for the preservation and transmission of knowledge; also that they regarded these written records not as the intellectual property of one person, but as a common reservoir of knowledge accessible to a group of physicians (who copied and used the same information more than once, as can be seen from the doublets in the Hippocratic writings) and admitting of additions and changes by this same group of physicians. The significance of this for our understanding of these texts can hardly be overstated. Rather than claiming that in the case of Hippocratic medicine the transition from orality to literacy *brought about* a change in mental attitude and even in thinking, as has been suggested by Miller and Lonie,[59] it seems more likely that, conversely, the development of prose writing, and the various forms in which the Hippocratic writers expressed themselves, is to be understood as a *consequence* of new ways of thinking – or rather as the result of a new attitude towards knowledge, resulting in a desire to store data gained by practical experience, to systematise them and to make them accessible for future use. It seems very likely that the Hippocratic authors regarded writing as an instrument for the *organisation* of knowledge concerning a great variety of phenomena, that is, not only in order to prevent knowledge from being forgotten – a desire they shared with, for example Herodotus – but also to keep knowledge available for

---

[56] *On Regimen in Acute Diseases* 3 (2.238 L.); 16 (2.254 L.); *On Joints* 10 (4.104 L.).
[57] For a discussion of this phrase, and in general of the material conditions for writing in the Hippocratic Corpus, see Langholf (1989a); Nieddu (1993); Althoff (1993). Cf. also the Hippocratic *Prorrheticon* 2.4 (9.20 L.).
[58] Langholf (1989a).
[59] G. L. Miller (1990); Lonie (1983); more in general Goody (1968) and Havelock (1982a).

practical application. And it seems entirely reasonable that medicine (rather than, say, mathematics or astronomy) should play this part: for, on the one hand, the empirical data reflected in case histories such as the *Epidemics* must soon have reached such unmanageable proportions and such a high degree of detail that it could not possibly be remembered; so there was a need for storage of information based on the belief that such information might remain useful. On the other hand, since medicine was incessantly confronted with new cases in which existing knowledge had to be applied or against which it had to be checked and, if necessary, modified, it had to be accessible in a conveniently retrievable form.

If all this is plausible, the emergence of the Hippocratic writings and especially the variety of forms they display can be seen as a result of the need for organisation of knowledge and research – a need arising also from the fact that their authors must have formed a community of scholars rather than being single scientists working independently. This might also suggest an alternative explanation of why all the Hippocratic writings are anonymous (cf. p. 23): while the works of Herodotus and Hecataeus of Miletus begin with a statement of the author's name, and this seems also to have been the case with medical writers such as Alcmaeon of Croton, the Hippocratic writings do not bear the name of their authors – which is not to deny that they are written by very self-conscious people who are much more prominently and explicitly present in the text (with personal pronouns and first-person verb forms) than, say, Aristotle.

In the course of the fourth century the collection and organisation of knowledge was further implemented and applied to a much broader area by Aristotle and his pupils (or colleagues), and a similar process of data preservation, common intellectual property and exchange of information evidently took place in the Lyceum.[60]

The above points illustrate in what respects a contextual approach to medical and philosophical texts allows a better understanding of a number of their formal features. More could be said from a contextual point of view about these and other features of medical and philosophical 'discourse'. For example, there is the formation of a scientific terminology and its relation to ordinary language, with stylistic and syntactic anomalies such as the use of 'shorthand' (brachylogy), 'aphoristic' style and formulaic language, or structural characteristics such as ring composition, paragraph division, use of introductory and concluding formulae and other structuring devices. Particularly interesting is the presence or absence of the author in

---

[60] See Ostwald and Lynch (1992).

the text, for example by means of the use of the first person singular in expressions like 'I state' or 'it seems to me', often lending great force to what is being claimed,[61] or by means of the presence of direct addresses to the reader or hearer. Furthermore, of great interest are the use of rhetorical questions, formulae for fictional objections, modes of argument used by the Hippocratic writers, Diocles and Aristotle, the use of metaphors and analogies, and patterns of thought, such as antithesis, binary or quaternary *schemata*, the various forms of *overstatement*, or the ways in which ancient scientific writers, just like orators, tried to convey a certain *ēthos* (in the ancient rhetorical sense of 'personality') to their audiences, for example by presenting themselves in a certain way or assuming a certain pose with regard to their audience and their subject matter.[62] We can think here of the exploratory style of some of Aristotle's works, where an impression of uncertainty on the author's part may be intended to suggest to the audience that the author knows just as little about the subject matter as they do and thus invite them to think along with him or to raise objections. Alternatively, the author may present himself as a venerable authority, as a schoolmaster ready to praise good suggestions and to castigate foolish answers, as a dispassionate self-deprecating seeker of the truth, or a committed human being who brings the whole of his life experience to bear on the subject he is dealing with, and so on. As many readers of this volume will be aware from their own experience with communication to academic audiences, these are different styles of discourse, with different stylistic registers, types of argument, appeals to the audience, commonplaces, and suchlike; what they were like in the ancient world deserves to be described, and the attempt should be made to detect patterns, and perhaps systematicity, in them. Ancient scientists, like orators, had an interest in *captatio benevolentiae* and were aware of the importance of strategies such as a 'rhetoric of modesty', a 'rhetoric of confidence'. In this respect the dialogues of Plato provide good examples of these attitudes, and they may serve as starting-points for similar analysis of scientific writing which is not in the form of a dialogue. The works of Galen present a particularly promising area of study, for one can hardly imagine a more self-conscious, rhetorical, argumentative, polemicising and manipulating ancient scientific writer than the doctor

---

[61] In chapter 1 we shall see an interesting example of a significant alternation of singular and plural by the author of *On the Sacred Disease*, where the author cleverly tries to make his audience feel involved in a course of religious action which he defends and indeed opposes to the magical one advocated by his opponents.

[62] See Lloyd (1987b) for a discussion of the alternation of dogmatism and uncertainty in ancient scientific writing.

from Pergamum. And, as I have shown elsewhere, the works of Caelius Aurelianus present a further example of medical literature full of rhetorical and argumentative fireworks.[63]

The topics discussed above may give some idea of the problems to be addressed in a study of the forms of ancient scientific writing and show how such a study should not focus exclusively on linguistic and textual matters, but take into account also the contexts and circumstances that influence the form a scientific speech act takes. At the same time, it will have become clear that these formal aspects of Greek and Latin medical writing are of great significance when it comes to the *use* of these texts as sources for what used to be seen as the primary jobs of the medical historian, namely the reconstruction of the nosological reality of the past and of the human response to this reality.

7 HISTORIOGRAPHY, TRADITION AND SELF-DEFINITION

When discussing the rhetoric of ancient medical, scientific and philosophical discourse, one further, related development in scholarship may finally be mentioned here briefly: the study of the 'self-definition' or *Selbstverständnis* of Greek and Roman scientific writers, especially their understanding of their own discipline and its historicity, and the way in which that understanding was expressed, both explicitly and implicitly, in their own work. I have dealt with this area more elaborately in a separate collaborative volume on medical doxography and historiography.[64] It has, of course, long been realised that reflection on the achievements of the past was, from the earliest stages of Greek thought up to late antiquity, an integral part of most intellectual projects of some ambition and profoundly influenced scientific and philosophical practice and research as well as theoretical reflection and rhetorical presentation of ideas. Many ancient medical writers, philosophers and scientists (as well as historians) regarded themselves as part of a long tradition, and they explicitly discussed the value of this tradition, and their own contribution to it, in a prominent part of their own written work, often in the preface. Yet, more recently, scholarship has drawn attention to the large variety of ways in which ancient scientific and philosophical discourse received and reused traditional material and to the many different purposes and strategies the description of this material served. Ancient writers on science and philosophy received and constructed particular *versions* of the

---

[63] See van der Eijk (1999c).   [64] See van der Eijk (1999a), especially ch. 1.

history of their own subject, which were the product of a sometimes long, possibly distorting and inevitably selective process of transmission, interpretation, 'recycling' and updating. The modalities of these processes have turned out to be very complicated indeed, and it has become clear that the subject of 'tradition' in ancient thought comprises much more than just one authoritative thinker exercising 'influence' on another.

Our understanding of 'doxography' and other genres of ancient 'intellectual historiography' has been significantly enhanced over the last two decades, and it has contributed to a greater appreciation of the various dimensions – textual, subtextual and intertextual – of much Greek and Roman philosophical and medical discourse. In particular, it has shed further light on the possible reasons behind the ways in which ideas are presented in texts and the modes in which ancient authors contextualise themselves, aspects which are of great relevance to the interpretation and evaluation of these ideas.

PART I

Hippocratic Corpus and Diocles of Carystus

CHAPTER I

The 'theology' of the Hippocratic treatise On the Sacred Disease

1 INTRODUCTION

The author of the Hippocratic treatise *On the Sacred Disease* is renowned for his criticism of magical and superstitious conceptions and modes of treatment of epilepsy. He has been credited with attempting a 'natural' or 'rational' explanation of a disease which was generally believed to be of divine origin and to be curable only by means of apotropaeic ritual and other magical instruments.[1] One interesting point is that he does not reject the divine character of the disease, but modifies the sense in which this disease (and, as a consequence of this conception, all diseases) may be regarded as divine: not in the sense that it is sent by a god, for example as a punishment,[2] and is to be cured by this same god,[3] but that it shares in the divine character of nature in showing a fixed pattern of cause and effect and in being subordinated to what may perhaps be called, somewhat anachronistically, a natural 'law' or regularity.[4]

On the basis of these positive statements on the divine character of the disease various interpreters have tried to deduce the writer's 'theology' or religious beliefs, and to relate this to the development of Greek religious thought in the fifth century.[5] The details of this reconstruction will concern us later; for the present purpose of clarifying the issue of this chapter it suffices to say that in this theology the divine is regarded as an immanent

---

This chapter was first published in *Apeiron* 23 (1990) 87–119.
[1] On the various possible reasons why epilepsy was regarded as a 'sacred' disease see Temkin (1971) 6–10.
[2] On the moral and non-moral aspects of pollution by a disease see Parker (1983) 235ff.
[3] On the principle that 'he who inflicted the injury will also provide the cure' (ὁ τρώσας καὶ ἰάσεται), as on other details of this belief, see Ducatillon (1977) 159–79. The identity, claims and practices of the magicians have also been studied by Lanata (1967); Temkin (1971) 10–15; Dölger (1922) 359–77; Moulinier (1952) 134–7; Nilsson (1955) 798–800.
[4] On the meaning of the word 'divine' (*theios*) and on the divinity of diseases see section 2 below.
[5] Edelstein (1967a) 205–46; Kudlien (1977) 268–74; Lain-Entralgo (1975) 315–19; Lloyd (1975c) 1–16; Lloyd (1979) ch. 1; H. W. Miller (1953) 1–15; Nestle (1938) 1–16; Nörenberg (1968); Thivel (1975); Vlastos (1945) 581.

45

natural principle (or as a certain group of concrete natural factors) and is no longer conceived as something supernatural. Consequently the influence, or the manifestations, of the divine are regarded as natural processes and no longer as supernatural interventions of gods within natural or human situations. On this view, the writer of *On the Sacred Disease* may be seen as the exponent of a 'rationalistic' or 'naturalistic' religiosity, or in any case as an adherent of a more advanced way of thinking about the divine, which can be observed in some of the Presocratic philosophers as well (e.g. Xenophanes, Anaximander; see n. 14 below), and which resembles opinions found in the Sophistic movement, in some of the tragedies of Euripides and in the *Histories* of Thucydides.

On the other hand, it has been recognised by several interpreters[6] that the author's criticism of the magicians, which occupies the entire first chapter of the treatise (and which is echoed several times later on),[7] reflects an authentic religious conviction. This applies particularly to his repeated accusations of impiety (*asebeia*) and even atheism (*atheos*) in sections 1.28–30 (6.358–60 L.) and 1.39ff. (6.362ff. L.). In these passages the author shows himself both a defender of religion and a critic of magic: he expresses definite opinions on what he believes to be the different domains of human action and divine action (1.25–31, 6.358–60 L.) and on the nature of the divine in its relation to man (1.45, 6.364 L.), and he makes stipulations concerning the truly pious manner of approaching the gods and making an appeal to their cleansing power (1.41, 6.362 L.; 1.42, 6.362 L.; 1.46, 6.364 L.). The religious belief which apparently underlies these passages is far more traditional and less 'advanced' than the naturalistic theology which is reflected in the statements on the divine character of the disease, since it appears that the author of *On the Sacred Disease* believes in a supreme divine power which cleanses men of their moral transgressions and which is accessible to cultic worship in sacred buildings by means of prayer and sacrifice.

The problem I intend to deal with in this chapter is how these two different sets of religious ideas are related to each other. For if it is true,

---

[6] See especially Ducatillon (1977) 163 and 180–5; cf. McGibbon (1965) 387–8 and the hesitant remarks of Nörenberg (1968) 74–6. None of these scholars, however, have satisfactorily solved the problem of this apparently 'double-faced' religiosity (see below).

[7] There is no sharp dividing line between the 'polemical' and the 'positive' part of the treatise: the polemical tone persists through the whole text (e.g. 2.6–7, 6.366 L.; 11.5, 6.382 L.; 12.2, 6.382 L.; 13.13, 6.386 L.; 17.1–10, 6.392–4 L.; 18.1–2 and 6, 6.394–6 L.), and in the polemical ch. 1 the author repeatedly expresses his own opinions (e.g. 1.2, 6.352 L.; 1.13–14, 6.356 L.; 1.25–6, 6.358 L.; 1.45–6, 6.364 L.). References to *On the Sacred Disease* follow the division into chapters and sections of H. Grensemann's edition (1968c). Compared to the Loeb edition by W. H. S. Jones (vol. 11, 1923), Grensemann's ch. 1 corresponds to Jones' chs. I–IV, then 2 to V, 3 to VI and so on up to ch. 16.1–5, which corresponds to Jones' ch. XIX; then 16.6–17.1–10 corresponds to Jones XX and 18 to XXI.

as Jeanne Ducatillon has claimed,[8] that the statements of the first chapter actually reveal an authentic religious conviction, we are obliged to define as accurately as possible how this conviction is related to the concept of the divine as an immanent natural law and of its workings as natural processes. But we must also consider the possibility (which Ducatillon appears to have overlooked) that the accusations of the first chapter are no more than rhetorical or occasional arguments *pour besoin de la cause* which need not imply the author's personal involvement, seeing that many of these statements have an obviously hypothetical character.[9] I may, for instance, criticise a person for acting contrarily to his own principles and I may even define how he should act according to these principles without endorsing either his principles or the corresponding behaviour. Yet such a hypothetical argument does reflect my opinion on the logical connection between the premise and the conclusion, since it shows what I believe to be a valid or a non-valid conclusion from a given premise (a premise which I need not believe to be true). Thus the argument reflects my sense of 'logic' or 'necessity' and the presuppositions underlying the stringency of my argument.

One might object that our apparent problem is not genuine, and that there is nothing strange about intellectuals participating in traditional cultic activities such as prayer and sacrifice, while at the same time holding 'advanced' religious or theological ideas which seem inconsistent with the presuppositions underlying these cultic practices.[10] However, the problem

---

[8] Ducatillon (1977) 180–5.

[9] Cf. the use of εἰ δέ in 1.23 (6.358 L.), of ὅπου γάρ in 1.25 (6.358 L.), of εἰ γάρ and εἰ δή in 1.31 (6.360 L.) as well as the modal imperfects ἐχρῆν in 1.41 (6.362 L.) and 1.43 (6.362 L.) (and ἔδει in 2.7, 6.366 L.). It is probably this hypothetical character which has led most interpreters to refrain from bringing these statements to bear on the discussion of the writer's theological ideas (e.g. Lloyd (1975c) 13 n. 19). Nörenberg (1968) 69 also claims that the sections 41–6 are put into the mouth of the magicians, although later on (74–6) he suddenly takes them seriously as reflecting the author's own opinion. However, his own 'hypothetical' remarks there on the 'moral significance' of the divine remain inconclusive and partly contradict his earlier views on the divinity of nature. As will become clear in the course of this chapter, I do not believe that 'the divine' (*to theion*) mentioned in 1.45 is identical with 'the divine' (sc. 'character') of natural laws or that both the 'moral' and the 'naturalistic' aspects of the divine are subordinated to a higher concept of divinity; nor do I see any textual grounds for denying that the author of *On the Sacred Disease* believes in 'personal' or 'anthropomorphic' gods (see section 4 below).

[10] This is apparently the view taken by H. W. Miller (1953) 2 n. 3: 'This passage [i.e. 1.44–5, PJvdE] as well as the following remarks concerning the true meaning of the use of purifications, suggests that the author would not refuse to accept and conform to the rituals of temple and civic religion – as would hardly be expected. His remarks reflect, indeed, a genuine belief in the Divine, but, as perhaps in the case of a Socrates or a Euripides, it is not simply a belief in the gods as traditionally and popularly conceived.' This is a complicated and controversial issue, and although I believe that it does not affect my argument, I am aware that 'nothing strange about it' does not do justice to this discussion. At least three questions are important: (i) To what extent did intellectuals try to harmonise their own theological conceptions with traditional beliefs and, if they did, then for what

does not concern a discrepancy between religious theory and religious practice or between theology and cult, but a tension between different ideas in one and the same text. For there is a difference between intellectuals simply participating (from habit or under social pressure) in cultic actions, and intellectuals, such as the author of *On the Sacred Disease*, making explicit statements and definitions about what they believe should be the right way of approaching the gods. Moreover, the author's assertions not only concern cult and ritual, but also characteristics of the divine and the way in which it manifests itself within human experience. Therefore the problem deserves to be considered, and we must try to find out how these two sets of religious opinions are related to each other.

I shall first deal with the statements on the divine character of the disease and consider whether these admit of being extrapolated into a 'theology'. This will for a substantial part consist in an attempt to evaluate and clarify the interpretative debate on the author's claim that 'all diseases are divine and all are human'. Then I shall deal with the statements in his chapter 1 and relate these to the assertions about the divine character of the disease. Finally I shall summarise my conclusions concerning the religious notions which can, with some degree of certainty, be attributed to the author of *On the Sacred Disease*.

2 THE DIVINITY OF DISEASES

In spite of the vast literature on this subject (see n. 5 above) we may say that basically there are two different interpretations of the use of the words 'divine' (*theios*) and 'human' (*anthrōpinos*) with regard to diseases in *On the Sacred Disease*, both of which have a strong textual basis.[11] I do not

---

reasons? On this question see Gigon (1952) 127–66, esp. 128–9 and 156–64, and Vlastos (1952) 104 and 112–13. (ii) To what extent were intellectuals at liberty to hold and propagate advanced ideas about religious matters? On the one hand it is often stated that there was no institutionalised orthodoxy in ancient Greece and no sacred books with authorised interpretations and that, consequently, many different religious beliefs were tolerated (see Lloyd (1979) 10–15). On the other hand it cannot be denied that at the end of the fifth century (in Attica at least) a growing intolerance manifests itself, e.g. in the trials of 'impiety' (*asebeia*). In this respect it is significant that it is the author of *On the Sacred Disease* himself who accuses his opponents of impiety and atheism (1.28ff.; 1.39ff.), charges which later (in the fourth century) were frequently connected with magic (e.g. in the trials of *asebeia* againt Ninos and Theoris). (iii) Did this apparent intolerance only concern participation in cult and ritual, or did it concern religious ideas as well? On all these matters see Bryant (1986); Dover (1975); Fahr (1969); Guthrie (1969) vol. III, 226–49; Meijer (1981); Mikalson (1983) 91–105; Sandvoss (1968) 312–29; Versnel (1990) 123–31.

[11] For this reason I shall not discuss as a separate alternative the view that the author of *On the Sacred Disease* has adopted the idea of the divinity of air from Diogenes of Apollonia (cf. H. W. Miller (1953) 9–15), though I shall say something about this in the course of my comments on interpretation (1). On the influence of Diogenes on this treatise see Grensemann (1968c) 29–30.

intend to offer a new one, but I believe that the debate would benefit from recognising that these interpretations are different and incompatible, and from acknowledging the presuppositions underlying both views. My second *a priori* remark is that the use of terminological oppositions such as 'rational versus irrational' and 'natural versus supernatural' in order to define the meaning of *theios* and *anthrōpinos* is confusing rather than illuminating.[12] The correct questions to ask are, first, in which respect (or, in what sense) a disease, according to the author, is to be regarded as divine or human, and, second, what connotations or associations of *theios* and *anthrōpinos* enable the author to apply these words to a disease.

The two interpretations are as follows:

(1) A disease is divine in virtue of being caused by factors (*prophasies*; on this term see below) which are themselves divine: the climatic factors heat, cold and winds. These can, on this view, be called divine because they are beyond human control (the author accepting *aporos*, 'hopeless', 'impossible to resolve', as a proper associate of *theios*, cf. 1.3–4, 6.352 L.).[13] The disease is human in virtue of being caused by other factors as well which are 'human', such as the particular constitution-type of an individual, the constitution of his brain, his age, and so on. These factors can be called human because they (or at least some of them) are capable of being controlled, or in any case influenced, by human agency.

(2) A disease is divine in virtue of having a *phusis*, a 'nature', that is, a definite character and a regular pattern of origin (cause) and growth (13.13, 6.368 L.: γίνεσθαι καὶ θάλλειν). The governing connotations of *theios*

---

[12] This is not to suggest that the oppositions 'rational–irrational' and 'natural–supernatural' are used by modern scholars as if they were equivalent, but rather to avoid the anachronistic associations these terms conjure up. Cf. the frequent use of 'rational–irrational' in Nörenberg (1968), e.g. 71: 'Damit bekommt das θεῖον wie die φύσις einen rationalen Charakter, der die Kritik an jeder irrationalen Auffassung und so auch an den θεοί des Mythos und des Volksglaubens, bzw. dem gänzlich irrationalen δαιμόνιον provozieren muss'; and Kudlien (1974) *passim*. A more cautious use of 'natural–supernatural' is to be found in Lloyd (1979) e.g. 26–7; but even with regard to the use of *phusis* in *On the Sacred Disease* this opposition creates a distinction which is not to the point, since the term 'supernatural' does not apply to the position that the author of *On the Sacred Disease* combats.

[13] In 1.3–4 (6.352 L.) the author discusses the possible reasons why people came to regard epilepsy as a sacred disease. One of these reasons, he says, may be the 'hopelessness' (ἀπορίη) with which the disease confronted them. But he proceeds to show that this only applies to a cognitive 'hopelessness' (ἀπορίη τοῦ μὴ γινώσκειν); as for the therapeutic aspect, he says, these people claim to be 'well provided' with means to cure (εὔποροι) rather than 'hopeless' (ἄποροι). Cf. the distinction between two respects of 'hopelessness' made in 13.13 (6.368 L.): καὶ οὐδέν ἐστι ἀπορωτέρη τῶν ἄλλων οὔτε ἰᾶσθαι οὔτε γνῶναι ('and it [i.e. the disease] is not more hopeless than the others, neither as far as curing nor as far as understanding it are concerned'). Apparently the author accepts *aporos* as a justified associate of *theios*, but he points out that these people are actually not *aporoi* at all. By showing that the disease is caused by 'human' factors as well (which are in their turn influenced by the divine factors mentioned) the author demonstrates that in his account a disease can be both divine and human (i.e. both divine and curable).

are here 'constant', 'unchanging', 'imperishable' – not in the sense that the disease itself is unchanging, but in that it shows a constant pattern of development. These connotations, in fact, also led the Presocratic philosophers to apply the word to their ultimate principles.[14] The disease is human in virtue of being capable of treatment and cure by human beings, but in a more abstract sense than in the first case (see below). Both interpretations are based upon the following passages:

1.2 (6.352 L.): οὐδέν τι δοκεῖ τῶν ἄλλων θειοτέρη εἶναι νούσων οὐδὲ ἱερωτέρη, ἀλλὰ φύσιν μὲν ἔχει καὶ τὰ λοιπὰ νοσήματα, ὅθεν γίνεται, φύσιν δὲ αὕτη καὶ πρόφασιν.[15]

[This disease] does not seem in any respect to be more divine or more holy than the others. It is rather that just as the other diseases have a nature from which they arise, likewise this one has a nature and a cause.

2.1–3 (6.364 L.): τὸ δὲ νόσημα τοῦτο οὐδέν τι μοι δοκεῖ θειότερον εἶναι τῶν λοιπῶν, ἀλλὰ φύσιν μὲν ἔχειν καὶ τὰ ἄλλα νοσήματα, ὅθεν ἕκαστα γίνεται, φύσιν δὲ τοῦτο καὶ πρόφασιν, καὶ ἀπὸ τοῦ αὐτοῦ θεῖον γίνεσθαι ἀφ' ὅτου καὶ τὰ ἄλλα πάντα, καὶ ἰητὸν εἶναι οὐδὲν ἧσσον ἑτέρων κτλ.[16]

It seems to me that this disease is in no respect more divine than the others, but rather that just as the other diseases have a nature from which each of them arises, likewise this one has a nature and a cause, and it derives its divinity from the same source from which all the others do, and it is in no respect less curable than the others ...

18.1–2 (6.394 L.): αὕτη δὲ ἡ νοῦσος ἡ ἱρὴ καλεομένη ἀπὸ τῶν αὐτῶν προφασίων γίνεται καὶ αἱ λοιπαί, ἀπὸ τῶν προσιόντων καὶ ἀπιόντων καὶ ψύχεος

---

[14] See Jaeger (1980) 204 (on Anaximander DK A 15, B 3): 'What happens in Anaximander's argument (and that of his successors in line) is that the predicate God, or rather the Divine, is transformed from the traditional deities to the first principle of Being (at which they arrived by rational investigations), on the ground that the predicates usually attributed to the gods of Homer and Hesiod are inherent in that principle to a higher degree or can be assigned to it with greater certainty.' The predicates in question are ἀγένητος ('ungenerated'), ἄφθαρτος ('imperishable'), ἀθάνατος ('immortal') and ἀνώλεθρος ('imperishable').

[15] This sentence is put between square brackets by Grensemann (1968c) *ad loc.* on the grounds that it is almost verbally repeated in 2.1–2 (6.364 L.), that αὕτη (instead of τοῦτο) is syntactically awkward and that the sentence οἱ ἄνθρωποι κτλ. (1.3) is in asyndeton with the preceding one. Each of these arguments may be questioned: repetition of this kind is quite frequent in *On the Sacred Disease* (e.g. 2.6, 6.366 L. and 5.1, 6.368 L.; 13.13, 6.386 L. and 18.1–2, 6.394 L.) and obviously serves an organising purpose; the word νοῦσος, to which αὕτη refers, is mentioned in the immediate context, and the alternation of νόσημα and νοῦσος is so frequent in this text that they seem practically synonymous; and the deletion of a whole sentence is more drastic than the insertion of δ'. Besides, after the opening sentence (περὶ τῆς ἱρῆς νούσου καλεομένης ὧδε ἔχει) it is more reasonable to expect an exposition of what the author believes than the rejection of what other people believe.

[16] On the sequel to this sentence, which contains an important qualification of the curability of the disease, see below, pp. 71–2.

καὶ ἡλίου καὶ πνευμάτων μεταβαλλομένων τε καὶ οὐδέποτε ἀτρεμιζόντων. ταῦτα δ'ἐστὶ θεῖα, ὥστε μὴ δεῖν ἀποκρίνοντα τὸ νόσημα θειότερον τῶν λοιπῶν νομίζειν, ἀλλὰ πάντα θεῖα καὶ πάντα ἀνθρώπινα, φύσιν δὲ ἕκαστον ἔχει καὶ δύναμιν ἐφ' ἑωυτοῦ, καὶ οὐδὲν ἄπορόν ἐστιν οὐδ' ἀμήχανον.

This disease which is called sacred arises from the same causes as the others, from the things that come and go away and from cold and sun and winds that change and never rest. These things are divine, so that one ought not to separate this disease and regard it as being more divine than the others; it is rather that all are divine and all are human, and each of them has a nature and a power of its own, and none is hopeless or impossible to deal with.

The first interpretation is mainly based upon the remark 'these things are divine' (ταῦτα δ'ἐστὶ θεῖα, 18.2); 'these things' is taken as a reference to the 'causes' (προφάσιες) mentioned in the previous sentence, 'the things that come and go away, etc.' (τῶν προσιόντων καὶ ἀπιόντων κτλ.). The author derives the divinity of the disease from the divinity of its causes, the climatic factors whose influence has been discussed in 10.2ff. (cold and heat; 6.378ff. L.) and chapter 13 (winds), and hinted at in 8.1 (6.374 L.), 8.7 (6.376 L.), 9.4 (6.378 L.) and 11.1 (6.380–2 L.). And since these factors are – as the author claims – the causes of *all* diseases, all diseases are equally divine, so that none of them should be distinguished from the others as being more divine.

At the same time all diseases are *anthrōpina*, 'human'. It is not stated explicitly in either of these passages in what sense they are human,[17] but it has been suggested that diseases are caused (or at least determined in their development) by human factors as well.[18] These factors are not mentioned here, probably for the very reason that they do not constitute the divine character of the disease, which is the important issue here, and, perhaps, because the importance of these factors varies from one disease to another, which explains why they cannot be included in 'the same causes' (τῶν αὐτῶν προφασίων). For these reasons, for instance, the brain (ὁ ἐγκέφαλος) is not mentioned in chapter 18, although the writer had stated earlier (3.1) that it is the brain which is causally responsible (αἴτιος) for this disease (and for all important diseases), a claim which he has substantiated at length in the preceding chapters 14–17 (on this, as on possible differences of meaning between πρόφασις and αἴτιος, see pp. 59–60

---

[17] This may be due to the polemical context: some diseases are called divine by the opponents, while others are therefore regarded as human. But in the author's view all diseases are both divine and human: the explanandum is not that all diseases are human, but in what sense all diseases are divine as well.
[18] Nörenberg (1968) 714; Nestle (1938) 3–4.

below). Among the 'human' factors determining the disease we should probably also reckon the individual's constitution (phlegmatic or choleric: 2.4–5, 6.364 L.; 5.1, 6.368 L.), which depends on peculiarities and degrees of prenatal and postnatal 'purgation' (ch. 5), the individual's age (chs. 8–9), the left or right side of the body (ch. 10), the length of time which has elapsed since the beginning of the disease (ch. 11), and a few minor variable factors which the author mentions in the course of his medical account of epilepsy.

A difficulty of this view is that not all of these factors seem to be accessible to human control or even influence, so that this connotation of *anthrōpinos* seems hardly applicable here. A man's constitution, for instance, is determined from his birth (5.1ff., 6.368ff. L.) and seems hardly capable of being influenced by human agency (although there is no reason why even this could not be thought to be changeable by means of diet – but the text does not discuss this). Yet perhaps another association of the opposition *theios–anthrōpinos* has prompted the author to use it here, namely the contrast 'universal–particular', which also seems to govern the use of *theios* in the Hippocratic treatise *On the Nature of the Woman*.[19]

However, this interpretation is based upon several assumptions and presuppositions deserving consideration.

Firstly, the meaning of the word *phusis* and the reason for mentioning it in all three passages remains unclear. If, as is generally supposed,[20] *phusis* and *prophasis* are related to each other in that *phusis* is the abstract concept and *prophasis* the concrete causing factor (*prophasies* being the concrete constituents of the *phusis* of a disease), then the mention of the word *phusis* does not suffice to explain the sense in which the disease is to be taken as divine, for the nature of a disease is constituted by human factors as well. It is the fact that some of the constituents of the nature of the disease are themselves divine which determines the divine character of the disease.

Secondly, in the sentence 'it derives its divinity from the same source from which all the others do' (2.1: καὶ ἀπὸ τοῦ αὐτοῦ θεῖον γίνεσθαι ἀφ'

---

[19] *On the Nature of the Woman* 1 (7.312 L.); cf. Ducatillon (1977) 202–3. I refrain from a systematic discussion of the concept of the divine in other Hippocratic writings, partly for reasons of space but also because such a discussion would have to be based on close analysis of each of these writings rather than a superficial comparison with other texts. Besides, it is unnecessary or even undesirable to strive to harmonise the doctrines of the various treatises in the heterogeneous collection which the Hippocratic Corpus represents, and it is dangerous to use the theological doctrine of one treatise (e.g. the supposedly divine character of climatic factors in *On the Sacred Disease*) as evidence in favour of an interpretation of the word *theios* in another treatise (e.g. *Prognostic*; on this see n. 30 below). For general discussions see Thivel (1975); Kudlien (1974); and Nörenberg (1968) 77–86.

[20] See Nörenberg (1968) 64–7; Lloyd (1979) 26.

ὅτου καὶ τὰ ἄλλα πάντα), we have to suppose, on this interpretation, that when writing 'the same source' (τοῦ αὐτοῦ) the author means the climatic factors, whose influence is explained later on in the text (see above) and whose divine character is not stated before the final chapter. Now if a writer says: 'this disease owes its divine character to the same thing to which all other diseases owe their divine character', it is rather unsatisfactory to suppose that the reader has to wait for an answer to the question of what this 'same thing' is until the end of the treatise. This need not be a serious objection against this interpretation, but it would no doubt be preferable to be able to find the referent of τοῦ αὐτοῦ in the immediate context.

Thirdly, this interpretation requires that in the sentence 'from the things that come and go away, and from cold and sun and winds that change and never rest' (18.1: ἀπὸ τῶν προσιόντων καὶ ἀπιόντων καὶ ψύχεος καὶ ἡλίου καὶ πνευμάτων μεταβαλλομένων τε καὶ οὐδέποτε ἀτρεμιζόντων) the second *kai* ('and') is taken in the explicative sense of 'that is to say'. In a sequence of four occurrences of *kai* this is a little awkward, since there is no textual indication for taking the second *kai* in a different sense from the others. Yet perhaps one could argue that this is indicated by the shift from plural to singular without article, and by the fact that the expression 'the things that come and those that go away' is itself quite general: it may denote everything which approaches the human body and everything which leaves it, such as food, water or air, as well as everything the body excretes.[21] On this line of reasoning, this expression would then be specified into the following items: cold, sun and winds; without this specification food, air and water as well as the corresponding excretions would be divine too, which seems unlikely.[22] Besides, it must be conceded that the specification of 'the things that come and go away' (τῶν προσιόντων καὶ ἀπιόντων) as the climatic factors mentioned is not without justification. At the end of

---

[21] τὰ ἀπιόντα is a common expression for excretions: cf. *Epidemics* 1.5 (2.632 L.) and 3.10 (3.90 L.; for other instances see Kühn and Fleischer, *Index Hippocraticus* s.v.); in this sense the word is used in *On the Sacred Disease* 5.8 (6.370 L.) as well (though this is Grensemann's emendation of the MSS reading ἀφίει). Against this specialised interpretation cf. Ducatillon (1977) 202: 'L'adjectif qui nous intéresse [i.e. *theios*, PJvdE] s'applique ici à de nombreux objets. Il caractérise d'une part ce qui entre dans le corps et ce qui en sort, c'est à dire l'air et les aliments, d'autre part le froid, le soleil, les vents, bref, les conditions climatiques et atmosphériques; c'est donc la nature entière, considérée comme une réalité matérielle qui est proclamée divine.'

[22] As G. E. R. Lloyd reminds me, it could be argued that the divinity of air, water and food need not be surprising in the light of the associations of bread with Demeter, and wine with Dionysus (cf. Prodicus DK B 5). But even if these associations apply here (which is not confirmed by any textual evidence), the unlikelihood of the divinity of the 'things that go out of the body' (τὰ ἀπιόντα) remains.

chapter 13 the same expression is used (the wording of the whole sentence 13.13 is closely similar to that of 18.1–2),[23] and since in chapter 13 the author has discussed the influence of winds, it seems safe to conclude that the same restriction is intended in 18.1.

Fourthly, this interpretation requires that the word *theios* in 18.2 is used in two different ways without this shift of use being marked explicitly in the text. First, in the sentence 'these things are divine', it indicates an essential characteristic of the things mentioned, but in the following sentence it is attributed to the disease in virtue of the disease's being related to divine factors. This need not be a problem, since *theios* in itself can be used in both ways; but it seems unlikely that in this text, in which the sense in which epilepsy may be called 'divine' is one of the central issues, the author permits himself such a shift without explicitly marking it. The point of this 'derived divinity' becomes even more striking as the role assigned to the factors mentioned here is, to be sure, not negligible but not very dominant either. Admittedly, the influence of winds is noted repeatedly and discussed at length (cf. 10.2, 6.378 L.; ch. 13); but the effects of heat and cold can hardly be said to play a dominant part in the author's explanation (see above). This may also help us to understand the use of the word *prophasis* here; for if the writer of *On the Sacred Disease* adheres to a distinction between *prophasis* and *aitios*, with *prophasis* playing only the part of an external catalyst producing change within the body (in this case particularly in the brain),[24] this usage corresponds to the subordinated part which these factors play in this disease. Then the statement about the divine character of the disease acquires an almost depreciatory note: the disease is divine only to the extent that climatic factors play a certain, if a modest part in

---

[23] 13.13: οὕτως αὕτη ἡ νοῦσος γίνεταί τε καὶ θάλλει ἀπὸ τῶν προσιόντων τε καὶ ἀπιόντων, καὶ οὐδέν ἐστιν ἀπορωτέρη τῶν ἄλλων οὔτε ἰᾶσθαι οὔτε γνῶναι οὐδὲ θειοτέρη ἢ αἱ ἄλλαι.

[24] This is suggested by the use of *aitios* and *prophasis* in 3.1: 'the brain is causally responsible (*aitios*) for this affection, as it is for the greatest of the other affections; in what manner and through what cause (*prophasis*) it occurs, I am going to tell you clearly' (ἀλλὰ γὰρ αἴτιος ὁ ἐγκέφαλος τούτου τοῦ πάθεος ὥσπερ τῶν ἄλλων νοσημάτων τῶν μεγίστων, ὅτῳ δὲ τρόπῳ καὶ ἐξ οἵης προφάσιος γίνεται, ἐγὼ φράσω σαφέως. Cf. 10.4, 6.378 L.; 10.7, 6.380 L.). But the whole question, especially the meaning of *prophasis*, is highly controversial. Nörenberg (1968), discussing the views of Deichgräber (1933c) and Weidauer (1954), rejects this distinction on the ground that, if *prophasis* had this restricted meaning, then 'dürfte der Verfasser bei seiner aufklärerischen Absicht und wissenschaftlichen Systematik gerade nicht so viel Gewicht auf die *prophasies* legen, sondern er müsste vielmehr von den "eigentlichen" *aitiai* sprechen' (67). However, I think that the use of *prophasis* here (apart from other considerations which follow below) strongly suggests that there are good reasons for questioning this 'aufklärerische Absicht'. On *prophasis* and *aitia* see also Lloyd (1979) 54 n. 31, and Rawlings (1975); Nikitas (1976); Robert (1976); Hunter (1982) 326–31.

its development. If this is true, it becomes difficult to read this statement as the propagation of a new theological doctrine.[25]

Fifthly, the remark that the climatic factors are divine is itself rather surprising and has not been anticipated in the preceding chapters.[26] Nor does the divinity of 'cold, sun and winds' appear to be a self-evident idea which the author can simply take for granted. Of the three factors mentioned, the sun is least problematic, since the divinity of the celestial bodies was hardly ever questioned throughout the classical period, even in intellectual circles[27] – although the focus of the text is not on the sun as a celestial body but rather on the heat it produces (see 10.2, 6.378 L.). The divinity of cold (*psuchos*) seems completely unprecedented, and the divinity of the winds could only be explained as the persistence of a mythological idea. This is, of course, not impossible, since the author has been shown to have adopted other 'primitive' notions as well.[28] Another possibility is to suppose that he is influenced on this point by Diogenes of Apollonia or by Anaximenes (on this see n. 11 above); but neither of these explicitly deduces from the divinity of 'air' (*aēr*) the divinity of winds, nor does the writer of *On the Sacred Disease* say that air is divine – although he does say that air is the source of human intelligence (*phronēsis*, 16.2, 6.390 L.).[29] Nor is the divinity of climatic factors attested in other Hippocratic writings.[30] In any case

---

[25] A derogatory tone of the words 'these things are divine' is also recognised by Thivel (1975) 66; however, as will become clear, I do not agree with Thivel's view that the author does not take the divine character of the disease seriously ('Vous cherchez du divin dans l'épilepsie, dit-il à peu près de ses adversaires, mais tout ce qu'il y a de divin dans cette maladie, c'est sa cause naturelle, c'est-à-dire qu'il n'y en a pas du tout'), nor with his general views on the religious belief of the author (see n. 59 below).

[26] See H. W. Miller (1953) 6–7: 'The basic question is why these forces or elements of Nature are described as divine.' I do not believe that the belief in the divinity of these factors can be derived from 1.31 ('for if a man by magic and sacrifices causes the moon to eclipse and the sun to disappear and storm and calm weather to occur, I would not call any of these things (τούτων) divine, but rather human, if indeed the power of the divine is controlled and subdued by human reasoning') for τούτων refers to the actions, not to the celestial and climatic factors.

[27] With the possible exception of Anaxagoras (DK A 42, A 35); on this see Guthrie (1965) vol. 11, 307–8.

[28] On this Lloyd (1979) 43–4; Parker (1983) 213ff.; on the divinity of winds in Greek religion see Nilsson (1955) 116–17, and D. Wachsmuth (1975) 1380–1. One objection, however, to this interpretation is the fact that this belief in the divinity of winds was frequently connected with magical claims and practices which the author of *On the Sacred Disease* explicitly rejects as blasphemous in 1.29–31 (6.358–60 L.).

[29] Contra H. W. Miller (1953) 7–8. On Diogenes see DK A 9; on Anaximenes' views on winds see DK A 5 and A 7. On the importance of air in *On the Sacred Disease* see also Miller (1948) 168–83.

[30] Kudlien (1977, 270) believes that in *Prognostic* 1 (p. 194,4 Alexanderson (2.212 L.)) the words 'something divine' (τι θεῖον) also refer to climatic factors, but this is apparently based on *On the Sacred Disease* 18.1–2 alone (on the danger of this sort of transference see n. 19 above). Moreover I am not sure whether the text of *Prognostic* can bear this interpretation. In the passage in question

the statement sounds too strange to be accepted as a self-evident idea not needing explanation.

Finally, as was already noted by Nestle,[31] the restricted interpretation of 'the divine' as the climatic factors is absent (and out of the question) in the parallel discussion of the divine character of diseases in chapter 22 of *Airs, Waters, Places*. Although the writer of *Airs, Waters, Places*, in accordance with the overall purpose of his treatise, generally assigns to climatic factors a fundamental role in his explanation of health and disease, he does not say anything about their allegedly divine character and surprisingly does not, in his discussion of the divinity of diseases in chapter 22, explain this with an appeal to climatic factors. In the case discussed there (the frequent occurrence of impotence among the Scythians) the *prophasies* of the disease are purely 'human' factors,[32] and no influence of climatic factors

(γνόντα οὖν χρὴ τῶν παθέων τῶν τοιούτων τὰς φύσιας, ὁκοσον ὑπὲρ τὴν δύναμιν εἰσιν τῶν σωμάτων, ἅμα δὲ καὶ εἴ τι θεῖον ἔνεστι ἐν τῇσι νούσοισιν, καὶ τούτων τὴν πρόνοιαν ἐκμανθάνειν), the distribution of πάθος (or νόσημα, which is the *varia lectio*) and νοῦσος suggests that in the author's opinion the first thing for the physician to do is to identify the nature of the pathological situation (which consists in diagnosis and, as the text says, in determining the extent to which the disease exceeds the strength of the patient's body) and at the same time to see whether 'something divine' is present in the disease in question. As the structure of the sentence (the use of the participle γνόντα and of the infinitive ἐκμανθάνειν) indicates, it cannot be maintained (as Kudlien believes) that a distinction is made here between diseases which result in death and diseases of divine, i.e. (in Kudlien's view) climatic, origin; as the context shows, the physician should check first whether the disease is capable of being cured lest, if not, he will be blamed for the patient's death (ἀναίτιος ἂν εἴη), thus τῇσι νούσοισι clearly refers to τοιούτων παθέων (the word νοῦσος being now used because the φύσις of the πάθος has been recognised), and τούτων can only refer to τοιούτων παθέων. Another objection to Kudlien's view is that the wording εἴ τι θεῖον ἔνεστι ἐν τῇσι νούσοισιν apparently implies that a certain disease may (but need not) contain a divine element, whereas if meteorological or environmental medicine were referred to here, it would only be possible to say that a disease has a climatic cause or that it has not. Nor is Kudlien's reference to ch. 25 convincing evidence for his view, for there the author is not concerned with causes of diseases, but with symptoms. Besides, we may wonder whether his claim that in different areas the significance of the symptoms remains the same is compatible with the principles of environmental medicine as stated in *Airs, Waters, Places*. I see no other possibility than to interpret the passage as a recognition (which may be quite perfunctory or just in order to be on the safe side) that in some cases a disease may be sent by a god and that, consequently, in these cases human treatment is useless (so that the physician cannot be blamed for therapeutic failure) and, perhaps (though this is not explicitly stated), that it can only be cured by divine agency; nor do I see why this interpretation would be inconceivable (for a similar case cf. *On the Nature of the Woman* 1, where the possibility that a divine element is present in diseases is recognised, without this possibility being specified or explained or taken into account in the course of the treatise).

[31] Nestle (1938) 4–5.
[32] The explanation of the Scythians' impotence is that owing to their habit of horse-riding they are afflicted with varicosity of the veins followed by lameness. Then they try to cure themselves by means of cutting the vein which runs behind each ear. It is this treatment which causes their impotence. Later on in the chapter (sections 11–12 Diller, 2.80 L.) it is only the practice of horse-riding (with the consequent swelling of the joints) which is mentioned as the *prophasis* of the disease, to which are added their wearing trousers, as well as cold and fatigue (here *psuchos* is mentioned, but it obviously refers to getting cold when riding on horseback for a long time).

is mentioned. Of course the validity of this argument depends on the assumption of a common author of *On the Sacred Disease* and *Airs, Waters, Places* and on the presumption that he has not changed his opinion on the subject – a long-standing issue which is still a matter of disagreement. It is evident that this question would have to be settled on other grounds as well, for possible divergencies in the concepts of the divine expressed in the two treatises might equally well be taken as ground for assuming two different authors.[33]

Perhaps none of these considerations can be regarded as genuine objections. But it can hardly be denied that the first interpretation necessarily presupposes all of them and that the champions of this interpretation should take account of them. It therefore remains to consider whether the second interpretation (2) rests on less complicated presuppositions.

On this interpretation the disease is divine in virtue of having a *phusis*, a 'nature' (in the sense defined above: a regular pattern of origin and growth). This appears to be closer to the text of the three passages quoted: the mention of *phusis* in 1.2 and 2.1–2 in the immediate context of the claim that epilepsy is not more divine than other diseases can easily be understood, since it is exactly its 'having a nature' which constitutes the divine character of the disease. A further advantage of this interpretation is that the referent of 'the same (i.e. origin)' (τοῦ αὐτοῦ) is immediately supplied by the context ('have a nature from which each of them arises', φύσιν ἔχειν ... ὅθεν ἕκαστα γίνεται) and that in 18.2 the sentence 'and each of them has a nature and a power of its own, and none is hopeless or impossible to deal with' (φύσιν δὲ ἕκαστον ... οὐδ' ἀμήχανον) can be taken as providing the explanation of 'all are divine and all are human' (πάντα θεῖα καὶ πάντα ἀνθρώπινα): all diseases are divine in virtue of having a nature and a power of their own, and all are human in virtue of being capable of human treatment and cure, with the phrase 'none is hopeless or impossible to deal with' (οὐδὲν ἄπορόν ἐστιν οὐδ' ἀμήχανον) answering 'it is in no respect less curable than the others ...' (καὶ ἰητὸν εἶναι οὐδὲν ἧσσον ἑτέρων) in 2.3 (6.364 L.). This corresponds very well with the use of 'human' (ἀνθρώπινος) in the author's criticism of the magicians (1.25, 6.358 L.; 1.31, 6.360 L.): whereas in their conception of the divinity of the disease 'divine' and 'human' exclude each other, the author regards it as one of his merits to have shown that

---

[33] On this question see, e.g., Heinimann (1945) 181–206; a useful summary of the discussion is given by Nörenberg (1968) 9–11; on the significance of similarities and discrepancies between the two treatises for the question of their authorship cf. Grensemann (1968c) 7–18 and the interesting analysis by Ducatillon (1977) 197–226; see also van der Eijk (1991).

in his conception the words can perfectly well be predicated of the same subject. *Theios* and *anthrōpinos* refer to aspects of diseases, but not, as in the first interpretation, in the sense of their being caused by divine factors and human factors (which would after all imply the incompatibility of the two words).[34] On this reading, the problem of the 'derived divinity' or of the 'shift' of the use of *theios*, as well as the need to take *kai* in 18.1 as explicative, disappears. Furthermore, on this view *On the Sacred Disease* and *Airs, Waters, Places* express the same doctrine concerning the divinity of diseases, and in both treatises the use of *theios* is justified by the connotations 'unchanging', 'imperishable' and 'eternal'. The fact that all diseases have a nature, a definite pattern of origin and growth or cause and effect, constitutes the element of 'constancy' which inheres in the word *theios*. Perhaps also the connotation of 'oneness' or 'definiteness' is present here, in that all the various and heterogeneous symptoms and expressions of the disease, which the magicians attributed to different gods (1.32–9, 6.360–2 L.), can be reduced to one fixed nature underlying them.[35]

There are, however, two difficulties involved in this interpretation, the first of which is precisely the basis of the other view: the phrase 'these things are divine' (ταῦτα δ' ἐστὶ θεῖα, 18.2). To be sure, the divine character of the factors mentioned in 18.1 might now, on the second interpretation, be better understood, as these factors too probably have a *phusis* and are therefore divine. But in order to understand the divinity of the disease the mention of the divine character of these factors is, strictly speaking, irrelevant, because it suffices for the author to have demonstrated that the disease is caused by natural factors which constitute its *phusis*. It is the fact of the disease having these causes (i.e. its having a *phusis*), not the allegedly divine character of these causes, which determines its divinity.

A possible solution to this problem is to adopt the reading of the manuscript Θ (which is in general not less reliable than the other authority

---

[34] As 1.25 (6.358 L.) and 1.31 (6.360 L.) show, the words *theios* and *anthrōpinos* are not applied to concrete factors, but to aspects which are expressed in the form of propositions: 'it belongs to divinity to ...' or 'we use the word divine when ...'.

[35] But it is dangerous to explain the author's connection of 'divine' with 'having a nature' by means of associations like 'rational' or 'the rationality of nature'. It is highly questionable whether the author of *On the Sacred Disease* can be credited with the identification of the divine with 'rational' or 'knowable': the only explicit statement which might support this association is his criticism of the idea that what is divine cannot be known or understood (1.4: 'their hopelessness of not knowing', ἀπορίη τοῦ μὴ γινώσκειν; 13.13: 'nor is it more hopeless [than other diseases] ... neither as far as curing nor as far as understanding it is concerned', οὐδὲν ἀπορωτέρη ... οὔτε ἰᾶσθαι οὔτε γνῶναι; cf. n. 13 above); but this does not imply that the divine is (in the Platonic sense) the knowable *par excellence*. Nor does the association of *theios* with the 'laws' of Nature have any textual basis (on the difference between the nature of the disease and Nature in general see below, pp. 60, 68–9).

M),³⁶ which has ταύτῃ instead of ταῦτα, and to take the diseases as the subject of ἐστί: 'in this way (or, in this respect) they are divine' (ταύτῃ δ' ἐστὶ θεῖα). On this reading, 'in this way' refers to their being caused by the causes (προφάσιες) just mentioned. Strictly speaking, this is syntactically awkward, as in the preceding sentence the word νοῦσος ('disease') is used, which would demand a plural verb form (εἰσί); but ἐστί might be defended by understanding τὰ νοσήματα ('the diseases') as its subject, the word νόσημα being used in the immediately following dependent clause.³⁷ On this reading the problem of the shift of the use of *theios* disappears as well.

One other problem remains, to which I see no completely satisfactory answer. Even if, as a consequence of this interpretation, the enumeration of causes in 18.1 is extended by understanding 'the things that come and go away' as referring to air, water and food, the absence of the brain, which was claimed to be the cause of the disease (3.1, 6.366 L.), is striking. We could suppose, as I have suggested above, that a distinction between *aitios* and *prophasis* is implicitly present here: for it is true that, for instance, chapters 13–16 explain how the winds affect the brain and so cause diseases, and the author's claim that the brain is *aitios* leaves open various possibilities for the account of the *prophasies*. But then the question remains why it is only these *prophasies* which are mentioned here in chapter 18, for it seems very improbable that they are more important as constitutive elements of the nature of the disease than the cause of the disease, the brain. Perhaps the point of mentioning them here is that they are the *prophasies* of *all* diseases, and that by showing this the author only strives to put epilepsy on an equal level with the other diseases. If this is correct, the reason for not mentioning the brain and other internal factors is not that they are not constitutive of the divine character of the disease (for on this interpretation they are) but that they do not play a part in all other diseases (3.1: 'the greatest', τῶν μεγίστων). Another possibility is to say that the divinity of the disease resides in the regular pattern of the process of its origin and

---

³⁶ See Grensemann (1968c) 31–9; Jones in Jones and Withington (1923–31) vol. IV, 135–7. [Postscript: See also Roselli (1996) 87 and 103 n. 105, who accepts this reading and translates 'quanto a questo (le malattie) sono divine' (though she does not print it in the Greek text on p. 86). Laskaris (2002, 122 n. 77) and Jouanna (2003, 130–1) discuss the problem but prefer to stick to the reading ταῦτα.]

³⁷ An anonymous referee has pointed to the use of νοσήματα in the final sentence of ch. 17. However, it is hard to believe that, on the reading ταῦτα, we should take this as referring to these νοσήματα, since in the intermediate sentence (18.1) several neuter terms have been used. Alternatively, one might perhaps even consider reading ταύτῃ δ' ἐστὶ θείη and understand αὕτη ἡ νοῦσος as the subject ('in this respect the disease is divine'). But this makes τὸ νόσημα difficult to account for, and it is, of course, not just choosing between two variant readings but emending the text as well.

growth, and that the *prophasies* are mentioned because they are simply the external starting-points of this process, which set the mechanism in motion.

It turns out that neither of the two interpretations is completely free from difficulties. Yet it seems that the problems involved in the first are more numerous and compelling than those inherent to the second; moreover, the second is closer to the wording of the text. Therefore, it is preferable to conclude that according to the author of *On the Sacred Disease* diseases are divine in virtue of having a nature, and that the supposedly divine status of their *prophasies* has nothing to do with it. But in any case, as far as the question of the 'theology' of the treatise is concerned, it suffices to say that on both views the divine character of the disease is based upon natural factors.

3 RECONSTRUCTIONS OF THE AUTHOR'S THEOLOGY

On the basis of either of these interpretations, or a combination of them, scholars have tried to reconstruct the author's theology or religious thought. These reconstructions have resulted in a conception in which 'the divine' (*to theion*) is regarded as an immanent natural principle or natural 'law' governing all natural processes and constituting the imperishable order within the ever flowing natural phenomena. It is sometimes stated that this 'divine' is identified with nature and that *to theion* is equal to *hē phusis* or *to kata phusin*.[38] As a consequence, it is claimed that the author of *On the Sacred Disease* does not believe in supernatural divine intervention within natural processes and human affairs. For the practical interest of the physician this conception has two important implications. First, diseases are no longer regarded as concrete effects of deliberate divine dispensation or as god-sent pollutions; second, for the treatment of the disease an appeal to the healing power of the gods (as made in temple medicine) is unnecessary or even useless, since the cure of the disease can be accomplished by ordinary natural means.

Both implications seem to obtain for the writer of *On the Sacred Disease*, for he explicitly denies the diseases are god-sent in the traditional sense (1.44, 6.362 L.) and he claims that the disease can be cured by means of dietetic measures (18.3–6, 6.394–6 L.). In this way his positive theological statements might be viewed as providing the general philosophical framework on which his aetiological and therapeutic views are based.

[38] Lloyd (1979) 31; Ducatillon (1977) 202.

However, this extrapolation of a 'theology' from the statements about the divine character of the disease presupposes three generalisations which are in themselves questionable, and which appear to be inconsistent with other assertions in the treatise. First, it is ignored that there is a difference between calling a particular phenomenon 'divine' in virtue of a certain aspect or characteristic, and speaking about 'the divine' (*to theion*) in a general and abstract way. As a result, it is tacitly assumed that by defining the divine character of the disease as its being caused by natural factors (or as its having a nature) the author implicitly confines the range of the divine to nature or to the regularity which natural phenomena show (as if he not only said 'Nature is divine', but also 'The divine is identical with nature'). Not only is such a generalisation of the use of the word *theios* dangerous in itself, but it also lacks any textual justification, for in none of the 'positive' statements does the writer use the expression *to theion* in an abstract way. In fact, the only instances of this use of *to theion* are 1.25 (6.358 L.), 1.27 (6.358 L.), 1.31 (6.360 L.) and 1.45 (6.364 L.), where the expression seems equivalent to *hoi theoi* ('the gods').[39]

Secondly, it is assumed that what the writer says about the divine character of diseases holds of every natural phenomenon or event ('natural' from our modern point of view, e.g. earthquakes, solar eclipses, etc.) and that in his view all these phenomena show a similarly regular pattern of origin and development and are therefore divine in the same sense as diseases.[40] But, strictly speaking, the author of *On the Sacred Disease* merely denies that epilepsy has a divine origin in the traditional sense (in which *theios* implies *theopemptos*, 'god-sent'), and he asserts that it is not more divine than other diseases. This need not imply that all other phenomena are divine in this new sense of 'being natural' (*panta*, 'all', in 18.2 refers to *nosēmata*, 'diseases'), nor that a particular phenomenon is divine only in this sense. The author leaves open the possibility that there are other things which may be the effect of divine dispensation (in the traditional sense), for example divine blessings, and the idea of divine dispensation or intervention as such is nowhere rejected. We may even wonder whether the author really rejects every appeal to divine healing, for in spite of his self-assurance concerning the curability of the disease (18.3–6, 6.394–6 L.), he admits that in some

---

[39] For other instances of τὸ θεῖον see 1.4 (6.352 L.), where the expression obviously means 'the divine character' (sc. 'of the disease'); 1.11 (6.354 L.) is ambiguous: τὸ θεῖον may be synonymous with οἱ θεοί, but it may also mean 'the (allegedly) divine character of the disease', as in 1.20 (6.356 L.) and 1.26 (6.358 L.); in 1.28 (6.360 L.) τὸ θεῖον αὐτῶν is best translated 'the divine character they talk about': there is no question of θεῖος meaning 'pious' here (contra Ducatillon (1977) 199).

[40] See Nörenberg (1968) 75: 'Insofern ist alles bis zu dem Grade göttlich, in dem es an diesen Naturgesetzen teilhat.'

cases the illness is too strong for medical drugs (2.3, 6.364 L.; 11.6, 6.382 L.). It may be doubted whether the author would regard an appeal to the gods in such cases as useless. Admittedly, one of his concerns is that epilepsy should be treated no differently from any other disease; but he nowhere categorically rejects any appeal to the gods for the healing of hopeless cases. These remarks may seem speculative and ill-founded, but I will qualify this issue below.

Thirdly, it is supposed that the word *phusis* is used here in the sense of 'Nature' or even 'the laws of Nature', or in any case of something general and universal, an all-pervading principle, comparable to the use of *phusis* in Presocratic philosophy, for example in treatises entitled 'On Nature' (*peri phuseōs*). But in the text of *On the Sacred Disease* the word *phusis* is used almost exclusively to denote the specific nature or character of the disease (18.2: 'each of them has a nature and a power of its own').[41] Admittedly in some cases the author makes more general claims concerning the items of his explanation,[42] but it cannot be maintained that his explanation of the disease makes explicit use of general patterns or principles like the *archai* of the Presocratic philosophers.

Apart from the question whether these generalisations are justified, there is evidence from the text itself that it is wrong to attribute such a 'naturalistic' theology to the author of *On the Sacred Disease*. In the polemical first chapter of the treatise, in his objections against the ideas and the practices of the magicians, we can find several implicit presuppositions which do not make sense within such a naturalistic conception of the divine. This applies particularly to the accusations of impiety (*asebeia*) and atheism (*atheos*) which begin in 1.28 (6.358 L.) and which are continued in 1.39ff. (6. 362 L.). First, the writer criticises his opponents for making impious claims, for example that they can influence the movements of sun and moon and the weather. This claim, the author says, amounts to believing that the gods neither exist nor have any power, and that what is said to be divine actually becomes human, since on this claim the power of the divine 'is overcome and has been enslaved' (1.31, 6.360 L.: κρατεῖται καὶ δεδούλωται) by human reason. I do not mean to say that we may infer from this that the author of *On the Sacred Disease* believes the movements of the sun and the moon and the weather-phenomena to be manifestations of divine agency (cf. note 26 above). The hypothetical sentences (note the use of εἰ γάρ in 1.29 and 1.31) show that he blames his opponents for behaving

---

[41] See Nörenberg (1968) 49–61, 80.
[42] For instance 2.4 (6.364 L.), 3.1 (6.366 L.), 18.5–6 (6.396 L.).

contrarily to their own principles: they pretend to be pious men and to rely on the gods for help, but in fact they make the impious claim to perform actions which a pious man believes to be reserved to the gods alone. Yet the author himself appears to have an explicit opinion on what is pious and what is not (or what a truly pious man should and should not do).

This becomes clearer in the second accusation of *asebeia* in 1.39ff. (6.362 L.). The impiety of his opponents, he points out, consists in their practising purificatory rites and incantations, and in their cleansing the diseased by means of blood as if they had a 'pollution' (*miasma*) or were possessed by a demon, or bewitched by other people. However, the writer proceeds (1.41, 6.362 L.), they should act in the opposite way: they should sacrifice and pray and, having brought the diseased into the temple, make supplications to the gods. Yet instead of this they practise purifications and conceal the polluted material lest anyone would get into contact with it. However, the author claims again (1.43, 6.362–4 L.), they should bring the material into the temple and hand it over to the god, if this god were the cause of it.

The remarks in sections 1.41 and 1.43 again show that the author has definite opinions on the pious course of action when dealing with a disease which is believed to be of divine origin and for which an appeal is made to divine healing. The contrast between sections 1.39–40 and 1.41 is clearly what we would call the contrast between magic and religion: in the first case man himself performs the purification by making the gods obey his incantations (*epaōidai*); in the latter case man approaches the gods in the temple and prays for help, but it is the god who performs the purification (cf. 1.44–5).[43] It has been suggested by Lanata that these precepts concerning piety (*eusebeia*) are characteristic of the holy prescriptions of temple medicine.[44] This is not inconceivable, since it is confirmed by our knowledge of the holy laws of Asclepieia[45] – although the precepts are so general that they can hardly be regarded as exclusively characteristic of temple medicine. Now, this is not to suggest that the author of *On the Sacred Disease*, who has always been hailed as one of the first champions of an emancipated science of medicine, actually was a physician serving in the cult of Asclepius[46] – even though the borderlines between secular

---

[43] See Nestle (1938) 2; Edelstein (1967a) 223, 237.
[44] Lanata (1967) 38 n. 86. Cf. Ducatillon (1977) 164 n. 3.
[45] On the ritual of temple medicine see Edelstein and Edelstein (1945) vol. II, 148–9; Parker (1983) 213 n. 31; Ginouvès (1962) 349–57; Krug (1985) 128–34.
[46] Contra Herzog (1931) 149–51, who ignores the hypothetical wording of the sentence and whose interpretation of the author's concept of the divinity of the disease is completely mistaken (cf. the criticism of Lloyd (1975c) 13 n. 19).

medicine and temple medicine never were as sharp as we tend to think, the co-operation of physicians in temple medicine being frequently attested;[47] nor does the suggestion itself seem unlikely, for it might well explain the vigour with which the author attacks magic and defends religion. The reason for not accepting this suggestion is simply that the text does not support it (on 1.44–6 see below). Yet what it does show is that the author has definite ideas on what one should do when invoking the help of the gods for the healing of a disease, and he may very well be thinking of the particular situation of temple medicine, with which he was no doubt familiar (which does not, of course, imply that he was involved in these practices or approved).

One may point to this hypothetical 'should' and object, as I suggested at the beginning of this chapter, that these remarks need not imply the author's personal involvement, but are solely used as arguments *ad hominem*. He may, for the purpose of criticising and discrediting his opponents, point out how a man *ought* to act when making an appeal to divine help for the cure of a disease, but this need not imply that he himself takes this way of healing seriously (after all, invoking the gods for healing presupposes the belief in a 'supernatural' intervention in natural processes). To a certain extent this objection is justified, for both sentences (1.41 and 1.43) are hypothetical and depend on premises to which the author himself need not subscribe. One of these premises is explicitly mentioned in 1.43: '*if* the god is the cause of the disease' (εἰ δὴ ὁ θεός ἐστιν αἴτιος). And one may point to the immediately following sentence (1.44), where the validity of this premise itself is denied by the author. In this way one might say that all the preceding stipulations about impiety and piety are just made for the sake of argument and do not reveal any of the author's own religious convictions: he may be perfectly aware of the truly pious thing to do without being himself a pious man.

Yet this hypothetical character is absent from the following passage (1.44–6, 6.362–4 L.), which has to be quoted in full:

οὐ μέντοι ἔγωγε ἀξιῶ ὑπὸ θεοῦ ἀνθρώπου σῶμα μιαίνεσθαι, τὸ ἐπικηρότατον ὑπὸ τοῦ ἁγνοτάτου, ἀλλὰ καὶ ἢν τυγχάνῃ ὑφ' ἑτέρου μεμιασμένον ἤ τι πεπονθός, ὑπὸ τοῦ θεοῦ καθαίρεσθαι ἂν αὐτὸ καὶ ἁγνίζεσθαι μᾶλλον ἢ μιαίνεσθαι. τὰ γ' οὖν μέγιστα τῶν ἁμαρτημάτων καὶ ἀνοσιώτατα τὸ θεῖόν ἐστι τὸ καθαῖρον καὶ ἁγνίζον καὶ ῥύμμα γινόμενον ἡμῖν, αὐτοί τε ὅρους τοῖσι θεοῖσι τῶν ἱρῶν καὶ τῶν τεμενέων ἀποδείκνυμεν, ὡς ἂν μηδεὶς ὑπερβαίνῃ ἢν μὴ ἁγνεύῃ, ἐσιόντες τε περιρραινόμεθα οὐχ ὡς μιαινόμενοι, ἀλλ' εἴ τι καὶ πρότερον ἔχομεν μύσος, τοῦτο ἀφαγνιούμενοι. καὶ περὶ μὲν τῶν καθαρμῶν οὕτω μοι δοκεῖ ἔχειν.

---

[47] See Lloyd (1979) 40–5; Edelstein and Edelstein (1945) vol. II, 139–41; Edelstein (1967a) 239; Krug (1985) 120f. and 159–63.

But I hold that the body of a man is not polluted by a god, that which is most corruptible by that which is most holy, but that even when it happens to be polluted or affected by something else, it is more likely to be cleansed from this by the god and sanctified than to be polluted by him. Concerning the greatest and most impious of our transgressions it is the divine which purifies and sanctifies us and washes them away from us; and we ourselves mark the boundaries of the sanctuaries and the precincts of the gods, lest anyone who is not pure would transgress them, and when we enter the temple we sprinkle ourselves, not as polluting ourselves thereby, but in order to be cleansed from an earlier pollution we might have contracted. Such is my opinion about the purifications.

It seems that if we are looking for the writer's religious convictions we may find them here. The first sentence shows that the author rejects the presuppositions of his opponents, namely that a god is the cause of a disease; on the contrary, he says, it is more likely that if a man is polluted by something else (ἕτερον, i.e. something different from a god), the god will cleanse him from it than pollute him with it. There is no reason to doubt the author's sincerity here: the belief that a god should pollute a man with a disease is obviously blasphemous to him; and the point of the apposition 'that which is most corruptible by that which is most holy' (τὸ ἐπικηρότατον ὑπὸ τοῦ ἁγνοτάτου) is clearly that no 'pollution' (*miasma*) can come from such a holy and pure being as a god. As for the positive part of the statement, that a god is more likely to cleanse people of their pollutions than to bestow these to them, one may still doubt whether this is just hypothetical ('*more* likely') or whether the author takes this as applying to a real situation.[48] But this doubt disappears with the next sentence (1.45–6), which evidently expresses the author's own opinion and in which his personal involvement is marked by the use of 'ourselves' (αὐτοί) and of the first person plural (ἡμῖν ... ἀποδείκνυμεν ... περιρραινόμεθα). This sentence shows that the author believes in the purifying and cleansing working of the divine. I do not think that the shift of 'the god' (ὁ θεός) to 'the divine' (τὸ θεῖον) is significant here as expressing a reluctance to believe in 'personal' or concrete gods, for in the course of the sentence he uses the expression 'the gods' (τοῖσι θεοῖσι).[49] The use of *to theion* is motivated by the contrast with *to anthrōpinon*: cleansing is performed by the divine, not – as the magicians believe (1.39, 6.362 L.) – by human beings. In fact, this whole sentence breathes an unmistakably polemical atmosphere: the marking off of sacred places for the worship of the gods was

---

[48] But ἂν καθαίρεσθαι represents a potential optative rather than an unfulfilled condition.
[49] Contra Nörenberg (1968) 69ff. The distribution of ὁ θεός, οἱ θεοί and τὸ θεῖον in this context does not admit of being used as proof that the author does not believe in 'personal' gods.

already hinted at in 1.41 and 1.43; apparently the magicians practised their purifications outside the official holy places. The use of the word 'sprinkle' (περιρραινόμεθα), which means ritual cleansing with water,[50] is opposed to the 'impious' use of blood in the purificatory rituals of the magicians (1.40);[51] and the obscure clause 'not as polluting ourselves thereby, but in order to be cleansed from an earlier pollution we might have contracted' (οὐχ ὡς μιαινόμενοι, ἀλλ᾽ ... ἀφαγνιούμενοι) probably contains a reaction against the strange idea held by the magicians that the use of water may entail pollution, which underlies their prohibition of the taking of baths (1.12, 6.354 L.).[52]

Thus interpreted, this sentence shows that the writer believes in the reality of divine purification. Does this mean that he believes, after all, in the divine healing of diseases as taking place in temple medicine? One cannot be sure here, for the divine purification is explicitly defined by the author as applying to moral trangressions (τῶν ἁμαρτημάτων), indeed to the greatest of these. This restriction is significant in that it may indicate that in the author's opinion an appeal to divine cleansing is only (or primarily) appropriate in cases of moral transgressions. I would suggest, as a hypothesis, that the author of *On the Sacred Disease* here aims at marking off the vague boundaries between medicine and religion: in his opinion it

[50] See Parker (1983) 19; Ginouvès (1962) 299–310.
[51] On the use of blood in cathartic ritual, and on the criticism it generally provoked, see Parker (1983) 371–3 and Temkin (1971), 12–13; cf. Theophrastus, *On Piety*, frs. 13–14 Pötscher (= fr. 584A Fortenbaugh, Sharples and Sollenberger). The emphasis in 1.40 is on αἵματι κτλ., but perhaps also on ὥσπερ μίασμά τι ἔχοντας.
[52] I am by no means sure that this is a correct interpretation of this difficult sentence (which is omitted, from ἀλλ᾽ εἴ τι onwards by MS Θ, which is perhaps, as Jones suggests, due to haplography of -μενοι but which may also indicate that the text is not completely reliable). At any rate, the phrase οὐχ ὡς μιαινόμενοι obviously expresses a reaction against the admittedly strange idea that the sprinkling of water entails pollution (on the prohibition to take baths see Ginouvès (1962) 395 n. 8; Lanata (1967) 51f.; Parker (1983) 215; Moulinier (1952) 136; Ducatillon (1977) 169). However, as Ginouvès points out, there is a difference between a λουτρόν and a περιρραντήριον. Perhaps it is preferable, as H. S. Versnel has suggested to me, to interpret the sentence as an extreme statement of the author's belief (expressed in 1.44–5) that a god does not pollute a man but rather purifies him from a pollution: 'while crossing the border between the sacred and the profane we sprinkle ourselves; this is, as I have said just now, not symbolic of a pollution which comes from the sacred [which is obvious to everyone, because:] it is a purification performed by God of the defilement that originates from something else [i.e. the secular]'. There is still another possible interpretation which might be considered, which makes the sentence apply to the practice of temple medicine: 'while entering the temple [for the healing of a disease], we sprinkle ourselves, not as if we were polluted [by the disease, i.e. as if the disease were a pollution – *quod non*: cf. 1.40] but in order to cleanse ourselves from an earlier pollution we may have contracted'. This would suit the author's aim of distinguishing between moral transgressions (which are, in his opinion, forms of pollution, μιάσματα) and physical diseases (which are not) and would make sense of the words ἤ τι πεπονθός in 1.44. However, on this interpretation πρότερον is difficult, and it would presumably require a perfect participle (μεμιασμένοι) instead of the present μιαινόμενοι.

is wrong to regard epilepsy (or any other disease) as a pollution (this seems to be the point of the words ὥσπερ μίασμά τι ἔχοντας in 1.40: 'as if a disease were a pollution – *quod non*'). He obviously thinks that no moral factor (punishment for crime or transgressions) is involved,[53] and that, as a consequence, one should not believe that it can be cured by the gods alone.

As for the author's religious notions, we may deduce from these passages that he believes in gods who grant men purification of their moral transgressions and who are to be worshipped in temples by means of prayer and sacrifice. It is difficult to see how this conception of 'the divine' (*to theion*) can be incorporated within the naturalistic theology with which he has often been credited.[54] If 'the divine' mentioned in 1.45 is to be identified with the divine Nature or natural laws, it cannot be seen how this moral purification should be conceived within such a theology (i.e., apart from the question of what would be the point of the writer making stipulations about ritual and cult if he held such a mechanistic conception of the divine). But instead of concluding, therefore, that the statements of the first chapter are merely rhetorical remarks which do not reflect the author's own religious opinion (which is apparently the course taken by most interpreters), I would throw doubt on the reality of this 'naturalistic theology' – for which I have given other reasons as well. It seems better to proceed in the opposite direction, which means starting from the religious assertions of the first chapter and then trying to understand the statements about the divine character of the disease. In this way, the text can be understood as motivated by two interrelated purposes. First, by claiming that epilepsy is not god-sent in the traditional sense, the author does not intend to reject the notion of divine dispensation as such; his statements are to be regarded as a form of corrective criticism of a traditional religious idea. The author claims that it is blasphemous to hold that a holy and pure being like a god would send diseases as a form of pollution; thus his remarks may be compared with statements by Plato which aim at correcting and modifying the traditional concept of divine dispensation (*theia moira*) without questioning the existence of this divine dispensation as such.[55] At the same time – and this is the second, but no doubt more urgent purpose of the treatise – the author strives to disengage epilepsy from the religious domain and to put it on an equal level, both in its aetiology and in its therapy, with all other diseases (an attempt which is easily understood from

[53] See Jaeger (1980) 158.
[54] Cf. the hesitant remarks of Nörenberg (1968) 76–7.
[55] Cf. *Republic* 379 a–380 c (e.g. 380 c 8–9: 'God is not the cause of everything but only of what is good') and *Phaedrus* 244 c.

the competitive character of early Greek medicine). To a certain extent this may be viewed as an attempt to 'secularise' the sacred disease; and from this point of view the positive statements about the divine character of the disease may be regarded as reluctant or even derogatory concessions rather than as proclamations of a new advanced theology. And from this perspective it can further be understood why the author states that epilepsy is *not more* divine than the other diseases instead of saying that all diseases are *just as* divine as epilepsy.[56] For the purpose of clarity one might paraphrase the author's intention, with some exaggeration, as follows (differentiating according to the two interpretations distinguished above): 'If epilepsy is divine, it is divine only in the sense in which all other diseases are divine; well, the only divine aspect of diseases which can be discerned is the fact that they are caused by factors which are themselves divine' (interpretation (1)) or, on interpretation (2), 'the only divine aspect of diseases which can be discerned is the fact that they have a nature'. As we have seen, on the first interpretation of the divine character of the disease (which posits its divine character in its being caused by climatic factors), this restricted conception of divinity may well be connected with the fact that the influence of these factors is rather limited (and with the use of the word *prophasis*). On the second interpretation (and on the reading ταύτῃ δ'ἐστὶ θεῖα, 'in this respect they [i.e. diseases] are divine') the emphasis is on ταύτῃ: 'it is (only) in *this* respect that they are divine'. On both views the derogatory tone of the statements can be understood from the author's attempt to mark off the boundaries between medicine and religion and to purify the concept of divine dispensation. And it can now also be understood why he defines the divinity of the disease only in those contexts where he tries to point out the difference between the sense in which his opponents believe it to be divine and the sense in which he himself believes it to be so.

This does not imply that the sincerity of the author's statements about the divine character of the disease should be doubted. Nor should their relationship with developments in natural philosophy and with other contemporary ideas on religion and the divine be questioned. It is precisely the philosophical search for unity and regularity in natural phenomena, the enquiry into cause and effect, and the belief, expressed by at least some of these philosophers, that in manifesting regularity and constancy these phenomena have a divine aspect, which may have led the author to assign a divine character to the disease in question. But the danger of stressing this relationship with natural philosophy is that we read into the text ideas

---

[56] Contra Nörenberg (1968) 26 and 49, who ignores the rhetorical impact of these statements. In 18.2 (πάντα θεῖα καὶ πάντα ἀνθρώπινα) the emphasis is on πάντα.

which simply are not there. This danger is increased when this reading is guided by modern ideas about what is 'primitive' or 'mythic' and what is 'advanced' and 'rational', so that by labelling an author as advanced or enlightened we are too much guided in our interpretation of the text by what we expect him to say. Nowhere in *On the Sacred Disease* do we find statements such as that 'Nature is divine'; nowhere do we find an explicit rejection of divine intervention in natural processes or of divine dispensation as such.[57] Caution is suggested not only by a consideration of the plurality and heterogeneity of opinions on religious matters in the second half of the fifth century,[58] but also by the different forms in which reflection on these matters has manifested itself. It is important to distinguish between the corrective, 'cathartic' criticism of traditional religious beliefs and the exposition of a positive theology. It seems that the author of *On the Sacred Disease* has been regarded too much as an exponent of the latter, and that he has been regarded more as a philosopher or a theologian than as a physician. Instead, I propose to regard as the author's primary concern the disengagement of epilepsy from the religious domain (which implies claiming it as an object of medicine) and his accusations of impiety as one rather successful way to achieve this goal; in this way the corrective criticism of a traditional idea (viz., that diseases are sent by the gods) is subordinated to a primarily medical purpose.

Even if this interpretation is convincing, it cannot be denied that there remains a tension between the author's belief in gods who cleanse men from their moral transgressions and his statements about the divine character of the disease. This tension becomes especially manifest when we confront his categorical rejection of the idea that holy beings like gods send diseases (which he labels as highly blasphemous) with his assertion, ten lines further down, that diseases are divine in virtue of having a nature. The problem is how this 'being divine' of diseases is related to the purifying influence of the gods mentioned in 1.44–6. The author does not explain this, and we may wonder whether he, if he was aware of this problem, would have been capable of solving it. Of course, there are several possible solutions which *we* might suggest, and we could speculate about the author's unexpressed ideas on theodicy and on the relation between the gods and the world in terms of providence, deism, determinism, and so on.[59] But I prefer to

---

[57] Contra H. W. Miller (1948) 2.   [58] On this Guthrie (1969) vol. III, 226–49.
[59] For such speculations cf. Thivel (1975) 67–8 and Nörenberg (1968) 75–6. Thivel draws an almost Aristotelian picture of the author's world-view: 'ces dieux...sont trop élevés pour intervenir dans les affaires humaines. Tout se passe comme si...l'univers était séparé en deux régions qui ne communiquent pas: le monde terrestre (en termes aristotéliciens on dirait: "sublunaire") où vivent les hommes, et qui est régi, y compris les maladies, par le déterminisme (la "nature", φύσιν καὶ

appreciate this tension and to accept it as a result of the polemical character of the treatise or even, perhaps, as one of those paradoxes and ambiguities which are characteristic of religious thought – even the religious thought of intellectuals.[60]

It may be thought that this view amounts, after all, to the position which I rejected at the end of the introduction, namely that we need not be surprised to find intellectuals holding or expressing religious ideas which seem incompatible with each other (either for social or for private reasons). But it will by now have become clear for what reasons (apart from those mentioned ad loc.) I did not accept that position. We have seen that the interpretation of the author's statements about the divine character of the disease, as well as the attempt to deduce his theological ideas from these statements, involved many problems. We have also seen the difficulties involved in the evaluation of the author's accusations of *asebeia*, and I have shown that it is possible to discern, in spite of the hypothetical character of most of these accusations, elements of the author's own conviction. If the results of this discussion (especially my views on the range and on the rhetorical impact of the assertions about the divinity of diseases) are convincing, the discrepancy noted at the beginning of this paper has decreased considerably, though it has not disappeared. Yet we are now in a much better position to formulate the problem more adequately and to look for an explanation that is more to the point than the one offered in section 1.

4 CONCLUSION

It will by now have become clear why the word 'theology' in the title of this chapter has been put between quotation marks. It is certainly wrong to hold that the author of *On the Sacred Disease* systematically exposes his religious beliefs and his ideas on the nature of divine causation in this text. Yet what he does show of these beliefs admits of the following conclusions. The writer believes in gods who grant men purification of their transgressions

---

πρόφασιν), et le monde céleste, séjour des dieux incorruptibles, qui habitent sans doute les astres. Ainsi les phénomènes naturels, pluie et sécheresse, vents et saisons, qui entrent pour une bonne part dans les causes des maladies, sont dus des enchaînements aveugles, où la responsabilité des dieux n'est nullement engagée.' But this view is a consequence of Thivel's interpretation of 18.1–2, which he takes as implying that natural phenomena have no divine aspect whatsoever (see n. 25 above). It will be clear that I cannot endorse this interpretation. As for Nörenberg see n. 9 above: his account of the problem is closer to the text, but it is confused because of his failure to distinguish between interpretations (1) and (2).

[60] Similar ambiguities may be found in the religious thought of, e.g., Plato and Aristotle; see Verdenius (1960); Babut (1974).

and who are to be worshipped in temples by means of prayer and sacrifice. The text is silent on the author's conception of the nature of these gods, but there is, at least, no textual evidence that he rejected the notion of 'personal' or even 'anthropomorphic' gods.[61] He has explicit opinions on how (and in what circumstances) these gods should be approached, and he definitely thinks it blasphemous to hold that these holy beings send diseases to men as pollutions. Diseases are not the effects of divine dispensation; nevertheless they have a divine aspect in that they show a constant and regular pattern of origin and development. How this 'being divine' is related to 'the divine' (or, the gods) which cleanses men from moral transgressions is not explained.

The idea of divine dispensation as such is nowhere questioned in the text of *On the Sacred Disease*. Gods are ruled out as causes of diseases; whether they are ruled out as healers as well is not certain, since the text is silent on this subject. As I remarked earlier, the author does not believe that epilepsy can be cured by natural means in all cases: on two occasions (2.3, 6.364 L.; 11.6, 6.382 L.) he recognises that in some cases the disease can no longer be cured. Of course we can only speculate what he would do in such cases, but it does not seem alien to Hippocratic medicine to make an appeal to the gods in such hopeless cases.[62] We have seen that the borderlines between secular medicine and temple medicine were vague and that the relationship between these was seldom hostile or antagonistic (see n. 47 above). Nor is the combination of 'natural' therapeutic measures with prayers and sacrifices unattested in the Hippocratic collection. Thus the writer of *On Regimen* explicitly recommends this combination, and among his therapeutic remarks dietetic precepts and instructions concerning the gods to whom one should pray are found side by side.[63] Of course, we should beware of generalisation and not try to harmonise divergent doctrines, for *On Regimen* has been claimed to reflect a religiosity which is rather exceptional in the Hippocratic corpus and which is, according to one critic, 'completely different' from that of *On the Sacred Disease*.[64] Now the 'theology' of *On*

---

[61] Contra Nörenberg (1968) 78, whose claim is probably prompted by the idea that this would be incompatible with the 'enlightening intention' ('aufklärerische Absicht') of the author of *On the Sacred Disease*.

[62] This is speculative, since it is nowhere stated explicitly that in these cases the patient should make an appeal to divine healing, though the case of *Prognostic* 1 (see n. 30 above) seems to imply this. But the recognition that in some cases medicine fails to help is frequently attested (see *On the Art of Medicine* 8). On hopeless cases see Edelstein (1967a) 243–5; Krug (1985) 120–1; Thivel (1975) 60.

[63] *On Regimen* 4.87 (6.642 L.): 'prayer is a good thing, but while calling on the gods one should also put in effort oneself' (καὶ τὸ μὲν εὔχεσθαι ἀγαθόν· δεῖ δὲ καὶ αὐτὸν συλλαμβάνοντα τοὺς θεοὺς ἐπικαλεῖσθαι); cf. 89.14 (6.652 L.), 90.7 (6.656 L.) and 93.6 (6.662 L.) (references are to the edition of R. Joly and S. Byl (1984)). [For a fuller discussion see van der Eijk (2004a).]

[64] Kudlien (1977) 274; cf. Nörenberg (1968) 77–8.

Regimen is another matter which cannot be discussed here – though here, too, interpreters have been misguided by *a priori* conceptions of 'mythic religiosity'.[65] It will be clear that on the above interpretation of *On the Sacred Disease* the positions advanced in the two treatises are not so far removed from each other. An important point is that the author of *On Regimen* recommends prayers in various sorts of diseases, whereas the writer of *On the Sacred Disease* would probably do so only – if ever – in hopeless cases. On the other hand it must be conceded that the author of *On Regimen* substantiates his claim to the ability to cure far more elaborately than the author of *On the Sacred Disease*, who confines himself to just a few general remarks on therapy which may apply to any disease.[66] But the treatises differ so widely in purpose and method that comparisons are problematic. The sole object of mentioning *On Regimen* is to show the danger of using apparent differences in 'theology' or 'religiosity' between the various Hippocratic treatises as evidence for establishing the relative dates of the treatises.[67]

Postscript

Major discussions of *On the Sacred Disease* that have come out since the original publication of this paper are Stol (1993), Roselli (1996), Hankinson (1998c), Wöhlers (1999), Laskaris (2002), Jouanna (2003) and Lloyd (2003) 43–50. While some scholars (Hankinson, Jouanna, Roselli) have accepted my position regarding the author's religious beliefs, others (Laskaris, Lloyd) prefer to read the author's arguments in chapter 1 predominantly as rhetorical and not necessarily expressing the author's own views. My suggestion to prefer the reading ταύτῃ in 18.2 has been adopted by Roselli, though

---

[65] See Nörenberg (1968) 78: 'Trotz seiner medizinischen Kenntnisse verschiedener Diäten und krankhafter Zustände unterliegt dieser Verfasser noch ganz dem Aberglauben'; and Thivel (1975) 64: 'Il existe probablement, dans la Collection hippocratique, peu de traités qui se tiennent aussi éloignés du véritable esprit scientifique.' Both Kudlien and Nörenberg point to the belief in divine dreams (4.87.1) as evidence of this; but this belief was hardly ever questioned throughout the classical period (with the exception of Aristotle). One of the interesting characteristics of *On Regimen* 4 is that the author states that he will not deal with divine dreams, but only with those dreams which have a physical origin, while at the same time incorporating religious instructions among his therapeutic remarks. This is, of course, not an inconsistency or a sign of the alleged 'compilatory' character of the book (as van Lieshout (1980, 186–7) seems to think), but an interesting example of the surprising relations between science and religion of which Greek medicine provides evidence (see Lloyd (1979) 42).

[66] This may be because his claims concerning the curability of the disease are actually quite weak (see Lloyd (1979) 22, 49 and 56–7), but it may just as well be due to the purpose of the treatise, which does not aim at giving therapeutic details. [It should further be noted that the author of *On Regimen* is first of all concerned with the prevention of disease rather than its cure; see van der Eijk (2004a).]

[67] Contra Kudlien (1977) 274 and Nörenberg (1968) 78.

Laskaris and Jouanna prefer to keep the other reading ταῦτα. According to Jouanna, the author in the course of his argument develops the notion of *prophasis* in the sense of external catalyst ('cause déclenchante due aux facteurs extérieurs') and in the end distinguishes it from that of *phusis*, the natural cause or 'law' determining the development of the disease ('cause naturelle et lois de développement de la maladie'). He concludes that there is no contradiction, since both external causal factors and the internal 'nature' of the disease are subject to the same natural laws and therefore divine ('Il n'y a aucune contradiction selon l'auteur entre une maladie divine à cause de sa *phusis* ou à cause de sa *prophasis*. Tout cela est de l'ordre du divin dans la mesure où tous ces phénomènes obéissent à des lois naturelles qui sont les mêmes aussi bien à l'extérieur de l'homme qu'en l'homme, lois qui sont indépendantes de l'intervention humaine' (2003, 130–1)). I still think that this does not fully address the problems I raise in my discussion of this passage and reads too many elements in the text which are not explicitly stated (e.g. the notion of 'natural law'), although I concede, as I did in my original paper, that my suggestion to read ταύτῃ is not free from difficulties either.

I have discussed the relationship between *On the Sacred Disease* and *Airs, Waters, Places* in van der Eijk (1991), arriving at the view that there is no reason to believe that the two treatises are by different authors; similar conclusions have been arrived at (apparently independently) by Bruun (1997); see also Jouanna (1996) 71–3 and (2003) lxx–lxxiv. I have discussed the similar structure of the argumentation in *On the Sacred Disease* and in Aristotle's *On Divination in Sleep* in van der Eijk (1994) 294–5 (see also Hankinson (1998c) making a similar point). I have dealt at greater length with the religious beliefs of the author of *On Regimen* in van der Eijk (2004a).

On the question of 'the divine' in other Hippocratic treatises see Lichtenthaeler (1992) on *Prognostic*, and Flemming and Hanson (1998) on *Diseases of Young Women*.

CHAPTER 2

Diocles and the Hippocratic writings on the method of dietetics and the limits of causal explanation

1 INTRODUCTION

In antiquity Diocles of Carystus enjoyed the reputation of being a 'younger Hippocrates', or 'second in fame and venerability to Hippocrates'.[1] Yet this did not prevent him from developing his own ideas and from writing medical treatises in his own style in the Attic dialect. To be sure, later reports on his doctrines often represent him as being in perfect agreement with 'Hippocrates' on various subjects;[2] but the fragments of his works that have been preserved, show that the authority of 'the great Coan' did not prevent him from taking issue with some ideas and practices that are similar to what is to be found in texts which we call Hippocratic.[3] Of course we do not know whether Diocles, if he had actually read these works, took them to be by Hippocrates – in fact, if we accept Wesley Smith's suggestion that the Hippocratic Corpus was created by third-century Alexandrian philologists who brought together a number of anonymous medical works into one collection under the name of Hippocrates,[4] we may wonder whether anything like Hippocratic authority already existed in Diocles' time (not to mention the fact that Diocles' date itself is the subject of another controversy). It is not even certain that Diocles had ever heard of Hippocrates or was familiar with any of his genuine works.[5]

This chapter was first published in R. Wittern and P. Pellegrin (eds.), *Hippokratische Medizin und antike Philosophie* (Hildesheim, 1996) 229–57.
[1] (Pseudo-)Vindicianus, *On the Seed* 2 (Diocles, fr. 3); Pliny, *Natural History* 26.10 (Diocles, fr. 4). The Diocles fragments are numbered according to my edition (2000a, 2001a), which replaces the edition by Wellmann (1901).
[2] See, for example, frs. 26, 27, 28, 33, 36 and 52.
[3] See, for example, frs. 55a, 55b and 57.   [4] Smith (1990a) 6–18.
[5] Notwithstanding Wellmann's view (1901, 64) that Diocles was familiar with many Hippocratic writings and even was the creator of the Hippocratic Corpus, there are no *verbatim* attestations that Diocles knew Hippocrates' name or that he took several writings to be Hippocratic. The only exception is fr. 55b (Stephanus of Athens, *Commentary on Hippocrates' Aphorisms* 2.33, p. 210,30ff. Westerink (*CMG* XI 1, 3, 1)), where Diocles is quoted as arguing explicitly against Hippocrates, but this seems to be a doxographic construction (Stephanus is generally believed to rely on Galen's commentary

This heaping up of uncertainties at the beginning of this chapter may appear a rather weak rhetorical strategy. Yet it throws some light on my reasons for selecting Diocles' fragment 176 for discussion in the context of an examination of the relationship between Hippocratic medicine and ancient philosophy, and it may serve to illustrate an approach to it which I would rather try to avoid. For the fragment in question – one of the few longer *verbatim* fragments of Diocles we possess – has repeatedly been interpreted as being related to, and perhaps even directed against, certain Hippocratic texts.[6] Moreover, it has fallen victim to what I believe to be exaggerated and unjustified interpretations of Diocles' own position. It has, for instance, been read as a foreshadowing of medical Empiricism or even Scepticism,[7] or as the culmination of the Aristotelian development from speculative philosophy to an empirically minded study of particular phenomena.[8] I shall be the last to deny that the fragment is important or that it testifies to Diocles' awareness of questions of methodology; and I shall argue that in this respect we may speak of an original contribution to dietetics by Diocles, which may be seen as a partial correction of the direction that dietetics had taken in the Hippocratic texts *On Regimen* and *On Ancient Medicine*; but it should not be seen as the 'great fragment on method' ('das große Methodenfragment') in which Diocles expounded his philosophy of science and from which extrapolations concerning his general medical outlook can be safely made.[9]

The chapter is structured as follows. First, I shall interpret the fragment itself in some detail (section 2).[10] Then I shall try to reconstruct the views Diocles is criticising and consider to what extent these correspond to what we find in the Hippocratic Corpus – and to what extent the critical elements

---

on the *Aphorisms* in which the *verbatim* quotation is not present); see Jaeger (1938a) 27 n. 1. In fr. 57 Galen has preserved a verbatim quotation of an argument used by Diocles against Hippocrates' assumption of the existence of fevers recurring every five, seven or nine days. However, although Diocles addresses someone in the second person singular, we cannot be certain that his objection was originally directed against Hippocrates. For caution with regard to Diocles' acquaintance with the name and reputation of Hippocrates see Smith (1979) 187ff.

[6] See Wellmann (1901) 163; Fredrich (1899) 169–73; Torraca (1965) 105–15 (with Italian translation of the fragment); Wöhrle (1990) 175ff.
[7] Kudlien (1963) and (1964), both reprinted in Flashar (1971) 192–201 and 280–95.
[8] See the publications by Werner Jaeger (1938a), (1938b), (1940) (reissued in German translation in [1951]), (1952) and (1959). The reactions Jaeger's views provoked are conveniently discussed by von Staden (1992).
[9] In this I endorse a view which was recently stated by von Staden (1992) 240.
[10] See also the commentary on the fragment in van der Eijk (2001a) 321–34. Further discussions of the fragment (other than the ones already mentioned) can be found in Deichgräber (1965) 274 n. 3; Bertier (1972) 32–3; Kullmann (1974) 350–3; Smith (1979) 183–6 (with an English translation), (1980) 439ff. and (1992) 267; Frede (1987a) 129 and 235, 238 and (1985) xxii; von Staden (1989) 120–1.

in Diocles' argument can be compared with the polemical remarks we find in such Hippocratic treatises as *On Regimen* and *On Ancient Medicine* (section 3). Finally, some remarks will be made about what I believe the fragment tells us (and what it does not tell us) about Diocles' own practice in dietetics and medical science as a whole (section 4).

2 INTERPRETATION OF FRAGMENT 176

The fragment is preserved by Galen in the introductory chapter of his voluminous dietetic work *On the Powers of Foodstuffs* (*De alimentorum facultatibus*, *De alim. facult.*). Having stated the importance of this subject, Galen says that it has generated great disagreement among medical writers, and that it is therefore necessary to judge which of these writers are right and which are wrong. The Greek text runs as follows:[11]

(1) ἐπεὶ δὲ τῶν ἀποδείξεων ἀρχαὶ διτταὶ κατὰ γένος εἰσὶν (ἢ γὰρ ἐξ αἰσθήσεως ἢ ἐκ νοήσεως ἐναργοῦς ἀπόδειξίς τε καὶ πίστις ἄρχεται πᾶσα), καὶ ἡμᾶς ἀναγκαῖόν ἐστιν ἢ θατέρῳ τούτων ἢ ἀμφοτέροις χρήσασθαι πρὸς τὴν τοῦ προκειμένου σκέμματος κρίσιν. (2) οὐσῶν δὲ τῶν διὰ τοῦ λόγου κρίσεων οὐχ ἅπασιν ὁμοίως εὐπετῶν, ἐπειδὴ καὶ συνετὸν εἶναι χρὴ φύσει καὶ γεγυμνάσθαι κατὰ τὴν παιδικὴν ἡλικίαν ἐν τοῖς θήγουσι μαθήμασι τὸν λογισμόν, ἄμεινον ἀπὸ τῆς πείρας ἄρξασθαι καὶ μάλισθ' ὅτι διὰ ταύτης μόνης εὑρῆσθαι τὰς δυνάμεις τῆς τροφῆς οὐκ ὀλίγοι τῶν ἰατρῶν ἀπεφήναντο. (3) τῶν μὲν οὖν ἐμπειρικῶν ἴσως ἄν τις καταφρονήσειεν ἔργον καὶ σπούδασμα πεποιημένων φιλοτίμως ἀντιλέγειν τοῖς εὑρισκομένοις διὰ τοῦ λόγου· (4) Διοκλῆς δὲ καίτοι δογματικὸς ὢν οὕτω κατὰ λέξιν ἔγραψεν ἐν τῷ πρώτῳ τῶν πρὸς Πλείσταρχον Ὑγιεινῶν·

> (5) 'οἱ μὲν οὖν ὑπολαμβάνοντες τὰ τοὺς ὁμοίους ἔχοντα χυλοὺς ἢ ὀσμὰς ἢ θερμότητας ἢ ἄλλο τι τῶν τοιούτων πάντα τὰς αὐτὰς ἔχειν δυνάμεις οὐ καλῶς οἴονται· πολλὰ γὰρ ἀπὸ τῶν οὕτως ὁμοίων ἀνόμοια δείξειεν ἄν τις γιγνόμενα. (6) οὐδὲ δὴ τῶν διαχωρητικῶν ἢ οὐρητικῶν ἢ ἄλλην τινὰ δύναμιν ἐχόντων ὑποληπτέον ἕκαστον εἶναι τοιοῦτον, διότι θερμὸν ἢ ψυχρὸν ἢ ἁλμυρόν ἐστιν, ἐπείπερ οὐ πάντα τὰ γλυκέα καὶ δριμέα καὶ ἁλμυρὰ καὶ τὰ λοιπὰ τῶν

---

[11] The text is reproduced from the edition by G. Helmreich (*CMG* v 4, 2), with one exception: at the end of section 1, I emend κρίσιν instead of the MSS readings εὕρεσιν and ἄθροισιν. See on this van der Eijk (1993c). Surprisingly, Jaeger seems not to have used Helmreich's edition, and his discussion of some textual problems (1938a, 25–6 and 37) should therefore be read with caution. [The translation printed here is the one printed in van der Eijk (2001a) 283–5.]

τοιούτων τὰς αὐτὰς ἔχει δυνάμεις, (7) ἀλλὰ τὴν ὅλην φύσιν αἰτίαν εἶναι νομιστέον τούτου, ὁτιδηποτοῦν ἀπ' αὐτῶν ἑκάστου συμβαίνειν εἴωθεν. οὕτω γὰρ ἂν ἥκιστα διαμαρτάνοι τις τῆς ἀληθείας.

(8) αἰτίαν δ' οἱ μὲν οἰόμενοι δεῖν ἐφ' ἑκάστου λέγειν, δι' ἣν τρόφιμον ἢ διαχωρητικὸν ἢ οὐρητικὸν ἢ ἄλλο τι τῶν τοιούτων ἕκαστόν ἐστιν, ἀγνοεῖν ἐοίκασι πρῶτον μέν, ὅτι πρὸς τὰς χρήσεις οὐ πολλάκις τὸ τοιοῦτον ἀναγκαῖόν ἐστιν, ἔπειθ' ὅτι πολλὰ τῶν ὄντων τρόπον τινὰ ἀρχαῖς τισιν ἔοικε κατὰ φύσιν, ὥστε μὴ παραδέχεσθαι τὸν ὑπὲρ αἰτίου λόγον· (9) πρὸς δὲ τούτοις διαμαρτάνουσιν ἐνίοτε, ὅταν ἀγνοούμενα καὶ μὴ ὁμολογούμενα καὶ ἀπίθανα λαμβάνοντες ἱκανῶς οἴωνται λέγειν τὴν αἰτίαν. (10) τοῖς μὲν οὖν οὕτως αἰτιολογοῦσι καὶ τοῖς πάντων οἰομένοις δεῖν λέγειν αἰτίαν οὐ δεῖ προσέχειν, πιστεύειν δὲ μᾶλλον τοῖς ἐκ τῆς πείρας ἐκ πολλοῦ χρόνου κατανενοημένοις· (11) αἰτίαν δὲ τῶν ἐνδεχομένων δεῖ ζητεῖν, ὅταν μέλλῃ παρ' αὐτὸ τοῦτο γνωριμώτερον ἢ πιστότερον γίγνεσθαι τὸ λεγόμενον.'

(12) αὕτη μὲν ἡ τοῦ Διοκλέους ῥῆσίς ἐστιν ἐκ πείρας μόνης ἐγνῶσθαι τὰς ἐν ταῖς τροφαῖς δυνάμεις ἡγουμένου καὶ μήτ' ἐκ τῆς κατὰ κρᾶσιν ἐνδείξεως μήτ' ἐκ τῆς κατὰ τοὺς χυμούς. (13) οὔσης δὲ καὶ ἄλλης τῆς κατὰ τὰ μόρια τῶν φυτῶν οὐκ ἐμνημόνευσεν αὐτῆς. (14) λέγω δὲ κατὰ τὰ μόρια τῶν φυτῶν ἔνδειξιν, ᾗ πρὸς ταῖς ἄλλαις ἐχρήσατο Μνησίθεος ἑτέρας μὲν δυνάμεις ἐν ταῖς ῥίζαις εἶναι τῶν φυτῶν ἀποδεικνύς, ἑτέρας δ' ἐν τοῖς καυλοῖς, ὥσπερ γε κἂν τοῖς φύλλοις καὶ καρποῖς καὶ σπέρμασιν ἄλλας.

(1) Since there are two different kinds of starting-points of scientific demonstrations (for every demonstration and argument starts from either perception or clear insight), it is necessary for us, too, to use either one of these or both for the purpose of judging the present problem. (2) Now, judgements through reason are not equally easy for all people, since one has to be intelligent by nature and to be trained during youth in the disciplines that sharpen reasoning. Therefore, it is better to start from experience, especially so because many doctors have declared that it is through experience only that the powers of food have been discovered. (3) Now, one might perhaps despise the Empiricists, who have taken great pains over arguing contentiously against the things which are discovered through reason; (4) however, Diocles, though being a Dogmatist, in the first book of his 'Matters of Health to Pleistarchus' writes the following, and I quote:

(5) 'Those, then, who suppose that [substances] that have similar flavours or smells or [degrees of] hotness or some other [quality] of this kind all

have the same powers, are mistaken; for it can be shown that from [substances] that are similar in these respects, many dissimilar [effects] result; (6) and indeed, one should also not suppose that every [substance] that is laxative or promotes urine or has some other power is like that for the reason that it is hot or cold or salt, seeing that not all [substances] that are sweet or pungent or salt or those having any other [quality] of this kind have the same powers; (7) rather must one think that the whole nature is the cause of whatever normally results from each of them; for in this way one will least fail to hit the truth.

(8) Those who believe that with every single [substance] one should state a cause why each one of such [substances] is nutritious or laxative or promotes urine or has some other similar power, apparently do not know, first, that for the use [of these substances] something like that is not often necessary, and further, that many of the [things] that are [the case] in some way look like some sort of starting-points by [their] nature, so that they do not admit of the [kind of] account that deals with [their] cause. (9) In addition, they sometimes make mistakes when, while accepting [things] that are not known or are disputed or implausible, they think that they state the cause sufficiently. (10) Therefore, one should not pay attention to those who state causes in this way or to those who believe that one should state a cause for all [things]; rather, one should give credence to the [things] that have been well grasped on the basis of experience over a long time. (11) One should look for a cause [only] of the [things] admitting one, whenever it is by this that what is said turns out to be better known or more reliable.'

(12) These are the words of Diocles, who believes that the powers contained in foodstuffs are known on the basis of experience only and not on the basis of an indication according to mixture or an indication according to humours. (13) There is still another [form of indication], namely the one according to the parts of plants, but he did not mention this. (14) By indication according to the parts of plants I mean the one used in addition to the others by Mnesitheus in his demonstration that powers in the roots of plants are different from those in the stems, just as those in the leaves are different, and those in the fruits, and those in the seeds.

It is important to note that both in the introduction to the fragment and immediately after the verbatim quotation Diocles' view is presented by Galen as advancing an *exclusively* empirical approach to the question of the powers of foodstuffs (section 2: 'through experience only', διὰ ταύτης μόνης; section 12: 'on the basis of experience only', ἐκ πείρας μόνης). I shall return to Galen's association of Diocles with Empiricism, and the apparent tension involved with his belonging to the 'Dogmatist' tradition, later on.

The first claim that Diocles attacks is that 'substances'[12] that have similar qualities have the same powers. I use the word 'quality' to refer to characteristics such as those mentioned in section 5 – being juicy or dry, having a particular smell, having a certain degree of hotness – although the Greek text has no separate term to denote this category. 'Power' is used for *dunamis*, which is the power to produce a certain effect in the body of the consumer (examples mentioned in the text are 'provoking urine' and 'laxative' in section 6 and 'nutritive' in section 8). This distinction will concern us later on. It is important to note that the claim Diocles criticises does not explicitly say that there is a causal connection between having a certain quality and having a certain power: it just states the combination of the two. Yet even this is shown by Diocles to be wrong on empirical grounds; he refutes the claim by means of a 'judgement based on experience' (a κρίσις ἀπὸ πείρας, to use the words with which Galen introduces the quotation from his work) by pointing out that not all substances that are similar in respect of having a certain quality, say, A (section 5: 'similar in these respects', οὕτως ὁμοίων), produce results that indicate the presence of a certain power, say, B.[13]

In section 6 this is immediately followed by the denial of a second claim, which Diocles does not explicitly put in the mouth of the same group, but which he presents as a consequence of the first claim ('and indeed, one should also not...', οὐδὲ δή). This consequence is easy to see. For claim one does not say, but by its wording at least suggests, that there is a causal connection between having a particular quality and the possession of a particular power. This connection may take various forms: for instance, sweetness may be the cause of being laxative; or (perhaps less likely) being laxative may be the cause of being sweet; or, thirdly, sweetness and being laxative may both be results or effects of an underlying cause (in which case sweetness could be regarded as a sign of being laxative). Diocles only mentions the first of these possible consequences – which is also the most obvious – and he refutes it by means of the same empirical evidence he adduced against the first claim: experience shows that not all things that have the same quality have the same powers.

---

[12] Throughout the fragment, Diocles' Greek does not specify what we have to think about; Galen's text suggests that 'foodstuffs' (τροφαί, σιτία, ἐδέσματα) are meant (see section 12), but drinks (πόματα) and possibly also drugs (φάρμακα) may also be included. [Hence I have now preferred 'substances' over the 'foodstuffs' of my (1996) translation.] Jaeger translates 'Dinge' or 'Mittel', Torraca 'sostanze', Smith 'foods'.

[13] Diocles' refutation ignores the possibility that a foodstuff may have a particular power but does not actualise it in a certain case (on this possibility cf. Aristotle, *Metaph.* 1071 b 19, 23).

Diocles does not deny that in all cases where a certain power B is present, quality A is present as well (his argument allows the possibility that, for instance, all things that are laxative are sweet as well). But he points out that not all foodstuffs with quality A have power B, and the consequence of this is that even in those cases in which power B and quality A are both present, we cannot say that quality A is the cause of power B. Such an explanation is not 'sufficient' (not ἱκανός, to use a word which Diocles mentions later on in the fragment in section 9), because it does not account for situations in which quality A is present but not power B. Nor does Diocles deny that qualities may play a part in the production of a certain effect; but he insists that they do not necessarily produce the effect in question, and that, if they incidentally do so, they need not be the only factors involved in this production. He thereby shows that claim one, apart from being sometimes counterfactual, is also misleadingly formulated – or to put it in Aristotelian terms: it is not *qua* being sweet that a foodstuff is laxative, and the statement 'sweet foodstuffs are laxative' is not true universally.

Instead, in section 7 Diocles alleges that 'what normally results from each of them' (i.e. the substances we are talking about) is caused by 'the whole nature'. The very fact that Diocles gives an explanation of this kind already indicates that any attempt to associate him with Empiricism or Scepticism is not very likely to be correct.[14] But what do these words 'the whole nature' (τὴν ὅλην φύσιν) refer to? Most likely, I believe, is that the nature of the substance is meant, the sum or total configuration of elements, constituents or qualities the foodstuff consists of and the way they are structured or interrelated – for instance, the proportion between qualities such as warm and cold, dry and wet by which it is characterised.[15]

---

[14] As will become clear below, this 'nature' is not something which can be perceived empirically: it is probably made up both from imperceptible entities such as humours, primary qualities, etc., and from perceptible qualities such as flavours, tastes, etc. Cf. the disjunction in Galen, *On the Natural Faculties* (*De naturalibus facultatibus*) 2.8 (p. 191,10–11 Helmreich): 'Some have discovered the power of the substance by indication from the very nature of it, while others have done so on the basis of experience only' (οἱ μὲν ἐκ τῆς φύσεως αὐτοῦ τὴν δύναμιν ἐνδειξαμένης εὑρόντες, οἱ δ' ἐκ τῆς πείρας μόνης).

[15] See Torraca (1965) 108: 'la composizione generale della sostanza ... non essendo possibile schematizzare e ridurre la causa ad una sola proprietà', and Kullmann (1974) 351, followed by Wöhrle (1990) 174. This interpretation is in accordance with Galen's use of the concept of 'the whole nature' (ὅλη ἡ φύσις) or 'the whole essence' (ὅλη ἡ οὐσία) to denote the cause of the power a foodstuff or drug has, for instance in *On the Mixtures and Powers of Simple Drugs* (*De simplicium medicamentorum temperamentis ac facultatibus, De simpl. med. fac.*) 5.1 (11.705 K.); *On the Composition of Drugs according to Kinds* (*De compositione medicamentorum secundum genera, De comp. med. sec. gen.*) 1.16 (13.435–6 K.); *On Mixtures* (*De temperamentis, De temper.*) 3.2 (1.655 K.). For other references see Harig (1974) 108–10; Röhr (1923) 118–20. Smith's translation is ambiguous on this point: 'Rather, one must consider that the whole nature (*physis*) is responsible (*aitios*) [for what usually occurs for each].'

This interpretation has the advantage that the referent of *phusis* is immediately supplied by the context; moreover, as we shall see below, it has some support from what follows in section 8. A second possible interpretation is that 'the whole nature' refers to the sum of natural factors that play a part in the production by a certain substance of a certain dietetic effect with a certain patient. Indeed, a number of such factors are mentioned by Galen in the pages following on the Diocles fragment: not only the 'peculiar essence' (οἰκεία οὐσία) of the substance itself, but also climate, geographical area, season, a patient's natural constitution, his way of life (τὰ ἐπιτηδεύματα), his age, particular characteristics of the stomach and the intestines determine the effect a foodstuff produces in a particular case.[16] Yet it may be objected against this interpretation that the words 'are used to occur' (συμβαίνειν εἴωθεν) indicate that Diocles is here concerned with the general rather than with the particular – although the very use of 'used to' (εἴωθεν), in combination with the words 'least fail to hit the truth' (ἥκιστα διαμαρτάνοι τῆς ἀληθείας) in section 7, suggests an awareness on Diocles' part that the effect a substance produces cannot be predicted for all cases. A third interpretation of 'the whole nature' has been proposed by Jaeger, who argued that the nature of the consuming organism is meant, that is, the constitution of its body, its age, and so on.[17] This interpretation introduces an element which is not provided by contextual evidence, for the consumer or his body is nowhere mentioned in the fragment. It therefore seems best to interpret the words 'the whole nature' as referring to the nature of the foodstuff.

In section 8 Diocles criticises a third claim, which is, like the first, presented as a view which is actually being held by a certain group ('those who believe ...', οἱ ... οἰόμενοι). The claim seems to be that in every particular case, one should state the cause why a thing (again we may think of a foodstuff) has a certain dietetic power. At first sight, this claim looks rather different from the ones discussed earlier, for what is at issue is not the identity or the kind of causes sought for but the search for causes itself. Moreover, there is a shift of attention from the universal ('all', πάντα in section 5) to the particular ('each', ἐφ' ἑκάστου in section 8). Diocles' refutation of it calls for close consideration. His first argument seems rather obvious: for practical purposes, causal explanation is not often 'necessary'. For instance, when we know that a certain foodstuff is profitable for people

---

[16] Galen, *De alim. facult.* 1.1.16ff. (pp. 207ff. Helmreich, 6.462ff. K.).
[17] Jaeger (1938a) 29; in the sequel to Galen's argument, this is referred to as 'the body of the living being that takes in the nourishment' (τὸ τοῦ τρεφομένου ζῴου σῶμα, see, e.g., 1.1.27, p. 210,13 Helmreich, 6.469 K.), but there is no indication for this in Diocles' words themselves.

suffering from a certain disease, that will do for the practical purpose of healing a patient suffering from this disease.

His second objection is that a causal explanation of a substance's having a certain power is in many cases not possible. As for the words 'many of the things that are', πολλὰ τῶν ὄντων, it seems that we have to think not only of things or separate entities (e.g. foodstuffs, drugs), but also of facts and states of affairs (e.g. honey is sweet; or, garlic affects the eyes).[18] The use of expressions such as 'in some way' (τρόπον τινά) and 'look like' (ἔοικε) seem to serve the same purpose of not committing oneself to a statement without qualification: Diocles does not say that many states of affairs *are* principles, but only that they *resemble* them, show some characteristics of them; nor does he say that this applies without qualification, but only *in a certain way* (a way which is explicated in the clause 'so that they do not admit...', ὥστε μὴ παραδέχεσθαι κτλ.). It is not clear from the text whether by 'starting-points' Diocles means fundamental physical states of affairs or logical postulates that should be accepted as valid without further demonstration, comparable to the logical postulates discussed by Aristotle in *Metaphysics* Γ,[19] but perhaps this is not relevant to the point he wants to make: 'honey is laxative' (to mention just an imaginary example) is similar to a postulate like 'a statement *p* and its negation not-*p* cannot both be true at the same time under the same conditions' in that it does not admit of demonstration.[20] This is not to say that the two have the same degree of fundamentality: the point of the use of ἔοικε is that there is a *similarity* between a statement like 'honey is laxative' and a logical postulate like the one mentioned, and this similarity is expressed in the sentence 'so that they do not admit of the [kind of] account that deals with [their] cause' (ὥστε μὴ παραδέχεσθαι ... λόγον). Whereas a real principle like a logical postulate is undemonstrable without qualification (ἁπλῶς, one is tempted to say), foodstuffs and their effects are so only 'in some way' (τρόπον τινά). What this 'some way' is, becomes clearer when we consider the words κατὰ φύσιν. These are usually translated in an Aristotelian-like way by 'naturally', 'by nature', or 'normally', suggesting as Diocles' intention that it is in the

---

[18] Cf. the translations by Jaeger ('vieles in der Wirklichkeit Gegebene'), Kullmann ('viele Gegebenheiten'); Torraca translates 'molti fenomeni reali', Smith 'many things'.

[19] Jaeger (1938a, 42) states without argument that 'Das Wort ἀρχαί weist hier nicht auf Prinzipien der Art hin, wie die Naturphilosophen sie gesucht hatten, die Urgründe der Physis, sondern auf Prinzipien im logischen Sinne oder oberste Beweisgründe.' Armelle Debru has suggested to me as an alternative that we may think here of basic or 'simple' (ἁπλῆ) foodstuffs (as against complex ones); but then it is difficult to see why Diocles says that many things (i.e. foodstuffs) *look like* basic entities, instead of saying that they *are* basic.

[20] Cf. Aristotle, *Gen. an.* 788 a 13: 'this is what it means to be a starting-point, being itself the cause of many things, without there being another cause for it higher up' (τοῦτο γάρ ἐστι τὸ ἀρχὴν εἶναι, τὸ αὐτὴν μὲν αἰτίαν εἶναι πολλῶν, ταύτης δ' ἄλλο ἄνωθεν μηθέν).

nature of things that many things look like, or are taken as, principles.[21] However, that would be a remarkable statement which would have no justification in the context. Yet if we connect the use of the word *phusis* here with that in section 7 above, a more comprehensible view emerges: *phusis* again refers to the nature of the substance in question, for example the foodstuff, and κατὰ φύσιν means 'according to their nature', 'in virtue of their nature'. In section 7 the 'whole nature' was said to be the cause of the effect the foodstuff normally produces; thus it is relatively easy to understand the statement that in virtue of their nature these foodstuffs and their producing such-and-such an effect are like principles. For the purpose of clarity, let me paraphrase what I think Diocles' line of thought in this whole fragment amounts to. A foodstuff has its effect due not to one of its particular qualities but to its nature as a whole; as soon as we descend to a level that is lower (e.g. more elemental) than this 'whole nature', for instance by considering the constituents or qualities of the foodstuff in isolation, we lose the 'wholeness', the total sum of these constituents or qualities and the structure or proportion according to which they are interrelated – whereas this very nature was said to be responsible for the effect in question. To be sure, we might be able to explain why honey is sweet (which is, after

[21] Jaeger: 'von Natur'; Torraca: 'secondo natura'. Kullmann takes κατὰ φύσιν as belonging to ἀρχαῖς: 'Viele Gegebenheiten gleichen in gewisser Weise bestimmten naturgemäßen Prinzipien, so daß sie keine Darlegung über die Ursache zulassen' (1974, 351) and he comments on p. 352: 'Es kommt Diokles gerade darauf an, daß diese Prinzipien naturgemäß und nicht künstlich sind, um die Frage nach abstrakten Letztursachen ein für allemal auszuschließen.' But this is difficult to accept because of the word order. Smith's translation ('many things are in some fashion like first principles in nature') is not explicit on this point, like Frede's paraphrase: 'He also maintained that we should treat many facts of nature as primitive, rather than try to explain them in terms of some questionable theory which would serve no further purpose' ('Introduction', 1985, xxii). Bertier's paraphrase goes too far beyond what is in the text: 'Apport insignifiant des théories explicatives, dans la mesure où les réalités contiennent en elles-mêmes le reflet de leurs principes, et où la théorie n'est qu'une répétition de la description du fait' (1972, 32). H. Gottschalk (private correspondence) understands the whole sentence as follows: '(a) *archai*, because they are *archai*, cannot be explained or demonstrated, and (b) any train of reasoning, even if it does not start from the most universal and ultimate *archai*, must start from something accepted as true for the purpose of that argument, a quasi-*arche* not subjected to further analysis or demonstration', and he takes the words κατὰ φύσιν as expressing that 'Our using such propositions [e.g. honey is laxative] as *archai* is arbitrary, yet it is in the nature of things that we reason in this way', but he admits that 'Diocles has not expressed himself very clearly, perhaps because he was trying to fit an Aristotelian idea into a context determined by older ways of thinking.' [After the original publication of this paper, I became aware of the paraphrase of fr. 176 by A. L. Peck in his 1928 Cambridge PhD thesis 'Pseudo-Hippocrates Philosophus; or the development of philosophical and other theories as illustrated by the Hippocratic writings, with special reference to De victu and De prisca medicina', pp. 116–17, of which the following parts are worth quoting: 'and that many of the substances we have bear a considerable resemblance in their nature to some of the first principles, so that there is no place left for an account of the cause (of their effects) ... when they think that they have given a satisfactory account of the cause by getting hold of something that is not known nor generally agreed upon nor even plausible'; in a footnote to the words 'so that there is no place left', Peck adds: 'Because it is not possible to trace out a cause further back than a first principle.' Peck further agrees that Hippocrates' *On Regimen* 'comes under Diocles' condemnation'.]

all, a question of elementary physics or pharmacology), but this does not contribute anything to our understanding of why honey produces certain dietetic effects. On the level of its nature and with regard to the effect it produces, a foodstuff 'resembles' (ἔοικε) a genuine undemonstrable starting-point – although it is not a starting-point in the absolute sense: the words 'in some way' serve the purpose of qualifying the resemblance that exists between a genuine starting-point and a foodstuff which, from a certain point of view, behaves like a starting-point. To say it with some exaggeration (which goes beyond what is in the text): there is a causal 'gap' between the nature of a foodstuff as being causally *responsible* for certain dietetic effects on the one hand, and the nature of the foodstuff as being the *result* of a certain sum of elements or qualities.

In section 9 Diocles states additional criticism. Since no subject of 'make mistakes' (διαμαρτάνουσιν) is specified, it seems that he is still referring to the same group as in section 8 (but see below). These people, he says, miss the truth (note the similarity to the wording at the end of section 7), because their explanations are ill-founded. 'Accept' (λαμβάνειν) is to be taken in the sense of 'postulate', 'take as a starting-point'.[22] It is not quite clear whether 'things that are not known' (ἀγνοούμενα) should be taken in the sense of 'invisibles' (the ἄδηλα), namely things unknown to human perception[23] (which, of course, would please those who read the fragment as an anticipation of Empiricism) or in the sense of 'not known to them', in which case Diocles means something like 'they do not know what they are talking about'.[24] The second objection is obvious: disputed things do not serve as an appropriate starting-point; apart from being wrong perhaps, they are unconvincing. The third objection of 'implausibility' introduces the notion of persuasiveness of the doctor's statements – an element which is also reflected in section 11 in the words 'more reliable' (πιστότερον) and which is familiar from the Hippocratic writings.[25]

In sections 10–11 Diocles summarises his criticism and states his own alternative. It is important to note the use of 'rather' (μᾶλλον), and to see to what exactly the habit of putting more trust in the results of long-term experience is said to be preferable: the ill-founded and undue

---

[22] Cf. Aristotle, *Mete.* 357 b 23–4: ἡμεῖς δὲ λέγωμεν ἀρχὴν λαβόντες τὴν αὐτὴν ἥν καὶ πρότερον ('let us discuss this adopting the same starting-point as we have adopted before') and *Pol.* 1290 b 22–3: διότι δὲ πλείους τῶν εἰρημένων καὶ τίνες καὶ διὰ τί λέγωμεν ἀρχὴν λαβόντες τὴν εἰρημένην πρότερον ('And because there are more [sc. forms of constitution] than those mentioned, let us discuss what they are and why they are different, adopting as starting-point the one we have mentioned earlier'). For other linguistic resemblances to Aristotle see n. 42 below.

[23] *On Ancient Medicine* 1.3 (p. 119,5 Jouanna, 1.572 L.): τὰ ἀφανέα τε καὶ ἀπορεόμενα ('the things that are invisible and difficult to know'). For Diocles' views on 'invisibles' see frs. 177 and 56b.

[24] In view of the use of γνωριμώτερον in section 11, the latter is perhaps more likely.

[25] Cf. *Prognostic* 1 (2.110 L.) and Langholf (1996).

causal explanations of the groups mentioned in the above.²⁶ There is no question of an absolute priority of experience over reasoning, and the last sentence (section 11) shows that Diocles acknowledges that causal explanation, in all those cases where it is possible,²⁷ may make the physician's account more informative and reliable. While 'those who believe that one should state a cause for all [things]' (τοῖς πάντων οἰομένοις δεῖν λέγειν αἰτίαν) clearly refers to the group criticised in section 8, it is less clear who are meant by the words 'those who state causes in this way' (τοῖς μὲν οὖν οὕτως αἰτιολογοῦσι). The most likely possibility is that it refers to those who are criticised in the sentence immediately preceding it, that is those who make mistakes because their causal explanations are ill-founded; but this is not quite compatible with section 9, where the lack of a change of subject suggests that Diocles' additional criticism ('in addition', πρὸς δὲ τούτοις) still applies to the same group. Another possibility is that 'those who state causes in this way' are the ones criticised in the first part of the fragment (the champions of claims one and two), although it is a bit awkward to take the phrase 'in this way' (οὕτως) as referring not to the ill-founded 'stating the cause' (λέγειν τὴν αἰτίαν) mentioned just before but to what was discussed in section 7.

Perhaps this difficulty becomes less urgent when we consider how the three claims Diocles criticises are interrelated. As I said, at first sight it seems that in his refutation of claim three in section 8, Diocles is arguing against a rather different group from the one which is his target in the earlier part of the fragment (claims one and two). Yet after reading the whole fragment, it is easy to see why he discusses these claims in the same context and in this order. The first claim is the weakest, in that it does not commit itself to the assumption of a causal nexus between quality and power; consequently, its empirical refutation is likewise easy. Subsequently, this empirical refutation is used by Diocles as an argument against the second claim, which is one of the possible implications of the first claim. Finally, this second claim can in its turn be seen as a possible instance of the third

---

[26] See Smith (1979) 184. The similarity of this sentence to *On Ancient Medicine* 2.1 (p. 119,13ff. Jouanna, 1.572. L.): καὶ τὰ εὑρημένα πολλά τε καὶ καλῶς ἔχοντα εὕρηται ἐν πολλῷ χρόνῳ ('and the things that have been discovered, which are manifold and are firmly established, have been discovered over a long time') was noted also by von Staden (1992) 240. Torraca ('a quelli che fondano le lore deduzioni sull' esperienza fatta per lungo tempo') and Smith ('those who reached understanding from experience through much time') wrongly take the participle as masculine; κατανοέω means 'observe', 'perceive', 'learn' (see LSJ s.v.). Bertier rightly concedes that Diocles does not reject causal explanation altogether (1972, 32).

[27] Following Jaeger (1938a) 38 and 40, I take ἐνδέχεσθαι in the same sense as παραδέχεσθαι in section 8: τὰ ἐνδεχόμενα are 'those things that admit of this, i.e. of being causally explained' (although I do not accept Jaeger's far-reaching conclusions drawn from linguistic resemblances to Aristotle on this point). I cannot endorse Smith's translation 'But we must seek a cause for what we accept.'

claim: it provides an example of what Diocles regards as an 'insufficient' causal explanation, because it is ill-founded and not based on knowledge of the facts (ἀγνοούμενα). It seems that Diocles is criticising views he believes to be erroneous rather than addressing distinct groups, each of which held one of the views in question. Thus we may understand why Diocles in section 10 syntactically presents the two groups as different, while at the same time marking a close connection between them ('those who state causes in this way', τοῖς μὲν **οὕτως** αἰτιολογοῦσι). Both claim one and claim two can easily be understood as manifestations or consequences of too strict an application of the quest for causes, which is what claim three amounts to. As for Diocles' own position, if the above explanation of the words 'the whole nature' and 'by nature' is acceptable, both sections of the fragment are closely interrelated and rooted in a consistent conviction.

3 THE IDENTITY OF DIOCLES' OPPONENTS

I turn now to the question of the identity of the group or groups Diocles is opposing – a problem which has attracted more attention than the text of the fragment itself, especially from scholars of ancient medicine at the end of the nineteenth century such as Carl Fredrich and Max Wellmann, who seemed to impose on Greek medicine a model which closely resembles the institutional organisation of the universities of their own time. The history of medicine was regarded as an ongoing process of exchange of ideas between members of the same 'school', of indiscriminate acceptance of the views of greater authorities ('influence') or of vigorous polemics against them. A striking example of this search for identification with regard to the Diocles fragment under discussion is provided by Fredrich.[28] He argued that Diocles, in his criticism of what I have called claim one (section 5 of the fragment), was opposing the same group as that against whom the writer (or, in Fredrich's words, the 'Compilator') of the Hippocratic work *On Regimen* (*De victu*) 2.39 was polemicising.[29] However, he also argued that Diocles' criticism of what I have called the third claim (section 8) was directed against

---

[28] Fredrich (1899) 171–3.
[29] *On Regimen* 2.39 (*CMG* I 2, 4, p. 162,9–18 Joly and Byl): 'All those who have undertaken to give a generalising account about the power of foods and drinks that are sweet or fatty or salt or any other of such nature, are wrong. For the foods and drinks that are sweet do not all have the same power, nor is this the case with the fatty or any other such things. Some sweet foods and drinks are laxative, others are stopping, yet others drying, yet others moistening. And in the same way, of those that are heating and all the others some have this power, some have another. It is impossible to give a general account of how these things are: but what power each of them individually has, I will set forth' (Σιτίων δὲ καὶ πομάτων δύναμιν ἑκάστων καὶ τὴν κατὰ φύσιν καὶ τὴν διὰ τέχνης ὧδε χρὴ γινώσκειν. ὅσοι μὲν **κατὰ παντὸς** ἐπεχείρησαν εἰπεῖν περὶ τῶν γλυκέων ἢ λιπαρῶν ἢ ἁλμυρῶν ἢ περὶ

the tendency of searching for causes at any cost which Fredrich found characteristic of the same 'Compilator'.[30] Now there is in itself nothing implausible about one person criticising another person in one respect but praising him in another; besides, not too much consistency can be expected from a 'Compilator'. But Fredrich's construction of the debate becomes problematic when he suggests that Diocles shows a common front with the Hippocratic author of *On Ancient Medicine*, who in his turn is said by Fredrich to be criticising the author of *On Regimen* for having the temerity 'to attribute to individual foods and drinks the properties cold, hot, dry or wet'.[31] Within the space of three pages and in a dazzling course of argument, Fredrich applied a complete metamorphosis to claim one, which was first said to be the claim that *On Regimen* is opposing, but which is later associated with what *On Ancient Medicine* and Diocles are opposing and which is identified by Fredrich as the view held by the compiler of *On Regimen*.

On this kind of identification it may be appropriate to quote Josef-Hans Kühn, who with regard to a similar question concerning the opponents of *On Ancient Medicine* made the following remark: 'The tendency to make connections between the few treatises from antiquity that have been preserved is understandable and justified. On the other hand, the sheer number of works dealing with medical topics must have been so large that it would be a great coincidence if the rather arbitrary selection of the tradition had preserved precisely those treatises which refer to each other.'[32] Kühn concludes that the best we can do is to regard the writings that have been preserved as examples of a no longer extant but presumably much broader spectrum of medical views, and to restrict ourselves to a reconstruction of the view that is being criticised without immediately putting a label on it or associating it with another treatise that has been preserved. Yet I would

---

ἄλλου τινὸς τῶν τοιούτων τῆς δυνάμιος, οὐκ ὀρθῶς γινώσκουσιν. οὐ γὰρ τὴν αὐτὴν δύναμιν ἔχουσιν οὔτε τὰ γλυκέα ἀλλήλοισιν οὔτε τὰ λιπαρὰ οὔτε τῶν ἄλλων τῶν τοιούτων οὐδέν. πολλὰ γὰρ τῶν γλυκέων διαχωρεῖ, τὰ δ' ἵστησι, τὰ δὲ ξηραίνει, τὰ δὲ ὑγραίνει. ὡσαύτως δὲ καὶ τῶν ἄλλων ἁπάντων· ἐστὶ δὲ ἄσσα στύφει καὶ διαχωρεῖται, τὰ δ' οὐρεῖται, τὰ δὲ οὐδέτερα τούτων. ὡσαύτως δὲ καὶ τῶν θερμαντικῶν καὶ τῶν ἄλλων ἁπάντων ἄλλην ἄλλα δύναμιν ἔχει. περὶ μὲν οὖν ἁπάντων οὐχ οἷόν τε δηλωθῆναι ὁποῖά τινά ἐστι· καθ' ἕκαστα δέ, ἥντινα δύναμιν ἔχει, διδάξω).

[30] Fredrich (1899) 171; this point has been misunderstood by Torraca (1965) 108.
[31] Fredrich (1899) 169: 'den einzelnen [Speisen und Getränken] die Eigenschaften Kalt, Warm, Trocken oder Feucht beizulegen'.
[32] J.-H. Kühn (1956) 84: 'Die Neigung, innerhalb der wenigen überlieferten Schriften der Antike immer wieder direkte Bezugsverhältnisse herstellen zu wollen, ist verständlich und berechtigt. Andererseits muß die Fülle der Arbeiten, die sich mit medizinischen Fragen beschäftigen, so groß gewesen sein, daß es ein großer Zufall wäre, wenn die mehr oder minder zufällige Auswahl unserer Überlieferung gerade die Schriften erhalten hätte, welche aufeinander Bezug nehmen.'

like to add a second *caveat*, which has to do with the nature of polemical writing in antiquity. Even if we can find a text A, the contents of which completely correspond with the ideas criticised by the author of another text, say, B, and a text C which only shows some similarities with what is criticised in B, the statement that B is consciously opposing A and not C can at best remain a plausible hypothesis. For we cannot rule out the possibility that B is actually aiming at C in a way which is – according to our standards – just unfair: he may represent the ideas of his opponent in a very distorted and caricaturist way by ignoring several important specifications or relevant details, or by isolating separate items from their context. Such a distortion need not be a manifestation of malevolence; it may also be a result of the fact that the way in which the author of B views text C is rather different from our perception of it. Especially in the case of an author, such as Diocles, whose writings have been lost, we should be very careful not to pretend that we can creep into his skin and perceive with his eyes the other text which is supposed to be criticised and which represents only a very small part of a literature that must have been of considerable size.

These remarks may appear unduly sceptical or a tedious example of stating the obvious. Yet the practice of ancient polemical writers in cases where they do mention their opponents by name and in which the writings of these opponents are preserved as well (e.g. the polemics of Christian writers such as Origen or Tertullian against the Gnostics), shows that fair polemics were the exception rather than the rule.[33]

Fredrich's identifications are, of course, an extreme example, and most scholars dealing with this fragment have expressed themselves in much more cautious terms. Yet the substantial similarity between Diocles' criticism of the first claim and the critical remarks of the author of the Hippocratic text *On Regimen* 2.39 is accepted, and it has been suggested that both *On Regimen* 2.39 and Diocles are arguing against generalisations of a type the physician Mnesitheus in fragment 22 Bertier (and perhaps also the writer of the Hippocratic text *On Affections* 55) provides evidence of – which is reinforced by the fact that Galen in the immediate context of this same fragment presents Diocles as disagreeing with Mnesitheus on a related subject (although it is not certain that chronology admits of the possibility that Mnesitheus actually was the target in either, or both, of these cases).[34]

---

[33] On Origen's polemics against the Gnostics see, for instance, Norelli (1992) and Castagno (1992).
[34] Mnesitheus, fr. 22 Bertier (Athenaeus 3.121 D): 'Salty and sweet flavours all have a relaxing effect on the belly, while those that are acid and sharp release urine. Those that are bitter are rather diuretic, while some of them also have a relaxing effect on the belly. Those that are sour, <retain> excretions' (Μνησίθεος δ' ὁ Ἀθηναῖος ἐν τῷ περὶ ἐδεστῶν· 'οἱ ἁλυκοί', φησίν, 'καὶ γλυκεῖς χυμοὶ πάντες

While it has also been argued very frequently that Diocles here shares the sceptical attitude towards theoretical approaches of dietetics found in the treatise *On Ancient Medicine*,[35] Fredrich's view that the third claim Diocles is criticising corresponds with the actual practice of the writer of *On Ancient Medicine* has been received with mixed feelings.[36]

However, it seems very questionable to me whether it is correct to present Diocles as making a common stand with the authors of *On Ancient Medicine* and *On Regimen*. As for *On Ancient Medicine*, this seems to misunderstand both the claims that Diocles is opposing (especially claim one) and Diocles' own position. The scope of the Diocles fragment is rather different from what is at issue in *On Ancient Medicine*. Diocles does not object to the postulation of warm and cold, nor does he object to referring to these postulates as causes *per se*: he simply warns against premature generalisations. His argument allows for cases in which a thing's having the quality hot causes it to produce such-and-such an effect, but he points out that this does not imply that all things that have that quality produce that effect (for instance because of the combination with other factors, or because it is only an incidental cause), nor that all cases where this effect is produced are due to this very quality. Diocles points out that one should look for the essential cause: sweet things may cause certain effects, but not necessarily so and not in so far as they are sweet. Nor does Diocles make the distinction between

---

ὑπάγουσι τὰς κοιλίας, οἱ δ' ὀξεῖς καὶ δριμεῖς λύουσι τὴν οὔρησιν. Οἱ δὲ πικροὶ μᾶλλον μέν εἰσιν οὐρητικοί, λύουσι δ' αὐτῶν ἔνιοι καὶ τὰς κοιλίας. οἱ δὲ στρυφνοὶ τὰς ἐκκρίσεις'). On Mnesitheus being a possible target see Smith (1980) 444, and von Staden (1992) 240; a more sceptical attitude is taken by Bertier (1972) 30–1.

[35] Apart from Fredrich (1899) 171 ('Kurz, Diokles vertritt denselben Standpunkt wie der Autor von περὶ ἀρχαίης ἰητρικῆς, der auch Praktiker ist') see also Wöhrle (1990) 175; Jaeger (1938a) 38; Kullmann (1974) 352; von Staden (1992) 240. The passage which comes closest to Diocles' views is *On Ancient Medicine* 17.1–2 (pp. 141,15–142,2 Jouanna; 1.612 L.), where the Hippocratic writer bluffs his way out of the problem of fever: 'I think personally that this is the most important proof that it is not simply through heat that people get fever, nor that this is the only cause of feeling unwell; rather it is the combination of bitterness and heat, or sharpness and heat, or saltiness and heat, and innumerable other things – and, again, the combination of cold with other properties' (Ἐγὼ δὲ τοῦτό μοι μέγιστον τεκμήριον ἡγεῦμαι εἶναι ὅτι οὐ διὰ τὸ θερμὸν ἁπλῶς πυρεταίνουσιν οἱ ἄνθρωποι οὐδὲ τοῦτ' εἴη τὸ αἴτιον τῆς κακώσεως μοῦνον, ἀλλ' ἔστι καὶ πικρὸν καὶ θερμὸν τὸ αὐτὸ καὶ ὀξὺ καὶ θερμὸν καὶ ἁλμυρὸν καὶ θερμὸν καὶ ἄλλα μύρια – καὶ πάλιν γε ψυχρὸν μετὰ δυναμίων ἑτέρων).

[36] See Wöhrle (1990) 175: 'Auch der zweite Teil des Textabschnittes, in dem sich Diokles gegen die Ätiologen wendet, kann sich kaum auf den Katalog des zweiten Buches von *De victu* beziehen. Denn erstens wird dort nur zu einem geringen Teil eine Erklärung für die Wirkung bestimmter Nahrungsmittel gegeben, und zweitens liegt diesen Ausführungen kein streng hypothetisches Schema zugrunde (im Gegensatz zur Feuer-Wasser-Theorie des ersten Buches).' On the other hand, Fredrich's view seems to have been accepted by Kullmann (1974) 352: 'Fredrich, der zugleich einleuchtend Polemik des Diokles gegen die hippokratische Schrift περὶ διαίτης vermutet') and by Düring (1966) 527 n. 105. On this see below.

primary and secondary qualities that is so important to the author of *On Ancient Medicine*; he rather distinguishes between qualities and powers, for it is the combination of these two that is supposed to be significant. Besides, there are more general reasons which should make us reluctant to associate Diocles with the author of *On Ancient Medicine*. The picture of Diocles that emerges not just from this single fragment, but from the more than two hundred that are preserved from him, shows that in matters of physiology and pathology Diocles' opinions display many speculative characteristics in whose company the author of *On Ancient Medicine* would have felt himself quite uncomfortable. Diocles' acceptance of the four primary qualities and of concepts such as innate pneuma and humours is frequently attested, and his use of them in the causal explanation of *diseases* in his work *Affection, Cause, Treatment* (Πάθος, αἰτία, θεραπεία) is well documented.[37] One may object that this information is based on testimonies (not on *verbatim* fragments such as fragment 176) supplied by sources which are perhaps not very reliable; but as far as this fragment is concerned, there is no reason for doubt concerning the validity of these reports, for they are perfectly compatible with it. Fragment 176 does not present itself as (nor claims to be) a methodological programme for medical science as a whole: it is concerned with dietetics, with the powers of foodstuffs and with the practical problems the physician has to face. It is far from self-evident that what Diocles says here also applies to anatomy, pathology and general physiology – or even if it would apply, what the implications of this would be.[38] Moreover, if the interpretation of the fragment given above is correct, we should say that even within the field of dietetics Diocles is not hostile towards causal explanations as such; he is just concerned with their limitations and with their correctness. He points out that there are many cases in which causal

---

[37] On Diocles' physiology see frs. 25–8; on his pathology see, e.g., frs. 109 (on which see Smith (1979) 186, and Flashar (1966) 50–3), 78, 95, 98, 117. A large number of Diocles' aetiological views on diseases are reported in the treatise on acute and chronic diseases by the so-called Anonymus Parisinus Fuchsii, edited by Garofalo (1997). It is remarkable that many of these aetiologies (e.g. frs. 72, 78, 98) are in the form of a definition stating the nature of the affection in question, while others describe the conditions under which (or the places where) the disease occurs (frs. 80, 87); moreover, fr. 98 seems to imply that Diocles distinguished different kinds of causes. Although we should take into account the possibility that in many cases it is the Anonymus who is responsible for the precise wording of the aetiologies, the testimonies nevertheless point to a sophisticated use of causal explanation by Diocles in dealing with diseases. The question of the reliability of the Anonymus (which is too often approached from an *a priori* negative point of view, for instance by Kudlien (1963) 462) can only be answered on the basis of an unbiased study of the whole text, which has only recently been made available in its entirety by Garofalo (1997); see also van der Eijk (1999b).

[38] An extreme example of this is Kudlien's view (1963, 461) that this fragment casts doubt on the reliability of doxographic reports that attribute to Diocles a doctrine of humours. On this see Flashar (1966) 54 n. 5; Schöner (1964) 72ff.; Smith (1979) 185–6 n. 12.

explanation is impossible, and that there are also cases in which it may be possible, but unnecessary for practical purposes – and one could imagine that *in this respect* the author of *On Ancient Medicine* would not have been too happy with Diocles' criticism of claim three, for *On Ancient Medicine* is one of the first among the Hippocratic treatises to proclaim the urgency of stating the cause in dietetics.[39] However, as sections 10–11 of the fragment show, Diocles recognises that there are also cases – albeit perhaps a minority – in which a causal explanation increases our understanding of the subject and adds to the plausibility of dietetic prescriptions.

As for *On Regimen*, I believe that Fredrich was right in detecting a very strong, almost indiscriminate application of the search for causes in the chapters on the powers of foodstuffs of this treatise (40–56). The use of words indicating causal links such as 'because', 'since', 'as a result of' (διότι, ἅτε, ὅτι, διά) in these sections is very frequent indeed. But it is especially the nature of these explanations which calls for consideration, for the fact is that many of them suffer from defects that might be interpreted as provoking the kind of criticism Diocles is expressing, such as circularity – no clear distinction being made between the level of qualities and that of powers – shifting the problem, and tautology – explanandum and explanation being stated in the same terms. Let us consider some of these explanations:

On Regimen 2.40 (p. 162,26 Joly and Byl): ψύχει [sc. μᾶζα] μὲν διότι ψυχρῷ ὕδατι ὑγρὴ ἐγένετο ('it [sc. maza] cools because it is moistened with cold water');[40]

2.42 (p. 164,22–26 Joly and Byl): διαχωρεῖ δὲ ὅτι ταχέως πέσσεται... διαχωρεῖ δὲ ὅτι τὸ γλυκὺ καὶ διαχωρητικὸν τοῦ πυροῦ συμμέμικται ('it passes, because it is soon digested... it passes because it is mixed with the sweet and laxative part of the wheat');

2.52 (p. 174, 6–8 Joly and Byl): ἕψημα θερμαίνει καὶ ὑγραίνει καὶ ὑπάγει· θερμαίνει μέν, ὅτι οἰνῶδες, ὑγραίνει δέ, ὅτι τρόφιμον, ὑπάγει δέ, ὅτι γλυκὺ καὶ πρὸς καθηψημένον ἐστίν ('Boiled-down wine warms, moistens, and sends to stool. It warms, because it is vinous, moistens because it is nutritious, and sends to stool because it is sweet and moreover boiled-down');

2.54 (p. 174,15 Joly and Byl): διαχωρεῖ δὲ καὶ οὐρεῖται διὰ τὸ καθαρτικόν ('It promotes stools and urine because of the purgative qualities it possesses');

---

[39] 'Science must therefore be causal or it is not science', J. Jouanna (1999, 255) comments on the well-known cheese example in ch. 20 of *On Ancient Medicine*. The most prominent instances where the importance of causal explanation is stated are: 20.3–4 (pp. 146,15–147,10 Jouanna; 1.622 L.); 21.2 (p. 148,7–13 Jouanna; 1.624 L.); 23.1 (p. 153,5–6 Jouanna; 1.634 L.); 2.3 (p. 120,7–11 Jouanna; 1.572–4 L.); 11.1 (p. 131,11–12 Jouanna; 1.594 L.).

[40] Translations adopted, with slight adaptations, from W. H. S. Jones in the Loeb Classical Library, *Hippocrates*, vol. IV.

2.56 (p. 178,13–14 Joly and Byl): ἐν ὄξει δὲ τεταριχευμένα θερμαίνει μὲν ἧσσον διὰ τὸ ὄξος ('When preserved in vinegar they [sc. meats] are less warming because of the vinegar').

Considering these examples, we may be inclined to say that Diocles' warnings against too automatic an application of causal explanation, as well as his prescription (in section 11 of fr. 176) that causal explanation must make the physician's account more informative (γνωριμώτερον), may well be understood as applying to the occasionally just truistic explanations found in *On Regimen*.

4 DIOCLES' POSITION IN DIETETICS AND IN THE PHILOSOPHY OF SCIENCE

It is not my intention to suggest that Diocles has the authors of the treatises *On Ancient Medicine* and *On Regimen* in mind as his targets, but only to state some objections against associating Diocles' own position with that of these two Hippocratic writers. It rather seems to me that Diocles is arguing against what he believes to be – in the context of dietetics – some undesirable consequences of the search for causes or principles, or to put it in other words, against too strict an application of what in itself – and in Diocles' opinion too – remains a sound scientific procedure. These consequences seem to have pervaded Greek scientific thought in the fourth century to such an extent that opposition to it was also expressed by Aristotle and Theophrastus (in their case, the opposition is probably directed against certain tendencies in the early Academy). There are a number of passages which reflect a similar awareness in Aristotle and Theophrastus of the limits of causal explanation.[41] Indeed the whole Diocles fragment shows

---

[41] Cf. Aristotle, *Metaph.* 1006 a 6–9: 'for it is characteristic of a lack of education not to know *of what things one should seek demonstration, and of what one should not*; for it is absolutely impossible for there to be a demonstration of everything (for that would go on indefinitely, so that there would be no demonstration)' (ἔστι γὰρ ἀπαιδευσία τὸ μὴ γιγνώσκειν τίνων δεῖ ζητεῖν ἀπόδειξιν καὶ τίνων οὐ δεῖ· ὅλως μὲν γὰρ ἁπάντων ἀδύνατον ἀπόδειξιν εἶναι (εἰς ἄπειρον γὰρ ἂν βαδίζοι, ὥστε μηδ' οὕτως εἶναι ἀπόδειξιν)). Theophrastus, *Metaphysics* 9 b 1–13: 'Wherefore this too is problematical or at any rate not easy to say, *up to which point and of which entities one should seek the cause*, in the objects of sense and in the objects of thought alike: for the infinite regress is foreign to their nature in both cases *and destroys our understanding*. Both of them are starting-points in some way: and perhaps the one for us, the other absolutely, or, on the one hand, the end and the other a starting-point of ours. Up to some point, then, we are capable of studying things causally, taking our starting-point from sense-perceptions in each case; but when we proceed to the extreme and primary entities, we are no longer capable of doing so, either owing to the fact that they do not have a cause, or through our lack of strength to look, one would say, at the brightest things' (ἧ καὶ τοῦτ' ἄπορον ἢ οὐ ῥᾴδιόν γε εἰπεῖν, μέχρι πόσου καὶ τίνων ζητητέον αἰτίας ὁμοίως ἔν τε τοῖς αἰσθητοῖς καὶ νοητοῖς· ἡ γὰρ εἰς ἄπειρον ὁδὸς ἐν ἀμφοῖν ἀλλοτρία καὶ ἀναιροῦσα τὸ φρονεῖν. ἀρχαὶ δὲ τρόπον τινὰ ἄμφω· τάχα δ' ἡ μὲν ἡμῖν ἡ δ' ἁπλῶς, ἢ τὸ μὲν τέλος ἡ δ'

Diocles of Carystus on the method of dietetics 93

many resemblances to Aristotelian and Peripatetic language and style of argument. For example, Diocles' way of expressing himself in section 8 certainly reminds us of Aristotle, who also often uses the combination of 'in a certain way' (τρόπον τινά) and 'look like' (ἔοικε) in order to qualify the similarities he sees between different entities or phenomena; the combination ἀρχαῖς ἔοικε ('look like starting-points') is also attested several times in Aristotle's works.[42] The sophisticated way in which Diocles argues

---

ἡμετέρα τις ἀρχή. μέχρι μὲν οὖν τινὸς δυνάμεθα δι' αἰτίου θεωρεῖν ἀρχὰς ἀπὸ τῶν αἰσθήσεων λαμβάνοντες· ὅταν δὲ ἐπ' αὐτὰ τὰ ἄκρα καὶ πρῶτα μεταβαίνωμεν οὐκέτι δυνάμεθα, εἴτε διὰ τὸ μὴ ἔχειν αἰτίαν εἴτε διὰ τὴν ἡμετέραν ἀσθένειαν ὥσπερ πρὸς τὰ φωτεινότατα βλέπειν; tr. van Raalte (1993) 57, slightly modified); Theophrastus, fr. 159 Fortenbaugh et al.: 'For just as the person who thinks that everything can be demonstrated does away above all with demonstration itself, in the same way *the person who looks for explanations of everything* turns completely upside down all the things there are, and their order which proceeds from a certain definite first principle' (ὥσπερ γὰρ ὁ πάντα ἀποδεικτὰ νενομικὼς αὐτὴν μάλιστα τὴν ἀπόδειξιν ἀναιρεῖ, τοῦτον τὸν τρόπον καὶ **ὁ πάντων αἰτίας ἐπιζητῶν** ἄρδην ἀνατρέπει τὰ ὄντα πάντα καὶ τὴν τάξιν αὐτῶν τὴν ἀπό τινος ὡρισμένης ἀρχῆς προϊοῦσαν, tr. Fortenbaugh et al. (1992) vol. 1, 321); Aristotle, *Ph.* 256 a 28–9: 'if, then, something causes movement by being itself moved, this must come to a standstill and not go on indefinitely' (εἰ οὖν κινούμενόν τι κινεῖ, ἀνάγκη στῆναι καὶ μὴ εἰς ἄπειρον ἰέναι); Aristotle, *Metaph.* 1070 a 2–4: 'it will go on to infinity, if it is not only the bronze that becomes round but also that which is round, or that bronze comes to be; it is necessary for this to come to a halt' (εἰς ἄπειρον οὖν εἶσιν, εἰ μὴ μόνον ὁ χαλκὸς γίγνεται στρογγύλος ἀλλὰ καὶ τὸ στρογγύλον ἢ ὁ χαλκός· ἀνάγκη δὴ στῆναι). On undemonstrable principles see Aristotle, *Top.* 158 b 1ff. On the limits of *teleological* explanation see Aristotle, *Part. an.* 677 a 16–17: 'for this reason, one should not seek a final cause of everything; rather, because some things are like that [i.e. having a final cause], many others occur of necessity as a result of these' (οὐ μὴν διὰ τοῦτο δεῖ ζητεῖν πάντα ἕνεκά τινος· ἀλλὰ τινῶν ὄντων τοιούτων ἕτερα ἐξ ἀνάγκης συμβαίνει διὰ ταῦτα πολλά). *Eth. Nic.* 1098 a 33–b 3: '*one should not ask for the cause in all cases in a similar way*; in some things it is sufficient that the fact is well established, as is the case with the principles; the fact is primary, and a principle' (**οὐκ ἀπαιτητέον δ' οὐδὲ τὴν αἰτίαν ἐν ἅπασιν ὁμοίως**, ἀλλ' ἱκανὸν ἔν τισι τὸ ὅτι δειχθῆναι καλῶς, οἷον καὶ περὶ τὰς ἀρχάς· τὸ δ' ὅτι πρῶτον καὶ ἀρχή).

[42] I performed Pandora complex searches on the Thesaurus Linguae Graecae CD Rom #D for combinations of forms of ἀρχή with forms of ἔοικα within three lines of context in the Hippocratic Corpus, Plato, Aristotle and Theophrastus and found the following results: Aristotle, *Hist. An.* 511 b 10–15: 'since the nature of the blood and that of the blood vessels *resembles a starting-point*... it is difficult to observe... the nature of the most principal blood vessels is invisible' (ἐπεὶ δ' **ἀρχῇ ἔοικεν** ἡ τοῦ αἵματος φύσις καὶ ἡ τῶν φλεβῶν... δυσθεώρητον... ἄδηλος ἡ φύσις τῶν κυριωτάτων φλεβῶν). Aristotle, *Metaph.* 1059 b 29–39: 'for these [i.e. the highest classes of things, i.e. being and unity] are supposed to contain everything that is and most *to resemble starting-points*, because they are naturally primary... but inasmuch as the species are destroyed together with the genera, it is rather the genera that *resemble starting-points*; for that which also causes destruction to something else, is a starting-point' (ταῦτα γὰρ μάλιστ' ἂν ὑποληφθείη περιέχειν τὰ ὄντα πάντα καὶ μάλιστα **ἀρχαῖς ἐοικέναι** διὰ τὸ εἶναι πρῶτα τῇ φύσει... ᾗ δὲ συναναιρεῖται τοῖς γένεσι τὰ εἴδη, τὰ γένη **ταῖς ἀρχαῖς ἔοικε** μᾶλλον· ἀρχὴ γὰρ τὸ συναναιροῦν). [Aristotle], *Mag. mor.* 1190 a 24: 'the end *looks like some sort of starting-point*, and every individual thing is for the sake of that' (τὸ δὲ τέλος **ἀρχῇ τινι ἔοικεν**, καὶ τούτου ἕνεκέν ἐστιν ἕκαστον). [Aristotle], *Mag. mor.* 1206 b 28: 'this is why an emotion that is in a good disposition towards virtue *looks more like a starting-point* than reason' (διὸ μᾶλλον **ἀρχῇ ἔοικεν** πρὸς τὴν ἀρετὴν τὸ πάθος εὖ διακείμενον ἢ ὁ λόγος).

Similar searches for combinations of τρόπον τινα and a form of ἔοικα yielded the following results: Aristotle, *Gen. an.* 758 a 30–b 3: 'That some of these animals come into being through copulation, others spontaneously, has been said before, and in addition that some produce grubs and for what reason. For pretty much all animals *in some way seem* to produce grubs to start with;

against claims one and two sounds very Aristotelian (although he does not use the typically Aristotelian terminology of καθ' αὑτό, κατὰ συμβεβηκός, or the qualifier ᾗ). The advice not to take unknown, disputed or implausible items as starting-points is perfectly in keeping with the principles and the practice of Aristotelian dialectic.[43]

the most imperfect embryo is of this kind, and also in all viviparous and oviparous animals the first embryo grows to perfection while being undifferentiated... in those animals that produce a living being within themselves the embryo *in some sort of way* becomes egg-like after its formation; for the moisture is contained within a fine membrane, as when one takes away the shell of an egg' (ὅτι μὲν οὖν τὰ μὲν ἐξ ὀχείας γίγνεται τῶν τοιούτων τὰ δ' αὐτόματα πρότερον ἐλέχθη, πρὸς δὲ τούτοις ὅτι σκωληκοτοκεῖ καὶ διὰ τίν' αἰτίαν σκωληκοτοκεῖ. σχεδὸν γὰρ **ἔοικε** πάντα **τρόπον τινὰ** σκωληκοτοκεῖν τὸ πρῶτον· τὸ γὰρ ἀτελέστατον κύημα τοιοῦτόν ἐστιν, ἐν πᾶσι δὲ καὶ τοῖς ζῳοτοκοῦσι καὶ τοῖς ᾠοτοκοῦσι τέλειον ᾠὸν τὸ κύημα τὸ πρῶτον ἀδιόριστον ὂν λαμβάνει τὴν αὔξησιν... τὰ δ' ἐν αὑτοῖς ζῳοτοκοῦντα **τρόπον τινὰ** μετὰ τὸ σύστημα τὸ ἐξ ἀρχῆς ᾠοειδὲς γίνεται· περιέχεται γὰρ τὸ ὑγρὸν ὑμένι λεπτῷ, καθάπερ ἂν εἴ τις ἀφέλοι τὸ τῶν ᾠῶν ὄστρακον). Theophrastus, *On the Causes of Plants* 2.9.8–9: 'Seeing that it is the opening of the fruit that makes it remain on the tree by producing ventilation and drainage, the process in the Egyptian mulberry *seems in some sort of way* similar; but some dispute this fact of opening and say that when the insects enter the fig they do not make it open but make it shut; and so one can give the opposite cause for retention and assert that caprification aims at closing the fruit. For once the fig is closed neither dew nor drizzle can make it miscarry, and it is dew and drizzle that get warmed and cause the drop, as with the pomegranate blossom. That these are responsible (and they are cited by some people) is indicated by what happens: there is more dropping of the fruit when light rain follows its first appearance' (**Ἔοικε** δ' εἴπερ ἡ ἄνοιξις ποιεῖ τὴν ἐπιμονὴν εὔνοιάν τε καὶ ἀπέρασιν ποιοῦσα παραπλήσιον **τρόπον τινὰ** [τὸ] συμβαῖνον καὶ ἐπὶ τῶν ἐν Αἰγύπτῳ συκαμίνων· ἀλλὰ τοῦτο διαμφισβητοῦσί τινες ὡς ἄρ' οὐκ ἀνοίγουσιν οἱ ψῆνες ἀλλὰ συμμύειν ποιοῦσιν ὅταν εἰσδύωσιν ὅθεν καὶ τὴν αἰτίαν ἐστὶν ἐκ τοῦ ἐναντίου φέρειν ὡς τούτου χάριν ἐριναζομένων· ἐὰν γὰρ συμμύωσιν οὔθ' ἡ δρόσος οὔτε τὰ ψακάδια δύναται διαφθείρειν ὑφ' ὧν ἀποπίπτουσι διυγραινόμενοι ὥσπερ καὶ οἱ κύτινοι τῶν ῥοῶν· ὅτι δὲ ταῦτα αἴτια μηνύει τὸ συμβαῖνον ὃ δὴ καὶ λέγουσί τινες· ἀποβάλλουσι γὰρ μᾶλλον ὑδατίων ἐπιγινομένων; tr. Einarson and Link, slightly modified); Theophrastus, *On the Causes of Plants* 5.2.5: 'What happens in plants that flower progressively from the lower parts upward closely *resembles in a way* what happens here' (**Ἔοικε** δὲ παραπλήσιον **τρόπον τινὰ** τὸ συμβαῖνον τοῖς κατὰ μέρος ἀνθοῦσιν ἀπὸ τῶν κάτωθεν ἀρχομένοις; tr. Einarson and Link, slightly modified); Theophrastus, *On the Causes of Plants* 6.9.4: 'by and large all fragrant substances are bitter. We shall deal with the reason for this later. It *seems* that of the two opposites, namely sweet and bitter, the sweet is the origin (as it were) of good flavour, whereas the bitter is the origin of fragrance and *in some way* the bitter is to a greater extent the origin of fragrance. For it is hard to find any fragrant thing that is not bitter, but many non-sweet things have excellent flavour' (Ὡς ἐπὶ πᾶν δὲ τά γ' εὔοσμα πάντα πικρά· τούτου μὲν οὖν τὴν αἰτίαν ὕστερον λεκτέον. **Ἔοικε** δὲ δυοῖν ὄντοιν ἐναντίων οἷον τοῦ τε γλυκέος καὶ πικροῦ τὸ μὲν οἷον εὐχυλίας ἀρχή τὸ δ' εὐοσμίας εἶναι καὶ **τρόπον τινὰ** μᾶλλον τὸ πικρὸν τῆς εὐοσμίας. Εὔοσμον γὰρ ἔργον λαβεῖν μὴ πικρὸν εὔχυμα δὲ πολλὰ καὶ μὴ γλυκέα, tr. Einarson and Link, slightly modified). I am aware that linguistic resemblances do not prove intellectual exchange or even similarity of doctrine (for the abuse of linguistic 'evidence' by Jaeger see von Staden (1992) 234–7) and that the Aristotelian corpus is so much larger than the Hippocratic that the significance of the fact that only occurrences in Aristotle and Theophrastus are found may be doubted (the computer also found Plato, *Phaedo* 100 e 6–a 1: ἴσως μὲν οὖν ᾧ εἰκάζω τρόπον τινὰ οὐκ ἔοικεν, but this passage is not quite comparable with the Diocles fragment). It will be clear that much linguistic work still needs to be done here. The resemblance (both linguistic and doctrinal) between Diocles, fr. 176, and a passage in ch. 9 of the Pseudo-Aristotelian text *De spiritu* (485 a 28ff.) was pointed out by Roselli (1992) 122.

[43] Cf., for instance, Aristotle's well-known definition of the 'common opinions' (ἔνδοξα) in *Top.* 100 b 20ff.

Diocles of Carystus on the method of dietetics

Connections of Diocles' views with Aristotle's have, of course, been made by earlier scholars, especially by Werner Jaeger, in whose picture of Diocles as a pupil of Aristotle fragment 176 played a central part. He argued that the fragment could not have been written without the influence of the great Stagirite on the Carystian physician, and from this and other considerations drew far-reaching conclusions concerning Diocles' date.[44] Jaeger's views have met with much criticism and opposition from various scholars, not just because of the authoritative way in which he presented them or because of the claim of inevitability he held with regard to the conclusions he drew from his observations.[45] Most of these criticisms appear completely justified to me, and I have little to add to them. Yet this should not make us *a priori* hostile to any attempt to associate Diocles with the Lyceum. The resemblance is not so much between Diocles' argument that knowledge of the cause is often not necessary for practical purposes and similar statements found in Aristotle's *Nicomachean Ethics* (which Jaeger emphasised) – it has been shown that what is at issue in those passages is rather different from what Diocles is concerned with.[46] More important in this respect is the point which Diocles makes in section 8 – and which is repeated in section 10 – that many things or states of affairs do not *admit* of a causal explanation. While, to my knowledge, no parallels of this idea can be found in the Hippocratic Corpus, it clearly resembles statements in Aristotle and Theophrastus (see note 41) to the effect that the search for causes should stop somewhere and that further analysis even 'destroys' our understanding. It will probably remain a matter of dispute whether this resemblance is actually to be interpreted as evidence of intellectual exchange between Diocles, Aristotle and Theophrastus.[47] Moreover, if the interpretation of section 8 given above is correct, Diocles' *reason* for saying that many things cannot be causally explained is slightly

---

[44] See n. 8 above; for earlier associations of Diocles with the Peripatos see von Staden (1992) 229 n. 11, 12 and 15. For a more recent attempt see Longrigg (1993) 161–75 and (1995).

[45] The most comprehensive and convincing refutation of Jaeger's arguments has been given by von Staden (1992). It should be noted, however, that Jaeger's views have been setting the agenda for Dioclean studies for quite a long time and are sometimes still determining the kind of questions asked by scholars who are at the same time in doubt concerning the validity of his conclusions (see, e.g., the article by Longrigg quoted in the previous note). For a plea for a study of Diocles in his own right (with the question of his date and his being 'influenced' by this or that particular 'school' being kept away from the study of the individual fragments as long as possible) see van der Eijk (1993b) and (2001a) xxi–xxxviii.

[46] See Kullmann (1974) 350ff.; von Staden (1992) 238.

[47] H. Gottschalk (private correspondence) points out to me that the doctrine of the limits of causal explanation, which is a very sophisticated piece of philosophy, is presented by Aristotle as his invention, whereas Diocles alludes to it very briefly: 'his sentence presupposes a knowledge of Aristotle or something very like it'.

different from the ones given by Aristotle and Theophrastus. The latter are either – in the case of real undemonstrable principles such as definitions or logical postulates – concerned with the avoidance of an infinite regress or with the consideration that *within the limits of a particular branch of study* some things should be accepted as starting-points, the demonstration of which belongs to another discipline: the ignorance of this is seen by them as a sign of 'being uneducated' (ἀπαιδευσία). While Aristotle's warnings against pursuing causal analysis too far in these latter contexts look like methodological prescriptions based on considerations of fruitfulness and economy (one *should* not ask for a cause here because it is useless – although it may be possible to state one), Diocles' point is that in the field of dietetics many things simply do not *allow* of explanation, because when pursuing the search for causes too far, one passes the level of the 'whole nature' of a foodstuff and loses the connection with the actual explanandum.

On the other hand, it is not unlikely that some sort of contact between Diocles and the Lyceum took place. Diocles enjoyed a good reputation in Athens – although our source for this does not specify in what times he did.[48] Moreover, there is the reference to a Diocles in Theophrastus' *On Stones* 5 (fr. 239a). It has been doubted whether this should be taken as applying to the Carystian physician, seeing that the name Diocles was very common in Greek and that several persons named Diocles in fourth-century Athens are known from literary and epigraphical sources.[49] Yet I do not see any compelling reason against assuming that the Diocles to whom Theophrastus refers is identical with the Carystian physician. The fact that he is credited by Theophrastus with an opinion on a mineralogical topic is a weak argument, which is based on doubtful presuppositions concerning a 'division of labour' between the sciences. Diocles may have had various interests, just as Theophrastus himself, or Aristotle, or the authors of such

---

[48] (Pseudo-)Vindicianus, *On the Seed* 2: 'Diocles, a follower of Hippocrates, whom the Athenians gave the name of younger Hippocrates' (*Diocles, sectator Hippocratis, quem Athenienses iuniorem Hippocratem vocaverunt*). The use of the Attic dialect may be an indication that Diocles lived or practised in Athens (although several fragments preserved in Oribasius also – in some manuscripts – show Ionic forms [see van der Eijk 2001a, xxiv n. 51]); but the characterisations by Kullmann (1974, 350: 'Der in Athen lebende Arzt Diokles') and Wöhrle (1990, 177: 'Die Weltstadt Athen, in der Diokles lebte') go beyond what is known with certainty.

[49] See Edelstein (1940) 483–9; Kudlien (1963) 462ff.; von Staden (1992) 252–4. The fact that Theophrastus refers to Diocles without further specification is regarded by Eichholz as evidence that the Carystian is meant (1965) 107–8; but this argument will not do, for two different people named Diocles are also mentioned in the will of the Peripatetic Strato (Diogenes Laertius 5.62–3). We can only say that it must have been evident to Theophrastus and his audience which Diocles was meant [see van der Eijk (2001a) 416–19].

Hippocratic writings as *On Fleshes* or *On Regimen* for that matter.[50] Nor are the words 'a certain Diocles' (*Diocli cuidam*) in Pliny's paraphrase of this Theophrastean testimony (fr. 239b) to be interpreted as evidence that Theophrastus referred to another Diocles:[51] they indicate that Pliny was (just as we are, and perhaps for similar reasons) in doubt whether the Diocles mentioned by his source Theophrastus was identical with the Diocles of Carystus known to him from other sources.[52] If Pliny knew for certain that another Diocles was meant – and how could he do so otherwise than because of autopsy of the text of this other Diocles or because he knew from other sources that Theophrastus referred to a text by another Diocles – he would never have expressed himself in this way. Of course we cannot prove that the Diocles mentioned by Theophrastus is the Carystian physician; but then there are a great number of other testimonies about a Diocles where this proof cannot be given.

What we can say, I think, is that Diocles marks a methodological awareness of the limits of causal explanation that was not anticipated in the Hippocratic Corpus and that showed several significant resemblances to remarks found in Aristotle and Theophrastus. These resemblances may have been the result of intellectual exchange and discussion between them (the existence of which is likely), but this cannot be proved, and we are in no position to decide who was 'influenced' by whom.

Finally, it seems that any association of Diocles with Empiricism or Scepticism should be abandoned once and for all. Those who have read the fragment in this way not only seem to have extrapolated Diocles' remarks about dietetics to all other branches of medicine (on the question whether this is justified, see above), but also, as far as dietetics itself is concerned, to have been guided by Galen's presentation of it, that is, as propaganda for an exclusively empirical approach to the search for the powers of

---

[50] It has been argued by von Staden (1992, 253) that there is no independent evidence of mineralogist interest by Diocles. But in fr. 22 Diocles displays a detailed interest in the cohesion between various sorts of objects, including wood and stones. The fragment is quoted by Galen in the context of embryology, but there is no evidence that in its original context it just served the purpose of analogy (as it does for Galen). Moreover, as von Staden concedes, in the immediate context of the Diocles fragment in *On Stones*, Theophrastus mentions dietetic and physiological factors affecting the magnetic force of the *lyngourion* – although I agree that this does not *prove* that the Diocles mentioned was Diocles of Carystus.

[51] Pliny, *Natural History* 27.53: 'what Theophrastus attributed to a certain Diocles' (*quod Diocli cuidam Theophrastus quoque credidit*).

[52] Contra Kudlien (1963, 462–3), who infers from this that the Theophrastus testimony 'mit aller Wahrscheinlichkeit' and 'offenbar' refers to another Diocles; and von Staden (1992, 253), who says that Pliny's wording implies 'that the two [i.e. the Diocles mentioned by Theophrastus and the Diocles of Carystus known to Pliny from other sources] are not identical'.

foodstuffs.⁵³ Compared with the *verbatim* fragment itself, Galen's introduction of Diocles as a champion of the view that the powers of foodstuffs are found by means of experience *only* (note the use of μόνος in sections 2 and 12, both just before and immediately after the quotation) is certainly a gross overstatement – just as his characterisation of Diocles as a 'Dogmatist' and his association with the Empiricists evidently suffers from anachronistic distortion. In fact, when reading Galen's own discussion of the right method of dietetics in the pages following on the fragment, it turns out that Diocles' position as reflected in the fragment (especially in his criticism of claims one and two) perfectly meets the requirements of what Galen himself calls 'qualified experience' (διωρισμένη πεῖρα; see chapter 10 below). By this concept, which Galen presents as his own innovation, he means an empirical approach which takes into account the conditions under which a dietetic statement like 'rock fish are difficult to digest' is true.⁵⁴ Some of the factors Galen enumerates as being relevant in this respect have already been mentioned above: climate, season, geographical area, the patient's natural constitution, age, way of life, and so on. All these should be considered, Galen points out, before any generalising statement about the power of a particular foodstuff is allowed. Galen represents Diocles as being completely unaware of these factors and as being more one-sided than he actually was – and it would seem that Galen is doing so not for lack of understanding but in order to articulate his own refined position as against Diocles' unqualified acceptance of experience as the only way to get to know the powers of foodstuffs.⁵⁵ That Galen is making forced efforts to distinguish himself from Diocles may also be indicated by the fact that later in the same introductory chapter of *On the Powers of Foodstuffs* Galen once more mentions Diocles,⁵⁶ and blames him for 'not even' having mentioned

---

⁵³ See Torraca (1965) 109; Smith (1979) 184.
⁵⁴ See *De alim. facult.* 1.1.45 (p. 216,5 Helmreich; 6.479 K.); 1.1.46 (p. 216,14 H.; 6.479 K.); 1.12.1 (p. 233,2–3 H.; 6.508 K.); *On the Method of Healing* (*De methodo medendi*) 2.7 (10.27 K.); 3.7 (10.204 K.); *De simpl. med. fac.* 2.7 (11.483 K.); 3.13 (11.573 K.); 4.19 (11.685 K.); 4.23 (11.703 K.); 6.1 (11.800 K.); 7.10 (12.38 K.).
⁵⁵ See Smith (1979) 184–6.
⁵⁶ Fr. 177 (Galen, *De alim. facult.* 1.1.27, p. 210,15 Helmreich (6.469 K.)) – a testimony which is not listed as such in Wellmann's collection but only referred to at the end of fr. 176 (Wellmann fr. 112) by 'vgl. Gal. VI 649', although there is little to be compared in the two passages: 'The [substances] that are even with respect to their mixtures and have no mastering quality are just foodstuffs, not drugs: they do not provoke emptying of the belly, nor do they stop, strengthen or relax the stomach, just as they do not stimulate or stop sweat or urine, nor do they bring about another state in the body characterised by hotness, coldness, dryness or wetness, but they preserve in every respect the body of the animal that is fed [by it] in the state in which they found it. But here too there is a highly useful qualification, itself, too, not mentioned by Diocles, just as also none of the others we have discussed until now [was mentioned by him]' (τὰ τοίνυν μέσα ταῖς κράσεσιν οὐδεμίαν ἐπικρατοῦσαν ἔχοντα ποιότητα

the 'highly useful distinction' (διορισμός) between 'foodstuffs' (τροφαί) and 'drugs' (φάρμακα) – that is to say, for not having pointed out under what circumstances a particular substance acts like a foodstuff (which only preserves the state of the body) or as a drug (which changes the state of the body) – just as he failed to deal, Galen adds maliciously, with the other distinctions discussed by him in the previous paragraphs.

In fact, in the context of another treatise, namely *On Medical Experience* (*De experientia medica*, *De exp. med.*),[57] Galen expresses himself in a much more positive way on Diocles' position, although his characterisation of it seems to be based on the same passage from Diocles' *Matters of Health to Pleistarchus*:

As for me, I am surprised at the sophists of our age, who are unwilling to listen to the word of Hippocrates when he says: 'In the case of food and drink experience is necessary', and are not content to accept for themselves and their followers an opinion concerning which the generality of men are completely unanimous, to say nothing of the *élite*. For if everything which is ascertained is ascertained only by reasoning, and nothing is ascertained by experience, how is it possible that the generality, who do not use reason, can know anything of what is known? And how was it that this was unanimously asserted among the elder doctors, not only by Hippocrates, but also by all those who came after him, Diogenes, Diocles, Praxagoras, Philotimus, and Erasistratus? For all of these acknowledge that what they know concerning medical practice they know by means of reasoning in conjunction with experience. In particular, Diogenes and Diocles argue at length that it is not possible in the case of food and drink to ascertain their ultimate effects but by way of experience.

In this testimony, the view of Diocles and the other ancient authorities is obviously referred to in order to support Galen's argument against an exclusively *theoretical* approach to medicine. And although we should not assign much independent value to this testimony – which, apart from its vagueness, is a typical example of Galen's bluffing with the aid of one of his lists of Dogmatic physicians – it is compatible both with the picture of Diocles' general medical outlook that emerges from the collection of fragments as a whole and with his approach to dietetics as reflected in our fragment 176. Diogenes and Diocles are mentioned by Galen in particular

τροφαὶ μόνον εἰσίν, οὐ φάρμακα, μήθ' ὑπάγοντα γαστέρα... διαφυλάττοντα δὲ πάντη τὸ τοῦ τρεφομένου ζῴου σῶμα τοιοῦτον, ὁποῖον παρέλαβεν. ἀλλὰ κἀνταῦθα διορισμός τίς ἐστι χρησιμώτατος οὐδ' αὐτὸς ὑπὸ τοῦ Διοκλέους εἰρημένος, ὥσπερ οὐδὲ τῶν ἄλλων τις, ὅσους ἄχρι τούτου διῆλθον).
[57] Fr. 16 (Galen, *De exp. med.* 13.4–5, p. 109 Walzer, whose translation I have adopted, except for the translation of *logos*, which Walzer leaves untranslated but which I have rendered by 'reason') [see n. 58]; this fragment is also (but obviously for different reasons) lacking in Wellmann.

for having pointed out that experience is an indispensable (but not necessarily the only) instrument for *ascertaining the ultimate effects* of food and drink. This reference to the 'ultimate effects'[58] is in accordance with the interpretation of section 8 given above: this ultimate effect does not admit of further causal explanation; we can only make sure what it is by experience, by applying the foodstuff in a given case and seeing how it works out.

Postscript
Discussions of this fragment that came out after the original publication of this paper can be found in Hankinson (1998a), (1999) and (2002), in van der Eijk (2001a) 321–34, and in Frede (forthcoming).

[58] [In the original version of this paper I suggested that the Greek original may have been something like ἡ ἐσχάτη διάθεσις, which could be related to what Diocles in fr. 176,21 says on 'the whole nature' (τὴν ὅλην φύσιν) of a foodstuff or drink: this 'whole nature', rather than the individual constituents of a foodstuff, should be held responsible for the effects it produces; and this can only be ascertained by experientially seeing how it works in practice. But a re-examination of the Arabic would seem to make this interpretation less plausible. A literal translation of the Arabic would read as follows: 'It is not possible to ascertain in the case of food and drink where their last things (*akhiriyatuha*?) return to/develop into (*ta'ûlu*) but by way of experience.' On this reading, it is the ultimate *effects* of foodstuffs which are meant, and this suggests that the Greek may have contained a word such as τελευταῖος or τελευτάω, or perhaps ἀποβαίνω (cf. Diocles, fr. 184,32). The idea is then that although a Dogmatist might speculate theoretically about the power (δύναμις) of a particular foodstuff, e.g. on the basis of its known constituents or on the basis of comparison or analogy with the known effects of other, similar foodstuffs, one can only *ascertain* the effects of any particular foodstuff by seeing experientially how it works out in practice. Thus the position attributed to Diocles here corresponds closely with that attributed to him by Galen in fr. 176; and it is plausible to assume that the fragment from Diocles' *Matters of Health* quoted in fr. 176 is also at least part of the basis of Galen's report on Diocles' position here. (I am indebted to Peter Pormann for his help here.) A different interpretation was proposed by Walzer, who translated the present phrase 'there is no way of ascertaining the ultimate disposal of foods and drinks except by experience'. This would suggest that Galen is referring to how foods and drinks are ultimately disposed of; but this would seem to be quite inappropriate to the context.]

CHAPTER 3

To help, or to do no harm.
Principles and practices of therapeutics
in the Hippocratic Corpus and in the work
of Diocles of Carystus

1 INTRODUCTION

In a well-known passage from the Hippocratic *Epidemics*, the doctor's duties are succinctly characterised as follows:

[The doctor should] declare what has happened before, understand what is present, and foretell what will happen in the future. This is what he should practise. As to diseases, he should strive to achieve two things: to help, or to do no harm. The (medical) art consists of three components: the disease, the patient, and the doctor. The doctor is servant of the art. The patient should combat the disease in co-operation with the doctor.[1]

The principle that the doctor is there to help, to refrain from anything that may be harmful, and to use his skill and knowledge and all the relevant information about the disease and the patient in order to assist the patient in his battle against the disease is an idea that frequently recurs in Greek medicine. It is succinctly summarised here in the words 'to help, or to do no harm' (ὠφελεῖν ἢ μὴ βλάπτειν), a formula which is often quoted or echoed both in the Hippocratic Corpus and in later Greek and Roman medical literature.[2]

This formula is interesting in that it reflects an early awareness of the possibility that medical treatment can also cause harm. The Hippocratic *Oath*, which explicitly mentions the well-being of the patient as the doctor's

---

This chapter was first published in slightly different form in I. Garofalo, D. Lami, D. Manetti and A. Roselli (eds.), *Aspetti della terapia nel Corpus Hippocraticum* (Florence, 1999) 389–404.

[1] λέγειν τὰ προγενόμενα, γινώσκειν τὰ παρεόντα, προλέγειν τὰ ἐσόμενα· μελετᾶν ταῦτα. ἀσκεῖν περὶ τὰ νοσήματα δύο, ὠφελεῖν ἢ μὴ βάπτειν· ἡ τέχνη διὰ τριῶν, τὸ νόσημα καὶ ὁ νοσέων καὶ ὁ ἰητρός· ὁ ἰητρὸς ὑπηρέτης τῆς τέχνης· ὑπεναντιοῦσθαι τῷ νοσήματι τὸν νοσέοντα μετὰ τοῦ ἰητροῦ. *Epidemics* 1.11 (2.634–6 L.).

[2] E.g. *On Affections* 47 (6.256 L.); 61 (6.270 L.); for a later echo see Scribonius Largus (first century CE), *Compositiones*, pref. 5: 'medicine is the science of healing, not of doing harm' (*scientia enim sanandi, non nocendi est medicina*).

guiding principle,³ understands this 'causing harm' in the sense of deliberately terminating a person's life or otherwise purposively causing disadvantage to his or her situation. Thus, according to the *Oath*, the doctor is not allowed to give a woman an abortive, nor to administer a lethal poison, not even when being asked to do so; and the doctor is instructed to refrain from every kind of abuse of the relation of trust that exists between him and the patient. Yet it is also possible – as the word 'or' suggests – to take the formula in the sense of unintended harm: 'To help, *or at least* to cause no harm', that is to say, the doctor should be careful when treating the patient not to aggravate the patient's condition, for example in cases that are so hopeless that treatment will only make matters worse, or in cases which are so difficult that the doctor may fail in the execution of his art; and as we shall see, there is evidence that Greek doctors considered this possibility too.

In this chapter I will examine how this principle 'to help, or to do no harm' is interpreted in Greek medical practice and applied in cases where it is not immediately obvious what 'helping' or 'causing harm' consists in. I will study this question by considering the therapeutic sections of a number of Hippocratic writings (most of which date from the period 425–350 BCE) and in the fragments of the fourth-century BCE medical writer Diocles of Carystus.

2 THE EARLY HISTORY OF THERAPEUTICS

In the preface to his *On Medicine* (*De medicina*), the Roman encyclopaedic writer Celsus (first century CE) gives an account of the early history of medical therapy from its beginnings in the Homeric era to the epistemological dispute between Dogmatists and Empiricists of his own time. This passage has received ample attention in scholarship, and it is not my intention to give a detailed interpretation or an assessment of its historical reliability.⁴ Instead, I will use it as a starting-point for a consideration of some aspects of therapeutics in classical Greek medicine that may be subsumed under the heading of what I would call the 'systematic status' of therapy in medicine. By this I mean the position and relative importance of therapeutics within the field of medicine as a whole, which gives rise to

---

³ 'I will use dietetic measures to the benefit of the patients ... I will keep them from harm and injustice' (διαιτήμασί τε χρήσομαι ἐπ' ὠφελείῃ τῶν καμνόντων ... ἐπὶ δηλήσει δὲ καὶ ἀδικίῃ εἴρξειν).
⁴ See the commentary by Mudry (1982); Serbat (1995) xxxviii–liii. For more general assessments of Celsus as a source for the history of medicine see Smith (1979) 226–30 and (1989) 74–80; von Staden (1994b) 77–101 and (1999b); Stok (1994) 63–75; Temkin (1935) 249–64.

questions such as the following: Are therapeutics and medicine identical? Or is therapeutics a part of medicine, or perhaps an aim (or even *the* aim) of medicine? Or is therapy just one among several different activities the doctor carries out? And how are the various components, or methods, of therapy interrelated? Do they all have the same purpose, and are they all considered to be equally important? Is there a special status for dietetics (which does not necessarily aim at *healing*)? The answers to these questions are by no means obvious, yet they are of fundamental importance to an understanding of what Greek doctors of this period were up to and what they believed the purposes of their activities to be.

As is well known, in sections 5–8 of the proem Celsus discusses the early period when the medical art was – in Celsus' view perniciously – incorporated within the theoretical study of the nature of things (*rerum naturae contemplatio*) and he presents, with obvious approval, Hippocrates as the one who emancipated medicine out of the bondage of philosophy (*studium sapientiae*), the pursuit of knowledge for its own sake, which Celsus claims to be so fundamentally harmful to the body:

Ergo etiam post eos de quibus rettuli, nulli clari uiri medicinam exercuerunt donec maiore studio litterarum disciplina agitari coepit (6) quae, ut animo praecipue omnium necessaria, sic corpori inimica est. Primoque medendi scientia sapientiae pars habebatur ut et morborum curatio et rerum naturae contemplatio sub isdem auctoribus nata sit, (7) scilicet iis hanc maxime requirentibus qui corporum suorum robora quieta cogitatione nocturnaque uigilia minuerant. Ideoque multos ex sapientiae professoribus peritos eius fuisse accipimus, clarissimos uero ex his Pythagoran et Empedoclen et Democritum. (8) Huius autem, ut quidam crediderunt, discipulus, Hippocrates Cous, primus ex omnibus memoria dignus, a studio sapientiae disciplinam hanc separauit, uir et arte et facundia insignis.[5]

After those, then, of whom I have just spoken, no man of any fame practised the art of medicine until literary activity began to be practised with greater zeal, (6) which, while being most necessary of all for the mind, is also harmful to the body. At first the knowledge of healing was regarded as a part of wisdom,[6] so that both the treatment of diseases and the study of natural things came into being under the same authorities, (7) clearly because those who most required it [i.e. medicine] were those who had weakened the strength of their bodies by their sedentary thinking and their wakeful nights. For this reason, as we hear, many of those who claimed expertise in wisdom were experienced in it [i.e. medicine], the most famous of them indeed being Pythagoras, Empedocles, and Democritus. (8) But a pupil of this last, as some believed him to be, Hippocrates of Cos, the

---

[5] Text according to Serbat (1995) 3–5.
[6] *Sapientia* clearly covers both science and philosophy.

first of all to deserve mention, separated this discipline from the study of wisdom; he was a man outstanding both for his skill [in medicine] and for his eloquence.[7]

In the sequel to this passage, Celsus describes a further stage in the development of the medical art. He presents Diocles, Praxagoras and Chrysippus, as well as Herophilus and Erasistratus, as men who exercised the art to such an extent that they developed different ways of healing, and he points out that 'also, in the same period' a divison of medicine took place into regimen, pharmacology, and surgery:

Post quem Diocles Carystius, deinde Praxagoras et Chrysippus, tum Herophilus et Erasistratus, sic artem hanc exercuerunt ut etiam in diuersas curandi uias processerint. (9) Isdemque temporibus in tres partes medicina diducta est ut una esset quae uictu, altera quae medicamentis, tertia quae manu mederetur. Primam διαιτητικήν, secundam φαρμακευτικήν, tertiam χειρουργίαν Graeci nominarunt.

After him Diocles of Carystus, and later Praxagoras and Chrysippus, and then Herophilus and Erasistratus practised the art in such a way that they even proceeded into diverse modes of treatment. (9) Also, in the same times, medicine was divided into three parts, so that there was one which healed by regimen, another by drugs, and a third manually. The Greeks named the first dietetics, the second pharmaceutics, the third surgery.

However, Celsus then seems to suggest that within dietetics (*eius autem quae uictu morbos curat*) a renewed interest in theoretical speculation took place: for he says that there were 'famous authorities' who, out of a desire for deeper understanding, claimed that for this purpose knowledge of nature was indispensable, because without it medicine was truncated and impotent (*trunca et debilis*).

Eius autem quae uictu morbos curat longe clarissimi auctores etiam altius quaedam agitare conati rerum quoque naturae sibi cognitionem uindicarunt, tamquam sine ea trunca et debilis medicina esset. (10) Post quos Serapion, primus omnium nihil hanc rationalem disciplinam pertinere ad medicinam professus, in usu tantum et experimentis eam posuit. Quem Apollonius et Glaucias et aliquanto post Heraclides Tarentinus et aliqui non mediocres uiri secuti ex ipsa professione se empiricos appellauerunt. (11) Sic in duas partes ea quoque quae uictu curat medicina diuisa est, aliis rationalem artem, aliis usum tantum sibi uindicantibus, nullo uero quicquam post eos qui supra comprehensi sunt agitante nisi quod acceperat donec Asclepiades medendi rationem ex magna parte mutauit.

Yet as for that part of medicine which cures diseases by regimen, by far the most famous authorities also tried to deal with some things at even greater depth and also claimed for themselves a knowledge of the nature of things as if, without this,

---

[7] Translation according to van der Eijk (2000a) 3–5.

medicine were incomplete and impotent. (10) After these, Serapion was the first to claim that this theoretical discipline had no bearing on medicine at all and that it [i.e. medicine] was a matter of practice and experience only. He was followed by Apollonius, Glaucias, and some time later by Heraclides of Tarentum and several other very distinguished men, who on the strength of the very claim they made gave themselves the name of Empiricists. (11) Thus that part of medicine which heals by regimen was also divided into two parts, some claiming for themselves that it was a theoretical art, others that it was a matter of practice only. After those who have just been dealt with, however, no one indeed added anything to what he had accepted from his precursors until Asclepiades made major changes to the method of healing.

Four brief comments on this passage are in order here:
(i) The art of medicine as practised by Hippocrates is presented by Celsus in a rather narrow sense of the art of healing (*curare*), namely treatment or therapy, which raises the question what place, if any, is left for anatomy, physiology, prognostics and pathology – areas which are well represented in the Hippocratic Corpus.
(ii) Progress in this art is said to have led to a differentiation of modes of treatment (*in diuersas curandi uias*) which occurred shortly *after* Hippocrates (8).
(iii) It is said (9) that 'in the same times' a tripartition of medicine occurred. It is unclear, however, what Celsus means by 'the same times', and whether this tripartition is identical to, or a consequence of, the differentiation mentioned in the previous sentence, or in other words, how the sentences *Post quem . . . processerint* and *isdemque temporibus . . . nominarunt* are related to one another.
(iv) The renewal of interest in the theoretical study of nature as well as the subsequent criticism this provoked among the Empiricists (9–11) is said to have taken place within the specific area of dietetics, which in its turn, and as a result of this development, was divided into two branches.

I shall be brief about point (i), for it may be, and often has been, argued that this perception of Hippocratic medicine reflects, to a much greater extent than the other three points, Celsus' personal view of the priorities in medicine.[8] Yet in at least one respect the surviving evidence does seem to agree with the picture he presents. The Hippocratic Corpus provides evidence of an increasingly self-conscious medical profession, which is reflecting on and promulgating its own principles, setting high standards

---

[8] On Celsus as a reporter of Rationalist medicine see von Staden (1994b); on Celsus' view of Hippocrates see Serbat (1995) liii–lvii; Mudry (1977) 345–52; Castiglioni (1940) 862–6.

to the execution of these principles and clearly trying to emancipate itself from philosophical speculation. Thus, as is well known, the author of the Hippocratic work *On Ancient Medicine* criticises what he calls 'philosophy'[9] and its influence on medical practice, and he refers disparagingly to the use of 'postulates' such as the elementary qualities hot and cold as all-pervading explanatory principles in the understanding and treatment of the human body.[10] The author of another Hippocratic work, *On the Art of Medicine*, defends medicine against accusations to the effect that it is not really a skill and that its successes are a matter of good luck. Interestingly, he counters the criticism that medicine is not in all cases capable of restoring health by pointing out that this is not due to lack of skill or poor performance of doctors (although this may of course be the case), but due either to lack of co-operation by the patient or to the fact that the disease is, or has become, incurable – and in such cases, he argues, it is actually to the doctor's credit to be realistic and to refrain from treatment.[11]

As far as point (ii) is concerned, what Celsus says here would again seem to receive confirmation from the surviving evidence of fifth- and fourth-century medical literature. For while the Hippocratic Corpus does not contain works specifically devoted to therapeutics as such, two leading medical writers of the subsequent generation, Diocles of Carystus and Praxagoras of Cos, are both reported to have written extensively on therapeutics *per se* in works entitled *On Treatments* (περὶ θεραπειῶν), at least four books being attested in the case of Diocles and three for Praxagoras;[12] and it may be noted that Aristotle, too, is credited with a work *On Remedies* (*De adiutoriis*, in Greek probably περὶ βοηθημάτων).[13] In the case of Diocles, we further know that this work *On Treatments* was different from the more frequently attested work *Affection, Cause, Treatment* (πάθος αἰτία θεραπεία, in one book).[14] Regrettably, our information on the nature of these two works and their possible differences is severely restricted by the fact that Diocles' works survive in fragments only; and in this particular case the problem is aggravated by the fact that all information about Diocles'

---

[9] *On Ancient Medicine* 20 (1.620 L.).   [10] *On Ancient Medicine* 1 (1.570 L.).
[11] *On the Art of Medicine* 8 (6.12–14 L.).
[12] Diocles, frs. 99 (*libro curationum*), 136 (*secundo libro curationum*), 100 (*tertio libro de curationibus*), 125 (*quarto libro de curationibus*) in van der Eijk's edition (2000a); Praxagoras, frs. 100, 101, 102, 103, 104, 105, 106, 107, 108, 109, 111, 112 in the edition of Steckerl (1958).
[13] Aristotle, fr. 360 (= Caelius Aurelianus, *Acute Affections* 2.13.87) in the edition of Gigon (1983).
[14] Diocles, frs. 49, 73, 79, 85, 92, 99, 100, 103, 109, 111a, 114, 116, 120, 123, 125, 128, 129, 131, 132a, 136, 139 in van der Eijk (2000a). To be sure, in frs. 116, 131 and 139 Caelius Aurelianus refers to the '*books*' (*libris*) Diocles wrote on diseases, causes, treatments, but the fact that in the overwhelming majority of references to this work he speaks of a 'book' (*libro*) and that Caelius, when he refers to this work, never specifies in which book Diocles said such and such, suggests that these three cases are just due to lack of accuracy on Caelius' part.

On Treatments is provided by the Methodist writer Caelius Aurelianus, who is not a very sympathetic reporter of Diocles' therapeutic views. Yet some fragments allow us to get some impression of the difference of emphasis between the two works. Thus in *Acute Affections* 3.17.159 (= Diocles, fr. 125), Caelius discusses Diocles' views on the treatment of ileus (intestinal disorder):

Diocles autem *libro, quo de passionibus atque causis et curationibus scribit*, phlebotomat in passione constitutos atque cataplasmatibus curat ex polline, quod Graeci omen lysin uocant, et adipe et uino et faece. tunc praepotat atque clysterizat ex abrotani semine cum mulsa ex aceto et aristolochia et cumino et nitro et foeniculi radice decocta ex uino admixta aqua marina uel passo uel acriore uino siue lacte cum decoctione lini seminis et mellis uel similibus. *Quarto autem libro de curationibus*

'Iuuenes', inquit, 'atque habitudine robustos et magis, quibus dolor ad latera fertur phlebotomandos probo ex manu dextera <uel> interiore[m] uena[m] et submittendos in aquam calidam, fotis uentri inicere admixto sale clysterem et rursum in aquam calidam deponere et fouere.'

praepotandos autem iubet etiam medicamentis, hoc est panacis dimidia drachma in mulso ex aceto tepido resoluta et myrrhae obolos duos cum peristereonis herbae foliis in uino albo uel cumino Aethiopico.

'Adiuuat etiam plurimos plumbi catapotium transuoratum, impellit enim pondere et excludit obtrudentia.'

diurnis inquit praeterea diebus sitientibus potandum uinum dulce uel aqua[m] temperatum aut marinam cum uino albo aut centauream herbam aut nitrum uel eius spumam, ut ea, quae potuerit, soluat.

'Danda etiam sorbilia uel cantabria lotura cum melle uel bromi sucus uel ptisanae aut cum farina olera cocta, alia ex adipe, alia ex alica atque sale; sorbendum etiam et iuscellum scari piscis et carabi et bucinarum et cancrorum. tunc resumptio', inquit, 'adhibenda',

cuius quidem materies percurrerit, quas superfluum est recensere. etenim ex supradictis uana atque iners commixtio materiarum demonstratur. Non enim solos oportet iuuenes phlebotomari, sed etiam alios in aliis aetatibus constitutos, neque semper e dextera manu uel interiore uena, sed etiam ex sinistra atque exteriore facta. detractio enim tumentia relaxat, usus autem <clysterum> acrimoniae causa erigit in feruorem tumentia. est praeterea uexabilis praebibendi medicaminis potio. etenim sunt acria atque mordentia et quae non sint mitigatiua celeritatis neque tumoris relaxantia. plumbum uero transuoratum premit quidem atque impellit pondere, sed tactu necessario frigidat atque intestina densitate coacta uexatione distendit. iuscella autem in corruptione<m> facilia et inflantia esse noscuntur, item ptisana[e] eadem perficere, uinum quoque in augmento inimicum.[15]

---

[15] Text according to Bendz and Pape (1990–3) vol. I, 386–8.

Diocles, in the book in which he writes on affections, causes and treatments, applies venesection to those in whom the affection [sc. ileus] has established itself and treats them with poultices from the flour which the Greeks call *ōmē lusis*, fat, wine and lees. Then he gives them something to drink first and applies a clyster consisting of the seed of abrotanum mixed with oxymel, and of birthwort, cumin, nitre, fennel root decocted in wine mixed with sea water, or raisin wine, or more acid wine, or milk with a decoction of linseed and honey, or similar things. Again, in the fourth book on treatments he says:

> 'For young people and those whose normal constitution is strong, and all the more for those in whom the pain stretches to the sides [of the body], I recommend venesection from the right hand, or from the internal vein, and bathing in hot water, and when they have got warm to inject in the belly a clyster mixed with salt, and then again to put them in hot water and to warm them.'

But he prescribes also that they should be given drugs to drink first, namely half a drachm of allheal dissolved in lukewarm oxymel, and two obols of myrrh with leaves of holy vervain in white wine, or with Ethiopian cumin.

> 'Most patients also benefit from swallowing a lead pill, for it drives the obstructing material away by its heaviness and expels it.'

Moreover, he says that patients who are thirsty should daily be given wine that is sweet or mixed with water, or sea water mixed with white wine, or centaury, or nitre, or soda, in order to dissolve as much as possible.

> 'One should also give soupy food, such as bran water with honey, or a gruel of oats or of pearl barley, or vegetables cooked with flour, some with fat, others with spelt groats and salt; the patient should also swallow a broth made from parrot wrasse, crayfish, bucinas and crabs. Then', he says, 'a convalescense cure should be applied',

of which he lists the materials, which it is superfluous to enumerate; for from the above it is evident that this mixture of stuffs is useless and unskilful. For one should venesect not only young people, but also people of other ages, and not always from the right hand or the interior vein, but also from the left hand and from the exterior vein. For after a withdrawal has been carried out, this gives relief to the swelling parts, but the use of clysters, due to their acid quality, causes the swelling parts to burn. Moreover, the drinking of drugs beforehand is irritating, for these are sharp and biting, and [are things] that do not soothe the acute state nor bring relief to the swelling parts. Swallowed lead, to be sure, presses and drives [the obstructing material] by its heaviness, but necessarily on contact cools and stretches the densely compacted intestines in an irritating manner. Broths are known to go off easily and to cause flatulency, and barley gruel to bring about the same effect; wine, too, is harmful when the disease is in its increasing phase.[16]

---

[16] Translation according to van der Eijk (2000a) 213–17.

A comparison between the two accounts shows that the therapeutic instructions derived from *On Treatments* are much more detailed and show greater differentiation according to the individual patient. The fact that a lead pill is not mentioned in the report of the therapeutic section of *Affection, Cause, Treatment* may be a matter of coincidence, or of Caelius' selectivity in reporting, but it may be significant that such a pill is also mentioned in another testimony where the two works are compared, in Caelius' discussion of Diocles' treatment of epilepsy (*Chronic Affections* 1.4.132).[17] Moreover, in this text, as in *Acute Affections* 3.8.87 (which deals with the treatment of tetanus), Caelius suggests that the therapeutic section of Diocles' *Affection, Cause, Treatment* differentiated according to the cause of the disease, as one would expect from a work with this title.[18]

---

[17] 'Again, Diocles, in the book in which he wrote on affections, recommends venesection for those who have caught this affection because of excessive drinking or eating of meat, [thereby] considering antecedent causes rather than present ones. Yet for those who have incurred this affection because of the usual state of their body, he recommends the withdrawal of a thick humour, which he called phlegma. He also applies drugs that stimulate the urinary passages, which people call diuretica, and also walking and being carried around. Yet even if these were real remedies, because of the smallness of their number and of their power it could hardly be said that they are strong enough against this great affection, or that they are sufficient for its destruction. Again, in the book of treatments he applies venesection and uses as medicine a pill which turns the stomach and causes vomiting after dinner by filling the head with exhalations. He gives vinegar to drink, and by causing sneezing before the patients fall asleep he troubles the sensory passages at a highly untimely moment. He also gives wormwood, centaury, ass's milk, and the scab of horses or mules not indicating the time these measures should be applied but afflicting the patients with dreadful things' (*Item Diocles* **libro, quo de passionibus** scripsit, in his, qui ex uinolentia uel carnali cibo istam passionem conceperint, phlebotomiam probat, antecedentes potius quam praesentes intuens causas. in his uero, qui ex corporis habitudine in istam uenerint passionem, humoris crassi detractionem probat adhibendam, quem appellauit phlegma. utitur etiam urinalibus medicamentis, quae diuretica uocant. item deambulatione ac gestatione, quae si etiam uera essent adiutoria, ob paruitatem tamen numeri et magnitudinis suae, magnae passioni difficile possent paria pronuntiari aut eius destructioni sufficere. Item **libro curationum** phlebotomans utitur medicamine catapotio, quod stomachum euertit atque post cenam uomitum facit, exhalationibus implens caput. potat etiam aceto <et> sternutamentum commouens priusquam in somnum ueniant aegrotantes, profecto intemporaliter commouet sensuales uias. dat etiam absinthium, centaurion et lac asininum et equorum impetigines uel mulorum neque tempus adiciens factis et odiosis aegrotantes afficiens rebus); Diocles, fr. 99 vdE; the title *de passionibus* is an abbreviation for *de passionibus atque causis earum et curationibus*; the singular *libro curationum* is not in accordance with the other references to the work (see n. 12 above), which is possibly, again, due to lack of precision on Caelius Aurelianus' part. On the relative infrequence of the use of pills in early Greek medicine see Goltz (1974) 206–7.

[18] 'Diocles, in the book in which he wrote on affections, causes and treatments, says that with people suffering from tetanus one should apply drugs that promote urine, which he called "diuretics", and then one should purge and evacuate the stomach. He also gives raisin wine mixed with water to drink to children or to those who have contracted the affection because of a wound. He also prohibits the giving of food and he prescribes the application of vapour baths to the [parts] that are stiffened by the affection and to make them flexible. Again, in the third book *On Treatments*, he similarly uses a clyster and gives sweet wine to drink and applies vapour baths, sometimes dry ones, sometimes wet ones, and he anoints the affected parts with wax-salve and covers them with wool' (*Diocles* **libro, quo passiones atque causas atque curationes scripsit**, tetanicis inquit adhibenda mictoria medicamina, quae appellauit diuretica, tum uentrem deducendum atque <e>uacuandum. dat etiam bibendum passum

It is hazardous, with so little information of such questionable reliability, to draw any firm conclusions, but there is some plausibility in the hypothesis that Diocles' *On Treatments* was a more specialised work, which paid more attention to therapeutic detail (apparently arranged by disease) but less to causal explanation or symptomatology, whereas his briefer pathological work *Affection, Cause, Treatment* dealt with the therapy of diseases in a wider, more general framework. Further titles and fragments of Diocles' works indicate that he wrote separate works on regimen in health, anatomy, physiology (digestion), external remedies, toxicology, prognostics, gynaecology, fevers, catarrhs, evacuations, bandages, surgery, vegetables, rootcutting, and possibly cookery and sexuality.[19] Although there may have been a substantial overlap in subject matter between some of these works, these titles suggest that by the time of Diocles medicine had increasingly become compartmentalised, and this well accords with Celsus' reference to Diocles 'proceeding into diverse ways of treatment'.[20]

As far as point (iii) in Celsus' text about the tripartition of medicine is concerned, some interpreters seem to take the words 'in the same times' (*isdemque temporibus*) as referring to the times of Diocles, Praxagoras and Chrysippus, Herophilus and Erasistratus, and this would mean that the division of medicine is presented as a post-Hippocratic development.[21]

---

*aquatum pueris uel his, qui ex uulnere in passionem ceciderunt. prohibet etiam cibum dari et iubet ea, quae passione tenduntur, uaporari et emolliri. item **tertio libro de curationibus** similiter clystere utitur et uinum dulce dat bibendum adhibens uaporationes nunc siccas, nunc humectas, et ungit cerotario atque lanis patientia contegit loca;* Diocles, fr. 100 vdE).

[19] See the list of preserved titles in van der Eijk (2000a) xxxiii–xxxiv. Apart from the titles mentioned, there is also a work by Diocles entitled *Archidamos* (fr. 185), which dealt, among other things, with the use of olive oil for hygienic purposes. Wellmann's assumption of a work by Diocles περὶ πυρὸς καὶ ἀέρος (fr. 20 W.) is based on the (highly doubtful) presupposition that the anonymous source to which (Ps.-)Vindicianus refers by means of formulae such as *inquit, ait*, is Diocles; a refutation of this view has been offered by Debru (1992); see also Debru (1996) 311–27 and van der Eijk (2001a) 79–91.

[20] I prefer to interpret this phrase as referring to variety *within* the healing practices of individual physicians rather than as suggesting that each physician developed his own peculiar method(s) of treatment as distinct from those of the others (von Staden (1999b) 268) or as referring to the divisions within the Dogmatist tradition between Erasistrateans, Herophileans, etc. (Smith (1989) 76: 'alludes, apparently, to the divisions between Erasistrateans and Herophileans, and perhaps to other dogmatic sects'; the latter seems unlikely as the difference is said to lie in methods of *treatment* rather than in theoretical justification for this). But many commentators have expressed uncertainty about the precise meaning of this phrase; cf. Smith (1989, 76): 'I am uncertain what differences Celsus may have had in mind' and Serbat (1995, xxxix: 'observation assez énigmatique'), and the translations by Spencer: 'so practiced this art that they made advances even towards various methods of treatment'; Serbat: 'pratiquèrent cet art en le faisant même progresser dans des voies thérapeutiques différentes'; and Mudry (1982, 67): 'pratiquèrent cet art de telle sorte qu'ils avancèrent encore dans des voies différentes').

[21] Mudry (1982) 67; von Staden (1989) 99; Serbat (1995, xxxix) takes it as a reference to the times of Herophilus and Erasistratus.

However, on this interpretation it is slightly strange to introduce a new paragraph at section 9, as Mudry does,[22] for this suggests that a new issue is to be discussed, whereas both sentences seem to be expressing more or less the same idea: progress leading to different methods of treatment and division of the art of medicine into three areas which are also defined by the way in which they provide treatment (*quae uictu... quae medicamentis... quae manu mederetur*) seem to amount to the same thing.[23] Instead, I would suggest taking *isdemque temporibus* as a less specific reference to the times mentioned in the previous section (thus including both Hippocratic and post-Hippocratic medicine) and reading the section from *isdemque temporibus* onwards as making a new point (as is indicated by the use of *que*), that is to say, a development running parallel to the events that were described in section 8 (Hippocrates' emancipation of the art of healing from the study of wisdom and the subsequent further refinement of medicine by Diocles and the others). It is important to see for what purpose Celsus has inserted the tripartition of healing into his argument.[24] It enables him to present the subsequent relapse into the theoretical study of nature as something taking place *within dietetics*,[25] thus arriving at the paradoxical, perhaps slightly tragic picture of medicine making fast progress towards greater refinement but this same differentiation allowing theoretical speculation to sneak in again through the back door of dietetics.[26] For although Celsus does not state whom he means when referring to 'by far the most famous authorities' (*longe clarissimi auctores*) in dietetics, it is hard not to think of Diocles and Erasistratus (and perhaps Mnesitheus, although he is not mentioned by Celsus), who had just been mentioned as those who had made further progress in medicine, but who are also known for their 'theoretical' outlook in general – and indeed it is hard not to think of the most philosophical treatise on dietetics that has come down to us, the Hippocratic *On Regimen*.

Thus interpreted, Celsus' report is consistent with the fact (which there was no reason for him to ignore) that the Hippocratic Corpus itself already provides evidence of a division of therapeutic activities roughly corresponding to the tripartition into dietetics, surgery and pharmacology. Although

---

[22] See also Spencer (1935) 6, and Serbat (1995) ad loc.
[23] On the interpretation of this phrase see n. 20 above.
[24] Surgery and pharmacology had already been identified as 'parts' of medicine in section 4 (dealing with the Homeric age). Dietetics is presented by Celsus as a more recent method of treatment.
[25] See Mudry (1982) 74.
[26] It may be disputed whether Celsus really values this development negatively (see von Staden (1994b) 85), considering his cautious approval of theory in section 47 of the proem; however, there the discussion is about fevers and wounds, not about dietetics, and theory is just presented as adding a special but not strictly necessary quality to medicine; and in section 59 (where the wording is strikingly similar to that of section 9) he is clearly being sarcastic about the value of theory.

this division is nowhere stated explicitly in either the texts of the Hippocratic writers[27] or the fragments of Diocles, Praxagoras or any other of the physicians mentioned,[28] nevertheless there is evidence that Hippocratic doctors regarded pharmacology and surgery as special types of treatment separate from the more regular dietetic measures.

As for pharmacology, the treatise *On Affections* (*Aff.*) frequently refers for further details about the drugs to be administered to a (lost) work entitled *Pharmakitis* or *Pharmaka*.[29] Judging from these references, this work not only dealt with the preparation of drugs,[30] but also with their workings and the conditions under which they were to be administered.[31] Furthermore, the author of *On Regimen in Acute Diseases* refers to a separate (not extant) discussion of composite drugs (σύνθετα φάρμακα).[32] Again, in other nosological works, such as *On Internal Affections* (*Int. Aff.*) and *Appendix to On Regimen in Acute Diseases*, it is frequently stated that in addition to a number of measures 'a drug (φάρμακον) should be given' or 'a treatment with drugs' (φαρμακεύειν) should, or should not, be adopted.[33]

Similarly, surgical measures are frequently referred to in a way suggesting that they are considered to belong to a separate category. Thus *On Diseases* 1.14 distinguishes between 'letting blood from the vessels of the arms' and 'a regimen'.[34] The author of *Appendix to On Regimen in Acute Diseases*

---

[27] The formulations that come closest are *Oath*: διαιτήμασι τε χρήσομαι... οὐ δώσω δὲ οὐδὲ φάρμακον... οὐ τεμέω ('I will use dietetic measures... I will not give a drug... nor will I use the knife'), and *On the Art of Medicine* 6 (6.10 L.) and 8 (6.14 L.): φάρμακα... διαιτήματα... τῶν ἐν ἰητρικῇ καιόντων... πῦρ... τῶν ἄλλων ὅσα τῇ ἰητρικῇ συνεργεῖ ('drugs... dietetic measures... medical instruments that burn... fire... all other instruments of the medical art').

[28] For the dubious evidence in the case of Diocles see the discussion in van der Eijk (2001a) 6 n. 15 and 80–1.

[29] E.g. in chs. 4 (6.212 L.), 9 (6.216 L.), 15 (6.224 L.) and 18 (6.226 L.).

[30] *Aff.* 4 (6.212 L.): 'one should at once give gargles, preparing them as has been described in the books on drugs' (παραχρῆμα μὲν τοῖσιν ἀναγαργαρίστοισι χρῆσθαι, σκευάζων ὡς γέγραπται ἐν τοῖς Φαρμάκοις).

[31] *Aff.* 27 (6.238 L.): 'In the case of cholera, if the patient has pain, one should give what has been described in the books on drugs as stopping pain' (τῇ δὲ χολέρῃ συμφέρει, ἢν μὲν ὀδύνη ἔχῃ, διδόναι ἃ γέγραπται ἐν τοῖς Φαρμάκοισι παύοντα τῆς ὀδύνης).

[32] *On Regimen in Acute Diseases* 64 (2.364 L.): 'this [i.e. the use of drinks and the correct time of their usage] will be described in relation to this disease, as will be done with the other composite drugs' (γεγράψεται παρ' αὐτῷ τῷ νοσήματι ὅπωσπερ καὶ τἆλλα τῶν συνθέτων φαρμάκων).

[33] E.g. *Int. Aff.* 15 (7.204 L.); 17 (7.208 L.). *Appendix to On Regimen in Acute Diseases* 8 (2.408 L.), 12 (2.418 L.), 27 (2.448 L.), 32 (2.462 L.); *Aff.* 20 (6.230 L.). Cf. *Aphorisms* 1.20 and 1.14 (4.464–6 L.). On Hippocratic pharmacology see Stannard (1961) 497–518. For the special status of drugs over dietetic measures cf. also Diocles, frs. 153,2–3 and fr. 183a, lines 25, 48 and 62–3 (although this fragment is of dubious authenticity); and Plato, *Timaeus* 89 b 3–4.

[34] *On Diseases* 1.14 (6.164 L.): 'It benefits such patients [i.e. those suffering from suppuration of the lung], when one undertakes to treat them in the beginning, to let blood from the vessels in the hands, and to give them a regimen that is most drying and bloodless' (ξυμφέρει δὲ τοῖσι τοιούτοισιν, ἢν κατ' ἀρχὰς λάβῃς ὥστε θεραπεύειν, φλέβες ἐξιέμεναι ἐκ τῶν χειρῶν καὶ δίαιτα ὑφ' ἧς ἔσται ὡς ξηρότατός τε καὶ ἀναιμότατος).

distinguishes between treatment by drugs, venesection and clystering,[35] and elsewhere between regimen, fomentations and drugs;[36] and the author of *On Internal Affections* distinguishes on one occasion between treatment by fomentations, drugs, foods and exercises,[37] and on another occasion between treatment by drugs, drink, food and exercises.[38]

With dietetics, matters seem to be more complicated. The verb *diaitan* (διαιτᾶν) is often used by Hippocratic authors to describe a treatment consisting of measures characteristic of what we would call dietetics, such as foods and drinks, walking, baths, exercise and sleep. But sometimes it just seems to be equivalent to 'treatment', as in a well-known statement of the doctor's primary requirements in *Epidemics* 3.16;[39] and indeed in the treatise *On Ancient Medicine* dietetics seems to be just what medicine is all about – although even here a brief reference to cupping instruments indicates that, to this author, medicine is not entirely a matter of food, drink and exercise.[40] At the same time this work, as well as the explicitly dietetic writings such as *On Regimen* and *On Regimen in Acute Diseases*, make it clear that dietetics is not only used for therapeutic purposes, that is, for the treatment of diseases, but also for the preservation and promotion of health (ὑγιεινά) and the prevention of disease.[41]

This raises the question whether it is correct to regard dietetics as a part or branch of therapeutics. It could be argued that it should rather be defined more generally as a care for the body *both* – and perhaps predominantly – in healthy states as well as (perhaps secondarily) in unhealthy states, or on the interface between the two, as seems to be the position of the author of *On Regimen*.[42] More importantly, as far as unhealthy states are concerned, dietetics seems to be a care for the body which does not necessarily aim

---

[35] *Appendix* 4 (2.400 L.): φαρμακεύειν ... φλεβοτομίη ... κλυσμόν.
[36] *Appendix* 56–7 (2.508–10 L.): αἷμα ... ἀφαιρέειν ... λιμοκτονέειν καὶ οἶνον ἀφαιρέειν αὐτῷ. ἔπειτα τῇ διαίτῃ τὰ ἐπίλοιπα αὐτὸν καὶ πυρίῃσιν ἐνίκμοισι θεράπευε ... κλύσματι ... φαρμακεῦσαι.
[37] *Int. Aff.* 50 (7.292 L.): μελετᾶν ... πυρίῃσι καὶ φαρμάκοισι καὶ ἐδέσμασι καὶ ταλαιπωρίῃσιν.
[38] *Int. Aff.* 24 (7.228 L.): φαρμάκοισι καὶ ποτοῖσι καὶ βρωτοῖσι καὶ ταλαιπωρίῃσι. Cf. the well-known Hippocratic *Aphorism* 7.87 (4.608 L.): 'Diseases that are not cured by drugs, the iron will cure; and those that are not cured by the iron, fire will cure; and those that are not cured by fire one should consider incurable.'
[39] *Epidemics* 3.16 (3.102 L.): 'To know about these things means to know whom one should treat by regimen and when and how' (εἰδότι περὶ τούτων ἐστιν εἰδέναι οὓς καὶ ὅτε καὶ ὡς δεῖ διαιτᾶν).
[40] *On Ancient Medicine* 22 (1.626 L.): 'On the other hand, cupping instruments, which are broad and tapering, have been designed for this purpose, that they withdraw and attract [material] from the flesh, and there are many other instruments of a similar kind' (τοῦτο δὲ αἱ σικύαι προσβαλλόμεναι ἐξ εὐρέος ἐς στενότερον συνηγμέναι πρὸς τοῦτο τετεχνέαται πρὸς τὸ ἕλκειν ἐκ τῆς σαρκὸς καὶ ἐπισπᾶσθαι, ἄλλα τε πολλὰ τοιουτότροπα). On this see Festugière (1948) 66–7. See also, in the same treatise, ch. 12 (1.596 L.), where the mention of 'many species of medicine' (πολλὰ εἴδεα κατ' ἰητρικήν) seems to envisage different parts of medicine.
[41] *On Ancient Medicine* 3, 5 and 7 (1.574, 580 and 584 L.).
[42] *On Regimen* 1.2 (6.470–2 L.); 3.67 (6.592 L.); 3.69 (6.606 L.).

at *restoring* the health of a sick body,[43] but rather at bringing about the least harmful, or least painful, state for a sick body, which may amount to combating symptoms such as pain[44] or, more generally, to making the disease more tolerable.

If Celsus is correct in portraying dietetics as a relatively late development in Greek therapeutics,[45] this must refer to dietetic *medicine*, the application of dietetic principles to the treatment of diseases. Rather than thinking that dietetics was originally a part of medicine and was only later, under the influence of changing social and cultural circumstances,[46] divided into a therapeutic part (the treatment of diseases) and a hygienic part (the preservation of health and hygiene), one may also defend the view that dietetics as a way of looking after the body was of an older origin and had, by the fifth century BCE, developed into an established corpus of knowledge primarily based on experience which was subsequently applied to the treatment of diseases.[47]

3 THE AIMS OF THERAPEUTIC ACTIVITY

With these considerations we are at the heart of what may be called, with the usual *caveats* and reservations about the diversity the Hippocratic writings display, 'Hippocratic medicine'. For the ambivalence just noted – preservation of health, or treatment of disease, or providing palliative care – is, in a way, characteristic of Hippocratic approaches to health and disease as a whole. Here the need for terminological clarification makes itself particularly felt, for neither the Greek θεραπεία nor its English derivative 'therapy' is specific with regard to this question about the aim(s) to be achieved. This brings us to a consideration of the terms in which the doctor's activities are referred to in the Hippocratic Corpus.

As Nadia van Brock has shown,[48] among the various words used to signify the doctor's activity – such as ἰῆσθαι ('cure'), θεραπεύειν ('treat'), μελετᾶν ('care'), ὠφελεῖν ('help, benefit'), βοηθεῖν ('remedy, assist'), μελεδαίνειν ('care'), μεταχειρίζεσθαι ('treat'), φυλάσσειν ('protect') – perhaps ἀπαλλάσσειν ('set free, release'), ὑγιάζειν ('make healthy'), and the passive ὑγιής

---

[43] See *On Regimen in Acute Diseases* 41 (2.310 L.) and 44 (2.316–18 L.).
[44] E.g. *On Diseases* 3.16 (7.150 L.): 'This also stops the pains' (τοῦτο καὶ τὰς ὀδύνας παύει).
[45] For other evidence to suggest that this was the case, see Longrigg (1999).
[46] On this see Edelstein (1967a) 303–16.
[47] See *On Ancient Medicine* 7 (1.586 L.): 'How do these two [i.e. development of a regimen in health and the use of regimen as treatment of disease] differ, except in that the latter has more different kinds and is more varied and requires more effort? But the former is the starting-point, and came before the latter (ἀρχὴ δὲ ἐκείνη ἡ πρότερον γενομένη).'
[48] N. van Brock (1961).

γίνεσθαι ('get healthy') and ὑπεκφυγγάνειν ('be released from') are the only terms that really indicate a full restoration of health;[49] and of the various translations available for these words (e.g. 'therapy', 'treatment', 'cure', 'care', 'attention', etc.), 'healing' is very often not the appropriate rendering. Accordingly, recommendations of particular modes of treatment are often expressed in terms such as συμφέρει ('it is profitable'), ἐπιτήδειόν ἐστι ('it is suitable'), ἀρήγει ('it is appropriate') and ἁρμόζει ('it is fitting').

As such, these terms and expressions provide a good illustration of the way in which the principle 'to help, or to do no harm' is interpreted in practice. We can see this principle at work particularly in the actual treatment advocated by the authors of the nosological works (*On Diseases* 1, 2, 3, *On Internal Affections*). In these works symptomatology, causal explanation and therapy of diseases are fairly consistently adopted as distinctive categories – and as such they resemble the apparently even more systematic discussion of diseases and their treatment as offered by Diocles in the work *Affection, Cause, Treatment* mentioned above. Reading through the therapeutic sections of these works, three points are particularly striking. The first is that on several occasions in *On Internal Affections* and *On Diseases* 2 and 3 a course of treatment is recommended in the full awareness of the lethal nature of the disease.[50] One of the reasons for doctors such as the author of *On Internal Affections* to adopt this attitude is clearly that they realise that it is very difficult to establish whether a particular case is hopeless or not, indeed that a certain mode of treatment may, by provoking a certain physical reaction, provide clarification on this,[51] or alternatively that by postponing treatment for too long, the disease may further exacerbate and become definitely incurable (though not necessarily fatal).[52] On the other hand, there are cases in which the doctor is advised to wait and see how the disease develops before deciding whether to treat it or not,[53] or to infer from certain symptoms whether the disease is curable or not.[54] Yet there are also several cases where the patient's chances of survival are considered to be negligibly small, but where treatment is nevertheless recommended.[55] The purpose of treatment in such cases is not always stated, but it may be, as

---

[49] An interesting collocation of the terms θεραπεύειν, ἀπαλλάσσειν, μελετᾶν and ἰῆσθαι is found in *Int. Aff.* 26 (7.234 L.).

[50] On degrees of 'mortality' see von Staden (1990) 79–80. The idea that Hippocratic doctors did not engage, or were reluctant to engage, in treatment of hopeless cases – though not without some textual support, e.g. *On the Art of Medicine* 8, *On Diseases* 2.48 – has been shown to be untenable in its generalising claims by Wittern (1979) and von Staden (1990). For a more recent discussion of this issue see also Prioreschi (1992).

[51] *Int. Aff.* 27 (7.238 L.); 41 (7.270 L.).   [52] *Int. Aff.* 26 (7. 236 L.); 47 (7. 284 L.).

[53] E.g. *On Diseases* 3.2 (7.120 L.).   [54] *Int. Aff.* 22 (7.220 L.).

[55] E.g. *On Diseases* 2.57 (7.88–90 L.); 3.1 (7.118 L.); 3.5 (7.122 L.); 3.6 (7.124 L.); 3.10 (7.130 L.); 3.11 (7.132 L.); 3.14 (7.134–6 L.); *Int. Aff.* 6 (7.182 L.); 29 (7.244 L.).

On Internal Affections 10 shows, in order to bring about the best condition or 'mode of living' (διαγωγή) of a patient who is almost certainly going to die:

> When the case is such, the patient wastes away sorrily for a year, and dies; you must treat him very actively and strengthen him ... If treated in such a way, the patient will fare best in the disease; the disease is usually mortal, and few escape it.[56]

Furthermore, in a passage from *On Diseases* 3.15 the doctor is even advised to tell the patient about the hopelessness of his case before engaging in treatment:

> If the sputum is not being cleaned out effectively, if respiration is rapid, and if expectoration is failing, announce that there is no hope of survival; unless the patient can help with the cleaning. But still treat as is appropriate for pneumonia, if the lower cavity cooperates with you.[57]

In these writings, then, treatment is recommended in virtually all cases whatever the outcome. The outcome is sometimes said to be that the patient will become healthy again;[58] but there are also several cases in which the result is left vague.[59]

A second, striking, fact is that it is often left at the doctor's discretion whether to follow a particular course of treatment, or even whether to engage in treatment at all. The tentative, by no means rigid character of Hippocratic treatment is indicated by expressions such as 'if you wish', 'if you think it is right', 'if you treat him', 'if you wish to treat him',[60] 'if you do not want to give him the drug'.[61] This is not to say that, for the Hippocratic doctors, treatment does not aim at restoring health; indeed, apart from the many cases where treatment is said to result in a recovery of health, there are several occasions where treatment is advocated not because lack of treatment would result in the patient's death but because it would cause the disease to become chronic and 'to age with' (συγκαταγηράσκειν),[62] or

---

[56] *Int. Aff.* 10 (7.190 L.): οὗτος ὁκόταν οὕτω ἔχει, ἐνιαυτῷ φθειρόμενος φαύλως θνῄσκει· μελετᾶν δὲ χρὴ ὡς μάλιστα καὶ ἀνακομίζειν ... οὗτος οὕτω μελετώμενος ῥήιστ' ἂν διάγοι ἐν τῷ νοσήματι. ἡ δὲ νοῦσος θανασίμη, καὶ παῦροι διαφυγγάνουσι (tr. Potter (1998) vol. VI, 105). See also *Int.* 27 (7.238 L.): τῆς δ' ὀδύνης ἕνεκα, and von Staden (1990) 108 (about *On Diseases* 1.6): 'easing the patient's condition or prolonging his or her life'; also *Int. Aff.* 12 (7.196 L.): ταῦτα ἢν ποιέῃ ῥήιον οἴσει τὴν νοῦσον (although this case is not hopeless).
[57] 7.140 L. (tr. Potter (1988) vol. VI, 37). On verbal intervention see von Staden (1990) 109–11.
[58] E.g. *Int. Aff.* 9 (7.188 L.); 12 (7.198 L.); 21 (7. 220 L.).
[59] E.g. *On Diseases* 2.15 (7.28 L.); 2.29 (7.46 L.).
[60] *On Diseases* 3.3 (7.122 L.); 3.7 (7.126 L.); 3.13 (7.134 L.); 3.17 (7.156 L.).
[61] *Int. Aff.* 10 (7.192 L.): ἢν δὲ μὴ βούλῃ δοῦναι τὸ φάρμακον.
[62] E.g. *On Diseases* 2.73 (7.112 L.).

'to die with' (συναποθνήσκειν),⁶³ the patient – which reminds one of what is sometimes said about incurable but non-fatal conditions (such as chronic fatigue syndrome): 'It is not that you die *of* it, you die *with* it.' It is clear that Hippocratic doctors regarded this as something highly undesirable: disease is something to be resisted and to be fought against, not something to resign onseself to.⁶⁴ But this has to be done in the awareness of the limitations of the art.⁶⁵

Thirdly, as a passage in *On Internal Affections* indicates, treatment does not stop after recovery: 'If the patient is not cared for after he has recovered, and does not keep a watch over himself, in many the disease has returned and killed them.'⁶⁶ The body needs to be looked after not only when it is healthy or when it is sick, but also when it has turned from sickness to health.

This comprehensive approach to therapeutics is continued and further developed by Diocles, whose dietetic fragments, in their meticulous attention to even the slightest detail, display an impressive degree of sophistication – some might say decadence.⁶⁷ Yet, as we have seen, in Diocles' work dietetics and therapeutics seem to constitute two distinct areas of the overarching category 'medicine'. This is further reflected in a fragment of Diocles' contemporary Mnesitheus of Athens, who divided medicine into two branches, the preservation of health and the dispelling of disease.⁶⁸ These classifications may be related to an increasing sense of unease in Greek society

---

⁶³ *Int. Aff.* 5 (7.180 L.); 46 (7.280 L.).
⁶⁴ *Epidemics* 1.11 (2.636 L.): ὑπεναντιοῦσθαι τῷ νοσήματι τὸν νοσέοντα μετὰ τοῦ ἰητροῦ.
⁶⁵ See *On the Art of Medicine* 8 (cf. Arist. *Rh.* 1355 b 12: 'nor is it the purpose of medicine to make a patient healthy, rather it is to promote this only in so far as is possible; for even those who are incapable of recovery can nevertheless be treated' (οὐδὲ γὰρ ἰατρικῆς [sc. τέλος] τὸ ὑγιᾶ ποιῆσαι, ἀλλὰ μέχρι οὗ ἐνδέχεται, μέχρι τούτου προαγαγεῖν· ἔστι γὰρ καὶ τοὺς ἀδυνάτους μεταλαβεῖν ὑγιείας ὅμως θεραπεῦσαι).
⁶⁶ *Int. Aff.* 1 (7.172 L.): ἢν δὲ μὴ θεραπεύηται ὑγιὴς γενόμενος καὶ ἢν μὴ ἐν φυλακῇ ἔχῃ ἑωυτόν, τοῖς πολλοῖς ὑποτροπάσασα, ἡ νοῦσος ἀπώλεσεν. Cf. *On Ancient Medicine* 14 (1.600 L.): 'and it is these things [i.e. food and drink] on which life completely depends, both for the healthy person and for the one that recovers from illness and for the sick person' (καὶ διὰ τούτων πᾶς ὁ βίος καὶ ὑγιαίνοντι καὶ ἐκ νούσου ἀναστρεφομένῳ καὶ κάμνοντι); *On Regimen* 2.76 (6.620 L.): 'and if the patient recovers in a month, one should subsequently treat him with what is proper; but if some (of the disease) remains, one should continue the treatment' (καὶ ἢν μὲν ἐν μηνὶ καθιστῆται, θεραπεύεσθω τὸ λοιπὸν τοῖσι προσήκουσιν· ἢν δέ τι ὑπόλοιπον ᾖ, χρήσθω τῇ θεραπείῃ).
⁶⁷ See Diocles 'Regimen in Health' in fr. 182, and the discussion by Edelstein (1967a) 303–16.
⁶⁸ Mnesitheus, fr. 11 Bertier: 'Mnesitheus said that the doctor either preserves health for those who are healthy or provides treatment of disease to those who are sick' (ἔλεγε τοίνυν ὁ Μνησίθεος ὅτι ὁ ἰατρὸς ἢ τοῖς ὑγιαίνουσι φυλάττει τὴν ὑγείαν, ἢ τοῖς νοσήσασι θεραπεύει τὰς νούσους). See also the Galenic *Definitiones medicae* 9 (19.351 K.): 'Medicine is the art that treats healthy people by regimen and sick people by therapeutics' (ἰατρικὴ ἐστι τέχνη διαιτητικὴ ὑγιαινόντων καὶ θεραπευτικὴ νοσούντων).

with regard to the claims of dietetics and indeed medicine as a whole in the fourth century – and, perhaps, with regard to the competence of the practitioners of dietetics. For the Hippocratic and Dioclean conception of medical care, combined with a growing awareness of the need for prevention of disease by means of a healthy lifestyle, seems to have led to a rapid expansion of the territory for which Greek physicians claimed expertise. Such a 'medicalisation' of daily life was strengthened by the intellectual cachet and rhetorical elegance of medicine which Celsus refers to, and to which the extant fragments of Diocles' works certainly testify; but it is easy to see how it may have met with resistance – an unease which is reflected, as far as the application of dietetic principles to the treatment of diseases is concerned, by Plato's well-known attack on dietetics in the *Republic*.[69]

In the light of such unease and doubts about the qualifications and competence of the practitioners of medical care, it is understandable that doctors started to specialise. This is illustrated by the fragment of Diocles' contemporary Mnesitheus just quoted, and also by a fragment of Erasistratus,[70] in which a distinction between medicine (ἰατρική) and the care for health (τὰ ὑγιεινά) is connected with a distinction between two different practitioners: the 'healer' (ἰατρός) and the 'health specialist' (ὑγιεινός). It is also illustrated five centuries later by Galen's treatise *Thrasybulus*, which deals with the question 'Whether the care for the healthy body belongs to medicine or to gymnastics'. But this specialisation, or indeed compartmentalisation, of medical care meant that the unity of therapeutics which the Hippocratic doctors had insisted on, was gradually lost: the distance between patient and doctor steadily increased – a development that has continued up to the present day, and which clearly goes against what I would still call the spirit of Hippocratic medicine.

[69] 403 e ff., on which see Wöhrle (1990) 122–4.
[70] Fr. 156 Garofalo.

CHAPTER 4

The heart, the brain, the blood and the pneuma: Hippocrates, Diocles and Aristotle on the location of cognitive processes

1 THE DEBATE IN ANTIQUITY ON THE LOCATION OF THE MIND: ORIGIN, DEVELOPMENT AND MISREPRESENTATION

In one of the first chapters of his systematic account of the treatment of acute and chronic diseases, the Latin medical author Caelius Aurelianus (fifth century CE) discusses *phrenitis*, a psychosomatic disorder with symptoms including acute fever, mental confusion, a weak and fast pulse and various forms of abnormal behaviour such as the picking of threads out of clothing.[1] Caelius Aurelianus, himself belonging to the medical school called the Methodists,[2] begins his argument, as usual, with a survey of the views on the nature and origin of this disease held by doctors belonging to other schools of thought, in particular their views on the question of which part of the body is affected by the disease. His main reason for doing so is to show the contrast between his own and only correct treatment of the disease and the general confusion among other doctors:

What part [of the body] is affected in phrenitis? This question has been raised particularly by leaders of other sects so that they may apply their treatments according to the different parts affected and prepare local remedies for the places in question... Now some say that the brain is affected, others its fundus or base, which we may translate *sessio* ['seat'], others its membranes, others both the brain and its membranes, others the heart, others the apex of the heart, others the membrane which incloses the heart, others the artery which the Greeks call *aorte*, others the thick vein (Greek *phleps pacheia*), others the diaphragm. But why continue in this way when we can easily clarify the matter by stating what these writers really had in mind? For in every case they hold that the part affected in phrenitis

---

This chapter was first published in Dutch in *Gewina* 18 (1995) 214–29.
[1] For the problem of identifying 'phrenitis' see Potter (1980) 110; Pigeaud (1981a) 72.
[2] For an outline of the Methodists' medical views see Edelstein (1967b); Pigeaud (1991); Gourevitch (1991); Pigeaud (1993) 565–99. The epistemological principles of the Methodists are discussed by Frede (1983) and by Lloyd (1983) 182–200. [On Caelius' version of Methodism see also ch. 11 below.]

is that in which they suspect the ruling part of the soul to be situated... Now we hold that in phrenitis there is a general affection of the whole body, for the whole body is shaken by fever. And fever is one of the signs that make up the general indication of phrenitis, and for that reason we treat the whole body. We do hold, however, that the head is more particularly affected, as the antecedent symptoms indicate, e.g., its heaviness, tension, and pain, head noises, ringing in the ears, dryness, and impairment of the senses... eyelids stiff, eyes bloodshot and bulging out, cheeks red, veins distended, face puffed up and full, and tongue rough. But there are those who argue as follows: 'We determine the part affected on the basis of the theory of nature (Greek *phusiologia*), for we know in advance that the ruling part of the soul is located in the head, and conclude that that must be the source of mental derangement.' Our answer to them is that, to begin with, the place of this ruling part is uncertain. But the number and variety of symptoms occurring in the head have shown us that this organ is more particularly affected than the rest of the body.[3]

In this fragment Caelius Aurelianus refers to a great variety of views on where to locate the affection of *phrenitis* in classical antiquity, which can be traced back to the fifth century BCE. This discussion was to a certain extent determined by a lack of clarity about the evidential value of the etymological relation between the name of the disease and the Greek word *phrenes*, which had been used since Homer to indicate the midriff (later, the common term for this became diaphragm, as used here by Caelius). Some advocates of the location in the diaphragm appealed to this etymology,[4] others were of the opinion that the name of the disease should not be related to any part of the body (be it affected or not), but to the faculty that was affected (*phronein, phronēsis*, standard terms in Greek for what we would call 'intelligence' or 'consciousness').[5] Others thought that the name given to a disease was arbitrary and did not offer any indication of its location.

Another significant fact is that Caelius Aurelianus criticises his predecessors' strong desire to locate the condition in one particular place in the body, and their presupposition that this place should also be the seat of the mind (the faculty affected in the case of *phrenitis*).[6] Following typically Methodist principles, Caelius is of the opinion that the disease cannot be located in

---

[3] Caelius Aurelianus, *On Acute Affections* 1.8.53–6, tr. Drabkin (1950).
[4] For this use of the term *phrenitis* on the basis of the affected part (*apo topou*) see Diocles, fr. 72 (all references to Diocles are to van der Eijk (2000a)); cf. Anonymus Londiniensis IV 13–15 (ed. Diels (1893a)); [Hippocrates], *On the Sacred Disease* 17 (6.394–6 L.); see Grensemann (1968c).
[5] Cf. the view of the medical writer Erasistratus (third century BCE), fr. 176 (ed. Garofalo (1988)).
[6] An example of a medical writer to whom this presupposition does not apply is Diocles of Carystus: according to the so-called Anonymus Parisinus (see Diocles, fr. 72 vdE), Diocles assumed that the disease affects the diaphragm but that the mind is seated in the heart. The psychological disorders arise as a result of *sumpatheia*, i.e. because the heart 'also suffers' from the fact that the diaphragm is heated.

any particular place, but that the entire body is ill and therefore the entire body requires treatment. Another characteristic of the Methodists is that speculations on the location of the mind are rejected for being pointless, as it is impossible to reach conclusions on the matter on empirical grounds, and the doctor should abstain from expressing any opinions ('first of all it is still uncertain which part of the body is the leading part'). This attitude is inspired by the close connection between the epistemological views of the Methodists and those of the philosophical school of the Sceptics, who on principle refuse to express opinions on any non-perceptible matters. In addition, the Methodists consider such questions irrelevant to therapeutic practice, which they regard as the focus of medical science.

Whether Caelius Aurelianus does justice to all his medical predecessors by presenting matters as he does is very much the question. Recent research into the principles and methods of doxography (the description of the *doxai*, the characteristic doctrines of authorities in a certain subject) has revealed that the question 'What is the leading principle in man and where is it located?' more or less assumed a life of its own in late antiquity, separate from the scientific context from which it originated. It became a favourite subject for practising argumentation techniques (comparable to questions such as 'Is an embryo a living being?'),[7] whereby contrasting views were taken in an artificial debate (sometimes even views that, although theoretically possible, have, as far as we know, never actually been supported), which were subsequently attributed to authorities in the field, and which served as exercise material for finding and using arguments both for and against. Such 'dialectic' staging of a debate bears little relation to a historically faithful rendition of a debate that actually took place in the past.

It is most probable that Caelius Aurelianus' summary of views as quoted above is part of such a doxographical tradition, and therefore highly schematised. In his presentation, the views of those to whom he refers – without mentioning their names[8] – imply a number of presuppositions regarding empirical evidence and theoretical concepts in respect of which it is questionable whether the authorities concerned actually held them. A question like 'What is the leading principle of the soul and where is it located?' presupposes that there is such a thing as a leading 'part' or principle in the soul and that it can be located somewhere. The debate to which Caelius

---

[7] On this see Mansfeld (1990), and for embryology Tieleman (1991).
[8] The doctors and philosophers to whom Caelius Aurelianus refers can be identified by studying other doxographic authors (for this purpose see the discussion by Mansfeld mentioned in n. 7). Further down in the same book Caelius Aurelianus discusses the therapeutic views on *phrenitis* held by Diocles, Erasistratus, Asclepiades, Themison and Heraclides.

Aurelianus is referring concerns the so-called *hēgemonikon* or *regale*. This term is probably of Stoic origin (*c.* 300 BCE) and refers to the 'leading' principle in the soul (commonly indicated as *nous* or *intellectus*, which is usually translated as 'thought' or 'intellect'). The use of this term implies the possibility of grading various psychic parts or faculties, some of which are subordinate to others, and presupposes an anatomical and physiological relationship underlying such a hierarchy. On the one hand such a presentation presupposes a rather elaborate psychological theory, free from the difficulties and obscurities that, for instance, Aristotle points out when he discusses the psychological views of his predecessors in the first book of his *On the Soul* (*De anima*). It will be clear that a presentation such as that by Caelius Aurelianus, in which all doctors and philosophers are called to the fore to express their views on the matter, puts opinions in their mouths that many of them (probably) never phrased in these terms. On the other hand, such a presentation does not do justice to thinkers such as Aristotle and some authors of the Hippocratic Corpus, as it often obscures the subtle differences in meaning between the various terms used for psychic faculties by these thinkers. We will see below that as early as the fifth and fourth centuries BCE, doctors and philosophers carefully differentiated between cognitive faculties such as 'practical', 'theoretical', and 'productive thinking'; 'insight'; 'understanding'; 'opinion'; and 'judgement'.[9] Indeed, the possibility of location was a matter of dispute too. Thus Aristotle was credited in late antiquity with the view that 'the soul', or at least its leading principle (the *archē*), is seated in the heart. We will see that this is a misrepresentation of Aristotle's views, which, strictly speaking, leave no room for location of the highest psychic faculty, the *nous*. Similarly, the author of the Hippocratic work *On Regimen* (at the start of the fourth century BCE) presupposes a view of the soul that does not specify where exactly it is located in the body; he even appears to assume that the location may vary. In short, this doxographic distortion attributes to doctors and philosophers answers to questions which some of them would not even be able or willing to answer as a matter of principle.

Finally, Caelius Aurelianus upholds a long tradition of contempt for the so-called *phusiologia*. This tradition dates back to the author of the Hippocratic writing *On Ancient Medicine* (*c.* 400 BCE). He was opposed to some of his colleagues' tendency to build their medical practice on general and theoretical principles or 'postulates' (*hupotheseis*) derived from

---

[9] Aristotle lists a range of terms for cognitive faculties (*nous, phronēsis, epistēmē, sophia, gnōmē, sunesis, doxa, hupolēpsis*) in book 6 of the *Nicomachean Ethics*; however, it remains uncertain to what extent the subtle differences in meaning that Aristotle ascribes to these terms are representative for Greek language in general.

natural philosophy, such as the so-called four primary qualities hot, cold, dry and wet. By contrast, he adopted a predominantly empirical approach to medicine, which in his view was tantamount to dietetics, the theory of healthy living. His approach was based on insights into the wholesome effects of food, insights that had been passed down from generation to generation and refined by experimentation. He even went so far as to claim that in reality physics does not form the basis for medicine, but medicine for physics.

The question of to what extent a doctor should be concerned with, or even build on, principles derived from physics (or metaphysics) remained a matter of dispute throughout antiquity. What made the problem even more urgent was that in many areas of controversy, such as that on the location of the mind, it remained unclear to what extent these could be resolved on empirical grounds. The doctor's desire to build views concerning the correct diagnosis and treatment of psychosomatic disorders such as *mania*, epilepsy, lethargy, *melancholia* and *phrenitis* on a presupposition about the location of the psychic faculties affected, which could not be proved empirically, differed according to his willingness to accept such principles, which were sometimes complimentarily, sometimes condescendingly labelled 'philosophical'.[10] This group of doctors with a profoundly philosophical interest included, for instance, Diocles of Carystus (fourth century BCE) and the author of the Hippocratic work *On the Sacred Disease* (end fifth century BCE). They corresponded to an ideal proclaimed first by Aristotle and later by Galen, namely that of the 'civilised' or 'distinguished' physician, who is both a competent doctor and a philosopher skilled in physics, logic, and rhetoric.[11] Caelius Aurelianus' derogatory remark shows that this ideal was by no means beyond dispute. Yet in this dispute, too, the variety of views on the matter was much wider than his general characterisation suggests. It is therefore highly likely that Caelius Aurelianus' presentation intends to exaggerate the differences in opinion between the doctors mentioned, in order to make his own view stand out more clearly and simply against the background of confusion generated by others.

These introductory observations may suffice to provide an outline of the debate on the seat of the mind, which was the subject of fierce dispute

---

[10] The first time the word *philosophia* is attested in Greek literature is in ch. 20 of the Hippocratic writing *On Ancient Medicine* (1.620 L.). The word is used in a clearly negative sense, to describe the practice of scrounging from physics, which is rejected by the author. The name Empedocles is mentioned in this context.

[11] For this Aristotelian ideal see below, ch. 6, pp. 193–7. Galen wrote a separate treatise entitled and devoted to the proposition that *The Best Physician is also a Philosopher* (i.e. skilled in logic, physics, and ethics; see 1.53–63 K.).

throughout classical antiquity (and remained so until the nineteenth century), and to which no definitive answer was found. In so far as antiquity is concerned, there were at least three causes for this: the reasons for asking the question (and the desire to answer it) differed depending on whether one's purposes were medical, philosophical or purely rhetorical; the status of the arguments for or against a certain answer (such as the evidential value of medical experiments) was subject to fluctuation; and the question itself posed numerous other problems related to the (to this day) disputed area of philosophical psychology or 'philosophy of the mind', such as the question of the relationship between body and soul, or of the difference between the various 'psychic' faculties, and so on. When following the debate from its inception until late antiquity, one gets the impression that the differences manifest themselves precisely in these three areas. Whereas the doctors of the Hippocratic Corpus were mainly interested in the question of the location of the mind in so far as they felt a need for a treatment of psychological disorders based on a theory of nature, later the situation changed and medical-physiological data were no more than one of the possible (but by no means decisive) factors to build arguments for one of the positions taken on.

In the section below I will pay particular attention to the early phase of the debate (fifth and fourth centuries BCE), concentrating on the main authors of the Hippocratic Corpus, Aristotle and Diocles, with brief references to Plato.

2 GREEK DOCTORS AND PHILOSOPHERS OF THE FIFTH AND FOURTH CENTURIES BCE

It can be inferred from remarks made by Plato, Aristotle and in the Hippocratic Corpus[12] that as early as the fifth century BCE doctors and natural philosophers disagreed on the question which bodily factors (organs, tissues or substances) played the most important part in performing faculties we would call 'psychic' or 'mental'. These include thinking, perception, feeling, remembering, and so on. Secondary literature on this issue usually distinguishes between the encephalocentric, cardiocentric and haematocentric view on the seat of the mind.[13] The encephalocentric view was allegedly

---

[12] Plato, *Phaedo* 96 b; Aristotle, *Metaph.* 1013 a 4ff. and 1035 b 25ff.; [Hippocrates], *On the Sacred Disease* 17 (6.392 L.).

[13] See, among others, Manuli and Vegetti (1977). A selection from the extensive range of literature on this subject: Bidez and Leboucq (1944); Byl (1968); Di Benedetto (1986) 35–69; Duminil (1983); Gundert (2000); Hankinson (1991b); Harris (1973); Manuli (1977); Pigeaud (1981b) 72; Pigeaud (1980); Pigeaud (1987); Revesz (1917); Rüsche (1930); B. Simon (1978); P. N. Singer (1992).

taken by the fifth-century medical writer Alcmaeon of Croton (South Italy), who was thought to be the first to discover the existence of the optic nerve, by the author of the Hippocratic work *On the Sacred Disease*, and by Plato (in the *Timaeus*). The cardiocentric view was represented in the Hippocratic writings *On Diseases* 2 (fifth century BCE), *On the Heart* (end of the fourth/start of the third century BCE) and by Aristotle, Diocles of Carystus and Praxagoras of Cos (fourth century BCE). The haematocentric view was taken by Empedocles and the authors of the Hippocratic writings *On Diseases* 1 and *On Breaths* (all fifth century BCE). Although this division may be largely appropriate in terms of the period concerned, it is already too much a product of the schematisation mentioned above, which became characteristic of the debate in later doxography. Strictly speaking, only the authors of *On the Sacred Disease* and *On the Heart* express an opinion on the *location* of what they consider the highest psychic faculty, the former choosing the brain, the latter the heart. Apart from this, the division into three areas presents the matter in too static a way: most of the authors mentioned appear to regard psychic activities mainly as *processes*, in which some parts of the body are more involved than others, but which are in principle based on the interaction between a number of anatomical and physiological factors.

It would be better to ask in which terms ancient doctors from the fifth and fourth centuries BCE thought about these matters, and which types of arguments they used to substantiate their views. The following categories can be discerned:

faculties (thought, perception, feeling, etc.)
parts of the body (heart, brain, diaphragm, etc.)
substances (blood, air, phlegm, etc.)
processes (decay, constipation, etc.)
relations/proportions (balance, mixture, etc.)

In the discussions which doctors devote to the subject, they employ terms that on the one hand refer to a certain part of the body or otherwise anatomical-physiological material, and on the other hand to an activity or faculty exercised or enabled by it: the part of the body 'contributes to', is 'the instrument of' or 'the material substrate of' a 'faculty' or 'ability'. It is not always immediately obvious to what extent the medical authors made a distinction between 'mental' processes as such and physiological processes.[14] Most authors of the Hippocratic Corpus appear to assume a kind of continuum between body and mind: in lists of symptoms, psychological phenomena are mentioned among purely physical ones without any

---

[14] See the discussion in Singer (1992) 131–43.

categorical difference, and the cause for mental disorders is virtually always sought in bodily factors.

Mental faculties are given a more independent role in the Hippocratic writing *On the Sacred Disease*, in which the function of the brain is characterised as 'interpreting' (*hermēneus*) what is derived from the air outside. This is in many respects a key text, not least because of the author's polemic stance to rival views:

> For these reasons I believe that the brain is the most powerful part in a human being. So long as it is healthy, it is the interpreter of what comes to the body from the air. Consciousness is provided by the air. The eyes, ears, tongue, hands and feet carry out what the brain knows, for throughout the body there is a degree of consciousness proportionate to the amount of air which it receives. As far as understanding is concerned, the brain is also the part that transmits this, for when a man draws in a breath it first arrives at the brain, and from there it is distributed over the rest of the body, having left behind in the brain its best portion and whatever contains consciousness and thought. For if the air went first to the body and subsequently to the brain, the power of discerning thinking would be left to the flesh and to the blood vessels; it would reach the brain in a hot and no longer pure state but mixed with moisture from the flesh and from the blood so that it would no longer be accurate. I therefore state that the brain is the interpreter of consciousness.
>
> The diaphragm (*phrenes*), however, does not have the right name, but it has got this by chance and through convention. I do not know in virtue of what the diaphragm can think and have consciousness (*phronein*), except that if a man suddenly feels pleasure or pain, the diaphragm leaps up and causes throbbing, because it is thin and under greater tension than any other part of the body, and it has no cavity into which it might receive anything good or bad that comes upon it, but because of the weakness of its structure it is subject to disturbance by either of these forces, since it does not perceive faster than any other part of the body. Rather, it has its name and reputation for no good reason, just as parts of the heart are called auricles though they make no contribution to hearing.
>
> Some say that we owe our consciousness to our hearts and that it is the heart which suffers pain and feels anxiety. But this is not the case; rather, it is torn just like the diaphragm, and even more than that for the same reasons: for blood vessels from all parts of the body run to the heart, and it encapsulates these, so that it can feel if any pain or tension occurs in a human being. Moreover, it is necessary for the body to shudder and to contract when it feels pain, and when it is overwhelmed by joy it experiences the same. This is why the heart and the diaphragm are particularly sensitive. Yet neither of these parts has any share in consciousness; rather, it is the brain which is responsible for all these. (16–17 [6.390–4 L.])[15]

---

[15] Translation Jones in Jones and Withington (1923–31) vol. 1, modified; section divisions according to Grensemann.

This passage is part of a rather complicated explanation of epilepsy (for details on this see the next paragraph). The brain plays a pivotal role in this explanation as it is the point from where bodily and psychic faculties are co-ordinated, but also because it is particularly sensitive to harmful influences from the environment, such as climate and season ('so long as it is healthy'). These influences can therefore be additional factors that contribute to the course the disease takes. The author emphasises this crucial role of the brain as part of his polemic against two rival factions which consider the diaphragm or the heart to be the central organ that is the source of consciousness. He dismisses the etymological argument of the first faction (*phrenes – phronēsis*) as invalid, and accommodates the empirical fact that both factions put forward – the heart's leaping in case of sudden gladness or sadness – into his own theory, which is also based on empirical observations (namely the delicacy of the diaphragm and the veins going to the heart). In a previous chapter he employed an empirical argument to support his conviction that the disease is caused by an accumulation of phlegm in or around the brain. He claimed that if one were to open the skull of a goat that died as a result of an epileptic fit, one would find a large amount of fluid (phlegm) around the brain.[16]

It is striking that a distinction is made here between 'consciousness' (*phronēsis*) and 'understanding' (*sunesis*): the latter is apparently related to the 'discerning thinking' (*diagnōsis*) which is mentioned later in the text, and which requires a certain degree of purity and precision that is adversely affected by contact with organs and tissues. In this context *phronēsis* clearly means more than 'thinking' or 'intelligence', as the word is commonly translated. It means 'having one's senses together' and refers to a universal force by which a living being can focus on its surroundings and can undertake activities; it also implies perception and movement.[17] *Phronēsis* can be found throughout the body, whereas 'understanding' is restricted to the brain. Another thing that is striking is that the author is of the opinion that the brain is also the source of feeling – although he admits that the heart and diaphragm take part in this as well.

A text in which mental phenomena are even more clearly classified as a separate category is the Hippocratic writing *On Regimen*.[18] The author, a particularly 'philosophically' inspired mind, presents *psuchē* (sometimes

---

[16] 11.3–5 (6.382 L.). As to the question whether this indeed concerns an experiment in the modern sense of the word, see Lloyd (1979) 23–4.
[17] See Hüffmeier (1961) 58. See too H. W. Miller (1948) 168–83.
[18] Edition with a translation and commentary by Joly and Byl (1984). There is a dispute about the date of this work: most scholars date it to the beginning of the fourth century BCE, but some argue in favour of a much later date (second half of the fourth century BCE).

also referred to as *dianoia*) as a distinct entity, separate from the body (*sōma*). This distinction manifests itself in particular during sleep (4.86–7). However, this does not imply that the soul is immaterial. The soul consists of water and fire (the elements which, according to this author, have the greatest influence on the constitution of the human body), which stand in a certain proportion to each other. Fluctuations in this proportion result in differences between individual people's cognitive skills, such as acuteness, a good memory, precision of the senses and proneness to certain emotions (1.35). When the balance between these two elements is seriously disturbed, it will give rise to psychological disorders, but these can be cured by changing eating and drinking habits and adopting a certain lifestyle (1.36). According to this author, the soul is therefore a material entity, yet it does not have a fixed location: it moves through the body via 'passages' (*poroi*). The condition of these passages (for instance their width or narrowness) is a further influential factor in someone's mental functioning. In the state of wakefulness, the soul distributes itself over the entire body and carries out certain tasks 'for the benefit of the body', including hearing, seeing, touching and movement. During sleep, or rather 'when the body is asleep', the soul remains awake and withdraws in its own 'home' (*oikos*), where it carries out the activities of the body independently. These include seeing, hearing, walking, touching, grieving, thinking: they are called *enhupnia* or 'dreams'. Yet the author does not venture an opinion on the location of the soul and its 'home'.

A presentation like this shows how inadequate terms like 'materialism' and 'dualism' are to describe ancient theories on body and mind. The author of *On Regimen* may be called a materialist to the extent that he holds an entirely material view on the soul; yet at the same time he assumes two separate entities which may normally co-operate and mutually influence each other, yet one of them (the 'soul') can also function independently, as, for instance, in sleep.[19]

The greatest refinement in the definition of the *status* of mental phenomena can be found in Aristotle, although his comments on the topic, too, show a certain amount of fluctuation. He expresses the view that the 'soul' is not a separate entity, which might exist independently of the body: 'soul' to Aristotle is 'the form of the body', that which causes a body to live, which gives it structure and enables it to exercise its faculties.[20] Yet this

[19] For the psychology of *On Regimen* see Palm (1933) 44–7; Joly and Byl (1984) 296–7; Hankinson (1991b) 200–6; Jouanna (1966) xv–xviii; Cambiano (1980) 87–96; Van Lieshout (1980) 100–3.

[20] For this interpretation of Aristotle's understanding of the soul see Sorabji (1974) 63–89 and Kahn (1966) 43–81, both reprinted in Barnes, Schofield and Sorabji (1979) 42–64 and 1–31; van der Eijk (2000b). For other attempts to reformulate Aristotle's view on the mind–body debate in modern terms see the volume by Nussbaum and Rorty (1992), with comprehensive bibliography.

does not prevent him from repeatedly speaking of 'experiences typical to the soul', activities a human being carries out 'with his soul', or perceptions which 'penetrate the soul'. According to Aristotle, the functioning of the dual entity that body and soul constitute is governed by a large number of organs and material factors. The heart is assigned the role of 'beginning' or 'origin' (*archē*), both as a source of essential bodily heat (required among other things for the digestion of food) and as the seat of the central sense organ, which is connected with the limbs and the separate sense organs and co-ordinates the data it receives from them.[21] Furthermore, in exercising this co-ordinating task the heart is supported by the blood (as a medium for transporting sensory information) and air (*pneuma*, for the transmission of motor signals). Their role is important, yet not fully defined.[22] The size of the heart, which differs in each species of animal, has an influence on certain character traits and on susceptibility to certain emotions;[23] the condition of the blood (pure, turbid, cold, hot) influences the quality and speed of sense perception.[24] The brain is not involved in all this: it has no cognitive faculties and serves only as a chilling element in the body, for tempering the heat that radiates from the heart.[25]

An even more elaborate physiological theory is presented by Diocles of Carystus (fourth century BCE). He assumes interaction between the heart (to him the real seat of the mind), the brain (which plays a pivotal role in sense perception) and the so-called 'psychic *pneuma*', a delicate substance that is responsible for transmitting sensory and motor signals.[26]

It is clear, then, that many medical authors of the fifth and fourth centuries BCE assume a cognitive centre somewhere in the body from where abilities such as perception and movement are 'transported' or 'transferred' to peripheral organs. Organs for perception, limbs and other parts of the body are assumed to be connected to each other and to a centre via certain 'passages' (*poroi, phlebes, neura*).[27] Through these passages air or blood are conducted; an accumulation of certain bodily fluids (such as phlegm or bile) can cause the passages to get blocked. The assumption of the existence of this network of passages and the ideas about their course and ramifications are highly speculative and hardly based on what we would

---

[21] *On Youth and Old Age* (*De iuventute et senectute, De iuv.*) 468 b 32ff.
[22] There is much debate on the question whether it is the blood or *pneuma* which, according to Aristotle, carries sensory information in the body. A summary and standpoint can be found in van der Eijk (1994) 81–7.
[23] *Part. an.* 667 a 10–20.   [24] *Part. an.* 656 b 5; 648 a 2ff.; 650 b 19ff.
[25] *Part. an.* 2.7.   [26] Diocles, frs. 78 and 80 vdE.
[27] In this respect it should be noted that nerves were not discovered until after Aristotle, in third-century Alexandria.

call focused anatomical research.[28] More elaborate views on the network of cognitive faculties in the body are only rarely based on empirical observations, as in the case with the above-mentioned Alcmaeon, who is believed to have arrived at an encephalocentric view on the mind on the basis of the connection between the eyes and the brain. Yet the fact that this observation was known both to the author of the Hippocratic work *On Fleshes* and to Aristotle, who nevertheless do not attribute any significant role in cognition to the brain, proves that it might equally give rise to other interpretations.

The authors mentioned do in fact employ rather sophisticated terminology for what we would call psychological, mental or spiritual faculties, but they assume a close connection between these faculties and anatomical and physiological factors. When speaking about exercising these faculties, they virtually always do so in terms of certain substances (such as blood, air or water) or qualities (hot, cold, dry, wet) and of processes such as flowing and distributing or, in case the psychic faculties have been disturbed, of stagnation, constipation, blockage, and so on. Another recurring element is the emphasis on balance (*isonomia, summetria, eukrasia*) and on the risk of an excess or shortage of a certain substance or quality.

An exception to this rule is Aristotle's idea that the highest cognitive faculty, thought, is not bound to a physical substrate. It is a kind of epiphenomenon that, although it is unable to function without sense perception (and therefore without physiological processes), cannot be located in a particular place of the body.[29] For this reason it is, strictly speaking, not correct to attribute a cardiocentric view on the mind to Aristotle, as has frequently been done both in antiquity and in modern literature.[30] The only text in which the mind is explicitly located in the heart is in the Hippocratic work *On the Heart*, which offers a remarkably detailed description of the anatomy of the heart. The author of this presumably post-Aristotelian writing claims that *gnōmē* ('mind', 'insight') has its seat in the left ventricle of the heart, from where it issues its decrees about 'the other (part of the) soul' (*allē psuchē*), which is situated in the rest of the body. To prove his stance, the author argues that if autopsy were carried out on a body of a living being that had just been killed, the aorta would still contain blood, but the left

---

[28] See Lloyd (1979) 146–9; for views on the vascular system see the studies mentioned in Harris (1973) and Duminil (1983).

[29] *De an.* 429 a 23–5, 27–8. As stated above, the heart is given a leading role in co-ordinating perception, movement and nutrition (see *Part. an.* 3.4 and *De iuv.* 3–4).

[30] For instance by Duminil (1983) 310; on the absence of statements by Aristotle on the location of the mind see, e.g., Mansfeld (1990) 3212–16. For the problems raised by Aristotle's view see Barnes (1971–2) 110–12, reprinted in Barnes, Schofield and Sorabji, vol. IV (1979) 39–40.

ventricle would not;[31] this maintains contact with the blood by means of a process of 'evaporation' and 'radiation'.

3 THREE APPROACHES TO EPILEPSY

I will conclude by discussing an example of the way in which various presuppositions about body and mind and about the location of the mind played a part in the medical debate on the disease of epilepsy. As we have seen before, the medical authors of the period we are discussing do not consider the question of the seat of the mind an isolated issue, but a matter that becomes relevant when treating diseases which, although they have a somatic cause like other diseases, also manifest themselves in psychic disorders. Of the four classic psychosomatic diseases, *mania* (a chronic disorder), *phrenitis*, *melancholia* and epilepsy, epilepsy was by far the most dreaded. It was also known as 'the big disease' or 'the sacred disease'; possession by the gods seemed the obvious explanation, but at the same time the physical aspects of the disease were so prominent that there could be no doubt as to its pathological status (as opposed to *mania* and *melancholia*, which were considered to manifest themselves in positive forms as well).[32]

The author of the Hippocratic writing *On the Sacred Disease* fiercely opposes the view that epilepsy is sent by the gods and can only be cured by applying magic (incantations, rituals involving blood, etc.) [see chapter 1 in this volume]. After a long philippic against those adhering to this view he expounds his own theory. Epilepsy is the result of an accumulation of phlegm (*phlegma*) in the passages that divide themselves from the brain throughout the body and enable the distribution of the vital *pneuma* (this air is indispensable for the functioning of the various organs). This accumulation is a result of insufficient prenatal or postnatal 'purification' (*katharsis*) of phlegm in the brain – according to the author this is a hereditary phenomenon. This obstruction can occur in different places in the body and, accordingly, manifest itself in different symptoms. Near the heart, it will result in palpitations and asthmatic complaints; in the abdomen, in diarrhoea; in the 'veins', in foaming at the mouth, grinding of teeth, clenched hands, rolling eyes, disorders in consciousness, and a lack of bowel control. This way the author explains the various symptoms that can present themselves during epileptic fits and which he describes in considerable detail in chapter 7 of the treatise.

---

[31] On this experiment see Harris (1973) 93ff.
[32] The classical, still very useful monograph on the history of epilepsy is Temkin (1971). Another useful book is Stol (1993). See also the discussion in ch. 1 above.

The structure of the explanation is clear: the disease is caused by a blockage of the passages which tentacle out from a cognitive centre over the rest of the body and which are responsible for transporting 'consciousness-bearing' material, in this case *pneuma*. The brain is the 'cause' (*aitios*) of the disease, and its condition can be influenced by a number of external causal factors (*prophaseis*) such as age, climate, season, the right or left side of the body, and the like.

A haematocentric approach to epilepsy can be found in the Hippocratic writing *On Breaths*. The author of this highly rhetorical treatise (probably written at the end of the fifth century BCE) assigns a pivotal role to air (*pneuma, phusa*) in the life of organisms. He takes the view that the main cause of diseases consists in a shortage or excess of air in the body or in the contaminated state of this air. This may either have external causes or be due to bad digestion of food, which also contains air, in the body (for instance because there is too much of it in the body) which causes all kinds of harmful gases to form. Such a disturbing effect of air due to a surplus of it is also what causes the 'so-called sacred disease'. It is again striking how the author incorporates the empirically perceptible phenomena of the disease in his own explanation:

In my view, the same cause is also responsible for the disease called sacred . . . I believe that none of the parts of the body that contribute to consciousness in anyone is more important than blood. So long as this remains in a stable condition, consciousness, too, remains stable; but when the blood undergoes change, consciousness also changes. There are many things that testify that this is the case. First of all, an affection which is common to all living beings, namely sleep, testifies to what has just been said. When sleep comes upon the body, the blood is chilled, for it is the nature of sleep to cause chill. When the blood is chilled, its passages become more sluggish. This is evident; the body leans and gets heavy . . . the eyes close, and consciousness is changed, and certain other thoughts remain present, which are called dreams . . . So if all of the blood is brought in a state of complete turmoil, consciousness is completely destroyed. . . . I state that the sacred disease is caused in the following way. When much wind has been mixed throughout the body with all the blood, many obstructions arise in many places in the blood vessels. Whenever therefore much air weighs, and continues to weigh, upon the thick, blood-filled blood vessels, the blood is prevented from passing on. So in one place it stops, in another it passes slowly, in another more quickly. When the progress of the blood through the body becomes irregular, all kinds of irregularities occur. The whole body is torn in all directions; the parts of the body are shaken in obedience to the troubling and disturbance of the blood; distortions of every kind occur in every manner. At this time the patients are unconscious of everything – deaf to what is spoken, blind to what is happening, and insensible to pain. So greatly does a disturbance of the air disturb and pollute the blood. Foam rises through the mouth, as is likely. For the air, passing through the vessels, itself rises and brings up with it the thinnest part of the blood. The moisture mixing with the air becomes white, for the air being pure is seen through thin membranes. For this reason the foam appears completely white. When then will the victims of this disease rid themselves of their disorder and the storm that attends it? When the body exercised by its exertions has warmed the blood, and the blood thoroughly warmed has warmed the breaths, and these thoroughly warmed are dispersed, breaking up the congestion of the blood, some go out along with the respiration, others with the phlegm. The disease finally ends when the foam has frothed itself away, the blood has re-established itself, and calm has arisen in the body.[33]

The structure of this explanation is very similar to the one found in *On the Sacred Disease*, yet there is a significant difference: air is not obstructed in its course, but air itself is the obstructing factor. Air causes the blood to become chilled, it flows more slowly and therefore it is less capable of providing the body with 'consciousness'. Another interesting factor is the comparison with sleep: a non-pathological state is employed to illustrate a more serious disorder resulting from the same physiological mechanism.[34]

The association with sleep returns in Aristotle, who dwells briefly on the subject of epilepsy in his treatise *On Sleep and Waking* (*De somno et vigilia*, *Somn. vig.*). Aristotle considers sleep a form of epilepsy, albeit not a pathological one. Sleep is a result of the digestion of food: after consumption food is carried to the centre of the body and 'cooked' or digested by the heat of the heart. The process of cooking gives rise to the evaporation (*anathumiasis*) of food; the air (*pneuma*), saturated by these hot vapours, is carried upwards from the heart to the brain and causes the head to become heavy. The brain causes these vapours to be chilled and return to the heart. Thus the heart is chilled, which is what actually causes the sensory faculties to fail (the 'formal cause', i.e. the definition of sleeping).[35]

> Sleep arises from the evaporation due to food... Young children sleep deeply, because all the food is borne upwards. An indication of this is that in early youth the upper parts of the body are larger in comparison with the lower, which is due to the fact that growth takes place in the upward direction. Hence too they are liable to epilepsy, for sleep is like epilepsy; indeed, in a sense, sleep is a type of epileptic fit. This is why in many people epilepsy begins in sleep, and they are regularly seized with it when asleep, but not when awake. For when a large amount of vapour is borne upwards and subsequently descends again, it causes the blood vessels to swell and it obstructs the passage through which respiration passes. (*Somn. vig.* 457 a 4–11)

[33] *On Breaths* 14.1–4 (6.110–12 L.), tr. Jones in Jones and Withington (1923–31) vol. 11, modified.
[34] For the ambivalent status of sleep in ancient medicine see Debru (1982) 30.
[35] For precise details of this process see Wiesner (1978) 241–80.

This explanation shows a strong similarity to the one in *On Breaths*, yet without mentioning blood. The main argument is that epilepsy is viewed as tightness of the chest or suffocation generated by the obstruction of the airways: the 'passage through which breath flows' is unlikely to refer to anything else but the windpipe. One air current, the air saturated by food vapours, obstructs the other, respiration. Aristotle does not speak about disorders in perception that are among the symptoms of epilepsy (and which apparently can be explained as analogous to the state of sleep, that is, as a result of the heat of the heart becoming chilled). Nor does he speak about other symptoms characteristic of epileptic fits. Yet he does make selective use of empirical data by stating that young children are particularly prone to the disease (a widely known fact in antiquity) and that the disease often manifests itself during sleep.

Lastly, the views of Diocles and his contemporary Praxagoras should be discussed. Both consider the heart to be the seat of the mind, but both also attribute an important role to the brain and to the mediation between the two by what they call 'psychic *pneuma*':

Praxagoras says that it [i.e. epilepsy] occurs around the thick artery, when phlegmatic humours form within it; these form bubbles and obstruct the passage of the psychic breath coming from the heart, and in this way this [the breath] causes the body to be agitated and seized by spasms; when the bubbles die down, the affection stops.

Diocles himself, too, thinks that it is an obstruction occurring around the same place, and that for the rest it happens in the same way as Praxagoras says it occurs...[36]

Compared to *On the Sacred Disease* it is significant that Diocles and Praxagoras consider the heart, not the brain, to be the starting-point for the psychic *pneuma*. In all other respects the explanations are virtually identical: the basic thought is that the passages through which the breath flows are obstructed or blocked; the obstruction is caused by phlegm (*phlegma*). Furthermore, Diocles and Praxagoras are the only doctors from the period concerned of whom we know some of the therapeutic measures they took in case the disease occurred. The authors of *On the Sacred Disease* and *On Breaths* restrict themselves to some very general remarks on curing the disease (by restoring the balance between the four primary qualities hot, cold, dry and wet; curing it by means of contrasting qualities). Diocles, on the other hand, is known to have based his treatment on the type of cause he established for the disease: purgative measures to remove *phlegma*, walking

---

[36] 'Anonymus Parisinus' 3 (published by I. Garofalo (1997)); tr. van der Eijk (2000a) 177.

and carrying around for those who contracted the disease due to their physical constitution, bleeding for those who contracted it by eating meat or due to dipsomania.[37] Our source of information is the above-mentioned Caelius Aurelianus (*Chronic Affections* 1.4.131–2), who remarks that these measures are far from adequate. On the other hand, Caelius Aurelianus is a sufficiently uncongenial informant for us to assume that Diocles provided more than just some vague indications. But in this respect the sources leave us in the dark.

The examples given show how each of the authors mentioned arrives at a different explanation of epilepsy, based on an *a priori* view on the physical aspects of cognitive processes, and how in their opinion the empirically perceptible symptoms of the disease can be fitted into this explanation. There is no empirical verification of such presuppositions in the modern sense of the word, apart from a rather haphazard use of empirical facts (yet not discovered in any targeted way), employed in the author's own defence or in his criticism of rival views. Much has been written about the reasons for this scientific attitude; in this respect it should be noted that systematic attempts at falsifying theories by gathering counter-examples in empirical reality were the exception rather than the rule in antiquity.[38] The pivotal role of the heart, both with respect to its position and with respect to its function, was a self-evident and undeniable fact; the same applies to the vital role of the blood. For this reason the encephalocentric view on the location of the mind needed quite some scientific and rhetorical force to secure its position in the debate.

---

[37] Fr. 99 vdE.
[38] The first thinker to appear to be aware of such a principle is Aristotle (see, for instance, *Gen. an.* 760 b 27ff.), yet he does not apply this in any way consistently either (see Lloyd (1979) 200–25).

PART II

Aristotle and his school

CHAPTER 5

Aristotle on melancholy

I INTRODUCTION

In a number of his writings Aristotle discusses a type of people he calls 'the melancholics' (*hoi melancholikoi*), without ever giving a definition of melancholy; indeed he does not even mention the term *melancholia*.[1] He only mentions, in passing, some typical features of a melancholic, sometimes adding a short psychological or physiological explanation, yet without relating these features to each other or to an underlying physiological theory. There is just one chapter (30.1) of the *Problemata physica* (*Pr.*), a collection of knowledge attributed to Aristotle, that contains a rather extensive discussion of melancholy. However, it is unlikely that the form in which this collection has come down to us dates back to Aristotle.[2] Recent scholarship has attributed the theory in this chapter to Theophrastus rather than Aristotle; according to Diogenes Laertius (5.44), Theophrastus wrote a treatise 'On Melancholy' (*Peri melancholias*) and the chapter in the *Problemata* is thought to be a summary or a revised version of this (lost) text.[3]

So far no attempt has been made to describe Aristotle's concept of melancholy as based on his undisputed works, and to compare it to the theory presented in *Pr.* 30.1.[4] Yet such an attempt could be useful, both because

---

This chapter was first published in German in *Mnemosyne* 43 (1990) 33–72.
[1] Literature on Aristotle's views on melancholy: Angelino & Salvaneschi (1982); Boyancé (1936) 185–94; Croissant (1932); Flashar (1956) 43ff.; Flashar (1962) 711ff.; Flashar (1966) 60–72; García Gual (1984) 41–50; Gravel (1982) 1, 129–45; S. W. Jackson (1986) 31–3; Klibansky, Panowsky and Saxl (1964) 15–40 [and (1990) 55–91]; Müri (1953) 21–38; Pigeaud (1978) 23–31; Pigeaud (1981a) 122–38; Pigeaud (1984) 501–10; Pigeaud (1988a); Simon (1978) 228–37; Tellenbach (1961) 1–15 [and Rütten (1992); Roussel (1988)].
[2] See on this subject the pioneering work by Flashar (1962) 303ff.; however, Marenghi (1966) [and Louis (1991–4) vol. III] consider Aristotle to be the author of the *Problemata*.
[3] Müri (1953) 31; Klibansky et al. (1964) 36–41; Flashar (1962) 711–14; Flashar (1966) 61 [and Sharples (1995) 5–6]; on the reasons for this attribution see n. 91 below.
[4] Aristotle's remarks are briefly discussed by Müri (1953) 38; Flashar (1966) 60; Flashar (1962) 712–13; Klibansky et al. (1964) 33–6; Croissant (1932) 35–8. On the influence of the theory of *Pr.* 30.1 see Flashar (1962) 715–17 and Klibansky et al. (1964).

139

it would be the only way to provide a solid basis for assessing the theory presented in the *Problemata,* and because attempts to relate this theory to pre-Aristotelian, especially medical views have proved unsuccessful.[5] Despite extensive research, the concept of melancholy in the Hippocratic Corpus remains a complicated issue.[6] Early Hippocratic writings describe melancholy only as a disease, sometimes very specifically as a pathological change of colour of the fluid bile. Significantly, these writings do refer to the so-called constitutional type of 'the melancholic' (*ho melancholikos*), yet without providing clarity on the underlying physiological theory, and in any case it is nowhere related to a bodily fluid called 'black bile'.[7] The Hippocratic writing *On the Nature of Man* (*c.* 400 BCE) seems to be the first to recognise black bile as a bodily fluid in its own right, but this recognition does not result in the concept of 'the melancholic'.[8] While the details of this recognition of black bile – in addition to yellow bile, blood and phlegm – as one of the four bodily fluids that form the basis for physical health are still open to dispute,[9] it is clear, as Müri and Flashar have shown, that in order to establish a link between the bodily fluid 'black bile' (*melaina cholē*) and the constitutional type of 'the melancholic', at least one further step is required. The problem is that, on the one hand, this step was supposedly first made in Aristotle's school (according to Jouanna (1975) 296), whereas on the other hand the Aristotelian use of 'the melancholics' as an established term seems to suggest that this step had already been taken. I say 'seems', for it is by no means certain that Aristotle actually associated the term *ho melancholikos* with this 'constitutional type' and its affiliated theory of the four humours.[10] There is even doubt as to whether Aristotle's use of the term has anything to do with a physiological theory on black bile.[11] There is some justification for this doubt in that the adjective *melancholikos* (just as *melancholōdēs* and the verb *melancholan*) was also used in non-medical discourse of the fifth and fourth centuries BCE and often

---

[5] Müri (1953) 38; Flashar (1962) 714; Flashar (1966) 62.
[6] In addition to the works by Müri and Flashar see Roy (1981) and Joly (1975) 107–28.
[7] See Flashar (1966) 32–5; Müri (1953) 30–2; Dittmer (1940) 95.
[8] Flashar (1966) 43; Jouanna (1975) 296.
[9] I am referring to the controversy between Joly (1969) 150–7; Joly (1975) 107–10; and Jouanna (1975) 48–9; also Roy (1981) 11–19; it concerns the date of this recognition and any differences between the humoral systems of the schools of Cos and Cnidos (cf. Grensemann (1968c) 103–4 and Lonie (1981) 54–62).
[10] Cf. the following statement by Lucas (1968) 284, which is entirely unfounded: 'Aristotle, who had been trained as a physician, accepted the Hippocratic theory of the human constitution, namely that health depends on the proper balance of the four humours present in the body, blood, phlegm, yellow bile, and black bile.' The fact that Aristotle knew the Hippocratic work *On the Nature of Man* (cf. *Hist. an.* 512 b 12) has no bearing on this question.
[11] Dirlmeier (1956) 491; W. D. Ross (1955) 252.

seems to mean virtually the same as *manikos* ('mad') or *mainesthai* ('be mad').[12]

In view of these issues it will be useful to clarify Aristotle's own concept of melancholy. This first of all requires an analysis of all occurrences of the words *melancholikos* and *melaina cholē* (sections 2 and 3) and an analysis of the role Aristotle assigns to (black) bile in human physiology (section 4). The results will enable us to gain a better insight into the relationship between Aristotle and the Hippocratic theory of humours. In the second part of this chapter (sections 5–7) I will discuss the theory set out in *Pr.* 30.1 and its relation to Aristotle's concept. This will also reveal the philosophical significance of the issue of melancholy: for Aristotle seems to use melancholics to illustrate the role played by the human *phusis*, both in the sense of 'natural predisposition' and of 'physiological constitution', in the moral, sensitive and intellectual behaviour of man, namely what the *Problemata* text calls the 'character-affecting aspect' (*to ēthopoion*) of *phusis*.

2 MELANCHOLY IN THE *PARVA NATURALIA* AND THE *EUDEMIAN ETHICS*

In the *Parva naturalia*, melancholics are mentioned a few times in relation to disorders in certain psychophysical processes. At the end of *On Memory and Recollection* (*De memoria et reminiscentia*, *Mem.* 453 a 14ff.) Aristotle briefly discusses the physiological aspect of recollection, saying that recollection is 'something physical' (*sōmatikon ti*). Proof of this is that certain people are disturbed by the fact that if they are unable to recollect something, despite making a strong effort, the process of recollecting continues even after they stop making the effort.[13] According to Aristotle melancholics are particularly prone to this disorder, 'for they are particularly affected by images' (τούτους γὰρ φαντάσματα κινεῖ μάλιστα). The cause of this disorder is that just as someone who throws something is unable to bring the thrown object to a halt, the process of recollection causes a bodily

---

[12] Müri (1953) 34; Flashar (1966) 37–8; Klibansky et al. (1964) 16. For the historical background to this use of the term, as well as the origin of the notion 'black bile', see also Kudlien (1967a) 75–88 and (1973) 53–8.

[13] τὸ παρενοχλεῖν ἐνίους, ἐπειδὰν μὴ δύνωνται ἀναμνησθῆναι καὶ πάνυ ἐπέχοντες τὴν διάνοιαν, καὶ οὐκέτ' ἐπιχειροῦντας ἀναμιμνήσκεσθαι οὐδὲν ἧττον (453 a 16–18). The subject of παρενοχλεῖν is ἀνάμνησις (this refers to the πάθος mentioned in line 25); οὐδὲν ἧττον belongs to ἀναμιμνήσκεσθαι. The 'disturbance' (παρενοχλεῖν) does not so much consist in the fact that these people are unable to remember something in particular (for how could this be an indication that memory is a physiological process?), but that they are unable to stop the process of recollection. The analogy in 20–1 (οὐκέτ' ἐπ' αὐτοῖς τὸ στῆσαι) clearly shows this. See Sorabji (1972a) 111–12.

movement which does not stop until the object of recollection is found. The disorder manifests itself particularly in people whose region of sensory perception is surrounded by moisture, 'for once moisture is set in motion, it does not readily stop moving until the sought object is found and the movement has taken a straight course'.

Melancholics are mentioned here in the context of a discussion of the bodily (physiological) aspect of recollection. Their characteristic feature is their disorder[14] in the process of recollection, in that they are unable to control this process. As causes for the disorder Aristotle first mentions the special movement by images (*phantasmata*) and secondly moisture (*hugrotēs*) located around the *aisthētikos topos*, the heart. Although it remains uncertain whether this sentence refers to melancholics, the structure of the argument seems to indicate that this moisture is the physiological cause of the previously mentioned special affection by images.[15] In the case of melancholics this moisture clearly is black bile;[16] thus it appears that they are characterised by a quantity of black bile around the heart, or at least they are prone to being affected by this.[17]

In the third chapter of his work *On Sleep and Waking* (*Somn. vig.*), Aristotle describes groups of people who are more prone to sleep and people who are less so. In 457 a 25 he discusses people with prominent blood vessels who, as a result of this width of their vessels (*poroi*), are not much given to sleep. Aristotle subsequently[18] states that melancholics are not prone to sleep (*hupnōtikoi*) either, for their inner parts are chilled, which results in limited 'evaporation' of food (according to Aristotle, this 'evaporation', *anathumiasis*, is the cause of sleep). This is also the reason why melancholics are on the one hand good eaters, yet on the other hand they are spare; their

---

[14] On (παρ)ενοχλεῖν see *On Divination in Sleep* (*De divinatione per somnum, Div. somn.*) 464 a 26.
[15] This is shown by the fact that the analogy argument in lines 20–2 is not finished until the general ὁ ἀναμιμνησκόμενος καὶ θηρεύων in the next sentence has been applied to the exceptional cases: thus the later καὶ μάλιστα in line 23 anaphorically picks up the earlier μάλιστα τοὺς μελαγχολικούς.
[16] See *Part. an.* 72 b 29, where a 'hot and residual moisture' (ὑγροτὴς θερμὴ καὶ περιττωματική) is mentioned, which is situated around the diaphragm and confuses the mind and sense perception. It is likely that this refers to black bile (cf. *Pr.* 954 a 34–8; see below). With regard to the complication that in Greek medicine melancholics were usually associated with dryness, I endorse Sorabji's solution (1972a, 113): black bile is of course a liquid (cf. *Part. an.* 647 b 11–13; *Hist. an.* 487 a 2–4), but it is dry compared to other liquids. In this passage melancholics are not characterised by the fact that they are particularly moist but by the fact that there is moisture around their heart (as is occasionally the case with other people), namely black bile.
[17] For similarities with Diocles' theory see Sorabji (1972) 113 and Flashar (1966) 50–9.
[18] See *Pr.* 954 a 7, where melancholics are said to have protruding veins (καὶ αἱ φλέβες ἐξέχουσιν). For the tendency in this chapter of the *Problemata* to take certain features, which Aristotle occasionally mentions in relation to melancholy, as part of a more fundamental basis of the melancholic nature, see n. 39 below.

body is in such a condition (*diakeitai*) that it seems as if they have not had any food at all:[19] 'for black bile is cold by nature and therefore chills the nutritive region (*threptikos topos*) of the body as well as any other parts that may contain this residue'.[20]

This passage, too, features in the context of a consideration of bodily (anatomical, physiological) influences on the psycho-physical phenomenon in question, namely sleep. First of all, it should be noted that Aristotle speaks not only of melancholics but also of 'black bile' (*melaina cholē*): underlying his use of the term *hoi melancholikoi* is a physiological concept that recognises black bile as a distinct fluid (i.e. apart from yellow bile or bile as such). The text implies that black bile is cold by nature and has a chilling effect on its environment. Cold as a natural elementary quality of black bile corresponds to the Hippocratic characterisation of black bile as dry and cold (see Flashar (1966) 39), although the phrase 'naturally' seems to leave open the possibility of heating.[21] Finally, there is the significant notion that black bile is a *perittōma*, a residue or remainder of food (this term will be discussed in section 4 below) and the remark that it can be located both near the nutritive region, that is, the heart (cf. *On Respiration* (*Resp.*) 474 b 3 and *On Youth and Old Age* (*De iuv.*) 469 a 5–7) and in other places in the body; this is an important addition to its localisation around the 'perceptive region' as stated in the above passage from *On Memory and Recollection*.[22]

The melancholic is given a particularly significant role in Aristotle's treatises on dreams (*De insomniis*) and on divination in sleep (*De divinatione per somnum*). At first there seems to be considerable discrepancy between the two writings: whilst melancholics are presented as an example of people with clear and prophetic dreams in *On Divination in Sleep* (*Div. somn.* 463 b 17ff.; 464 a 32ff.), in *On Dreams* (*Insomn.* 461 a 22), by contrast, the images they see in their dreams are said to be cloudy and confused. Closer analysis of the relevant passages should reveal whether they are indeed inconsistent.

To start with the passages in *On Divination in Sleep*, at the beginning of chapter 2 (463 b 12ff.) Aristotle argues that dreams are not sent by the gods, but that their origin lies in human nature. For this reason dreams are not divine, albeit beyond human control, for nature is beyond human control

---

[19] See *Pr.* 954 a 7–11 (I endorse Flashar's reading σκληφροί instead of σκληροί here).
[20] ἡ δὲ μέλαινα χολὴ φύσει ψυχρὰ οὖσα καὶ τὸν θρεπτικὸν τόπον ψυχρὸν ποιεῖ καὶ τὰ ἄλλα μόρια, ὅπου ἂν ὑπάρχῃ τὸ τοιοῦτον περίττωμα (457 a 31–3).
[21] This possibility is explicitly recognised in *Part. an.* 649 a 24ff., and the author of *Pr.* 30.1 clearly uses it (954 a 14ff., in particular line 21, which refers to *Somn. vig.* 457 a 31).
[22] It is possible to interpret this in the sense that the location of black bile in the region of the heart is a characteristic feature of the melancholics, whereas its occurrence in other places may happen to all people.

but not divine.²³ To prove the truth of this conclusion Aristotle argues that quite common people have vivid and prophetic dreams (εὐθυόνειροί εἰσι καὶ προορατικοί). The only explanation for this is that these dreams are not sent by a god, but it is in the nature (*phusis*) of garrulous and melancholic people to see all kinds of images (in their dreams), as these people are subject to a large number and variety of movements, which cause them to chance upon 'images similar to events' (ὁμοίοις θεωρήμασιν). Their good fortune in this respect can be compared to that of people who in a game of chance have a better chance of winning because they just keep trying.

Aristotle speaks here of people with a 'garrulous and melancholic nature' (λάλος καὶ μελαγχολικὴ φύσις),²⁴ who apparently serve as an example of the general rule that 'quite common' people (πάνυ εὐτελεῖς ἄνθρωποι) have prophetic dreams. This is used to prove that prophetic dreams are not sent by the gods. Melancholics are therefore implicitly contrasted with the group of 'the best and most intelligent' (see 462 b 21–2), for these would typically be expected to be the recipients of divine provision, if any such thing exists.²⁵ The ability to foresee the future in sleep is particularly strong in people whose abilities to apply reason and rational thought are for some reason weak or impaired. Aristotle explains the *euthuoneiria* of melancholics (463 b 18ff.) here as a combination of their natural (physiological) sensitivity to a large number and variety of movements or images (*phantasmata*), and a kind of statistical probability: the more images one sees, the greater the chance of seeing an image that resembles a future event.

Later on in the text (464 a 32ff.) there is one further mention of melancholics, this time not in a polemical context but as part of a discussion of various groups of people with special prophetic powers. This rather obscure passage is made even more difficult to interpret, as the explanation it gives for the prophetic dreams of melancholics seems to differ considerably from the one given in 463 b 17ff.²⁶ A determining factor for the divination of melancholics is said to be not only the number of images that they are confronted with, but also a certain ability for making connections by association between objects that are far apart. This ability is based on a similarity (*homoiotēs*) between the objects concerned. A further factor is the strength and intensity (*sphodrotēs*) of their imagination, which prevents the process

---

²³ For a discussion of the numerous difficulties involved in the interpretation of this paragraph see van der Eijk (1994) 289–301 [see also ch. 6 below]. For other interpretations of this passage see Barra (1957) 75–84; Boyancé (1936) 192; Croissant (1932) 36; Détienne (1963) 140–69; Effe (1970) 82 n. 41; A. Mansion (1946) 268 n. 46; Nolte (1940) 92–3; Verdenius (1960) 61.
²⁴ Cf. *Pr.* 954 a 34, in which garrulousness (*lalia*) is considered to be caused by a heating of black bile.
²⁵ For the background to this argumentation see ch. 6, below.
²⁶ See Pigeaud (1978) 28–9 and Croissant (1932) 38–40.

of association from being disturbed by other bodily movements. The *euthuoneiria* of melancholics (referred to here as *eustochia*, ability to make the right conjecture, which suggests a greater degree of activity)[27] seems to be based on the ability to 'perceive similarities' (τὰς ὁμοιότητας θεωρεῖν); on other occasions Aristotle relates this ability to a special natural disposition (*phusis* or *euphuia*) and considers it an important principle for poetry and philosophy.[28] Aristotle's explanation of the prophetic dreams of melancholics is therefore in line with his remark in *Mem.* 453 a 15 (quoted above).

It is difficult to see how these statements can be reconciled with *Insomn.* 461 a 22–3. In this passage Aristotle brackets melancholics together with the feverish and the intoxicated as examples of people who see confused and monstrous images in their sleep and whose dreams themselves are not coherent (οὐκ ἐρρωμένα). The cause of this blurriness is that all these affections contain air (πνευματώδη) and therefore produce much movement and confusion.[29] It is clear that these remarks are in stark contrast with the characterisation of melancholics as 'having clear dreams' (*euthuoneiroi*) in *Div. somn.* 463 b 15–17 and as 'hitting the mark' (*eustochoi*) in 464 a 33, where the clear dreams of the melancholics are explained as a result of their sensitivity to 'being subjected to many and manifold movements'!

Given the close connection between both treatises (*Div. somn.* 464 b 9–10 even refers to *Insomn.* 461 a 14ff., i.e. to the direct context of the passage on melancholics), it is highly unlikely that Aristotle was unaware of this contradiction. To solve this problem, B. Effe (1970, 85 n. 49) has suggested a different interpretation of the word *euthuoneiros*: not 'dreaming clearly', but 'dreaming rightly', that is to say, 'dreaming the truth'. Yet even if this interpretation of *euthuoneiros* is adopted, it remains impossible to square Aristotle's remark in *Insomn.* 461 a 22–3 (with its context of distortion of images in dreams)[30] with the possibility to dream rightly.

---

[27] To interpret the difference between the two passages as an antithesis between passive susceptibility and active seeking is to a certain extent misleading, for this more active ability also escapes conscious rational control (cf. *Mem.* 453 a 14ff., in which the word θηρεύειν is used, but with the explicit note that recollection in these people is 'beyond their control', οὐκ ἐπ' αὐτοῖς). The 'daemonic' nature of the effect of the human *phusis* actually consists in the fact that it escapes rational control, i.e. it is οὐκ εφ' ἡμῖν (cf. *Somn. vig.* 453 b 23–4; *Eth. Nic.* 1179 b 21ff.)

[28] 464 b 1: καὶ διὰ τὸ μεταβλητικὸν ταχὺ τὸ ἐχόμενον φαντάζεται αὐτοῖς... ἐχόμενα τοῦ ὁμοίου λέγουσι καὶ διανοοῦνται... συνείρουσιν εἰς τὸ πρόσω. 464 b 7 explicitly mentions the perception of similarities (τὸ τὰς ὁμοιότητας θεωρεῖν), but the purpose of this passage is to portray the ability of the interpreter of dreams to determine the resemblance between dream and reality in cases in which the dreams are not actually clear. See below (section 6) for the significance of this principle in Aristotle's views on cognitive psychology.

[29] πάντα γὰρ τὰ τοιαῦτα πάθη πνευματώδη ὄντα πολλὴν ποιεῖ κίνησιν καὶ ταραχήν.

[30] 461 a 10ff.: πολλάκις μὲν ὁμοίας, πολλάκις δὲ διαλυομένας εἰς ἄλλα σχήματα ... (15) φαίνεται μέν, διεστραμμένον δὲ πάμπαν, ὥστε φαίνεσθαι ἀλλοῖον ἢ οἷόν ἐστιν.

Moreover, a check of all the occurrences of *euthuoneiros* and *euthuoneiria*[31] in Greek literature proves Effe's interpretation to be wrong. The fact that *euthuoneiriai* are opposed to 'confused and disturbed images' (εἴδωλα διαπεφορημένα καὶ διεστραμμένα) in 464 b 9ff. shows that *euthuoneiria* refers to 'lucid' and 'clear' dreams, which come about because the way taken by the movement of sensory perception from the sensory organ to the heart has been *straight* (*euthus*).[32] Consequently, the relation between these dreams and reality is immediately clear (this explains the remark in 464 b 10 that anyone can interpret such dreams; cf. 463 a 25). For this reason these dreams *can* in fact be right or prophetic, yet this possibility *also* applies to the distorted and blurred images in dreams, for, Aristotle says, assessing *their* relation to reality clearly is the work of a professional interpreter of dreams.

Another option is to assume that the confusing effect of air (*pneuma*) mentioned in *On Dreams* apparently does not apply in the cases referred to in *On Divination in Sleep*. This is either due to the large number of images (for, in *On Divination in Sleep* images seen in dreams are a result of movement, whereas *On Dreams* speaks about the influence of bodily movement on images that have already been formed),[33] or because other psycho-physical processes or states neutralise, as it were, the confusing effect. If one attempts to solve the problem in this way (supported by J. Croissant),[34] one has to assume that the contradiction is only apparent, but it must be admitted that Aristotle did not make an effort to avoid the impression of contradicting himself. Yet it is very well possible that this is partly due to the differences in aim and method between the more technical and programmatic *On Dreams* and the more polemical *On Divination in*

---

[31] The noun εὐθυονειρία occurs in 463 a 25 and 464 b 7 and 16, the adjective εὐθυόνειρος in 463 b 16 and 464 a 27 as well as in the passage *Eth. Eud.* 1248 a 39–40, which will be discussed below. Apart from the Aristotelian Corpus, the word does not occur until in Plutarch (*De def. or.* 437 d–e, a passage that does not offer much of an explanation as it clearly refers to *Div. somn.* 463 b 16ff.). As to the meaning of this word, similar combinations with εὐθύς are to be mentioned, such as εὐθυωρία (cf. Geurts (1943) 108–14).

[32] Cf. the use of εὐθυπορεῖν in *Mem.* 453 a 25.

[33] The 'many and manifold movements' (πολλαὶ καὶ παντοδαπαὶ κινήσεις) from *Div. somn.* 463 b 18 are clearly 'movements that produce images' (κινήσεις φανταστικαί), whereas the 'huge movement' (πολλὴ κίνησις) from *Insomn.* 461 a 24 refers to the 'resistance' (ἀντίκρουσις) against these movements, as mentioned in 461 a 11.

[34] Croissant (1932) 38–9. According to Croissant, the effect of the lack of rational activity in melancholics is that the movements can reach the central sense organ, despite strong resistance of the air in the blood. However, this interpretation presupposes the identity of 'the ecstatic people' (οἱ ἐκστατικοί) and the melancholics (οἱ μελαγχολικοί). Although Croissant bases this identity on *Pr.* 953 b 14–15 (and probably also *Eth. Nic.* 1151 a 1–5; see below), it does not do justice to the separate discussion of 'the ecstatics' in *Div. somn.* 464 a 24–7 and 'the melancholics' in 464 a 32ff., as well as the differences between the explanations Aristotle gives for each group.

Sleep (which makes no mention of *pneuma* and blood at all and which otherwise shows a lack of physiological details too).

However, close analysis of the text of *On Dreams* reveals a clear connection between both occurrences. At the start of the third chapter Aristotle explains what causes dreams to appear: due to their weakness, sensory movements are obscured by stronger movements during the day; yet by night, when the individual senses are inactive, they flow to the central sensory organ (the 'principle of perception' or the 'authoritative sense-organ' that is situated in the heart) as a result of a flow of heat. These movements often still resemble the object originally perceived, but equally often they take on different shapes due to resistance (for this reason no dreams occur after a meal).

Hence, just as in a liquid, if one disturbs it violently, sometimes no image appears, and sometimes it appears but is entirely distorted, so that it seems quite different from what it really is, *although when the movement has ceased, the reflections are clear and plain*; so also in sleep, the images or residuary movements that arise from the sense-impressions are altogether obscured owing to the aforesaid movement when it is too great, and sometimes the images appear confused and monstrous, and the dreams are morbid, as is the case with the melancholic, the feverish and the intoxicated; for all these affections, being full of air, produce much movement and confusion. In animals that have blood, *as the blood becomes quiet and its purer elements separate*, the persistence of the sensory stimulus derived from each of the sense organs makes the dreams healthy.

The analogy thus has to be considered to apply to the whole process: the phrase 'when the movement has ceased, the reflections are clear and plain' (17) corresponds to 'as the blood becomes quiet and its purer elements separate' in line 25. It shows that the process does not stop at the confused images in dreams: if the movement is preserved (σῳζομένη), it will eventually reach the heart. It seems that *Div. somn.* 464 a 32ff. refers in particular to this 'preservation' of movements, for the 'intensity' of the melancholics that is emphasised there is responsible for this preservation, and the 'other movement' discussed here seems to refer to the 'resistance' (*ekkrousis*) mentioned in *Insomn.* 461 a 11. The advantage of this interpretation is that in the later treatise (*On Divination in Sleep*) Aristotle explicitly refers to the earlier one (*On Dreams*), using it to try to explain two facts and characteristics of melancholics that at first sight seem difficult to square with each other. It appears that melancholics can have both vague and clear dreams; and which one of both affections manifests itself most strongly in a particular case apparently depends on the person's physiological state at the time (volume of air and heat, intensity of images), which in the case of unstable people like melancholics must be considered a variable factor.

Another notable remark on the physiology of the melancholic (*Insomn.* 461 a 23–4) is that melancholy, fever and drunkenness are 'spirituous affections', with *pneumatōdēs* probably meaning 'containing/producing air' (cf. *On Sense Perception* (*De sensu, Sens.*) 445 a 26). The fact that drunkenness and melancholy are mentioned together, and are both said to be 'pneumatic' in character, will be discussed below, when I deal with *Pr.* 30.1 (for the connection between wine and *pneuma* also cf. *Somn. vig.* 457 a 16). With regard to the question of the melancholic 'constitution', it is worth noting that the use of the word *pathos* points to melancholy as a disease rather than a natural predisposition. However, it may well be that Aristotle chose the word *pathos* to refer to fever and drunkenness, without considering the difference (viz. that both are affections that occur sporadically, whereas melancholy is a predisposition) relevant in this context, and therefore did not discuss it.

There is a direct relation between the passages from *On Divination in Sleep* and the remark in the *Eudemian Ethics* (1248 a 39–40) about the *euthuoneiria* of melancholics. It is mentioned as an example of the way in which people who lack reason and deliberation (*logos* and *bouleusis*), by means of divine movement in their soul can still be successful in their actions and do the right thing.[35] This divine movement is probably identical to the mechanism that Aristotle called *daimonia phusis* in *Div. somn.* 463 b 15.[36] It is again striking that melancholics are categorised as belonging to the group of 'irrational people' (*alogoi, aphrones*) and that a relation is perceived between their lack of reason and their prophetic powers.

3 MELANCHOLY IN THE *NICOMACHEAN ETHICS*

In the seventh book of the *Nicomachean Ethics,* melancholics are mentioned on three occasions. In his treatment of lack of self-control (*akrasia,* 1150 b 19)

---

[35] *Eth. Eud.* 1248 a 39–40: 'This entity [i.e. God] sees both the future and the present well, even in people whose reasoning faculty is disengaged; this is why melancholics have clear dreams, for it seems that the principle works more strongly when reason is disengaged' (τοῦτο [i.e. ὁ θεός] καὶ εὖ ὁρᾷ καὶ τὸ μέλλον καὶ τὸ ὄν, καὶ ὧν ἀπολύεται ὁ λόγος οὗτος. διὸ οἱ μελαγχολικοὶ καὶ εὐθυόνειροι. ἔοικε γὰρ ἡ ἀρχὴ ἀπολυομένου τοῦ λόγου ἰσχύειν μᾶλλον).

[36] For the interpretation of this difficult chapter, and for an assessment of the differences between the views in *Eth. Eud.* 8.2 and *Div. somn.*, see ch. 8 below. With regard to the passage *Eth. Eud.* 1248 a 39–40, the remarks made by Flashar (1962, 713 and 1966, 60 n. 2) should be noted. Flashar argues that there is a contradiction between *Eth. Eud.* 1248 a 39–40 and *Insomn.* 461 a 22–4 with regard to the 'clear' and 'vague' images melancholics see in their dreams. However, he does not seem to have noticed that the relationship between *Eudemian Ethics* and *On Dreams* is the same as between *On Divination in Sleep* and *On Dreams*. His explanation is that this contradiction may have something to do with the fact that Aristotle later, in the *Parva naturalia*, denies that dreams could be of divine origin, something Aristotle considered possible in the *Eudemian Ethics*, which may well be earlier. In my opinion this explanation is not correct, as *On Divination in Sleep* also says that melancholics have clear dreams.

Aristotle distinguishes between two types of lack of self-control: on the one hand recklessness (*propeteia*), and on the other hand weakness (*astheneia*). According to Aristotle the difference is that the weak person thinks and deliberates, yet does not persist with the conclusions of his deliberations, whereas the reckless person does not think or deliberate at all. In both cases this failure is caused by passion (*pathos*). As examples of the reckless type of lack of self-control Aristotle mentions 'the irritable' (*hoi oxeis*) and 'the melancholics' (*hoi melancholikoi*) in lines 25ff.; both 'do not wait for rational deliberation'. In the case of the former (*hoi oxeis*) this is due to their speed (*tachutēs*), in the case of the latter (*hoi melancholikoi*) it is due to their intensity (*sphodrotēs*), that is, their inclination to follow their imagination (τὸ ἀκολουθητικοὶ εἶναι τῇ φαντασίᾳ).

The argument that melancholics lack rational thought corresponds to statements of the same nature in the *Parva naturalia* (in particular *On Divination in Sleep*) and the *Eudemian Ethics*. The 'intensity'[37] that Aristotle mentions as explanation here was mentioned in *On Divination in Sleep*, where it was called typical for their strong imagination; in the next sentence it is specified in the sense of their inclination 'to follow imagination' (cf. for this *Mem.* 453 a 15). The relationship between imagination and passion is not made explicit in the text of the *Nicomachean Ethics*, but it consists in the fact that *phantasia* presents the perceived object as something to be pursued or avoided (and therefore it can produce pleasure or pain).[38] Melancholics are inclined to act upon the objects of their imagination without first holding them against the light of reason (οὐκ ἀναμένουσι τὸν λόγον).

This typology of lack of self-control returns in 1151 a 1–5, where the reckless are simply called *hoi ekstatikoi*, 'those who are prone to get beside themselves'.[39] Recklessness is said to be better than weakness, for a weak person is susceptible to even slighter passions and, unlike the reckless person, does not act without prior deliberation. Further on (in 1152 a 17ff.) it is argued that someone who lacks self-control is not really evil or unjust (despite his evil and unjust actions), for he has no evil intentions: 'for the one does not follow his intentions, yet, by contrast, the melancholic does not deliberate at all'. In this text *ho melancholikos* is therefore prototypical

---

[37] The translation by Dirlmeier (1956) 157, 'ein unheimlich brodelndes Temperament' is entirely unfounded.
[38] Cf. Tracy (1969) 251–3 and Nussbaum (1978) 232–41.
[39] The *ekstatikoi* are also discussed in *Div. somn.* 464 a 25, i.e. in the same context as the melancholics, yet without being identified with them (see n. 34 above; on the relation between ecstatics and melancholics see Croissant (1932) 38–41); *ekstasis*, however, is mentioned in *Pr.* 30.1 (953 b 14–15) as an expression of the heating of black bile. For this tendency in the chapter from the *Problemata* see n. 18 above.

for the reckless type. In lines 27–8, the lack of self-control of melancholics (i.e. their recklessness) is said to be easier to cure (*euiatotera*) than the lack of self-control of those who deliberate but who do not act upon their deliberations (i.e. the weak). This corresponds to 1151 a 1–5;[40] yet the next sentence is confusing, for Aristotle continues by saying that those who lack self-control out of habit (*ethismos*) are easier to cure than those who lack self-control by nature (*tōn phusikōn*). Does this new differentiation (habit vs. nature) correspond to the recklessness – weakness we already know? Yet that would imply that melancholy is not a natural predisposition (as the remark on the *melancholikē phusis* in *Div. somn.* 463 b 17 suggests) but an attitude (*hexis*) acquired by habit, and that the characterisation *hoi melancholikoi* would not refer to the nature but to the character of the person. But this text may in fact refer to a subcategory of the reckless type in which melancholics are to be regarded as 'reckless by nature'.[41] Anyhow, Aristotle's argumentation is not entirely clear here, and it may well be that the classification of melancholics as belonging to the second type (weakness) in the pseudo-Aristotelian *Great Ethics* (*Magna moralia, Mag. mor.* 1203 b 1–2) is based on this passage.[42]

The last occurrence of the melancholics can be found in the section that follows (*Eth. Nic.* 7.12–15), in which Aristotle discusses pleasure (*hēdonē*). In 1154 a 26 he asks the question why physical pleasure seems more desirable than other pleasures. The first reason he gives is that it drives away pain (*lupē*) and functions, as it were, as a cure against it. The second reason (1154 b 3) is that because of its intensity (*sphodra*) it is pursued by people who are unable to enjoy any other pleasure and who perceive even their normal state (in which there is neither pleasure nor pain) as painful.

---

[40] Croissant's remark (1932, 41 n. 2) that the melancholics are categorised as the other type (*astheneia*) is based on an incorrect interpretation: τῶν βουλευομένων μὲν μὴ ἐμμενόντων δέ is a genitive of comparison. This incorrect interpretation may also be the reason why melancholics are said to belong to the weakness category by the author of *Mag. mor.* 1203 b 1–2 (see below).

[41] In this respect the remark by Plato (*Republic* 573 c 7–9) is worth noting: the tyrant can become 'prone to drinking, sex and melancholy either by nature, or by his activities, or by both' (ἢ φύσει ἢ ἐπιτηδεύμασιν ἢ ἀμφοτέροις μεθυστικός τε καὶ ἐρωτικός καὶ μελαγχολικός).

[42] 'This type of weakness of will [i.e. recklessness, *propeteia*] would seem to be not altogether blameworthy, for it is also found in respectable people, in those who are hot and those who are naturally gifted (ἐν τοῖς θερμοῖς καὶ εὐφυέσιν); the other type occurs in people who are cold and melancholic (ἐν τοῖς ψυχροῖς καὶ μελαγχολικοῖς), and these are blameworthy.' This contradiction can only be solved by taking into account the fluctuations in the temperature of black bile which are possible according to *Pr.* 954 a 14ff. However, this offers no explanation for the prototypical use of *hoi melancholikoi* to refer to both the reckless type in *Eth. Nic.* 7 (which, incidentally, does not mention heat and cold) and the weak type in *Magna moralia*. Dirlmeier (1958, 390) and Flashar (1962, 713) discuss this issue. As the authenticity of the *Magna moralia* is still disputed (see for the latest debate the works of Cooper (1973) 327–49 and Rowe (1975) 160–72), I will not go into this complication here (for the possible origin of the contradiction see n. 40 above).

For people constantly feel pleasure in their youth because they are growing; conversely, melancholics by nature constantly need to be cured (τὴν φύσιν ἀεὶ ἰατρείας δέονται), for the 'mixture' of their bodies keeps them in a constant state of stimulation (τὸ σῶμα δακνόμενον διατελεῖ τὴν κρᾶσιν) and they are always subject to intense desires (καὶ ἀεὶ ἐν σφοδρᾷ ὀρέξει εἰσίν).

According to Aristotle the pain is driven out by pleasure, once it has gained sufficient strength, and therefore these people are undisciplined and bad (*akolastoi kai phauloi*) in the way they act.

This is again a context in which the influence of the body on people's moral behaviour is discussed (hence the remark about lack of discipline). Aristotle speaks about people who even perceive the normal state as painful *due to their nature* (*dia tēn phusin*), their physiological constitution.[43] Apparently, melancholics serve as an example for this group: they constantly require cures *by nature*, that is, in their normal state. They might be said to be permanently ill,[44] for their bodies are permanently 'bitten' (*daknomenon*) as a result of their 'mixture' (*krasis*). The word *krasis*, which plays an important part in Greek medicine and physiology,[45] clearly refers to a physiological state. As Aristotle makes no mention of a mixture of *humours* anywhere else, but does mention a particular mixture of heat and cold as the basis for a healthy physical constitution,[46] it is appropriate to think of a mixture of *qualities*. In this theory, melancholics are characterised by a mixture of heat and cold (either too cold or too hot) that is permanently out of balance, something which Aristotle clearly regards as a sign of *disease*. Thus this passage confirms the remark in *Somn. vig.* 457 a 29ff., as quoted above; it also becomes clear that the difference between constitution and disease,[47] which is problematic in any case, fails because of the nature of the Aristotelian concept of melancholy: the melancholic is, so to say, constitutionally ill.[48]

---

[43] This explains Aristotle's parenthetic remark about the testimony of the *phusiologoi* (see Dirlmeier (1956) 506).

[44] See the use of *euiatotera* in *Eth. Nic.* 1152 a 27.

[45] See den Dulk (1934) 67–95 and Tracy (1969) *passim* (in particular 35–8; 167–72; 175–6).

[46] *Ph.* 246 b 4–5: 'the virtues of the body, such as health and handsomeness, we posit in a mixture and balance of hot and cold' (ἐν κράσει καὶ συμμετρίᾳ θερμῶν καὶ ψυχρῶν); on this see Tracy (1969) 161–2. Cf. *Pr.* 954 a 15: 'the melancholic humour is a mixture of hot and cold, for from these two the nature (of the body) is constituted' (θερμοῦ καὶ ψυχροῦ κρᾶσίς ἐστιν· ἐκ τούτων γὰρ τῶν δυοῖν ἡ φύσις συνέστηκεν). On this question see also den Dulk (1934) 75f.

[47] See Dittmer (1940) 76–80; and Müri (1953) 30 n. 11.

[48] See the remark made by Klibansky et al. (1964) 30: 'The natural melancholic, however, even when perfectly well, possessed a quite special "ethos", which, however it chose to manifest itself, made him fundamentally and permanently different from "ordinary" men; he was, as it were, normally abnormal.'

The remark about the strong desires of melancholics, with their resulting lack of discipline, is confirmed by the results so far.[49] Some final points of interest are Aristotle's remark about youth and the influence of physical growth on the human character (*ēthos*), as well as the comparison with drunks.[50] Aristotle uses youth and old age as typical examples to elucidate the close connection between mental and physical states (*Rh.* 2.12–13, in particular 1389 a 18–19 and b 29–32); and the use of these examples as an analogy for the 'character-affecting' influence (*to ēthopoion*) of the melancholic mixture will return in *Pr.* 30.1 (954 b 8–11).

4 BLACK BILE IN PHYSIOLOGY

We have seen that Aristotle credits the melancholics with several psychophysical and moral deviations or weaknesses, sometimes adding brief references to their physiological causes. Further details about this physiological basis can be found in the only passage entirely devoted to bile (*cholē*), in *Part. an.* 4.2. The chapter begins by listing animals which have bile and animals which do not.[51] Aristotle remarkably claims that not all people possess bile (676 b 31–2) and that, contrary to popular belief, bile is not the cause of acute diseases. So why does bile exist? According to Aristotle, bile is a residue (*perittōma*) without purpose (οὐχ ἕνεκά τινος), and although nature sometimes makes good use of residues, this does not imply that we should expect everything to have a purpose. After all, there are many things that are necessarily by-products of things that do serve a purpose, but are themselves without purpose. On bile as a *perittōma* Aristotle says a few lines further on (677 a 25): 'when the blood is not entirely pure, bile will be generated as a residue, for residue is the opposite of food'. Bile appears to be a 'purifying secretion' (*apokatharma*), which is confirmed by the saying in antiquity that people live longer if they do not have bile.

---

[49] The complication that in the discussion of lack of self-control melancholics were considered to be lacking in self-control, whereas the relevant passages (*Eth. Nic.* 1150 a 16ff.; 1150 b 29ff.) differentiate between *akrasia* and *akolasia* can be resolved by assuming that the difference is probably irrelevant in the other context.

[50] 'Likewise in youth, because of the process of growth, people are in a state similar to drunk, and youth is pleasant' (ὁμοίως δ' ἐν μὲν τῇ νεότητι διὰ τὴν αὔξησιν ὥσπερ οἱ οἰνωμένοι διάκεινται, καὶ ἡδὺ ἡ νεότης) (*Eth. Nic.* 1154 b 10–12).

[51] The question is whether J. Ogle (1910) is correct in translating *cholē* as 'gall bladder' and whether it should not be understood as 'bile' until later. The Greek text does not differentiate between the two. In *Part. an.* 676 b 11–13 Aristotle does differentiate between bile situated near the liver and bile that is situated in the other parts of the body (cf. 677 b 9–10), but it is possible that the former refers to the liquid in the gall bladder. [Cf. Lennox (2001) 288.]

It is not certain, but neither is it impossible, that the bile 'that is situated in the other parts of the body' (ἡ κατὰ τὸ ἄλλο σῶμα γινομένη [sc. χολή]) is black bile, as P. Louis suggests.[52] In any case this passage confirms the characterisation of black bile as a residue in *Somn. vig.* 457 a 31. This characterisation returns several times in Aristotle's writings on biology: *Part. an.* 649 a 26 (just bile), *Hist. an.* 511 b 10 (which mentions both black bile and yellow bile, together with phlegm (*phlegma*) and faeces (*kopros*); on phlegm as a *perittōma* cf. *Part. an.* 653 a 2, *Gen. an.* 725 a 15–16, *Pr.* 878 b 16 and *Somn. vig.* 458 a 3). The chapter in *Parts of Animals* clearly states that the residues are themselves without purpose, but that nature sometimes uses them for a good purpose.[53] This statement is complemented by *Gen. an.* 724 a 4ff., where Aristotle calls phlegm an example of those residues which can be of benefit to the body when combined with other substances, as opposed to the worthless residues that can even harm physical health.

This characterisation of yellow and black bile and phlegm[54] as *perittōmata* plays a pivotal part in the question whether Aristotle adopted the Hippocratic theory of the four humours.[55] It is clear that Aristotle knew both black and yellow bile,[56] as well as blood and phlegm. However, there is no indication that these fluids in any combination form a kind of humoral system similar to the theory of the four humours in *On the Nature of Man*; the only place where three are mentioned together (viz. yellow bile, black bile and phlegm) is in the above quoted *Hist. an.* 511 b 10, where they are listed as residues, together with faeces. This itself shows that it is unlikely that Aristotle assigned them a role as important bodily fluids on which human health depends. In addition, it should be pointed out that the notion of *perittōma* does not appear in the Hippocratic Corpus and was probably not introduced into Greek medicine until the second half of the fourth century BCE (perhaps by Aristotle himself, or by one of his students), after

---

[52] Louis (1956) 189 n. 5.
[53] On this remark and the use of the word καταχρῆται, see Preus (1975) 227–33.
[54] Bonitz's claim (1870; 586 b 17) that Aristotle considered blood as a *perittōma* as well is not confirmed by the two passages he cites (*Part. an.* 650 b 5; *Gen. an.* 738 a 8) and seems rather unlikely in view of the statements made in the chapter (*Part. an.* 2.3) that discusses the blood (650 a 34: 'It is evident that blood is the ultimate nourishment for animals that have blood'; b 2: 'blood is present in blooded animals for the purpose of nutrition'; b 12: 'blood is present for the purpose of nutrition and the nutriment of the parts').
[55] See Schöner (1964) 67. Cf. n. 10 above.
[56] With regard to yellow bile, see *Part. an.* 649 b 34, *De an.* 425 b 1 and *Metaph.* 1044 a 19. Aristotle uses the Hippocratic typology *phlegmatōdēs – cholōdēs* once, though not in a biological context (and in a passage of dubious authenticity: *Metaph.* 981 a 12). This typology occasionally occurs in the *Problemata* (860 a 27; 860 b 15; cf. 862 a 28).

which it began to play an important part in nosology.[57] Therefore, both in its thought and in its terminology the Aristotelian concept is such a far cry from the Hippocratic theory of four humours that one can hardly speak of Hippocratic *influence*.

We may conclude that the texts do not give detailed information on the physiological basis of Aristotle's use of the term *hoi melancholikoi*. Yet it seems clear that such a concept does exist in Aristotle's work: *hoi melancholikoi* are melancholics *by nature* (*tēn phusin*), that is, as a result of a physiological constitution, which, however, is diseased and permanently in need of a cure. It is impossible to say with certainty whether melancholics are characterised (1) by the very presence of black bile in them (for, as *Part. an.* 676 b 31–2 shows, not every human being has bile); (2) by the fact that the mixture of heat and cold in them is special and abnormal (*Eth. Nic.* 1154 b 13); (3) by the fact that black bile is localised in a particular part of the body, namely the heart (*Mem.* 453 a 24; cf. *Part. an.* 672 b 29); or (4) by the particularly high quantity of black bile in their body (if one interprets *krasis* in *Eth. Nic.* 1154 b 13 as a mixture of bodily fluids). This is probably due to the fact that Aristotle pays limited attention to medical matters when he writes in his capacity of *phusikos*: he only discusses the principles of health and disease, that is to say, the role of heat and cold in the body and the balance between them.[58] Consistent with this method and its consequent limitations is Aristotle's tendency to discuss medical views on anatomy and physiology occasionally, but without examining them systematically; any views he considers correct are reformulated in the terminology and concepts of his own philosophical system.[59] This obviously makes it even more

---

[57] See Thivel (1965) 266–82 (in particular 271) and Jouanna (1974) 507–8. Thivel states that in Aristotle, by contrast to the later Anonymus Londiniensis, the *perittōma* has not yet become a 'principe de maladie'. In fact, this notion can be found occasionally in the *Problemata* (e.g. 865 a 1; 884 a 23; 959 b 29), which Thivel apparently considers post-Aristotelian; however, it seems to appear as early as in *Somn. vig.* 457 a 2 and in *Gen. an.* 738 a 29. For the notion of *perittōma* in Aristotle see also *On Length and Shortness of Life* (*De longitudine et brevitate vitae*) 466 b 5–9 and Peck's Loeb edition of *On the Generation of Animals*, lxv–lxvii, as well as Harig (1977) 81–7.

[58] Cf. *Sens.* 436 a 17ff.; *Resp.* 480 b 22ff.; *Div. somn.* 463 a 5–7; see also the limiting remarks made in *Long. et brev. vitae* 464 b 32f. and *Part. an.* 653 a 10. [See also ch. 6 below.] Flashar (1962, 318) writes that Aristotle states about himself that he is not a medical expert and only considers medical questions from a philosophical or scientific point of view. However, the objection must be made that Aristotle's statement may well refer only to the methodical process employed in his writings on physics (*phusikē philosophia*, including his clearly planned but perhaps never written *On Health and Disease*). Aristotle may have discussed medical facts in greater detail elsewhere, for instance in the *Iatrika* which Diogenes Laertius (5.25) ascribes to him, or in his own *Problemata* (now lost). On this possibility see Marenghi (1961) 141–61 [and ch. 9 below].

[59] A clear example of this process is Aristotle's judgement on the use of dreams as a prognostic tool in *Div. somn.* 463 a 3–21, which he adopted from the 'distinguished physicians'. For a more extensive discussion of this passage see van der Eijk (1994) 271–80 [and ch. 6 below].

difficult to assess his dependence on sources in general and his attitude towards the Hippocratic writings in particular. For this reason, and in view of our limited knowledge of fourth-century medicine in general, it is virtually impossible to say anything with certainty on the sources of Aristotle's concept of melancholy. At any rate, there is no indication that Aristotle made a connection between the 'constitutional type' of the melancholic, well-known from the early writings of the Hippocratic Corpus, and the later, similarly Hippocratic embedding of black bile in the theory of the four humours of *On the Nature of Man* (which, after all, does not mention the melancholic type). In fact, the notion of melancholy as an abnormal predisposition and a disease, and the fact that black bile is considered a *perittōma*, makes any possible Hippocratic influence rather unlikely. The concept of the melancholic, with the associated psycho-physical and ethical characteristics seems to be a predominantly independent and genuine invention of Aristotelian philosophy.

5 THE THEORY ON MELANCHOLY IN *PROBLEMATA* 30.1

Let us proceed with the theory on melancholy and 'genius' in *Pr.* 30.1 mentioned at the beginning. In view of the extensive scholarly literature on this chapter[60] I will, rather than giving a summary, start with some interpretative observations that I consider of paramount importance for assessing the Aristotelian character of the theory. First of all, it should be said that I certainly do not intend to reinstate Aristotle as the *author* of this text: as far as the issue of the authorship of the *Problemata* is concerned I concur entirely with Hellmut Flashar's view (1962, 303–16) that the *Problemata* are most probably not the same as the *Problemata* that Aristotle wrote (or planned to write). What matters is to define the relationship between the theory elaborated in *Pr.* 30.1 and Aristotle's own views on melancholy more precisely, and to examine any possible reasons for ruling out Aristotle's views as a *source* for the selection made by the author of the *Problemata*.

With regard to the opening question, 'Why is it that all men who have made extraordinary achievements in the fields of philosophy or politics or poetry or the arts turn out to be melancholics?', scholars have long observed that this question contains part of its answer, for it states as a fact

---

[60] The works quoted in n. 1 above form the basis for the interpretation of the text, in particular the works by Flashar (1962), Klibansky et al. (1964) and Pigeaud (1988a). However, there are still numerous passages in this text that have not been fully explained in the existing interpretations. I will make some remarks on these in the footnotes.

the idea that *all* (*pantes*) 'extraordinary' (*perittoi*) men are melancholics. The subsequent discussion of the heroes Heracles, Aias and Bellerophontes and the poets and philosophers Empedocles, Socrates and Plato shows that the presupposition implied in the question is apparently based on a rather specific notion of melancholy. Epilepsy, bouts of ecstasy, prophetic powers, but also depressions, extreme fear of people, and suicidal inclinations are all attributed to the same disease.[61] It is very important here to establish clearly the actual aim of the author. Apparently, this aim lies first of all in the explanation that this attribution actually has a physiological justification, that is, that the very different, at times even contrasting characteristics of the melancholic are all based on one coherent physiological condition; secondly, the author intends to explain the in itself paradoxical connection between melancholy as a *disease* (953 a 13, 15: *arrōsthēma*; 16: *nosos*; 18: *helkē*; 29: *nosēmata*; 31: *pathē*) and the extraordinary political, philosophical and poetic achievements (*ta peritta*) by means of this physiological basis. This second aim has correctly been understood as readopting the Platonic theory of *mania*.[62] Yet whereas Plato, in his discussion on the origin of *mania*, distinguished between divine enthusiasm and pathological madness (*Phaedrus* 265 a), the Peripatetic discussion of this topic not only takes a much larger range of mental and physical afflictions into consideration, but also relates them all to one physical condition, and in the explanation all divine influence is disregarded (even without fierce opposition against this, as we find this in the Hippocratic writing *On the Sacred Disease* and in Aristotle's *On Divination in Sleep*[63]).

Answering the opening question of the chapter is in fact only attempted in the context of the second aim; the largest part of the text is devoted to answering the other question of why the ways in which melancholy manifests itself differ so much. The opening question is referred to on just two occasions: in 954 a 39–b 4 and, very briefly, in 954 b 27–8. This division is also followed in the structure of the final summary of the chapter (955 a 29ff.), which first recapitulates the explanation of the instability (*anōmalia*) and the variety of aspects to the nature of the melancholic character, followed by the summary of the explanation of the relationship

---

[61] On a number of occasions, although never in a systematic order, these features are indeed associated with melancholic diseases in the Hippocratic writings (see Müri (1953) and the commentary of Flashar (1962) on the particular occurrences).
[62] Flashar (1966) 62; Tellenbach (1961) 9; Klibansky et al. (1964) 17.
[63] See Tellenbach (1961) 10, Pigeaud (1988a) 51. Boyancé (1936, 191) presumes that a certain divine influence is implied in the role of the *pneuma*, yet there is no indication of this in the text of the chapter (on the role of the *pneuma* see n. 68 below).

Aristotle on melancholy

between melancholy and extraordinary achievement (36ff.).[64] The possible grounds for this arrangement will be discussed below.

The basis for achieving both aims lies in the fact that the author distinguishes between disease (*nosos, nosēma, arrōsthēma*) and natural disposition (*phusis*); in this respect it is striking that the 'natural melancholics' are also affected by 'melancholic diseases' and that they apparently are more prone to this than other people (953 a 12–15 and 29–31).[65] In 953 a 20 this *phusis* is referred to as a 'bodily mixture' (*krasis tōi sōmati*), more closely defined in 954 a 13 as a 'mixture of hot and cold'. To explain its effects, the author employs the analogy between the melancholic nature and wine (this analogy returns in statements made by Aristotle).[66] The objective of using this analogy is twofold: firstly, it is evidence for the fact that the physical condition of people not only influences their state of mind, but it can also

---

[64] It seems that scholars have hardly recognised the problem in the last sentence (955 a 36–40; see translation below). Müri (1953, 25) only implicitly alludes to it when he states 'indem die Disposition da, wo es not tut (z.B. in der Furcht), wärmer ist, und da, wo es not tut, kälter ...'. The text says: ἐπεὶ δ' ἔστι καὶ εὔκρατον εἶναι τὴν ἀνωμαλίαν καὶ καλῶς πως ἔχειν, καὶ ὅπου δεῖ θερμοτέραν εἶναι τὴν διάθεσιν καὶ πάλιν ψυχράν, ἢ τοὐναντίον διὰ τὸ ὑπερβολὴν ἔχειν, περιττοὶ μέν εἰσι πάντες οἱ μελαγχολικοί, οὐ διὰ νόσον, ἀλλὰ διὰ φύσιν. As the author presents this sentence as a summary of something previously discussed, the question arises what καὶ ὅπου δεῖ refers to, for in this sentence the *eukrasia* that underlies the melancholic's *peritton* does not seem to be referring to a balance of heat and cold (as in 954 b 1), but to a certain ability to *adapt* this balance to the conditions required by each individual situation (*hopou dei*). There is, however, no parallel for such a flexibility in the prior treatise. Significant in this context are the differences between the translations of Klibansky et al. (1964) ('since it is possible for this variable mixture to be well tempered and well adjusted in a certain respect – that is to say, to be now in a warmer and then again a colder condition, or vice versa, just as required, owing to its tendency to extremes – therefore ...') and Flashar (1962) ('Da es aber auch möglich ist, dass die Ungleichmässigkeit gut gemischt sein und sich in gewisser Weise richtig verhalten kann, und, wo es nötig ist, unser Zustand wärmer und wieder kalt ist oder umgekehrt, weil er [bestimmte Eigenschaften] in Übermass besitzt, deshalb ...'). Klibansky et al. interpret the text as an explication ('that is to say') whereas Flashar apparently sees this as an analogy ('*unser* Zustand'). Another difficulty here is the interpretation of διὰ τὴν ὑπερβολὴν ἔχειν: what would this 'surfeit' precisely be? And what exactly does it explain? – Finally, a difference between the opening question and the final sentence should be noted: at the beginning all *perittoi* were said to be melancholics, but at the end the author writes that all melancholics are *perittoi*. This contradiction could only be solved by understanding *perittos* here in the final sentence as a neutral notion and therefore synonymous with *ektopos* ('eccentric'). This is to a certain extent justified by the fact that no specification as to the precise field (ἢ φιλοσοφίαν κτλ.) is presented in this passage. However, as the causal subclause refers to a healthy balance (*eukraton*), *perittos* must be understood in a positive sense. I do not see a solution to these problems (cf. the explanations by Pigeaud (1988a) 127).

[65] See Tellenbach (1961) 9; Pigeaud (1988a) 42–3. At first sight it seems that 953 a 29–31 speaks about a difference between 'disease' (*nosēma*) and 'nature' (*phusis*), but in fact it says that many melancholics actually get melancholy-related diseases, while others are only very prone to getting these disorders. Nevertheless, as the next sentence shows, both groups belong to the 'natural melancholics' (*phusei melancholikoi*).

[66] *Insomn*. 461 a 22; *Eth. Nic.* 1154 b 10; cf. also the role of drunkenness as an analogy in the treatise about lack of self-control (1147 a 13–14; 1147 b 7, 12; 1152 a 15).

to a large extent determine it (the so-called 'character-affecting aspect', *to ēthopoion*, of human physiology, 953 a 35; cf. Pigeaud (1988a) 25ff.). Secondly, it explains that wine, depending on the quantity consumed, has the ability to provoke very *different* (*pantodapous*, 953 a 38) and even contrasting states of mind. In 953 b 17 this analogy is applied to the problem of melancholy: both wine and the melancholic nature 'affect character', yet the difference is that wine does so only occasionally and for a brief period of time, whereas the melancholic nature does so permanently and persistently (*aei*). For some people are aggressive, taciturn or sentimental by nature – they are in a state of mind that affects other people only occasionally and for a brief period of time, under the influence of wine. Yet in both cases the cause of this *ēthopoion* remains the same: it is the heat that controls[67] the body and causes the development of breath (*pneuma*) (the connection between heat and breath is made again in 955 a 35).[68] In the ensuing passage the breath-containing properties of wine and black bile, as well as aphrodisiacs, are discussed. In 954 a 11, the author returns to the notion of the melancholic nature: his remark that black bile is a mixture of heat and cold (954 a 13) ties in with line 953 b 22, but it also allows him to continue his train of thought, as this mixture is said to allow for variation: although black bile is cold by nature (954 a 21; cf. *Somn. vig.* 457 a 31), it can be heated and invoke various states of mind, depending on the mixture of heat and cold (954 a 28–30: ὅσοις δὲ ἐν τῇ φύσει συνέστη κρᾶσις τοιαύτη, εὐθὺς οὗτοι τὰ ἤθη γίνονται παντοδαποί, ἄλλος κατ' ἄλλην κρᾶσιν): this way, the second objective of the analogy with wine is met.[69] Those in whom cold predominates are numb and obtuse, yet those in whom heat predominates get beside themselves (*manikoi*),[70] or they become astute, horny or prone

---

[67] Flashar's translation 'all dies nämlich wird durch die Veränderung des Wärmehaushaltes bewirkt' does not do justice to the use of ταμιεύεσθαι (cf. 954 a 14; 955 a 32–3).

[68] As to the role of *pneuma*, cf. Klibansky et al. (1964) 30: 'In this "pneuma" there dwells a singularly stimulating driving-force which sets the whole organism in a state of tension (*orexis*), strongly affects the mind and tries, above all in sexual intercourse, literally "to vent itself"; hence both the aphrodisiac effect of wine and the lack of sexual restraint, proper, in the author's view, to the man of melancholic temperament.' On *pneuma* as physiological principle of movement cf. *Somn. vig.* 456 a 7ff.

[69] This paragraph also gives further information on the physiology of the melancholic: the typical feature of the melancholic is apparently not the mixture of heat and cold within the black bile (as might be concluded from 954 a 13), for this balance may vary. Rather, the typical feature is that he has an excess of black bile by nature, as 954 a 22–3 shows.

[70] Flashar states that the word *manikos* cannot be right here, as it is indicated in line 36 'as a further increase' of the heat and as it does not fit well with the other predicates. Against the latter it has to be said that the combination of *manikos* and *euphuēs* (curiously translated 'gutmütig' by Flashar) is known from *Poet.* 1455 a 32 and *Rh.* 1390 b 28. As to the former difficulty, it should be noted that 35–6 does not speak about 'a further increase' at all: in fact it deals again with those

Aristotle on melancholy 159

to mood changes and desires, and some become more talkative. Those, however, who have reached a 'mean' (*meson*) in the mixture between heat and cold, come closer to reason and are less abnormal. They are the people who have reached outstanding achievements in the arts, culture and politics (954 a 39–b 4). Thus here for the first time, the opening question of the chapter is answered. However, and this is very important, it is striking that this conclusion is immediately followed by the remark that this balance of heat and cold is uncertain and unstable (*anōmalos*). The author repeats this remark later, in 954 b 26–8 (after a digression). This is followed by interesting and rather elaborate observations on *euthumia* and *dusthumia* as the effects of excessive heat and cold of the black bile, and on the melancholic's inclination to commit suicide. Here, too, the analogy with wine is made, and a second analogy, with youth and old age, is added.[71] The chapter ends with the summary discussed above (see note 64).

With regard to the physiological disposition of the melancholic this chapter reveals precisely those details on which the scattered remarks in the Aristotelian writings did not allow us to gain full clarity. It appears that the 'natural melancholic' is characterised by an excess of black bile in his body which is constantly and permanently present (954 a 22–3: ἐὰν ὑπερβάλλῃ ἐν τῷ σώματι; and Klibansky et al. (1964) 29). This does not mean, however, that underlying this text is the humoral system of the Hippocratic theory of the four humours, for a mixture of *humours* is nowhere mentioned: wherever the word *krasis* is used (953 a 30; 954 a 13, 29, 30; 954 b 8, 12, 25, 33; 955 a 14) it refers to a mixture of heat and cold.[72] The place where black bile can normally be found is not defined; only the presence of heat near the 'place where thinking takes place' (*noeros topos*) is mentioned

---

disorders of the black bile that are *not* constitution-related (hence the word *nosēmata*), which are contrasted with the cases of Sibyls and Bakides and such people who are not enthusiastic because of a *nosēma*, but as a consequence of their *phusis*. Both the *polloi* and the other group suffer from heat (*thermotēs*) around the 'region where thinking takes place' (*noeros topos*) (this is what *hothen* refers to); yet with the *polloi* it is not nature but illness, whereas with the other group (Sibyls, Bakides and the 'naturally inspired') it is nature. That this is the correct interpretation is shown by the sentence ὅταν μὴ νοσήματι γένωνται, for in Flashar's interpretation this sentence would be a negation of what was confirmed in line 35. Cf. Tellenbach (1961) 9 and Pigeaud (1988a) 41–2 on this interpretation.

[71] On youth and old age as 'ethopoietic' factors cf. *Rh.* 2.12–13 and the remark on youth in *Eth. Nic.* 1154 b 9–11.

[72] See above section 3 on *Eth. Nic.* 1154 b 13 and Pigeaud (1988a) 19. Incidentally, the fact that Aristotle refers to black bile as a *perittōma* in the chapter from the *Probl.* is unparalleled (the term *perittōma* is only used in 955 a 24–5, but in that passage without referring to black bile). Therefore Pigeaud's association of the *peritton* of the melancholic with the *perittōma* of black bile is not to the point (1988, 20: 'L'homme exceptionnel est l'homme du résidu par excellence').

(954 a 34ff.),[73] yet this seems to leave room for the possibility of bile being in other places (cf. *Somn. vig.* 457 a 33). The lack of clarity as to whether the defining feature of melancholics is cold (*Somn. vig.* 457 a 31) or heat (*Part. an.* 672 b 29; and implicitly (probably) the passages on recklessness and lack of self-control from *Eth. Nic.* 7) is solved here by attributing to black bile the possibility of great changes in temperature (954 a 14–15: διὸ καὶ ἡ μέλαινα χολὴ καὶ θερμότατον καὶ ψυχρότατον γίνεται). Lastly, the question whether *melancholikos* characterises the human *phusis* or the human *ēthos* receives an answer here, which is: both; for melancholics appear to illustrate how the human character is influenced by the physiological constitution. The text of the *Problemata* uses the term *ēthopoios*, 'affecting character', to describe this influence.

6 THE ARISTOTELIAN CHARACTER OF THE THEORY IN THE *PROBLEMATA*

When considering the Aristotelian character of the theory presented in this chapter, it should first of all be said that whereas the psycho-physical and moral features of melancholics that Aristotle mentions do not occur in the exact same words in the text of the *Problemata*, most of them easily fit into the theory. The melancholic's sensitivity to a large number of movements and images, repeatedly discussed in the *Parva naturalia* and *Eudemian Ethics*, and the resulting divination in sleep can readily be related to the effects of heat in the melancholic nature as mentioned in 954 a 31–8. The use of the example of the melancholic in the context of lack of self-control and physical lust (*Nicomachean Ethics*) in the *Problemata* theory could equally be understood as an expression of a mixture of black bile dominated by heat (954 a 33: καὶ εὐκίνητοι πρὸς τοὺς θυμοὺς καὶ τὰς ἐπιθυμίας). However, it cannot be denied that the chapter in the *Problemata* relates the melancholic nature to a much larger number and variety of mental and physical afflictions (as shown above); in addition, an important question is whether there are elements in this process which cannot be reconciled with Aristotle's statements (see below).

Secondly, it should be noted that the author of the text apparently is very well informed about Aristotle's statements on melancholy, and even seems to make an effort to take the Aristotelian concept into account

---

[73] Cf. *Mem.* 453 b 23–4, which mentions the presence of black bile around the 'perceptive region' (*aisthētikos topos*, i.e. the heart, which to Aristotle is also the 'place where thinking takes place', *noeros topos*). [See also ch. 4 and ch. 7, p. 224.]

wherever possible. The thoughts that are expressed and sometimes even their literal wording show a number of parallels with Aristotelian writings.[74] However, as this applies to many parts of the *Problemata*, the fact in itself does not substantiate the claim that Aristotle would have adopted the whole theory (as Croissant argues (1932) 78–9), and neither does the use of the typical Aristotelian notion of the mean (*mesotēs*), long recognised by scholars, in the explanation of the melancholics' 'extraordinariness' (*perittōn*).[75]

It seems more important to examine the reasons that have been given to demonstrate that the Aristotelian concept of melancholy cannot be reconciled with the theory presented in *Pr.* 30.1. Some scholars claim[76] that Aristotle only speaks about melancholics in terms of their deviations (considering them pathological or plainly negative), and that in his view a melancholic is ill *by nature* and needs to be cured. This would be irreconcilable with the characterisation of melancholics as 'extraordinary' (*perittoi*) in the respectable fields of philosophy, politics and poetry. However, this negative assessment corresponds to the idea – which is expressed frequently in the chapter from the *Problemata* – that melancholics are 'abnormal' or 'deviant' (*ektopoi*) *by nature*.[77] It is true to say that Aristotle does not refer to the extraordinary achievements of melancholics, apart from their 'clear dreams' (*euthuoneiria*), which, however, are not related to the *peritton* in the field of philosophy or politics;[78] but this is in line with the view expressed in *Pr.* 30.1, that the extraordinary achievements of melancholics are an *exception* rather than a rule. As stated above, the chapter is largely devoted to explaining the diversity and variety of expressions of the melancholic nature. The opening question is merely touched upon and the author seems

---

[74] Most of the parallels have been listed in Flashar's notes. The complete list of all occurrences is: 953 b 23–6 ∼ *Insomn.* 461 a 23–5; 953 b 27–30 ∼ *Somn. vig.* 457 a 16–17; 953 b 33–954 a 4 ∼ *Gen. an.* 728 a 10ff. and 736 a 19; 954 a 2 ∼ *Hist. an.* 586 a 16; 954 a 7 ∼ *Somn. vig.* 457 a 29; 954 a 18–20 ∼ *Part. an.* 648 b 34ff.; 954 a 21–2 ∼ *Somn. vig.* 457 a 31; 954 a 32 ∼ *Div. somn.* 463 b 17 and *Rh.* 1390 b 28; 954 a 34–6 ∼ *Part. an.* 672 b 28–33; 954 b 13 ∼ *Part. an.* 650 b 27 and 692 a 23 as well as *Rh.* 1389 b 29ff.; 954 b 39–40 ∼ *Eth. Eud.* 1229 a 20; 955 a 3 ∼ *Eth. Eud.* 1229 a 20; 955 a 4 ∼ *Rh.* 1389 a 19ff. and *Eth. Nic.* 1154 b 9ff.; 955 a 22–9 ∼ *Gen. an.* 725 b 6–18; 955 a 25–8 ∼ *Gen. an.* 783 b 29–30.
[75] Müri (1953) 24–6; Klibansky et al. (1964) 33–6.
[76] Flashar (1962) 713; Klibansky et al. (1964) 37.
[77] 954 b 2 (ἧττον ἔκτοποι); 954 b 26 (ἀνόμοιοι τοῖς πολλοῖς). Cf. the remark quoted above in n. 48 made by Klibansky et al. (1964) and their observations on the word *perittos* (31).
[78] The gift of divination in sleep which melancholics possess is not mentioned at all in *Pr.* 30.1, but in view of the remarks on enthusiasm in 954 a 35–6, the author would certainly categorise it among the 'manic' expressions of the melancholic blend, i.e. those caused by excessive heat; it would not be related to the *peritton* that is close to the 'intelligence' (*phronēsis*) and based on the 'mean' (*meson*) of heat and cold. In *Div. somn.* 464 b 2–3 the melancholics are compared to 'people who are possessed' (οἱ ἐμμανεῖς) because of their *euthuoneiria*. Cf. Klibansky et al. (1964) 37.

to use it as a starting point for a discussion on the instability (*anōmalia*) of the melancholic nature rather than for any other purpose.[79] In addition, the text explicitly states that the physiological balance which forms the basis of extraordinary achievements is uncertain and unstable.[80] These two facts underline the exceptional nature of the melancholic *peritton*; they clearly show that this notion was apparently considered a negligible factor and as such played no part in Aristotle's theory of virtue, and as a philosophically insignificant empirical phenomenon was only discussed in a text such as the *Problemata*.[81]

The fact that the medical observations that are so typical of the *Problemata* are absent from Aristotle's statements on melancholics and the fact that Aristotle only discusses the 'manic' or 'passionate' expressions of melancholy (Flashar (1962) 713) therefore do not, in my opinion, have any implication for the relationship between Aristotle and *Pr.* 30.1. The difference in objectives between these texts, and in particular Aristotle's fundamentally limited interest in medical issues in his works on natural science (and *a fortiori* those on ethics), seem largely to explain this lack of balance or at least make it understandable. In Aristotle's work, the number of passages in which the 'manic' expressions of the melancholic nature are worth mentioning as illustrative examples (for instance contexts that mention its sensitivity to desires and passions) outnumber the passages that would be suitable for mentioning its 'depressive' manifestations. On a total of nine occurrences, this might prove a sufficient explanation. In addition, it should be noted that Aristotle fully takes into account the effects of cold that are typical to melancholy, as is shown in *Somn. vig.* 457 a 31 (i.e. disregarding *Mag. mor.* 1203 b 1, which is probably not written by Aristotle and therefore does not constitute proof).

The most important reason for any irreconcilability between Aristotle's view on melancholy and the theory presented in *Pr.* 30.1 has so far been given little attention by scholars. This reason would be that Aristotle denies

---

[79] This observation is very much in accordance with the fact that the structure of the text differs greatly from the other *Problemata*. Similarly, it fits in well with the suggestion (see Flashar (1962) 711, 714; Flashar (1966) 61; Müri (1953) 21) that this chapter consists of an editorial combination of a typical *Problemata* question and an excerpt of a treatise on melancholy, in which answering the question posed at the start of the chapter was perhaps not the main objective of the author. For a different explanation for the structure of this chapter see section 7 below.

[80] Tellenbach (1961, 9) correctly states that these *perittoi* are characterised by an above-average instability.

[81] In this respect the *peritton* of melancholics can be compared to the phenomenon of *eutuchia*, discussed in *Eth. Eud.* 8.2 (see ch. 8 below), with divination in sleep as discussed in *On Divination in Sleep* (see ch. 6 below) [and the *peritton* mentioned in *Part. an.* 4.10, 686 b 26]. Although Aristotle considers both to be results of experience, they play no part in his ethics and psychology, perhaps because of their uncontrollable nature and instability.

melancholics the ability of deliberation and rational thought (see the passages from *Nicomachean Ethics* and *Eudemian Ethics*), and that he attributes their special mental ability (divination in dreams) only to the fact that for some reason their reasoning faculty is inactive or powerless (*On Divination in Sleep* and *Eudemian Ethics*): as a result they are classified in these texts under the group of 'simple-minded people', as opposed to the 'best and most intelligent'. This seems to be in stark contrast to the thought expressed in *Pr.* 30.1, namely that the *peritton* of melancholics is connected to reason (954 b 1: φρονιμώτεροι δέ), for without this connection it would in Aristotelian terms have been impossible to apply the *peritton* in the fields of philosophy, politics and poetry, which in Aristotle's view are unthinkable without reason (*phronēsis*). It is impossible to see how Aristotle's statements are supposed to tie in with the existence of a 'wise melancholic' (*melancholikos sophos*) as recognised in the chapter from the *Problemata* (cf. the references to Socrates, Plato and Empedocles).

However, apart from the exceptional nature of the melancholic *peritton* and the fact that the *euthuoneiria* of melancholics is unrelated to this (see note 78), the text in the *Problemata* does in fact allow for some positive remarks on this contradiction. The way in which the relevant passage in the chapter is phrased shows that the author was apparently aware of the fact that the connection between *phronēsis* and melancholy implies a paradox in an Aristotelian context. To quote the passage: 'All those, however, in whom the excessive heat is moderated towards a mean, these people are, to be sure, melancholics, but they are more intelligent, and they are, to be sure, less eccentric, but different from the others in many aspects, some in culture, others etc.' (ὅσοις δ' ἂν ἐπανεθῇ τὴν ἄγαν θερμότητα πρὸς τὸ μέσον, οὗτοι μελαγχολικοὶ μέν εἰσι, φρονιμώτεροι δέ, καὶ ἧττον μὲν ἔκτοποι, πρὸς πολλὰ δέ διαφέροντες τῶν ἄλλων, οἱ μὲν πρὸς παιδείαν, οἱ δὲ κτλ.).[82] The use of μέν...δέ ('to be sure...but') and the comparatives may well indicate that the author was aware of the paradoxical nature of his statement: *although* they are melancholics, *yet* they are relatively close to reason; *although* they are less abnormal, *yet* they are outstanding. The comparatives φρονιμώτεροι and ἧττον show that these people are not rational and normal *per se* (that would really contradict Aristotle's statements), but only in comparison to other melancholics (or to those moments when their own balance between hot and cold, which is after all unstable, is disturbed or absent). They are not really 'intelligent', but

---

[82] For this reading (instead of the transmitted but incomprehensible ἐπανθῇ) see Klibansky et al. (1964) 24 n. 58; Flashar (1962) 720; Müri (1953) 25 n. 5 (against Pigeaud (1988a) 123).

only closer to reason than other melancholics; they remain 'eccentric' (for melancholics are *fundamentally* abnormal), but to a lesser degree than other melancholics; yet rather than implying that they are similar to ordinary people, it means that they distinguish themselves from other people, but this time in a positive rather than a negative sense. The sentence is construed in such a way that each clause, so to speak, corrects a possible implication of the previous one, and this construal may well be interpreted as an explicit acknowledgement of Aristotle's concept of melancholy.

As to the question about where to place the melancholic *peritton* in Aristotle's theory of virtue, little can be said with any certainty, due to a lack of explicit statements on the subject. However, a good starting-point for the debate would be the principle on which the discussion in the chapter of the *Problemata* is built, namely that of the *ēthopoion* of the *phusis*, the influence which the human *phusis* (in the sense of a 'natural predisposition' and a 'physiological constitution') exerts on the formation of the human character. It is a fact that the role of nature as a condition or prerequisite for man's moral and cognitive behaviour in Aristotle's ethics and psychology is limited.[83] On the other hand, Aristotle repeatedly recognises and refers to the importance of a physiological balance (an *eukrasia* between heat and cold in the body) for the proper functioning of sensory perception, practical deliberation and intellectual thought; the typical notion of *mesotēs* (which is derived from physiology) plays an important part here.[84] The effect of physical conditions on the psychological and moral state is usually only mentioned in a negative context, namely that of disorders resulting from a lack of physiological balance: the fact that melancholics are repeatedly mentioned in the *Ethics* and the *Parva naturalia* can be explained by the fact that they are particularly suitable for illustrating these negative effects of the physiological constitution, as they lack this balance *by nature* (see Tracy (1969) 226–7, 256). However, this example implies that what disturbs melancholics on a permanent basis can occur to every person occasionally and periodically (hence the analogy with wine and drunkenness).

Yet the effect of nature in these areas can also manifest itself in a positive way, in outstanding expressions of a special predisposition, which cannot be achieved in what Aristotle considers the usual way, namely by force of habit (*ethismos* or *askēsis*) and teaching (*didachē* or *mathēsis*). To describe this special predisposition and its expression in 'particularly mental shrewdness',

[83] See the general statements on this theme in *Eth. Nic.* 10.9, *Eth. Nic.* 2.1 and *Eud. Eth.* 1.1, as well as Gigon (1971) 100ff.; Gigon (1985) 135–8; Verbeke (1985) 247–58.
[84] Of fundamental importance on this theme is the work by Tracy (1969) in particular 197–282.

Aristotle frequently uses the word *euphuia*. An illuminating example of this notion is Aristotle's frequent reference to metaphors; see the remark in the *Poetics* (1459 a 5–7), 'The most important thing is the ability to use metaphors. For this is the only thing that cannot be learned from someone else and a sign of natural genius; for to produce good metaphors is a matter of perceiving similarities' (πολὺ δὲ μέγιστον τὸ μεταφορικὸν εἶναι· μόνον γὰρ τοῦτο οὔτε παρ' ἄλλου ἐστὶ λαβεῖν εὐφυίας τε σημεῖόν ἐστι· τὸ γὰρ εὖ μεταφέρειν τὸ τὸ ὅμοιον θεωρεῖν ἐστιν). Other passages on this feature of metaphor (its being incapable of being taught) can be found in *Rhetoric* (1405 a 8) and *Poet.* 1455 a 29ff., which states that the best poet is either a genius (*euphuēs*) or a madman (*manikos*; cf. *Pr.* 954 a 32). Aristotle explains his use of the word *euphuia* in this passage in the *Poetics* (1459 a 7) by saying that good use of metaphor is based on the ability 'to see similarities' (*to homoion theōrein*). This corresponds to the fact that Aristotle (as discussed above in section 2 ad *Div.* 464 a 32ff.) relates the *eustochia* of melancholics to this very principle: therefore this passage, too, shows the connection between the ability to perceive similarities and a special natural predisposition.

It seems to be this connection that enables the melancholic *peritton* in the areas of philosophy, politics and poetry. For to Aristotle, the principle of 'perceiving similarities' not only plays a part in the use of metaphor[85] and in divination in sleep, but also in several intellectual activities such as induction, definition and indeed philosophy itself.[86] It recognises relevant similarities (both similar properties and similar relations and structures) that are not evident or noticeable to everyone, and as such it is able to see relationships between matters that are far apart.[87] The explicit connection of this principle with a targeted approach led by intuition (*eustochia*, *Rh.* 1412 a 12) and a special predisposition (*euphuia*, *Poet.* 1459 a 7) indicates that the *peritton* of melancholics in the areas mentioned should be sought in a certain intuition and creativity which does not impede reason, but rather enhances it, with *phantasia* playing an important mediatory role.[88]

At first it seemed peculiar that the great philosophers Plato, Socrates and Empedocles are taken as examples of the 'extraordinary melancholics'

---

[85] See Bremer (1980) 350–76; Swiggers (1984) 40–5.
[86] Cf. *Rh.* 1394 a 5; 1412 a 10 (with the use of the word *eustochia*); *Top.* 108 a 7–14; 108 b 7, 24; *Metaph.* 981 a 7. On the principle see Lambert (1966) 169–85.
[87] *Rh.* 1412 a 12: τὸ ὅμοιον ἐν πολὺ διέχουσι θεωρεῖν; *Top.* 108 b 21: ἐν τοῖς πολὺ διεστῶσι χρήσιμος πρὸς τοὺς ὁρισμοὺς ἡ τοῦ ὁμοίου θεωρία.
[88] See Tracy (1969), *passim* (in particular 261–4).

(*Pr.* 953 a 27), but in this interpretation this becomes more easy to understand: *phusis* presents Aristotle with a possibility to explain the fact that a certain creativity is required in the intellectual area of philosophy as well, and that in this respect there is a difference between great minds (the *perittoi*) and average minds (the *mesoi*, cf. *Pr.* 954 b 24). This explanation is actually used in the text of the *Problemata*, but can also be found in several short statements in Aristotle's authentic writings. A direct relationship between bodily constitution and intelligence is for instance made in *De. an.* 421 a 23ff., where Aristotle states that people with soft flesh (*malakosarkoi*) are more intelligent (*euphueis*) than people with hard flesh (*sklērosarkoi*); and in two instances in *Parts of Animals* (648 a 2ff. and 650 b 18ff.), where he writes that the quality of the blood determines the degree of intelligence. In this respect chapters 12–15 of the second book of the *Rhetoric* are of particular importance, in which the 'ethopoietic' effects of youth and old age and 'noble descent' (*eugeneia*) are discussed; in particular chapter 15 on *eugeneia* (with its clear relationship to *phusis* in the sense of a 'natural predisposition') is significant. Melancholics are not mentioned in this passage, but it demonstrates precisely the same thought structure as that used to describe melancholics: most of the people of noble descent (*eugeneis*) belong to the category of 'the simple-minded' (*euteleis*, 1390 b 24; cf. the use of melancholics as an example of *euteleis* in *Div. somn.* 463 b 17), but some become 'exceptional' (*perittoi*): 'There is a change in the generations of men as in those who move from one place to another, and sometimes the generation is good, and during certain intervals the men are exceptional, and then they decline again' (φορὰ γάρ τίς ἐστιν ἐν τοῖς γένεσιν ἀνδρῶν ὥσπερ ἐν τοῖς κατὰ τὰς χώρας γιγνομένοις, καὶ ἐνίοτε ἂν ᾖ ἀγαθὸν τὸ γένος, ἐγγίνονται διά τινος χρόνου ἄνδρες περιττοί, κἄπειτα πάλιν ἀναδίδωσιν).

In this passage, similarly to the melancholic's 'instability', reference is made to the quick decline of the *eugeneis*, either to 'those who are by character more inclined to madness' (examples for this are the descendants of Alcibiades and Dionysus) or to stupidity and obtuseness (ἀβελτερία καὶ νωθρότης; 1390 b 27–30). It appears that these two forms of degeneration correspond very well with both the 'manic-passionate' and 'depressive-cold' expressions of the melancholic nature in *Pr.* 30.1 (see in particular 954 b 28–34).

A consideration of the physiological aspect to people's mental processes and ethical behaviour, as is done frequently in the *Problemata*,[89] turns out

---

[89] On this tendency of the *Problemata,* which is sometimes unfortunately referred to as 'materialistic', see Flashar (1962) 329ff.

to be an approach that Aristotle fully recognises and which he provides with a methodological foundation; it is by no means incompatible with the more 'psychological' approach demonstrated in particular in the *Ethics*, and Aristotle considers it rather as complementary.[90] Explaining deviations in the domain of the psyche, whether they are valued as positive or negative, by pointing to an equally deviant physiological state can very well be considered a consequence of Aristotle's conviction that psyche and body are closely connected.

7 CONCLUSION

It has transpired that the theory of *Pr.* 30.1 corresponds quite well to the Aristotelian concept of melancholy and that there are insufficient grounds to claim that Aristotle did not support this theory. Whether the text of the chapter goes back to a treatise on melancholy that may have been part of Aristotle's lost *Problemata* or whether it goes back to an attempt made by a later Peripatetic (perhaps Theophrastus)[91] to systematise the scattered statements of the Master, will remain unknown. In any case, our analysis of the chapter, in particular of the author's two different objectives, and of the prima facie disproportionate discussion of these objectives, has shown that it is *possible* to read the text as a deliberate attempt to explain an observation that would at first sight be unthinkable in Aristotle's philosophy (i.e. the *peritton* of melancholics in intellectual areas) – an attempt which is achieved by means of statements on melancholy and psycho-physiology

---

[90] For further examples of this consideration see Tracy (1969) 247–61. For the methodological basis see *De an.* 403 a 3–b 16 and Tracy (1969) 247ff. and 224 n. 80, as well as Sorabji (1974) 63–89.

[91] No argument can be made for ascribing this theory to Theophrastus; virtually nothing is known about the views of Theophrastus on melancholy and enthusiasm. Ascription can only be based on the statement in 954 a 20–1 (εἴρηται δὲ σαφέστερον περὶ τούτων ἐν τοῖς περὶ πυρός) and the fact that Diogenes Laertius (5.44) says that Theophrastus has written a treatise 'On Melancholy' (περὶ μελαγχολίας). The former argument has proved to be rather weak: as Flashar (1962, 671) must admit, the statement is not really in line with Theophrastus' writing *De igne*. One might point to chapter 35, but precisely at the relevant point the text of the passage is uncertain, and even if one accepts Gercke's conjecture ⟨διὸ καὶ τοιαῦτα θερμότατα⟩ τὰ πυρωθέντα καθάπερ σίδηρος, the parallel is not very specific (σαφέστερον). The statement would make more sense as a reference to a lost book on fire in the *Problemata* (see Flashar (1962) 671) or the Aristotelian treatment of heat and fire in *Part. an.* 648 b 34ff. (although the phrase ἐν τοῖς περὶ πυρός is more likely to refer to a separate treatise; cf. Croissant (1932) 78). Yet even if one is prepared to accept the statement as referring to Theophrastus' *De igne*, there is the possibility that the Peripatetic editor/compilator of the *Problemata* collection is responsible for this, and it need not imply that the theory presented in the chapter is originally from Theophrastus (see Flashar (1956) 45 n. 3). – With respect to the title περὶ μελαγχολίας, it should be noted that the word μελαγχολία does not appear in the text of the chapter of the *Problemata*: only μελαγχολικὴ φύσις, μελαγχολικὴ κρᾶσις, μέλαινα χολή and μελαγχολικὸς χυμός are mentioned. These terms correspond to Aristotle's usage, whereas the word μελαγχολία reminds one either of the Hippocratic names for melancholic diseases (for instance *Airs, Waters, Places* 10, 12; 52, 7 Diller) or of Theophrastus' theory on character.

made by Aristotle himself. This way, the explanation of the *anōmalia* and the variety of expressions of the melancholic nature serves to answer the chapter's opening question, which at the end should not look quite so un-Aristotelian (and indeed no longer does) as at the start. In any event, as the theory of *Pr.* 30.1 has proved to depend strongly on Aristotle's own statements on melancholics, it has become much less isolated within the history of ideas.

Finally, this chapter should hopefully provide a starting-point for a renewed testing of the working hypothesis that those parts of the *Problemata* that have been passed on to us can be used as testimonies of Aristotle's views, on the understanding that these passages do not contradict the authentic texts.[92] Obviously, one single piece of research does not suffice to prove the value of this hypothesis in general, and further study into the so far too neglected *Problemata* is required.

---

[92] When examining this working hypothesis, the other scattered statements on melancholics in the *Problemata* should be taken into account as well (1.12; 3.25a; 4.30; 11.38; 18.1 and 7; 30.14). These occurrences do not really seem to contradict the statements made by Aristotle (perhaps with the exception of 860 b 21ff., which is difficult to reconcile with *Part. an.* 676 b 5ff.). The characteristics of the melancholic mentioned are partly affirmative (4.30: strong drive for sexual intercourse), and partly supplementary to the characteristics mentioned by Aristotle, and the physiological explanations can be reconciled with Aristotle's statements very well (11.38: 'following one's imagination'; 18.1 and 7 as well as 4.30: connection with *pneuma*; 30.14: very strong movement of the soul). However, only an in-depth analysis of these at times very difficult passages can more clearly define the precise relationship with Aristotle's concept. For the moment, the brief yet valuable remarks made by Flashar (1962) 303ff. and Marenghi's (1966) commentary on the medical problems should be noted. For a rather sceptical view on the working hypothesis see Flashar (1962) 303 and 315.

CHAPTER 6

Theoretical and empirical elements in Aristotle's treatment of sleep, dreams and divination in sleep

1 PRE-ARISTOTELIAN VIEWS ON SLEEP AND DREAMS

'Anyone who has a correct understanding of the signs that occur in sleep, will discover that they have great significance for everything.'[1] This is the opening sentence of the fourth book of the Hippocratic work *On Regimen*, a treatise dating probably from the first half of the fourth century BCE and dealing with the interpretation of dreams from a medical point of view, that is, as signs pointing to the (future) state of the body of the dreamer.[2] The passage reflects the general opinion in ancient Greece that dreams are of great importance as 'signs' (*sēmeia*) or 'indications' (*tekmēria*), not only of the physical constitution of the dreamer and of imminent diseases or mental disturbances befalling him/her, but also of divine intentions, of things that may happen in the future, things hidden to normal human understanding.[3] Dreams played an important part in Greek divination and religion, especially in the healing cult of Asclepius, because they were believed to contain important therapeutic indications or even to bring about healing themselves.[4] The belief in the divine origin of dreams and in their prophetic power was widespread, even among intellectuals. As a result, dreams were mostly approached with caution because of their ambiguous nature. The Greeks realised that dreams, while often presenting many similarities with daytime experiences, may at the same time be bizarre or monstrous. This ambiguity gave rise to questions such as: is what appears to us in the dream real or not, and, if it is real, in what sense? What kind

---

[1] περὶ δὲ τῶν τεκμηρίων τῶν ἐν τοῖσιν ὕπνοισιν ὅστις ὀρθῶς ἔγνωκε, μεγάλην ἔχοντα δύναμιν εὑρήσει πρὸς ἅπαντα, *On Regimen* 4.86 (6.640 L.).
[2] For a full bibliography of discussions of this work see van der Eijk (2004a).
[3] For a bibliography on Greek views on dreams see van der Eijk (1994) 106–32, to which should be added Byl (1998); Hubert (1999); Holowchak (1996) and (2001); Jori (1994); Liatsi (2002); Oberhelman (1993); Pigeaud (1995); Repici (2003); Sharples (2001). For general surveys of Greek thought on dreams see van Lieshout (1980) and Guidorizzi (1988); for discussions of early and classical Greek thought on sleep see Calabi (1984); Marelli (1979–80) and (1983), Wöhrle (1995) and Byl (1998).
[4] See Edelstein and Edelstein (1945, reissued in 1998).

of experience is dreaming, and how is it related to other mental processes such as thinking and perceiving?

In the fifth and the fourth centuries BCE we can see a growing concern with the nature of dreams and with the kind of information they were believed to provide among philosophers (Heraclitus, Plato, Democritus), physicians (such as the Hippocratic author just quoted), poets (Pindar) and historians (Herodotus). In this context of intellectual and theoretical reflection on the phenomenon of dreaming, Aristotle's two works *On Dreams* (*Insomn.*) and *On Divination in Sleep* (*Div. somn.*) stand out for containing the only systematic account of dreams and of prophecy in sleep that has been transmitted to us from antiquity.[5] Short as they are (covering not more than six pages in the Bekker edition), these works are extremely rich and condensed, and they are very valuable sources for our knowledge of the ways in which Aristotle applies some of his more prominent theoretical notions about the soul and its various 'parts' or 'powers' (such as 'imagination', the 'common sense', etc.) to the analysis of specific psychic phenomena. At the same time, Aristotle's style in these treatises is characteristically elliptical, and they present numerous problems of interpretation.

In this chapter I will of course say something about the contents of this theory and its connection with other parts of Aristotle's work; but the emphasis will be on the methodology which Aristotle adopts in these writings. First, I will deal with how Aristotle arrived at his theory, with particular consideration of the relation between theoretical presuppositions and empirical observations in both works. We know that Aristotle in his biological works often insists on the importance of collecting empirical evidence in order to substantiate 'theories' or 'accounts' (*logoi*) of nature. He sometimes takes other thinkers to task for their lack of concern with empirical corroboration of their theories, or he even accuses his opponents of manipulating the facts in order to make them consistent with their theories.[6] But we also know that Aristotle is often to be blamed for the very defects he is criticising in other thinkers.[7] Hence it may be proper to examine what empirical claims Aristotle makes concerning dreams and what part they play in the course of his argument.

My second question concerns the *ratio* underlying Aristotle's treatment, especially the selection of topics he deals with and the order in which they are

---

[5] For a translation with introduction and commentary of these works see van der Eijk (1994); see also Pigeaud (1995); Gallop (1996) (a revised edition of his [1990]); Dönt (1997); Morel (2000); Repici (2003).

[6] See, e.g., *Gen. an.* 760 b 27–32. [7] See Lloyd (1978) and (1979).

discussed. For although Aristotle, within the scope of these short treatises, covers an admirable amount of topics and aspects of the phenomenon of dreaming with a sometimes striking degree of sophistication, it is at the same time remarkable that some important aspects of dreaming are not treated at all – aspects which are of interest not only to us, but also to Aristotle's contemporaries. Let me give two examples. (i) Aristotle does not appear to be interested in the contents of dreams, in their narrative structure or in the mechanism responsible for the sequence of events and experiences that occur to the dreamer in a certain order. Nor does he pay serious attention to the interpretation of dreams: he only makes some very general remarks about this towards the end (464 b 9–16); he does not specify the rules for a correct interpretation of dreams. Yet the *meaning* of dreams was what the Greeks were most concerned with, and we know that in Aristotle's time there existed professional dream interpreters who used highly elaborated techniques to establish the meaning of dreams.[8] (ii) A further striking fact is that Aristotle hardly discusses the relation of dreams with other mental processes during sleep, such as thinking and recollection. He has little to say on questions such as: can we think in sleep? can we solve mathematical problems in sleep? (a problem that attracted much attention in later thought on dreams, e.g. in medieval Arabic dream theory). This lack of interest calls for an explanation, for not only does experience evidently suggest that these mental operations are possible in sleep, but there was also a powerful tradition in Greek thought, widespread in Aristotle's time, that some mental operations, such as abstract thinking (*nous*), could function better and more accurately in sleep than in the waking state, because they were believed to be 'set free' in sleep from the restrictions posed by the soul's incorporation in the body. Why does Aristotle not address this issue?

Now, in response to this, one could argue that Aristotle was under no constraint from earlier traditions to discuss these points, for early and classical Greek thought tends to display rather ambivalent attitudes to the phenomenon of sleep, and in particular to whether we can exercise our cognitive faculties in sleep. On the one hand, there was a strand in Greek thought, especially in some medical circles, in which sleep was defined negatively as the absence of a number of activities and abilities that are characteristic of the waking life, such as sense-perception, movement, consciousness and thinking. And as we shall see in a moment, Aristotle's theory of sleep shows strong similarities to this tradition. On the other hand, there was also a strand in Greek thought, represented both in Orphic circles but

---

[8] See del Corno (1982).

also in philosophers like Democritus and, perhaps, Heraclitus, in which sleep was viewed positively as a state in which humans, or at least some of us, are capable of modes of cognition not open to us in the waking state and in which we enjoy a special receptivity to experiences, impulses or, as Aristotle would put it, 'movements' (*kinēseis*) that we do not receive, or at least are not aware of, during the waking state; and there are elements of this in Aristotle's theory too. These experiences and impulses can be subdivided into stimuli that have their origin within the dreamer and those that come from outside.[9] The internal stimuli are the ones arising from the dreamer's body, or from his/her internal experiences, memories, thoughts, imaginations or emotions; and these are the stimuli that were of particular interest to medical writers, such as the author of the Hippocratic work *On Regimen* just mentioned, and to philosophers (like Aristotle) interested in the relation between the psychological and the physiological aspects of sleep. The external stimuli can in their turn be subdivided into two categories: those that have their origin in the natural world, and those that come from the supernatural (gods, demons, etc.);[10] and this group of external stimuli was of particular interest to thinkers such as Democritus (and, again, Aristotle) trying to find an explanation for the phenomenon of prophecy in sleep concerning events that lie beyond the dreamer's direct experience.

A similar, related ambivalence surrounded the question whether the sleeping life of an individual presents a complete negation of the character and personality of his/her waking life, or whether there is some connection or continuity between the two states. It would seem that if one defines sleep negatively (as Aristotle does) as an incapacitation of our powers of consciousness, the consequence would be that in the sleeping state the characteristics of our individual personalities are somehow inactivated: it would be as if, in sleep, we lose our identity and temporarily become like a plant. Yet, paradoxically, this negative view also allowed a positive valuation of the state of sleep. For it can be argued that in sleep our souls or minds are released from our bodies (and from experiences associated with the body, such as perception and emotion) and acquire a temporary state of detachedness and purity, thus anticipating the state of the immortal soul after its definitive detachment from the body after death. This latter view – that in sleep the soul is set free from the body and regains its 'proper nature' (*idia phusis*) – was especially found in Orphic and Pythagorean thought, with its negative view of the body and its dualistic concept of the relation between soul and body, and found its expression in stories

---

[9] See Aristotle, *Insomn.* 460 b 29–30; *Div. somn.* 463 a 3–30; 463 b 1–2; 463 b 22–3; 464 a 15–16.
[10] See *On Regimen* 4.87 (6.640–2 L.); cf. Arist., *Somn. vig.* 453 b 22–4 (but on the interpretation of the term *daimonios* there see below, pp. 187, 191, and 246–7 with n. 30).

about 'ecstatic', clairvoyant experiences such as told about Hermotimus of Clazomenae and other 'shamans'.[11] It seems to have appealed also to Plato and even, if the indirect tradition can be trusted, to Aristotle in his early years.[12] Yet both thinkers seem to have emancipated themselves from this position. For, at other places in his work, Plato seems to allow that our sleeping lives somehow reflect our mental state in the waking life. Thus in a well-known passage in the *Republic*, he suggests that dreams reflect an individual's spiritual state in that they show whether the soul is calm and orderly, guided by reason, or subjected to emotions and desires:

> (I mean) those desires that are awakened in sleep, when the rest of the soul – the rational, gentle, and ruling part – slumbers. Then the beastly and savage part, full of food and drink, casts off sleep and seeks to find a way to gratify itself. You know that there is nothing it won't dare to do at such a time, free of all control by shame or reason. It doesn't shrink from trying to have sex with a mother, as it supposes, or with anyone else at all, whether man, god, or beast. It will commit any foul murder, and there is no food it refuses to eat. In a word, it omits no act of folly or shamelessness... On the other hand, I suppose that someone who is healthy and moderate with himself goes to sleep only after having done the following: First, he rouses his rational part and feasts it on fine arguments and speculations; second, he neither starves nor feasts his appetites, so that they will slumber and not disturb his best part with either their pleasure or their pain, but they'll leave it alone, pure and by itself, to get on with its investigations, to yearn after and perceive something... whether it is past, present or future; third, he soothes his spirited part in the same way, for example, by not falling asleep with his spirit still aroused after an outburst of anger. And when he has quieted these two parts and aroused the third, in which reason resides, and so takes rest, you know that it is then that he best grasps the truth and that the visions that appear in his dreams are least lawless.[13]

As for Aristotle, the view that in sleep our souls regain their 'proper nature' seems, at best, to have been a Platonic relic appealing to him in his early years, soon to be abandoned in favour of his characteristic 'hylomorphic' theory of the soul as the formal aspect of the natural soul–body composite that makes up a living being.[14] In this view, soul and body are jointly affected by experiences (*pathē*) such as sleep; but how this works out with regard to whether our sleeping lives somehow reflect our waking lives, is not immediately obvious. Thus a passage in Aristotle's *Nicomachean Ethics* presents a certain ambivalence:

---

[11] Apollonius, *Mirabilia* 3; see the discussion by Bremmer (1983) 24–53.
[12] For a discussion of the fragments from his lost works *On Philosophy* and *Eudemus* see van der Eijk (1994) 89–93.
[13] Plato, *Republic* 571 c ff., tr. Grube and Reeve (1997) 1180.
[14] See the discussion in van der Eijk (2000b).

ταύτης μὲν οὖν κοινή τις ἀρετὴ καὶ οὐκ ἀνθρωπίνη φαίνεται· δοκεῖ γὰρ ἐν τοῖς ὕπνοις ἐνεργεῖν μάλιστα τὸ μόριον τοῦτο καὶ ἡ δύναμις αὕτη, ὁ δ' ἀγαθὸς καὶ κακὸς ἥκιστα διάδηλοι καθ' ὕπνον (ὅθεν φασιν οὐδὲν διαφέρειν τὸ ἥμισυ τοῦ βίου τοὺς εὐδαίμονας τῶν ἀθλίων· συμβαίνει δὲ τοῦτο εἰκότως· ἀργία γάρ ἐστιν ὁ ὕπνος τῆς ψυχῆς ᾗ λέγεται σπουδαία καὶ φαύλη), πλὴν εἴ πῃ[15] κατὰ μικρὸν καὶ διικνοῦνταί τινες τῶν κινήσεων, καὶ ταύτῃ βελτίω γίνεται τὰ φαντάσματα τῶν ἐπιεικῶν ἢ τῶν τυχόντων. (1102 b 2–10)

The excellence of this part [i.e. the vegetative part] of the soul seems to be common to all living beings and not peculiar to humans; for it is generally believed that this part and this faculty [nutrition] is particularly active in sleep, and that the difference between a good and a bad person is least evident in sleep (which is why people say that for half of their lives, there is no difference between happy people and miserable people; this is a reasonable conclusion, for sleep is a kind of inactivity of that [part of the] soul in virtue of which it [the soul] is called good or bad), unless in a certain way, and to a small extent, certain sense-movements penetrate to [the soul during sleep], and in this way the dream images of good people are superior to those of common people.

The possibility envisaged here towards the end in the clause 'unless in a certain way...' is precisely what Aristotle is exploring in much greater detail in his investigations of sleep and dreams in the two works already mentioned *On Dreams* and *On Divination in Sleep* (see esp. 463 a 21ff.), and in the work *On Sleep and Waking* which precedes them.[16] Yet, as we shall see later, these treatises make it clear that the connection between what we perceive in the daytime and what appears to us in sleep is rarely straightforward or direct (*euthuoneiria*), and often dreams are confused as a result of physiological turbulence that disturbs the transmission of sensory images in the body (461 a 9ff.). And the tentative way in which, in the *Ethics* passage, the possibility of a connection between waking and sleeping life is introduced (πλὴν εἴ πῃ κατὰ μικρόν... τινες τῶν κινήσεων) does not suggest that Aristotle attached great relevance to it in the context of his moral philosophy.

2 THE CONTEXT OF ARISTOTLE'S TREATISES ON SLEEP AND DREAMS

In order to appreciate Aristotle's approach to these issues better, it is important to consider the context in which his views on dreams are expounded.

---

[15] Some MSS read μή here instead of πῃ.
[16] Although these three treatises are presented in the preface of *On Sleep and Waking* as parts of one continuous investigation and follow on each other in the MS tradition, the precise relationship between them poses considerable problems. See van der Eijk (1994) 62–7.

That is explicitly and emphatically the context of natural science: the theoretical study of *nature* as Aristotle conceives it. They belong to a series of treatises which are usually called *Parva naturalia*. Although this title does not originate from Aristotle but from the Middle Ages, it rightly indicates that psychology means for Aristotle psycho-*physiology*, an analysis both of the formal ('mental') and of the material ('physical') aspects of what it means for a natural entity to be a living being.[17] At the beginning of this series of treatises (which Aristotle seems to have conceived as a continuing discussion of connected topics), Aristotle says that he will be concerned with the most important 'activities and experiences' of living beings (man, animals, plants), in particular with those that are 'common to the soul and the body': sense-perception, memory and recollection, sleep and waking, youth and old age, growth and decay, breathing, life and death, health and disease. These are, Aristotle says, the most important functions living beings can realise or experience *qua* living beings, and it is for the purpose of these functions that the bodily structures such as described in *History of Animals* and *Parts of Animals* (and in the lost work *On Plants*) exist. The *Parva naturalia* are closely linked to Aristotle's work *On the Soul*, and the psycho-physiological explanation of dreams which Aristotle expounds in *On Dreams* (and which, in the enumeration listed above, is subordinated to and included in the discussion of sleeping and waking) heavily draws upon Aristotle's general theory of the soul, especially his views on sense-perception, 'imagination' (*phantasia*), and on the so-called 'central sense faculty' (*kurion aisthētērion*). This context of the study of nature should make clear from the outset that the interest taken by Aristotle in dreams is neither epistemological nor practical, hermeneutic or therapeutic – as it is, for example, in the Hippocratic work *On Regimen* quoted above, of which Aristotle was aware.

Against this background, the questions Aristotle is pursuing in the three works in question make perfect sense. Thus in the preface to *On Sleep and Waking* (453 b 11–24), which in a way serves as an introduction to all three of the treatises, he says that he is going to consider whether sleeping and waking are 'peculiar to the soul' or 'common to soul and body', and, if common to both, what parts of soul and body are involved; whether sleep occurs in all living beings or only in some; and through what cause (*aitia*) it occurs.[18]

Considering this psycho-physiological context, one would expect Aristotle to pay some attention to the question of the possibility of cognition

---

[17] On the structure and underlying rationale of the series of treatises assembled under the heading *Parva naturalia* see van der Eijk (1994) 68–72; see also Morel (2000) 10–24 and (2002b).

[18] For a discussion of this 'Preface' see van der Eijk (1994) 68–72.

(either perceptual or intellectual, and either 'normal' or extraordinary) in sleep. But this question is not explicitly raised, and his relevant remarks are scattered, nuanced and complicated, so that an answer unfolds only gradually through the continuous discussion in the three works; and it is not free from apparent contradictions. In *On Sleep and Waking*, Aristotle begins by defining sleep negatively as the inability of the sense faculty to be activated (*adunamia tou energein*, 454 b 5, 458 a 29). Sleep is said to be a 'fetter and immobilisation' (*desmos kai akinēsia*, 454 b 10) an 'inactivity' (*argia*) or 'incapacitation' (*adunamia*) of the sensitive faculty (455 b 3ff.). It is a state in which the vegetative part of the soul gains the upper hand (455 a 1–2), and it is caused by various physiological processes that are connected with the digestion of food (such as heating, cooling, evaporation of food, and sifting of the blood).[19] There is no sensation in sleep, he says, because the central sense-organ, the *kurion aisthētērion*, which is located in the heart, is affected by these processes and thus incapacitated, and as a result of this the peripheral sense-organs (eyes, ears, nose, etc.) cannot function either (455 a 13ff.). Whether these physiological processes also affect the ability to think and the operations of the intellectual part of the soul, is a question which Aristotle does not address explicitly. Strictly speaking, since Aristotle's supreme intellectual faculty, the *nous*, is said to be incorporeal and not to require simultaneous perception in order to be active,[20] there is, at least in principle, no reason why we should not be able to think while being asleep.[21] There are a few hints to this in the text, for example in *Insomn.* 459 a 6–8 and 462 a 29–30, which speak of an activity of 'judgement' (*doxa*) and of the presence of 'true thoughts' (*alētheis ennoiai*) in sleep, but it remains vague (see below).

Aristotle's negative definition of sleep does not, however, imply a negative evaluation of this 'affection' (*pathos*). Sleep is a good thing and serves a purpose, for it provides rest (*anapausis*) to the sense-organs, which would otherwise become overstretched, since they are unable to be active without interruption (454 a 27, 455 b 18ff.). Here, again, one may note a difference compared with thinking; for one of the differences between perception and thinking, according to Aristotle, is that perception cannot go on forever, indeed if we overstretch our sense-organs, we damage them; thinking, on

---

[19] For a discussion of Aristotle's physiological explanation of sleep see Wiesner (1978).
[20] *De an.* 430 a 17–18, 22–3; *Gen. an.* 736 b 28–9; see also ch. 7 below.
[21] In *De an.* 429 a 7–8 Aristotle mentions the possibility that the intellect (*nous*) may be 'overshadowed' (*epikaluptesthai*) by sleep, but it is unclear from this passage whether this is always the case in sleep or only in exceptional circumstances.

the other hand, does not know fatigue and the harder we exercise our intellectual faculty, the better it functions.[22]

The way in which Aristotle arrives at these views is largely theoretical and by *a priori* reasoning. Sleep, he argues in chapter 1 of *On Sleep and Waking*, is the opposite of waking; and since waking consists in the exercise of the sensitive faculty, sleep must be the inactivity of this faculty. Sleep affects all animals, because sensation is characteristic of animals. Plants do not sleep, because they have no perception. In fact, sleep is nothing but a state of what Aristotle elsewhere calls 'first entelechy',[23] a state of having a faculty without using it, which may be beneficial in order to provide rest to the bodily parts involved in its exercise. Furthermore, Aristotle is characteristically keen to specify that sleep is a particular kind of incapacitation of the sense faculty as distinct from other kinds of incapacitation, such as faint and epileptic seizure (456 b 9–16). He also applies his explanatory model of the four causes (which he reminds us of in 455 b 14–16) to the phenomenon of sleep, listing its formal, final, material and efficient causes, and leading up to two complementary definitions stating the material and the formal cause of sleep:

the upward movement of the solid part of nutriment caused by innate heat, and its subsequent condensation and return to the primary sense organ. And the definition of sleep is that it is a seizure of the primary sense organ which prevents it from being activated, and which is necessary for the preservation of the living being; for a living being cannot continue to exist without the presence of those things that contribute to its perfection; and rest (*anapausis*) secures preservation (*sōtēria*). (458 a 25–32)

By contrast, there is little consideration, let alone evidence of systematic gathering and interpreting, of empirical evidence to back up the theory arrived at. It is true that, in the course of his argument, Aristotle occasionally refers to empirical observations, or at least he makes a number of empirical claims, which can be listed as follows:

1. Most animals have their eyes closed when they sleep (454 b 15ff.).
2. Nutrition and growth are more active in sleep than in the waking state (455 a 1–2).
3. All animals have a sense of touch (455 a 6).
4. In fainting fits, people lose sensation (455 b 6).
5. Those who have the veins in the neck compressed become unconscious (455 b 7).
6. Breathing and cooling take place in the heart (456 a 5).
7. Insects that do not respire are seen to expand and contract (456 a 12).

[22] *De an.* 429 a 30–b 6. [23] *De an.* 412 a 25–6.

8. Insects buzz (456 a 18).
9. Some people move and perform various activities in sleep, and some of these people remember their dreams, though they fail to remember the 'waking' acts they perform in sleep (456 a 25).
10. The blood vessels have their origin in the heart (456 b 1).
11. Words are spoken by people who are in a state of trance and seemingly dead (456 b 16).
12. Several narcotics make the head heavy (456 b 23).
13. Children sleep more than other people (457 a 4).
14. In many epileptic patients, epileptic seizure begins in sleep (457 a 10).
15. The embryo lies quiet in the womb at first (457 a 20).
16. People with inconspicuous veins, dwarfish people, and people with big heads are inclined to much sleep (457 a 20).
17. People with marked veins do not sleep much; nor do melancholics, who in spite of eating much remain slight (457 a 26).
18. The brain is the coldest part of the body (457 b 30).
19. The heart has three chambers (458 a 15ff.).

Yet while some of these claims are interesting as testifying either to Aristotle's own observational capacities or to his considerable knowledge of medico-physiological views on sleeping, as a whole they can hardly be regarded as impressive for their wide range or systematicity; and in the argument, most of these empirical claims have at best only a marginal relevance to the topic of sleep. They are mentioned only in passing, and none are presented by Aristotle as guiding the investigation inductively to a general theory or as playing a decisive role in settling potentially controversial issues. Nor does Aristotle explain how observations that seem to be in conflict with the theoretical views he has expounded can nevertheless be accommodated within that theory. Thus, in spite of his definition of sleep as the absence of sensation, Aristotle on several occasions acknowledges that various things may occur to us while we are in a state of sleep. This is obviously relevant for the discussion of dreams and divination in sleep that follows after *On Sleep and Waking*; but already in *On Sleep and Waking* we find certain anticipations of this idea, for example in 456 a 25–9, where he acknowledges that people may perform waking acts while asleep on the basis of an 'image or sensation' (nos. 9 and 11). And on two occasions, the wording of *On Sleep and Waking* seems to open the door to sensations of some kind experienced in sleep: 'Activity of sense perception in the strict and unqualified sense (*kuriōs kai haplōs*) is impossible while asleep' (454 b 13–14), and 'we have said that sleep is in some way (*tropon tina*) the immobilisation of sense perception' (454 b 26). These specifications suggest that more may be at stake than just an unqualified absence of sensation. Yet how the phenomena referred to are to be explained within the overall theory, he does not make clear.

3 ON DREAMS

In his treatment of dreams, the approach is likewise psycho-physiological, as emerges clearly from the questions Aristotle asks in the course of his discussion:
(i) To what part of the soul does dreaming belong (i.e. how is dreaming related to other mental faculties such as sense-perception and thinking)? (458 b 1)
(ii) How do dreams originate? (459 a 23)
(iii) What is a dream, what is its definition? (459 a 23)

In these questions, we can again detect the typically Aristotelian pattern of the four causes; only the final cause is lacking, and this has to do with the fact that Aristotle does not attribute any natural purpose or end to dreams. This absence of a teleological explanation of dreams is significant, and I shall come back to it at the end of this chapter.

In *On Dreams*, as in *On Sleep and Waking*, Aristotle again begins by stating rather bluntly that dreams cannot be an activity of the sense faculty, since there is no sense-perception in sleep (458 b 5–10). However, in the course of the argument he recognises that the fact that sense-perception cannot be activated (*energein*) does not mean that it is incapable of being 'affected' (*paschein*):

ἆρ' οὖν τὸ μὲν μὴ ὁρᾶν μηδὲν ἀληθές, τὸ δὲ μηδὲν πάσχειν τὴν αἴσθησιν οὐκ ἀληθές, ἀλλ' ἐνδέχεται καὶ τὴν ὄψιν πάσχειν τι καὶ τὰς ἄλλας αἰσθήσεις, ἕκαστον δὲ τούτων ὥσπερ ἐγρηγορότος προσβάλλει μέν πως τῇ αἰσθήσει, οὐχ οὕτω δὲ ὥσπερ ἐγρηγορότος· καὶ ὅτε μὲν ἡ δόξα λέγει ὅτι ψεῦδος, ὥσπερ ἐγρηγορόσιν, ὅτε δὲ κατέχεται καὶ ἀκολουθεῖ τῷ φαντάσματι. (459 a 1–8)

But perhaps it is true that we do not see anything [in sleep], but not true that sense perception is not affected, and perhaps it is possible that sight and the other senses are somehow affected, and that each of these affections makes some impression on sense perception as it does in the waking state, but not in the same way as in the waking state; and sometimes our judgement tells us that this is false, as it does when we are awake, but sometimes it is withheld from doing this and follows what it is presented with.

He goes on to say that dreams are the result of 'imagination' (*phantasia*), a faculty closely associated with, but not identical to sense perception. The way this works is explained in chapters 2 and 3 of *On Dreams*. This time, though, Aristotle presents his account much more emphatically as being built on observation of 'the facts surrounding sleep' (459 a 24), and his claims are backed up by a much more considerable amount of empirical evidence:

1. There is no sense-perception in sleep (458 b 7; but see nos. 23 and 24 below).
2. During sleep, we often have thoughts accompanying the dream-images (458 b 13–15); this appears most clearly when we try to remember our dreams immediately after awakening (458 b 18–23).
3. When one moves from a sunny place into the shade, one cannot see anything for some time (459 b 10–11).
4. When one looks at a particular colour for a long time and then turns one's glance to another object, this object seems to have the colour one has been looking at (459 b 11–13).
5. When one has looked into the sun or at a brilliant object and subsequently closes one's eyes, one still sees the light for some time: at first, it still has the original colour, then it becomes crimson, then purple, then black, and then it disappears (459 b 13–18).
6. When one turns one's gaze from moving objects (e.g. fast flowing rivers), objects that are at rest seem to be moving (459 b 18–20).
7. When one has been exposed to strong sounds for a long time, one becomes deaf, and after smelling very strong odours one's power of smelling is impaired (459 b 20–2).
8. When a menstruating woman looks into a mirror, a red stain occurs on the surface of the mirror, which is difficult to remove, especially from new mirrors (459 b 23–460 a 23).[24]
9. Wine and unguents quickly acquire the odours of objects near to them (460 a 26–32).

---

[24] For a full discussion of this extraordinary claim see van der Eijk (1994) 167–93 with more detailed bibliographical references (to which should now be added Woolf (1999), who arrives at a very similar view to mine about the passage being illuminating for Aristotle's views on material alteration in sense-perception). While in earlier scholarship the authenticity of the passage was disputed, the discussion now focuses on the following issues: (1) the problem of the passage's obvious counterfactuality; (2) is the theory of menstruation as expounded here in accordance with what Aristotle says elsewhere? (3) is the theory of something emanating from the eye not inconsistent with Aristotle's views on visual perception as stated elsewhere? (4) What is the point of the passage for the discussion of the way in which dreams come into existence? Briefly summarised, my view is (1) that what seems to be underlying the passage is a traditional belief (perhaps derived from magic or midwives' tales) in the dangerous and polluting effects of menstrual blood, and that Aristotle must have accepted this story without checking it because he felt able to provide an explanation for it; such beliefs were not uncommon regarding menstruation (although most of the evidence dates from the Roman period); (2) there is no inconsistency regarding the cause of menstruation, for in 460 a 6–7 the words διὰ ταραχὴν καὶ φλεγμασίαν αἱματικήν must be connected with ἡ διαφορά ... ἄδηλος ἡμῖν (pace Dean-Jones (1987) 256–7); (3) there is no inconsistency, for Aristotle is not discussing perception but reflection, in which the eye is not the perceiving subject but the object that sets the process in motion and brings the reflection about; (4) the passage illustrates (a) the swiftness and acuteness of the senses, which allows them to register even the tiniest differences and changes, and (b) the lingering of such tiny perceptions after the impression has been made. It is these lingering, tiny movements that constitute the material for dreams.

10. When one is under the influence of strong emotions, one is very susceptible to sensitive illusions (460 b 4–16).
11. When one crosses two fingers and puts an object between them, it is as if one feels two objects (460 b 22–3).
12. When one is on a ship which is moved by the sea and looks at the land, it is as if the land moves (460 b 26–7).
13. Weak stimuli of pleasure and pain are extruded by stronger ones and escape our attention (461 a 1–3).
14. When one gets to sleep immediately after dinner, one has no dreams (461 a 11–12).
15. Very young children do not dream at all (461 a 12; cf. *Gen. an.* 779 a 13).
16. Dreams occur in a later stage of sleep; they are often distorted and unclear, but sometimes they are strong (461 a 18–27).
17. Melancholics, drunk people and those suffering from fever have confused and monstrous dream images (461 a 21–2).
18. The dream image is judged by the dreaming subject (461 b 3–7).
19. When one presses a finger under one's eye, one single object appears double (462 a 1).
20. Sometimes, during sleep, one is aware of the fact that one is dreaming (462 a 2–8).
21. At the moment of falling asleep and of awakening, one often sees images (462 a 10–11).
22. Young people see in the dark all kinds of appearances when their eyes are wide open (462 a 12–15).
23. In situations of half-sleep, one can have weak perceptions of light and sounds from one's environment (462 a 19–25).
24. One may even give answers to questions when one is asleep (462 a 25–6).
25. Many people never had a dream in their whole lives; others first got them after considerable advance in age (464 b 1–11; cf. *Hist. an.* 537 b 13 ff.).

This is a substantial list of empirical claims, some of which testify to Aristotle's sharp observational capacities (for example, nos. 2, 4, 20). However, we also find claims that are highly questionable from a modern point of view or for which the empirical basis can only be said to be very weak (e.g. 8, 11, 14, 15). It is difficult to decide to what extent these 'data' (*phainomena* or *sumbainonta*, as Aristotle would call them) are derived from deliberate and purposeful observation by Aristotle and his pupils themselves, or just from common human experience (on the list, observations 15 and 25 are also found in other biological works of Aristotle, but they are evidently only a minority). Moreover, we should certainly take into account the possibility that Aristotle has borrowed some of these data from other scientific writings, for example the psychological works of Democritus (whom Aristotle mentions in *Div. somn.* 464 a 4) and medical literature (to which he refers explicitly in 463 a 4–5), and perhaps also from literary descriptions of dreams such as were found in Homer and the epic tradition. However, since this tradition has only been preserved in fragments, it is difficult to assess the extent of his dependence on earlier sources.

Yet when looking more closely at the way in which these empirical 'data' are used in Aristotle's argument in *On Dreams*, it becomes clear that the treatise goes far beyond the level of empirical fact-finding. Aristotle does not present his theory as being built up, so to speak, inductively on the basis of a number of observations; on the contrary, the three research questions mentioned above ((i), (ii) and (iii)) are treated in a systematical and deductive way, and empirical 'data' are mentioned in the course of this theoretical argument – often in the form of examples or analogies – in order to support or clarify opinions and presuppositions which Aristotle already seems to take for granted. And although Aristotle's style of reasoning seems very cautious and essayistic – the first chapter, for example, is highly aporetic[25] – it is, in fact, rather dogmatic. The general impression one gets is that empirical evidence is primarily mentioned when it suits the argument – and if not, it is either ignored or explained away in a questionable manner.

Thus at the end of *On Dreams*, it turns out that the three questions raised at the beginning are to be answered as follows:

(i) Dreams belong to the sensitive part of the soul *qua* imaginative part (459 a 21); dreaming is not an operation of sense-perception but of 'imagination', which is defined by Aristotle as 'the movement which occurs as a result of actual perception' (459 a 17–18). This definition, together with Aristotle's use of the words *phantasia*, *phantasma*, and *phainesthai*, is in broad agreement with his general theory of 'imagination' in *On the Soul*, to which he explicitly refers (459 a 15). In the course of the long argument which leads to this conclusion, only claims (1) and (2) play a part; for the rest, the argument is purely theoretical and logical.

(ii) How do dreams come into being? Aristotle assumes the following mechanism: During the waking state, the sense-organs are stimulated by a great quantity of sense-movements (stimuli brought about by sensible objects); but not all of these movements are equally strong. The stronger movements overrule the weaker, so that the weaker are 'not noticed' by the perceiving subject (460 b 28–461 a 8). Aristotle assumes, however, that the remnants of these weaker movements remain present in the sense-organs in the form of traces. When in sleep the sense-organs have stopped being active – and as a result of this cannot receive new stimuli – the remnants of

---

[25] For an analysis see van der Eijk (1994) 36–8.

these weaker movements, which escaped our attention in the waking state, get, so to speak, a second chance to 'present themselves' to the perceiving subject. They are 'reactivated' and 'come to the surface' (461 a 3, 7). This is an operation of the faculty of 'imagination'. The physiological picture to be drawn for this process is not completely clear, but seems to be roughly as follows. Aristotle thinks that apart from the peripheral sense-organs (eyes, ears, nose, etc.) there is also a central, co-ordinating sense-organ located in the heart (the so-called 'principle of perception', 461 a 6, 31; 461 b 4). His view seems to be that, normally speaking, a sensitive impulse is transmitted from the peripheral sense-organs to the heart, where it is received, recorded and noticed, and co-ordinated with movements from other senses (461 a 31). The transmitting agency is probably the blood (although this is not quite clear from the text).[26] In the waking state, the weaker sense-movements, which have arrived at the peripheral sense-organs during the waking state, are prevented from reaching the heart because of the competition with stronger movements; it is only in sleep, when the blood withdraws from the outer parts of the body to the inner parts, that they penetrate to the heart. The 'perception' or 'noticing' of these movements is dreaming in the strict sense. Thus dreams originate from weak sense-movements, which have entered the sense-organs in the waking state, but which were not noticed by the perceiving subject because of their weakness in comparison with stronger movements.

By explaining the occurrence of dreams in this way, Aristotle manages to account for the fact that dreams often display many similarities with what the dreamer has experienced in the waking state (because they consist of movements received during the waking state), but that these elements often appear in a distorted, completely 'unrealistic' configuration due to the physiological conditions that influence the transmission to the heart. In order to substantiate this explanation, Aristotle has to presuppose, first, that the sense-organs actually receive very slight movements and, second, that these small movements are being 'preserved' (*sōizesthai*, 461 a 25) in the sense-organs from the moment of their arrival (in the waking state) to the moment of their transport to the heart and subsequent appearance in sleep.

When we look at our list of empirical 'data', we can see that numbers 3–9 are used by Aristotle in order to illustrate the mechanism of 'lingering' or 'persisting' sense-movements after the actual perception has disappeared; numbers 8–9 point to the receptivity of the sense-organs to small

---

[26] See 461 a 25 and b 11, 27. See van der Eijk (1994) 81–7 and, with reservations, Johansen (1998).

sense-movements. Number 13 serves as an illustration of the 'extrusion' of weak movements through stronger ones. Numbers 14–17 are concerned with the physiological conditions that influence or disturb the transport of sense-movements from the peripheral sense-organs to the central sense-organ. Numbers 10–12 and 18–20 illustrate the 'experiencing' or 'noticing' of the sense-movements by the dreaming subject: the experiences of illusion in the waking state serve as analogy for the fact that the dreaming subject often does not notice that what (s)he experiences is only a dream.

(iii) Aristotle's answer to the third question of the definition of the dream is best studied through a quotation from the last chapter of *On Dreams* (462 a 15–31):

ἐκ δὴ τούτων ἁπάντων δεῖ συλλογίσασθαι ὅτι ἐστὶ τὸ ἐνύπνιον φάντασμα μέν τι καὶ ἐν ὕπνῳ· τὰ γὰρ ἄρτι λεχθέντα εἴδωλα οὐκ ἔστιν ἐνύπνια, οὐδ' εἴ τι ἄλλο λελυμένων τῶν αἰσθήσεων φαίνεται· οὐδὲ τὸ ἐν ὕπνῳ φάντασμα πᾶν. πρῶτον μὲν γὰρ ἐνίοις συμβαίνει καὶ αἰσθάνεσθαί πῃ καὶ ψόφων καὶ φωτὸς καὶ χυμοῦ καὶ ἁφῆς, ἀσθενικῶς μέντοι καὶ οἷον πόρρωθεν· ἤδη γὰρ ἐν τῷ καθεύδειν ὑποβλέποντες, ὃ ἠρέμα ἑώρων φῶς τοῦ λύχνου καθεύδοντες, ὡς ᾤοντο, ἐπεγερθέντες εὐθὺς ἐγνώρισαν τὸ τοῦ λύχνου ὄν, καὶ ἀλεκτρυόνων καὶ κυνῶν φωνὴν ἠρέμα ἀκούοντες ἐγερθέντες σαφῶς ἐγνώρισαν. ἔνιοι δὲ καὶ ἀποκρίνονται ἐρωτώμενοι· ἐνδέχεται γὰρ τοῦ ἐγρηγορέναι καὶ καθεύδειν ἁπλῶς, θατέρου ὑπάρχοντος θάτερόν πῃ ὑπάρχειν. ὧν οὐδὲν ἐνύπνιον φατέον, οὐδ' ὅσαι δὴ ἐν τῷ ὕπνῳ γίνονται ἀληθεῖς ἔννοιαι παρὰ τὰ φαντάσματα, ἀλλὰ τὸ φάντασμα τὸ ἀπὸ τῆς κινήσεως τῶν αἰσθημάτων, ὅταν ἐν τῷ καθεύδειν ᾖ, ᾗ καθεύδει, τοῦτ' ἐστὶν ἐνύπνιον.

From all this we have to conclude that the dream is a sort of appearance, and, more particularly, one which occurs in sleep; for the images just mentioned are not dreams, nor is any other image which presents itself when the senses are free [i.e. when we are awake]; nor is every image which occurs in sleep a dream. For, in the first place, some persons actually, in a certain way, perceive sounds and light and taste and contact [while asleep], albeit faintly and as it were from far away. For during sleep people who had their eyes half open have recognised what they believed they were seeing in their sleep faintly as the light of the lamp, as the real light of the lamp, and what they believed they were hearing faintly as the voice of cocks and dogs, they recognised these clearly on awakening. Some even give answers when being asked questions. The fact is with being awake and being asleep that it is possible that when one of them is present without qualification, the other is also present in a certain way. None of these [experiences] should be called dreams, nor should the true thoughts that occur in sleep as distinct from the appearances, but the appearance which results from the movement of the sense-effects, when one is asleep, in so far as one is asleep, this is a dream.

Thus the dream is defined as 'the appearance which results from the movement of the sense-effects, when one is asleep, in so far as one is asleep.' The qualification 'when one is asleep and in so far as one is asleep' is necessary in order to distinguish the dream from other experiences one may have in and around sleep; and there is a pun here, for the Greek word *enhupnion*, which Aristotle uses throughout for 'dream', literally means '(something) in sleep', *en hupnōi*. These 'other experiences' have been discussed by Aristotle in the preceding lines with the aid of examples (462 a 9–15): in sleep we sometimes perceive things which on awakening we recognise as being caused by sense-movements that actually present themselves to our sense-organs, and children often see frightening visions in the dark with their eyes open; and as he says in the passage quoted, in transitional states of half-sleep we may perceive weak impressions of light and sound, we may even give answers to questions which are being asked, and we may have thoughts in sleep about the dream image. How these experiences are physiologically possible is not explained by Aristotle, but what he says about them is highly significant in theoretical respect. Sleep and waking are not absolute opposites: when one of them is present 'without qualification' (*haplōs*), the other may also be present 'in a certain way' (*pēi*). In these transitional states between sleeping and waking, we may, after all, have some sort of direct perception of the actual state of affairs in the external world. Aristotle's recognition of this possibility entails an implicit modification of his earlier assertions in the first chapter of *On Sleep and Waking*, where he defined sleep and waking as opposites and sleep as the privation of waking (453 b 26–27), and in chapter 1 of *On Dreams*, where he said that we cannot perceive anything in sleep. It now turns out that we *may* actually perceive in sleep, though faintly and unclearly. In accordance with his dream theory, Aristotle here insists that none of these experiences 'in sleep' (*en hupnōi*) are 'dreams', that is, *enhupnia* in the strict sense.

A remarkably modern consequence of this view is that according to Aristotle the state of sleeping can be divided into different stages. Aristotle does not show any awareness of 'rapid eye movements'; but on theoretical grounds he assumes that the beginning of sleep is characterised by an absence of dreams, because then, as a result of the process of digestion, there is too much confusion and 'turbulence' in the body, which disturbs the transport of sense-movements through the blood (461 a 8ff.). Appearances that manifest themselves in that early stage are not dreams, Aristotle points out: dreams occur later, when the blood is separated into a thinner, clearer part and a thicker, troubled part; when this process of separation of the blood is completed, we wake up (458 a 10–25). Thus dreams are experiences which we have when in fact we are on our way to awakening. Experiences, however, which we have *just before or simultaneously with* awakening and which are caused by actual perceptions – not, such as in dreams, by lingering sense-movements which derive from *previous* perceptions in the waking state – are not dreams, because we do not have these experiences 'in so far as' (*hēi*) we are asleep, but in so far as we are, in a sense, already awake.

This typically Aristotelian usage of the qualifier *hēi* also provides us with an answer to the other question I raised earlier in this chapter, namely why Aristotle does not explicitly address the possibility of other mental experiences during sleep such as thinking and recollection. The answer seems to be that thoughts, beliefs, perceptions, hallucinations, recollections and indeed 'waking acts' (*egrēgorikai praxeis*) performed while sleepwalking (456 a 25–6) are not characteristic of the sleeping state: they do not happen to the sleeper 'in so far as' (*hēi*) (s)he is sleeping. They do not form part of the dream, but they exist 'over and above' the dream (*para to enhupnion*). We cannot say, in Aristotle's theory, that we 'think in our dream', although we can say that we think in our *sleep*. The role of thought in sleep is apparently not essentially different from that in the waking state,[27] although there is nothing in what Aristotle says here to suggest that we might have clearer, 'purer' thoughts in sleep than in the waking state.

The definition of dreams that Aristotle presents here is, as I said, in accordance with his views in *On Sleep and Waking*. Dreams are not actual perceptions, rather they are, as it were, reactivated perceptions which we received during the waking state; they are 'movements of sense-effects' (τῆς κινήσεως τῶν αἰσθημάτων). Aristotle, again, differentiates between various kinds of experience in sleep. And although the recognition that we may after all have perceptions in sleep constitutes an important qualification of Aristotle's initial, and repeatedly reiterated view that there is no sense-perception in sleep, Aristotle avoids contradicting himself by saying that although we have these perceptions while we are asleep, we do not have them in so far as we are asleep. The point of the specifications *kuriōs kai haplōs* in *Somn. vig.* 454 b 13 and *tropon tina* in 454 b 26 has now become clear, and they are answered here by the specifications *pēi* and *hēi*.

4 ON DIVINATION IN SLEEP

When we turn to the third treatise, *On Divination in Sleep*, however, it is becoming increasingly less clear how Aristotle manages to accommodate the phenomena he recognises within his theory without getting involved in contradictions. In this work, he does accept that we sometimes foresee the future in sleep; but his theory of dreams as expounded so far does not give much in the way of help to explain how this can happen.

---

[27] But see no. 20–1 above.

Aristotle on sleep and dreams

Before considering the difficulties that arise here, let us first consider Aristotle's methodology in this short work. Basically, Aristotle tackles the mysterious phenomenon in three ways:
  (i) by considering the causal relation between the dream in which a certain event is foreseen, and the event that later actually happens
  (ii) by considering the kinds of events that can be foreseen in sleep
  (iii) by considering the kinds of people who have prophetic dreams.

He does not explicitly present these research questions at the beginning of the treatise itself in the way he does in *On Sleep* and *On Dreams*, although questions (i) and (ii) are included in the summary of questions at the beginning of *On Sleep and Waking*, where he says that he is going to consider

καὶ πότερον ἐνδέχεται τὰ μέλλοντα προορᾶν ἢ οὐκ ἐνδέχεται, καὶ τίνα τρόπον εἰ ἐνδέχεται, καὶ πότερον τὰ μέλλοντα ὑπ' ἀνθρώπων πράσσεσθαι μόνον ἢ καὶ ὧν τὸ δαιμόνιον ἔχει τὴν αἰτίαν καὶ φύσει γίνεται ἢ ἀπὸ ταὐτομάτου. (453 b 22–4)

[We also need to examine] whether it is possible to foresee the future in sleep or not, and if it is possible, in what way; and whether [it is possible to foresee] only what will be done by human beings, or also things whose cause belongs to the domain of what is beyond human control (*to daimonion*)[28] and which occur naturally or spontaneously.

In his discussion of these issues, he once again makes a number of empirical claims:

1. Some people foresee what will happen at the Pillars of Heracles or at the Borysthenes (462 b 24–6).
2. When one is asleep, weak impulses appear stronger: weak sounds are perceived as thunder, a tiny bit of phlegm is perceived as honey, local warmth brings about the illusion that one goes through a fire; only after awakening, one recognises the real nature of these impulses (463 a 11–18).
3. In sleep one often dreams of things one has experienced in the waking state (463 a 22–4).
4. One often thinks of a person who shortly later appears (463 b 1–4).
5. Not only man, but also some other animals dream (463 b 12; cf. *Hist. an.* 536 b 27 ff. and 537 b 13).
6. Garrulous people and melancholics often have clear and prophetic dreams (463 b 17–22).
7. Many dreams do not come true (463 b 22).
8. Foresight of things happening beyond the dreamer's control does not occur with intelligent people, but with those of mediocre mental capacities (463 a 19–20).

[28] For a discussion of this expression see van der Eijk (1994) 291–6.

9. Foresight is characteristic of people who are prone to anger or to melancholics (464 a 24–7; 464 a 32–b 5).
10. Prophetic dreams mostly concern people who are related to the dreamer (464 a 27–32).
11. Images in moving water are often distorted and difficult to reconstruct (464 b 10–12).

In his treatment of question (i), Aristotle in turn distinguishes three possibilities:

(a) The dream may be a sign (*sēmeion*) of the event, in that it is caused by the same factor or starting-point which also causes the future event itself. In order to illustrate this possibility, he refers to the prognostic use of dreams as signs in medicine, and he uses several empirical data as evidence (no. 2), to which I shall turn shortly.

(b) The dream is a cause (*aition*), or indeed *the* cause, of the event, in that it causes the event to happen. For example, it may happen that we dream about an action which we actually perform the following day. Again, empirical evidence of this is produced (no. 3): Aristotle points out that it often happens that we dream of an action we have performed previously, and this action is the starting-point of the dream. Conversely, he argues, we can also in our actions be motivated by a dream we have had before.

(c) The dream coincides (*sumptōma*) with the event without there being any real connection between the occurrence of both. Aristotle compares this with the general experience many people have that we think of a person and that a few minutes later this person suddenly turns up (cf. no. 4).

In his discussion of question (ii), Aristotle makes a further, fundamental distinction between events whose origins lie within the dreamer him/herself and events whose origins do not lie within the dreamer. A similar distinction between human agency and things happening beyond human control was already alluded to in the preface to *On Sleep and Waking* quoted above. Diseases which may affect the dreamer, and actions the dreamer himself performs, obviously belong to the category of things whose origin (*archē*) is within the dreamer; but events that are 'extravagant in time, place or magnitude' (464 a 1–4) such as things occurring at the 'Pillars of Heracles' (462 b 24–6) obviously belong to the latter category. Aristotle connects this distinction with the results of his earlier distinction between causes, signs and coincidences: in cases where the origin of the event lies within the dreamer, it can be reasonably assumed that an explanation by reference to 'cause' or 'sign' is plausible, but in the latter (the origin of the event lying outside the dreamer) it is very likely that all we are dealing with is a coincidence of two occurrences without any physical relation (463 b 1–11).

As for question (iii), we need to look more closely at one of the most famous – but also rather controversial – passages from *On Divination in Sleep* (463 b 12–18)

ὅλως δὲ ἐπεὶ καὶ τῶν ἄλλων ζῴων ὀνειρώττει τινά, θεόπεμπτα οὐκ ἂν εἴη τὰ ἐνύπνια, οὐδὲ γέγονε τούτου χάριν, δαιμόνια μέντοι· ἡ γὰρ φύσις δαιμονία, ἀλλ' οὐ θεία. σημεῖον δέ· πάνυ γὰρ εὐτελεῖς ἄνθρωποι προορατικοί εἰσι καὶ εὐθυόνειροι, ὡς οὐ θεοῦ πέμποντος, ἀλλ' ὅσων ὥσπερ ἂν εἰ λάλος ἡ φυσις ἐστι καὶ μελαγχολική, παντοδαπὰς ὄψεις ὁρῶσιν.

In general, since some other animals have dreams too, dreams are not sent by a god, nor do they exist for this purpose; however, they are beyond human control, for the nature [of the dreamer] is beyond human control, though not divine. A sign of this is that quite simple people are inclined to having foresight and to having clear dreams, which suggests that it is not a god who sends them, but rather that all people who have, so to speak, a garrulous and melancholic nature, see all kinds of visions [in their sleep].

This passage is very characteristic of Aristotle's method in tackling the phenomenon of dreams and prophecy in sleep. He firmly rejects the belief – which was generally accepted in his time, even in intellectual circles – that dreams are sent by a god. The argument he produces against this belief consists of an intriguing combination of two empirical claims with an *a priori* presupposition. The empirical claims are that some other animals (apart from human beings) also dream (no. 5) – an inference based on the observation that dogs often bark during their sleep, as we learn from *Hist. An.* 536 b 27ff. – and that prophecy in sleep particularly occurs with people of mediocre intellectual capacities (no. 6). These two claims are combined with a rather sophisticated belief about the conditions of divine dispensation of mantic knowledge. Aristotle silently presupposes that gods, if they sent foreknowledge of the future to humans, would not send this to simple-minded people but rather (or even exclusively) to the best and most intelligent of people. This appears from another passage further on in the treatise (464 a 19–21):

καὶ διὰ ταῦτα συμβαίνει τὸ πάθος τοῦτο τοῖς τυχοῦσι καὶ οὐ τοῖς φρονιμωτά-τοις· μεθ' ἡμέραν τε γὰρ ἐγίνετ' ἂν καὶ τοῖς σοφοῖς, εἰ θεὸς ἦν ὁ πέμπων.

And for this reason this experience [i.e. foresight of the future concerning events whose origins lie outside the dreamer] occurs with simple people and not with the most intelligent; for it would present itself both during the day and with intelligent people, if it were a god who sends them.

The rationale for this seems to be as follows. If the gods really granted knowledge of the future to humans, they would distribute this knowledge according to the extent to which people meet the criterion of 'being beloved by the gods', and this means for Aristotle that a person should realise his/her moral and intellectual virtues to the highest degree and thus approach the divine level.[29] However, Aristotle argues, we can observe that prophetic dreams in reality occur also (or, exclusively) with simple-minded people, who stand on a lower moral level, and even to animals, who do not even have reason and thus lack the capacity to realise virtue. *Ergo*: dreams cannot be sent by a god.[30]

Aristotle thus presupposes that people with low moral and intellectual capacities are particularly susceptible to prophetic dreams. His favourite example is the melancholics, whom he mentions twice because of their remarkable foresight (cf. chapter 5 above). He explains this by reference to their physiological constitution, which brings about a certain receptivity to a large number and variety of appearances: the chance that they meet with a phantasm which resembles an actual future state of affairs is, from a statistical point of view, greater than with other people. It is entirely unclear how Aristotle arrived at this view (there are no antecedents of this characteristic of the melancholics in medical literature).[31] It seems, rather, that we have a case of 'wishful thinking' on the part of Aristotle here (and perhaps an extrapolation of his own dreaming experiences). Of course, his theory allows for prophecy in sleep to occur with intelligent people as well, but then we are dealing with cases where the origin of the event foreseen in the dream lies *within the dreamer* (for example, an action (s)he is going to perform, a physical disturbance which is going to befall him/her and which announces itself through another physical manifestation, namely, a dream). But in those cases where the future event foreseen in the dream occurs, for example, at the other end of the world, this must be a coincidence due to the multiplicity of images befalling the melancholics in their sleep, he seems to say.

The second presupposition underlying Aristotle's reasoning here is of a teleological kind: if some dreams can be shown not to be of divine origin, then this applies to all dreams. In this way, Aristotle anticipates two possible counter-arguments one might raise, namely that it is not necessary that *all* dreams are god-sent, or that it is not necessary that *all* dreams are prophetic. This kind of classification of various types of dreams is already found in

---

[29] Cf. *Eth. Nic.* 1179 a 21–30, discussed below in ch. 8.
[30] For a parallel argument concerning 'good fortune' (εὐτυχία) see ch. 8 below.
[31] See ch. 5 above.

Homer, in the well-known metaphor of the gates of horn and ivory in the *Odyssey* (19.560ff.), which distinguishes between true and false dreams, and in the Hippocratic work *On Regimen* quoted above, which differentiates between dreams of a divine origin and dreams that have a physical origin.[32] However, these counter-arguments based on a classification of dreams into different categories would not impress Aristotle: it is clearly inconceivable for him that a god incidentally and *ad hoc* uses a natural phenomenon to serve a purpose which is different from its normal, natural goal.

On the other hand, the passage also shows that Aristotle does not simply confine himself to a rejection of a divine origin of dreams: his criticism is directed against the specific assumption of dreams being 'sent' by the gods, of divine messages being 'sent' through the medium of dreams. But that does not imply that the phenomenon is deprived of any divine aspect whatsoever. In the sentence 'they are beyond human control, for the nature (of the dreamer) is beyond human control, though not divine' he recognises that dreams still have something 'super-human' because the natural constitution of the dreamer, which is the cause of the dream, is itself something beyond human control. It appears from another passage, in the preface to *On Sleep and Waking* quoted above, that the word *daimonios* is not to be understood in the sense of 'sent by demons', but in the sense of 'beyond human control' (the opposite, so to speak, of 'human', *anthrōpinos*): what appears to us in a dream is beyond our control, just as it is beyond our control what kind of natural, physiological constitution we have.

It may incidentally be observed that the structure of Aristotle's argument here is strikingly similar to that found in the Hippocratic works *On the Sacred Disease* and *Airs, Waters, Places* (see chapter 1 above). In the former treatise, the author rejects the view that epilepsy is sent by the gods, and one of the arguments he produces is concerned with the distribution of the disease among different kinds of people, which he claims is different from what one would expect if it were sent by a god. Thus in 2.4–5 he says: 'Here is another indication that this disease is in no way more divine than the others: it affects the naturally phlegmatic, but not those who are choleric. Yet if it were more divine than other diseases, it would have to occur with all sorts of people in equal manner and make no distinction between phlegmatic and choleric.' And in *Airs, Waters, Places* 22, the author argues against the belief in the supernatural origin of impotence among the Scythians, again by pointing out that the actual distribution of the affliction (predominantly among wealthy people, who can afford horses) is exactly

---

[32] On this distinction see van der Eijk (2004a).

the opposite from what one would expect if it were sent by a god, that is, among the poor, who are unable to please the gods by abundant sacrifice and who complain about this.[33] Again, the view expounded in both treatises that epilepsy and impotence *are* divine, but in the sense in which all diseases are divine, namely in 'having a nature', is strikingly similar to Aristotle's concession here that dreams, though not divine in the traditional sense, are nevertheless 'beyond human control' because the nature that produces them is *daimonios*.

5 A MEDICAL *ENDOXON*

In producing examples for all this from the empirical domain, however, Aristotle manoeuvres himself into considerable difficulties, for he cites evidence that, on closer inspection, falls short of fulfilling the strict requirements for dreams he had set out in *On Dreams*. In what follows, I will present two examples of this, which are case studies of his adoption and transformation of a view borrowed from others, which is accommodated in Aristotle's theory (and explained in a different way from the context from which he derived them) and backed up by empirical evidence. I will conclude by making some more general observations about the nature of these difficulties and possible explanations as to how they may have arisen.

First, in his explanation of how dreams can be signs, Aristotle begins by referring to the view attributed to 'the more distinguished among medical writers' that dreams deserve careful attention – a further indication that Aristotle was well aware of the medical views of this time:

ἆρ' οὖν ἐστι τῶν ἐνυπνίων τὰ μὲν αἴτια, τὰ δὲ σημεῖα, οἷον τῶν περὶ τὸ σῶμα συμβαινόντων; λέγουσι γοῦν καὶ τῶν ἰατρῶν οἱ χαρίεντες ὅτι δεῖ σφόδρα προσέχειν τοῖς ἐνυπνίοις· εὔλογον δὲ οὕτως ὑπολαβεῖν καὶ τοῖς μὴ τεχνίταις μέν, σκοπουμένοις δέ τι καὶ φιλοσοφοῦσιν. (*Div. somn.* 463 a 3–7)

Are some dreams, then, causes and others signs, for example of things happening in the region of the body? At any rate the distinguished among doctors, too, say that close attention should be paid to dreams. And it is reasonable for those to think so, too, who are no experts, but inquire the matter to a certain extent and have a general interest.

The wording of this passage sheds an interesting light on Aristotle's view on the relationship between medicine and the study of nature. The difference between the two groups referred to here (the *technitai* and the *philosophountes*) signifies a distinction between a specialised, practical as

---

[33] For a full discussion of the argument here see van der Eijk (1991) and (1994) 294–5. See also Hankinson (1998c), who makes the same point.

Aristotle on sleep and dreams

opposed to a non-expert, theoretical approach, that is, between knowledge being pursued with a view to its *use* or application in a particular case, and knowledge being pursued for its own sake.[34] The verb *philosophein* does not have the narrow meaning of 'practising philosophy'; it rather means 'be interested in, want to know, study',[35] and as such it seems almost equivalent to the verb *skopeisthai* ('inquire') in the same context.[36] *Philosophountes* here denotes people with a theoretical and a more general, non-specialised interest.

The view mentioned here is attributed to 'the distinguished among physicians' (*charientes tōn iatrōn*). This expression calls for some explanation.[37] *Charieis* basically means 'pleasing, charming, appealing to someone's taste', but the word is frequently used to refer to an intrinsic quality in virtue of which someone is pleasing: hence we may consider translations such as 'elegant, refined, sophisticated, cultivated, civilised, liberal-minded'. Perhaps 'distinguished' covers both aspects most appropriately. In Aristotle's works, we sometimes find the expression *hoi charientes*,[38] which denotes a group of people who are distinguished from *hoi polloi* ('the crowd') and *hoi phortikōtatoi* ('the vulgar' or 'the mean').[39] There are also instances where the word seems to refer to intellectual qualities such as cleverness and skilfulness.[40] The question is, therefore, in what sense the doctors mentioned here are 'distinguished' from other doctors.

The point of this reference to medical writers and the terminology in which it is cast become clearer from a comparison with two other passages from the *Parva naturalia*, namely from the treatises *On Sense Perception and Perceptible Objects* and *On Respiration*:

---

[34] Cf. the distinction between *epistēmē* and *technē* in *Metaph.* 981 b 14–982 a 3 and between practical and theoretical sciences in *Eth. Nic.* 1139 b 19–1140 a 24. Strictly speaking, medicine counts as a 'productive art' (*poiētikē technē*), since its purpose, i.e. health, is distinct from the activity of healing (cf. *Eth. Nic.* 1140 a 1–23; *Mag. mor.* 1197 a 3; *Pol.* 1254 a 2), but the difference between practical and productive arts, not always being relevant for Aristotle's purposes, is not always clearly explained (cf. *Rh.* 1362 b 4; *Pol.* 1325 b 18).

[35] For numerous examples see H. Bonitz, *Index Aristotelicus*, 820 b 25ff.; a number of instances are listed by Bonitz under the heading 'angustiore sensu, i q philosophari', but many of these may be questioned: there is, for instance, no distinction in Aristotle between natural science and natural philosophy (e.g. *Part. an.* 640 b 5).

[36] Cf. the use of *periergos* in the passage from *On Respiration* (quoted below).

[37] There is great variety in translations of this expression; some examples: 'accomplished physicians' (Hett); 'scientific physicians' (Beare); 'les médecins les plus distingués' (Mugnier); 'les plus habiles médecins' (Tricot); 'die tiefer angelegten Ärzte' (Rolfes); 'ii qui inter medicos sunt peritiores' (Siwek); 'medici elegantiores' (Bussemaker); 'clever doctors' (Ross); 'i medici più accorti' (Lanza).

[38] E.g. *Eth. Nic.* 1095 a 18; 1095 b 22.

[39] See *Eth. Nic.* 1127 b 23; 1128 a 15; 1128 a 31; *Pol.* 1320 b 7.

[40] See *Eth. Nic.* 1128 a 15; *Pol.* 1320 b 7; other instances are listed by LSJ, s.v. II, who render by 'accomplished'.

It is further the task of the student of nature to study the first principles of health and disease; for neither health nor disease can occur with that which is deprived of life. For this reason one can say that most of those people who study nature end with a discussion of medicine, just as those doctors who practise their discipline in a more inquisitive way (*philosophōteros*) start dealing with medicine on the basis of principles derived from the study of nature. (*Sens.* 436 a 17–b 2)

Concerning life and death and the subjects kindred to this inquiry our discussion is practically complete. As for health and disease, it is the business not only of the doctor but also of the student of nature to discuss their causes up to a certain point. However, in what sense they are different and study different things, should not be ignored, since the facts prove that their discussions are to a certain extent contiguous: those doctors who are ingenious and inquisitive do have something to say about nature and think it important to derive the principles of their discipline from the study of nature; and concerning those students of nature who are most distinguished, one may well say that they end with the principles of medicine. (*Resp.* 480 b 22–31)

In these passages Aristotle says that it belongs to the task of the student of nature (*phusikos*) to deal also with health and disease, because health and disease are characteristics of living beings.[41] However, this interest is limited to a discussion of the *principles* or the *causes* of health and disease.[42] Those who do so are called the 'most distinguished students of nature'; the same word *charieis* is used here as in the passage from *On Divination in Sleep*, where it is said of doctors. He further remarks that there are doctors who base their medical practice on the principles of the study of nature in general: these are called the doctors who 'practise their discipline in a more inquisitive way (*philosophōteros*)' and who are 'ingenious and inquisitive'. This is reasonable, he says, because natural science and medicine, though being different and studying different things, are 'contiguous' (*sunoroi*): up to a certain point their procedures run parallel or even overlap.

In a passage from the *Nicomachean Ethics* we find the same expression as in *On Divination in Sleep*:

clearly it is the task of the student of politics to have some acquaintance with the study of the soul, just as the doctor who is to heal the eye should also know about the body as a whole, and all the more since politics is a higher and more honourable art than medicine; and among doctors those who are distinguished devote much

---

[41] I.e. animals and plants. The scope of the *Parva naturalia* is the 'affections' experienced by beings that possess soul, e.g. life and death, youth and old age, respiration, sense-perception, sleep, dreaming, memory, recollection. See the preface to *On Sense Perception* and the discussion in van der Eijk (1994) 68–72.

[42] Similar remarks about the limited interest of medicine for the student of nature are to be found in *Long. et brev. vitae* 464 b 32ff. and *Part. an.* 653 a 8ff.

attention to the study of the human body. Therefore the student of politics should also study the nature of the soul, though he will do so with a view to these subjects, and only so far as is sufficient for the objects he is discussing; for further precision is perhaps more laborious than our purposes require. (1102 a 18–26)

It turns out that both doctors and natural scientists are called 'distinguished' by Aristotle in virtue of their tendency to cross the boundaries of their own discipline. For the doctors, this means that they take an interest in the body as a whole[43] and build their procedures on theoretical knowledge of the causes of bodily processes and the structures and functions of the parts the body consists of. Aristotle praises them for this and, as a consequence, acknowledges that these doctors may even contribute to the study of nature.[44] This is probably the 'overlap' mentioned in the passage in *On Respiration*. It is at least one of the reasons why he takes their view about the relevance of dreams for his discussion of prophecy in sleep quite seriously. It is not difficult to imagine the candidates to whom these expressions may refer: the writers of *On Regimen* and *On Fleshes* would no doubt come into the picture, and outside the Hippocratic corpus perhaps Diocles.[45]

The wording of the passage further implies that according to Aristotle not *all* doctors belong to this group: there are also doctors who primarily or exclusively rely on experience and who are ignorant of – or even explicitly hostile towards – theoretical presuppositions. A similar distinction between more or less theoretical approaches in the sciences is made in *Metaphysics* 1.1, where Aristotle uses the example of medicine to distinguish between the 'master craftsmen' (*architektones*) and the 'handworkers' (*cheirotechnai*); the former are the real possessors of a *technē* in that they know (in the case of medicine) the causes of diseases and of the effects of therapeutic measures, so that they can give an account of why they are curing a patient in a particular way, but the latter only work on the basis of experience[46] – although

---

[43] The background of this passage is provided by a passage in Plato's *Charmides* (156 b 3–c 5), where mention is made of the 'good physicians' (*hoi agathoi iatroi*) who practise their discipline from a broader, more theoretical perspective.

[44] This is a remarkably generous statement, but it remains a far cry from the opinion of the author of the Hippocratic treatise *On Ancient Medicine* ch. 20, who says that medicine is the *only* way to arrive at knowledge of nature.

[45] See Diocles, fragments 52 and 61 vdE.

[46] *Metaph.* 981 a 12–b 14. Perhaps the distinction of *charientes iatroi* also has a social aspect, in that they belong to a higher class. As for a 'class distinction' of doctors as made by Aristotle in *Pol.* 1282 a 3–4 (on which see Kudlien 1985), however, it seems to me – for the reasons mentioned – that they are closer to the *iatroi architektonikoi* than to the *iatroi pepaideumenoi*, for the latter are generalists with an encyclopaedic knowledge of medicine rather than experienced practitioners. The use of the word *pepaideumenos* by Aristotle usually has to do with an awareness of the methodological limits of a certain discipline (see Jori 1995), whereas the word *charieis* is used to refer to people who enrich their discipline by crossing its boundaries; on the other hand, in the passage from *Nicomachean Ethics*

Aristotle also recognises that the latter are often more successful in practical therapy than the former.

The passage from *On Respiration* further mentions differences between distinguished doctors and distinguished students of nature. These are not explained by Aristotle, but they probably have to do with the difference between theoretical and practical sciences mentioned above (differences of interest, such as the lack of therapeutic details in the account of the natural scientist, as well as different degrees of accuracy). Moreover, his remark that the more distinguished natural philosophers '*end* by studying the principles of health and disease', whereas distinguished doctors are praised for *starting* with principles derived from natural science, seems to imply a certain hierarchy or priority of importance, which is hardly surprising given Aristotle's general preference for theoretical knowledge. This would correspond with the fact that the discussion of health and disease (*Peri hugieias kai nosou*) was apparently planned by Aristotle at the end of the series of treatises which we know as the *Parva naturalia*. The treatise has not survived, and it is not even certain that it was ever written.[47] It is at any rate clear that in this treatise medical topics were, or would have been, discussed from the point of view of the study of nature: the treatise would probably deal with the principles of physiology, the causes of disturbances of the equilibrium between warm and cold, and the formation and the role of the residues (*perittōmata*). But it would no doubt refrain from worked-out nosological descriptions and from extended and detailed prescriptions on prognostics and therapeutics.[48]

Thus Aristotle's views on the relation between natural science and medicine are quite specific. He obviously approves of doctors who build their practice on principles of natural science, but he also acknowledges that more empirically minded doctors often have greater therapeutic success. He further praises those liberal-minded students of nature (among whom he implicitly counts himself) who deal with the principles of health and disease. He obviously prefers the study of nature rather than medicine, because the former is concerned with universals, the latter with particulars, and because the former reaches a higher degree of accuracy, but he

---

quoted above Aristotle credits the liberal-minded student of politics with a similar awareness of a limited degree of accuracy in his interest in psychology: one might say that this implies a comparable awareness with the distinguished doctors with regard to their use of principles derived from the study of nature.

[47] On this see Marenghi (1961) 145ff.; Tracy (1969) 161ff.; Strohmaier (1983); Longrigg (1995); R. A. H. King (2001); see also ch. 9 below.

[48] It should be stressed that this does not imply that Aristotle did not devote more specialised treatises to medical questions. See ch. 9 below.

also recognises that even medicine may contribute to the study of nature (a fact he hardly could ignore, given the large amount of anatomical and physiological information preserved in the Hippocratic writings). This explains his readiness to incorporate medical views into his own writings.

Having considered his theoretical position on the relationship between medicine and the study of nature, let us now turn to the practice of the 'inquisitive non-specialist' Aristotle in his discussion of the prognostic value of dreams. For although the distinguished doctors' opinion is a reputable view and as such an important indication that there are, in fact, dreams which play the part of signs of bodily events, the rational justification (*eulogon*) for the natural scientist's sharing this view does not lie in the doctors' authority, but in the fact that he can give an explanation for it. The explanation which follows makes use of empirical claims but is also based on Aristotle's own theory of dreams.

For the fact is that movements occurring in the daytime, if they are not very great and powerful, escape our notice in comparison with greater movements occurring in the waking state. But in sleep the opposite happens: then it is even the case that small movements appear to be great. This is evident from what often happens during sleep: people think that it is lightning and thundering, when there are only faint sounds in their ears, and that they are enjoying honey and sweet flavours when a tiny bit of phlegm is running down their throats, and that they go through a fire and are tremendously hot when a little warmth is occurring around certain parts of the body. But when they wake up, they plainly recognise that these things are of this nature. Consequently, since of all things the beginnings are small, it is evident that also of diseases and of other affections which are going to occur in the body, the beginnings are small. It is obvious, then, that these are necessarily more clearly visible in sleep than in the waking state. (*Div. somn.* 463 a 7–21)

It would seem that Aristotle's account perfectly meets his requirements for the dream being a sign of the event, that is, the disease. We have a starting-point (e.g. a physical disturbance which causes pain) which is going to produce a disease in the future and which also, at present, causes a dream image. If the dream is correctly interpreted, it can be reduced to its cause, which can be recognised as the cause of an imminent disease. Aristotle pays no attention to the rules for such a correct interpretation of dreams; he only analyses the causal structure of the relationship between the dream and the event foreseen in it. This analysis is based on two principles. The first is one of the corner stones of his theory of dreams as set out in *On Dreams* (460 b 28ff.), namely that small movements become manifest more clearly in sleep than in waking; this is because in the waking state these small movements escape our notice because they are overruled by more powerful ones, whereas in sleep, as a result of the lack of input of strong actual movements, the small ones get a chance to present themselves. This principle is demonstrated by means of a number of examples derived from common experience (no. 2 on the list above). The second principle is that the origins of all things (including diseases) are small and therefore belong to the category of small movements. The two principles are combined in the form of a syllogism at the end of the paragraph.

These points are most relevant for an assessment of what Aristotle is doing in the passage under discussion. It has, of course, long been recognised by commentators that the sentence 463 a 4–5 may very well be a reference to the Hippocratic treatise *On Regimen*, the fourth book of which deals with dreams and which I quoted at the beginning of this chapter. Although the Hippocratic Corpus contains several examples of the use of dreams as prognostic or diagnostic clues,[49] we nowhere find such an explicit theoretical foundation of this as in this book. It is chronologically possible and plausible that Aristotle knew this treatise, because other places in the *Parva naturalia* show a close similarity of doctrine to *On Regimen*.[50] That he is referring to it here becomes more likely when we consider that the writer of *On Regimen* certainly meets Aristotle's requirements for being a *charieis iatros*. Moreover, the author's approach must have appealed to Aristotle for the very fact that the interest of dreams is that they reveal the *causes* of diseases.

However, these similarities should not conceal the fundamental difference of approach between the medical writer and Aristotle. This difference not only manifests itself in that Aristotle, as a natural scientist, is only interested in the causal relationship between the dream and the event, whereas *On Regimen* is primarily a text about regimen (both from a preventive and from a therapeutic point of view), which explains the great amount of detailed attention paid to the interpretation of the contents of dreams and to prescriptions about preventive dietetic measures. The most important difference lies in the psycho-physiological explanation of the significance of dreams given by the two authors. The author of *On Regimen* appeals to a rather 'dualistic' conception of the relation between soul and body, of the type referred to earlier on in this chapter:

---

[49] See the instances listed in van der Eijk (1994) 279. The most explicit statement apart from *On Regimen* 86 is ch. 45 of the treatise *On Sevens*, but this is considered by most scholars to be post-Aristotelian.

[50] On this see W. D. Ross (1955) 56–7, who points out that Aristotle's 'comparison of the heart-lung system to a double bellows [in *De respiratione* 480 a 20–3] is clearly borrowed from *Vict.*'; see also Byl (1980) 321 n. 32 and 325, and Lefèvre (1972) 203–14.

For when the body is awake, the soul is its servant: it is divided among many parts of the body and is never on its own, but assigns a part of itself to each part of the body: to hearing, sight, touch, walking, and to acts of the whole body; but the mind is never on its own. However, when the body is at rest, the soul, being set in motion and awake, administers its own household and of itself performs all the acts of the body. For the body when asleep has no perception; but the soul, which is awake, cognises all things: it sees what is visible, hears what is audible, walks, touches, feels pain, ponders, though being only in a small space. All functions of the body or of the soul are performed by the soul during sleep. Whoever, therefore, knows how to interpret these acts correctly, knows a great part of wisdom. (*On Regimen* 4.86)

He presents soul and body as two separate entities which co-operate in the waking state but whose co-operation ends in sleep.[51] Aristotle, however, views the soul as the principle of organisation of all bodily functions, the formal apparatus which enables every organism to live and to realise its various functions. It would be impossible for Aristotle to say – as the writer of *On Regimen* does – that in sleep the body is at rest but that the soul works. Sleep is for Aristotle an affection of *the complex* of soul and body due to the heating and cooling of food and preventing the animal from perceiving actual sense movements.

It is obvious, therefore, that we cannot say that Aristotle is *influenced* here by the medical writer's views on dreams. It would be more appropriate to say that the non-specialised student of nature gives a theoretical explanation or even a justification of the view held by the distinguished doctors; this justification is given entirely in Aristotle's own terminology and based on his own presuppositions (the two principles mentioned above). This procedure is completely in accordance with his general views on the relation between natural science and medicine discussed above.

However, the incorporation of the medical view on the prognostic value of dreams into his own theory of sleep and dreams does confront Aristotle with a difficulty which he does not seem to address very successfully. For, as we have seen above, in *On Dreams* Aristotle says that dreams are based on the remnants of small sensitive movements which we receive in the waking state but do not notice at the time, because they are overruled by more powerful movements which claim all our attention. Yet during sleep, when the input of stronger competing sensitive movements has stopped, the remnants of these small movements come to the surface and present themselves to us in the form of dreams. As I have already said, it is exactly this mechanism to which Aristotle seems to refer in *Div. somn.* 463 a 7–11.

[51] On this conception see Cambiano (1980) 87–96.

But the problem is that the empirical examples of this mechanism given in the following lines seem to belong to a different category. The experiences of hearing thunder, tasting sweet flavours and going through a fire are apparently the result of movements in the body which present themselves *at the time of sleep*. These movements are not the remnants of movements which have occurred during the daytime but which were overruled then, but they are *actual* movements which take place at the moment of sleep and which are noticed at the moment that they occur.

Now, as we have seen, Aristotle in *On Dreams* acknowledges that this kind of perception may take place in sleep; but he immediately adds the qualification that this kind of perception is not a dream (an *enhupnion*) in the strict sense of the word, whereas that is the word he is using here in *On Divination in Sleep*. Moreover, in the present passage Aristotle states that we perceive these movements 'more clearly' in sleep than in the waking state, whereas the examples of the borderline experiences he gives in *On Dreams* are said to be perceived 'faintly and as it were from far away'.

There are several ways to cope with this problem, none of which, however, are free from difficulties.[52] We might consider the possibility that the experiences mentioned here are not examples of dreams, but effects of a more general mechanism which is operative in sleep, and of which dreams are a different species. In this respect the transition from line 10 to 11 may be understood – and paraphrased with some exaggeration – as follows: 'for then it even happens that small movements (no matter whether they are remnants of earlier perceptions or actual impressions) appear stronger than they really are'. The word 'even' (*kai*) may then be taken as pointing to the fact that the examples which follow demonstrate more than is really necessary for Aristotle's purpose. What is necessary for the argument is that the small movements which escaped our notice in the waking state become manifest to us in sleep. What is redundant in it is, first, that *all kinds* of small movements (i.e. both remnants of small movements from the waking state and small movements which actually occur to us when we are asleep) manifest themselves more clearly in sleep than in the waking state and, secondly, that these small movements appear stronger than they really are.

---

[52] I leave aside the interpretation according to which the experiences mentioned here *are*, after all, remnants of actual sense impressions received during the waking state, in which case there would be no inconsistency with *On Dreams*. This interpretation, however, seems unlikely: the present participles *gignomenōn, katarrheontos, gignomenēs*, as well as the fact that no example from the visual domain is given, surely indicate that the occurrence of the stimulus and its experience by the sleeper are simultaneous.

However, a similar problem presents itself further down in the text, when Aristotle considers yet another possible explanation for the phenomenon of divination in sleep; and again the difficulty arises while accommodating the view of another thinker, in this case the atomist philosopher Democritus.

6 A DEMOCRITEAN ELEMENT

As for dreams that do not have origins of the nature we just described, but origins that are extravagant in time, place or size, or in none of these respects but without those who see the dream having the origin in themselves – if foresight of the future [in these cases] does not occur as a result of coincidence, the explanation is more likely to be as follows than as Democritus says, who adduces idols and emanations as causes. Just as when something sets water in motion or air, and this moves something else, and when the one has stopped exercising motion, such a movement continues until it reaches a certain point where the original moving agent is not present, likewise nothing prevents a certain movement and sense-perception from arriving at the dreaming souls, proceeding from the objects from which Democritus says the idols and the emanations proceed, and in whatever way they arrive, [nothing prevents them from being] more clearly perceptible at night because during the day they are scattered more easily – for at night the air is less turbulent because there is less wind at night – and from bringing about sense-perception in the body because of sleep, for the same reason that we also perceive small movements inside us better when we are asleep than when we are awake. These movements cause appearances, on the basis of which people foresee the future even about these things. (*Div. somn.* 464 a 6–19)

Unfortunately, we do not have much information on Democritus' views on prophetic dreams that would allow us to check what Aristotle is attributing to him,[53] but it seems that Aristotle is largely sympathetic to it, though with the adaptation that instead of Democritus' 'idols and emanations' (*eidōla kai aporrhoiai*) he favours 'movements' (*kinēseis*) as the mediating factors. Furthermore, Aristotle says explicitly that the explanation offered for these 'extravagant' cases of foresight is built on the assumption that they are not due to coincidence (εἰ μὴ ἀπὸ συμπτώματος γίνεται τὸ προορᾶν). Thus he is offering an alternative explanation for cases of foresight which earlier on he attributed to coincidence (463 b 1–11) – and this was apparently also what Democritus was doing. The experiences mentioned here are clearly derived from sources outside the dreamer's body, which emit 'movements' that, after travelling over a great distance, reach the soul in sleep; and they can do so more easily at night because, Aristotle says, there is less wind

---

[53] See van der Eijk (1994) 310–12 for a discussion and fuller references.

at night and because in sleep we perceive these slight movements more clearly than in the waking state. Aristotle does not say to which category the dreams discussed here belong, but it seems that, if the category of 'coincidence' (*sumptōma*) is eliminated, these dreams stand to the events they predict in a relationship of signs (*sēmeia*), and that both the event and the dream go back to a common cause.

It is difficult, however, to see how the experiences described here can be accommodated within Aristotle's theory of sleep and dreams. They clearly do not fulfil the requirements for dreams as posited in *On Dreams*; nor do they seem to belong to the category of borderline experiences, because, again, Aristotle stipulates that they appear to us stronger than in the waking state. Unless we were to assume that Aristotle is contradicting himself, we might prefer to accept that in addition to dreams and to the borderline experiences of hearing faint sounds and suchlike, he recognises yet another kind of experience during sleep and that, by calling these experiences *enhupnia*, he uses the term in a less specific, more general sense than the strict sense in which it was used in *On Dreams*. After all, as I have said, the word *enhupnion* basically means 'something in sleep', and this could be used both at a more general and at a more specific level. But in that case, very little is left of Aristotle's initial, *a priori* assumption that sleep is an incapacitation of the sensitive part of the soul, for it turns out that we are perfectly well capable of perceiving these movements while asleep, provided that the atmospheric conditions are favourable. Nor is it open here to Aristotle to say that these movements originating from remote places such as the Pillars of Heracles are perceived by us not 'in so far as' we are asleep but in so far as we are, in a certain way, already awake: in fact, Aristotle explicitly says that we receive these stimuli 'because' we are asleep – indeed, they 'cause perception because of sleep' (αἴσθησιν ποιοῦσιν διὰ τὸν ὕπνον), which seems in blatant contradiction to everything he has said in *On Sleep*.

A different approach to this problem is to seek an explanation for these apparent inconsistencies in what Charles Kahn has called 'the progressive nature of the exposition' in Aristotle's argument.[54] In the course of his argument, Aristotle sometimes arrives at explanations or conclusions which implicitly modify or qualify things he has said earlier on without recognising this explicitly or revising his earlier formulations. Instead, he simply goes on, eager to explain as much as he can and carried away by the subtlety and explanatory power of his theories, but without bothering to tell us how these explanations fit in with what he has said earlier on. This may be

[54] Kahn (1966).

an argumentative, 'dialectic' or perhaps even didactic strategy (we should not forget that Aristotle's extant works derive from the teaching practice, and that they are very likely to have been supplemented by additional oral elucidation). Alternatively, it may be a matter of intellectual temperament or style. However this may be, it is undeniable that Aristotle in his works on sleep and dreams, as in his biological works at large, sometimes shows himself an improviser of *ad hoc* explanations, constantly prepared to adapt his theories to what the phenomena suggest. This inevitably means a lower degree of systematicity than we would perhaps regard as desirable; on the other hand, the elasticity of his explanations, and his readiness to accommodate new empirical observations, are things for which he is to be commended.

Lack of systematicity is, to a varying extent, characteristic of many Aristotelian works and can also be observed in other parts of the *Parva naturalia*, both within and between the individual treatises that make up the series. But it seems to obtain particularly to *On Divination in Sleep*,[55] which is in general a less technical treatise whose degree of accuracy, both in scientific terminology[56] and in the description of psycho-physiological details, is rather low in comparison with the other two works. Instead, it shows what could be called a more 'dialectical' character. Aristotle approaches the problem of divination in sleep from different perspectives, but he offers neither a definition nor a comprehensive explanatory account. The text has a strongly polemical tone and is for a substantial part devoted to an assessment of current views on the subject, such as the view (referred to and criticised three times) that dreams are sent by the gods, or the view held by the 'distinguished doctors', or the theory of Democritus.

---

[55] As for systematicity, it is of course true that a discussion of the topic of prophecy in sleep is announced, as we have seen above, in the preface to *On Sleep and Waking* (453 b 22–4), and that *On Divination in Sleep* refers, at one point (464 b 9–10), back to *On Dreams* (461 a 14ff.). Yet not too much weight should be attached to these cross-references, as they may easily have been added at a later, editorial stage; besides, the preface to *On Sleep and Waking* presents a programme of questions that is somewhat different from what is actually being offered in what follows, and this also applies to *On Dreams*. Thus the beginning of *On Sleep and Waking* announces a discussion of the question 'why people who sleep sometimes dream and sometimes do not dream, or, alternatively, if they always dream, why they cannot always remember their dreams' (453 b 18–20); but these questions can hardly be regarded as central to *On Dreams*, where they are addressed only in passing (in 461 a 13) and incompletely (in 462 a 31–b 11, a passage that itself, too, shows signs of a hastily added appendix). Such discrepancies between programme and execution need not, however, be due to later editorial additions, for it is, again, not uncharacteristic of Aristotle's works for there to be discrepancies between programme and execution.

[56] E.g. the use of *aisthanesthai* in the wide sense of 'notice', 'be aware of' (464 a 10, 15, 17), or the reference to 'perception arriving at the dreaming souls' (αἴσθησιν ἀφικνεῖσθαι πρὸς τὰς ψυχὰς τὰς ἐνυπνιαζούσας) in 464 a 10.

This polemical nature may also be related to the fact that Aristotle has a rather low estimation of the importance or value of dreams. As his discussion shows, and in particular the passage from 463 b 12–18 quoted above, dreams do not have any cognitive or moral significance and do not contribute in any way to the full realisation of human virtues. True, Aristotle concedes that in some cases foresight in sleep is possible, but this is not to be taken in the sense of a special kind of *knowledge* which some people possess, but rather in the straightforward sense of 'foreseeing', in a somewhat accidental and uncontrollable manner, what later actually happens. He does not assign a final cause to dreaming, and the answer to the question of the purpose of dreams is only given in a negative way. In the passage 463 b 14 discussed above, Aristotle says that dreams 'do not exist for this purpose', to serve as a kind of medium for divine messages. His own view seems to be that dreams simply exist as a necessary (i.e. non-purposive) side-effect of two other 'activities and experiences' of living beings, namely sense-perception and sleeping, both of which do have a purpose, sense-perception being essential to living beings, and sleep serving the purpose of providing the necessary rest from the continuous activity of the sense-organs.

This lack of a teleological explanation is not something to be surprised at, for as Aristotle himself says, one should not ask for a final cause with everything, for some things simply exist or occur as a result of other things or occurrences.[57] The only conceivable candidate for being the final cause of dreams – divination – meets with scepticism on Aristotle's part. Foresight in sleep is not an intellectual or cognitive *virtue* in the sense of the Aristotelian notion of excellence (*aretē*); on the contrary, it occurs with people whose intellectual powers are, for some reason, weakened or inactive. Prophecy in sleep is a matter of luck and belongs to the domain of chance: it escapes human control, and its correctness can only be established afterwards, when the event that was foreseen has actually taken place. Mantic knowledge is not knowledge in the strict sense (for many dreams do not come true, 463 b 22–31), and the insights gained by it, if correct, are at best 'accidental insights', which only concern the 'that', not the 'because': they only point to the existence or occurrence of something without providing an explanation for this.

This low estimation provides an additional reason why Aristotle shows so little interest in the contents and the meaning of dreams, which was one of the questions with which this investigation started. It will have become clear that the 'omissions' in Aristotle's discussion of dreams that I mentioned at

---

[57] *Part. an.* 677 a 16–19.

the beginning can better be understood both in the light of the framework of the study of nature in which his discussion takes place and in the light of his overall attitude towards the phenomenon in the wider context of his psychology and ethical theory. From this point of view, we can arrive at a more appropriate assessment of Aristotle's achievement in the study of sleep and dreams. The strength of Aristotle's treatment lies, in my view, in his highly intelligent and systematic approach, as it is reflected in the shrewd and original questions he asks. His use of empirical material does not, to be sure, always concord with all criteria that we, from a modern point of view, might think desirable for a truly scientific investigation; and his optimistic tone throughout both treatises, suggesting that everything is clear and only waiting to be explained by the master, does not quite do justice to his struggle with the perplexing phenomenon of prophecy in sleep – which he, not surprisingly, is unable to explain satisfactorily. Yet when measuring Aristotle's achievement in comparison with what was known and believed in his own time, we have good reasons to be impressed. His works on sleep and dreams are without any doubt the most intelligent extant treatment of the subject in classical literature.

CHAPTER 7

The matter of mind: Aristotle on the biology of 'psychic' processes and the bodily aspects of thinking

I PSYCHOLOGY, BIOLOGY, AND VARIATIONS IN COGNITIVE PERFORMANCES

Although Aristotle's *On the Soul* (*De anima*) has for centuries been regarded as a 'metaphysical' rather than a 'physical', or as a 'philosophical' rather than a 'scientific', work, there seems nowadays to be a consensus among students of his psychology as to the thoroughly biological status of the theory set forth there.[1] This may have to do with recent developments in the philosophy of mind, but it is probably also related to a reassessment of the importance of Aristotle's zoological writings (i.e. *History of Animals* (*Hist. an.*), *Parts of Animals* (*Part. an.*), *Generation of Animals* (*Gen. an.*), *Progression of Animals* (*De incessu animalium*, *IA*) and *Movement of Animals* (*De motu an.*)) and to a growing conviction among students of Aristotle's biology concerning the interrelatedness of what were traditionally called the 'psychological writings' of Aristotle (i.e. *On the Soul* and parts of the *Parva naturalia*) and the zoological works. There also seems to be a general agreement as to the basic consistency of Aristotle's psychological theory, or at least a tendency to explain apparent contradictions between *On the Soul* and the *Parva naturalia* on the one hand, and statements related to the soul in the zoological writings on the other (or between *On the Soul* and the *Parva naturalia*, or between different sections of the *Parva naturalia*) as the result of differences of method, approach, or argumentative strategy of particular treatises or contexts rather than in terms of a development in Aristotle's psychological ideas.[2]

This chapter was first published in W. Kullmann and S. Föllinger (eds.), *Aristotelische Biologie. Intentionen, Methoden, Ergebnisse* (Stuttgart, 1997) 221–58.

[1] See, e.g., Kahn (1966) 46ff.; Sorabji (1974) 65–6.

[2] For a convenient summary of the older discussion – initiated by Nuyens (1948) and applied to the *Parva naturalia* by Drossaart Lulofs (1947) and Block (1961a) – see Fortenbaugh (1967) 316–27. The compatibility of 'instrumentalism' and 'hylomorphism' was stressed by Kahn (1966); Lefèvre (1972) and (1978); and for the *Parva naturalia* by Wiesner (1978); and Wijsenbeek-Wijler (1976). See also

This consensus might easily give rise to the view that there is no such thing as an Aristotelian 'psychology', or at least that psychology more or less coincides with, or forms part of, biology in that it represents an investigation of animals (and plants) *qua* living beings, that is, ensouled natural things. Although this view is, in my opinion, not entirely correct (see below), it is in general accordance with Aristotle's belief that the study of soul 'contributes greatly' to the study of nature,[3] his definition of soul as 'the form of the body'[4] and his programmatic statement that all psychic 'affections' (παθήματα) are 'forms embedded in matter' (λόγοι ἔνυλοι).[5] For these statements clearly imply that psychology, in Aristotle's view, amounts to psycho-*physiology*, an analysis of both the formal and the material (i.e. bodily) aspects of psychic functions. The fact that in *On the Soul* itself we hear relatively little of these bodily aspects[6] might then be explained as a result of a deliberate distribution and arrangement of information over *On the soul* and the *Parva naturalia*, which should be seen as complementary parts of a continuous psycho-physiological account which is in its turn complementary to the zoological works.[7]

A very welcome consequence of this point of view could be that students of Aristotle's psychology pay more systematic attention to what the zoological works have to say on the (bodily) conditions for the actual functioning of the psychic powers identified in *On the Soul* (nutrition, growth, locomotion, desire, sense-perception, imagination, thinking). Thus the present chapter will deal with Aristotle's views on the bodily aspects of thinking, and it will attempt to show that although thinking, according to Aristotle, is perhaps itself a non-physical process, bodily factors have a much more significant part to play in it than has hitherto been recognised. In their turn, students of Aristotle's zoological writings might feel an increasing need to relate Aristotle's views on bodily parts and structures of organisms explicitly to the psychic functions they are supposed to serve,

---

Hardie (1964); Tracy (1969) and (1983); Verbeke (1978); Hartman (1977); Modrak (1987). This is not to say that developmental approaches to Aristotle's psychology have entirely disappeared; on certain specific topics, such as the various discussions in *On the Soul* and the *Parva naturalia* of the 'common sense' and its physiological aspects, there is still disagreement about how to account for the discrepancies; a developmental explanation is offered by Welsch (1987), a very important book which seems to have gone virtually unnoticed by Anglo-American scholarship on Aristotle's psychology, and by Block (1988).

[3] *De an.* 402 a 5–6. [4] *De an.* 412 a 19–21. [5] *De an.* 403 a 25.
[6] To be sure, physical aspects of the various psychic powers are referred to occasionally in *De an.*, e.g. in 417 a 4–5; 420 a 9ff.; 421 b 27–422 a 7; 422 b 1; 423 a 2ff. Brief references in *De an.* to the heart as centre of psychic activity are discussed by Tracy (1983).
[7] See Kahn (1966) 68: 'Thus the physiology of the *Parts of Animals* and the psychology of the *De Anima* are fully compatible, and they are in fact united in the psychophysiology of the *Parva Naturalia*.'

and to take into account the overarching framework of 'principal activities and affections' (πράξεις καὶ πάθη) of living beings for the sake of which, according to Aristotle, these parts and processes exist or occur.[8]

The result might well be a more *complete* picture of Aristotle's views on what it means to be a living being, that is to say, on how the various constituents that make up a living entity are interrelated. For, as Aristotle himself indicates, a purely formal description of psychic powers and processes is insufficient for at least two reasons. First, as he repeatedly stresses (apparently in polemics against the Pythagoreans), the connection of a certain psychic function with a certain bodily structure (an organ such as the eye, a process such as heating) is by no means coincidental; on the contrary, the bodily basis should have a certain nature or be in a certain condition in order to enable the exercise of a certain psychic power (e.g. perception).[9] Secondly, the material, bodily embedding of psychic functions accounts for the occurrence of *variations* (διαφοραί) both in the distribution of these functions over various kinds of animals and in their exercise. These variations may exist, or occur, among different species, but also among individual members of one species, or among *types* of individuals within one species, or even within one individual organism at different moments or states (e.g. sleep versus waking, drunkenness versus sobriety). As this chapter will try to show, variations in *intellectual* capacities and performances among different kinds of animals, among different members of one kind or even within one individual on different occasions are explained by Aristotle with a reference to *bodily* factors.[10] This raises the interesting question of the causal relationship between these intellectual performances and the bodily conditions corresponding to them, both in abnormal cases and in normal ones, and how the form–matter distinction is to be applied in these various circumstances: does form fail to 'master' matter in these cases, and if so, why? Should we speak of *one* form (e.g. rationality) being present in different pieces of matter, or should we say that there are different levels on which the form–matter distinction can be made (as in typological variations)? Are the variations to be explained mechanically or teleologically, and are defects compensated for by other skills?

In spite of this pronouncedly biological context, however, there *are* indications that the study of the soul has, for Aristotle, a special status and is

---

[8] See *Part. an.* 645 b 15–28. This approach is illustrated by Lloyd (1992).
[9] See *De an.* 412 a 15, 21; 412 b 5, 12; 414 a 22, 26.
[10] This is not to say that other factors, such as habit and education (ἐθισμός, διδαχή) play no role here; on the extent to which, according to Aristotle, cultural factors (education, local customs) may account for variations in the degree of perfection of these capacities, see below.

not completely reducible to the study of nature. His consideration of the – perhaps no more than potential – existence of 'affections that are peculiar to the soul' (ἴδια τῆς ψυχῆς) in *De an.* 1.1 and *Part. an.* 1.1 does suggest that there are areas, or at least aspects, of the study of the soul which biology does not cover (because no bodily factor appears to be involved).[11] Thus the assumption that *On the Soul* is, in fact, a biological treatise becomes problematic when one considers that it contains an extended, although notoriously sketchy, discussion of thinking (νοῦς, 3.4–8); for *if* thinking is really a non-physical process – an issue on which Aristotle's remarks are tentative and not always quite clear[12] – one would rather expect its treatment to belong somewhere else, for example in the *Metaphysics*.

Likewise unclear is the status of the *Parva naturalia*, which seem to occupy a kind of middle position between *On the Soul* and the zoological works and which, as a result, have traditionally, although rather unfortunately, been divided into a 'psychological' and a 'biological' section.[13] Their subject matter is intriguingly defined by Aristotle as 'the affections that are common to the soul and the body'[14] – which, again, at least *suggests* the existence of affections *peculiar* to the soul, just like affections peculiar to the *body*, such as diseases.

Hence it would perhaps be more appropriate to say that for Aristotle psychology and biology, as far as their subject matter is concerned, overlap

---

[11] *De an.* 402 a 9; 403 a 8ff.; *Part. an.* 641 a 32-b 10. Cf. Frede (1992) 106.
[12] The clearest statements are *De an.* 430 a 17–18, 22–3, and *Gen. an.* 736 b 28–9.
[13] See Kahn (1966) p. 49; Balme (1987) 9–20; Hett (1957) 388.
[14] See *Sens.* 436 a 8. On the method and scope of the *Parva naturalia* see van der Eijk (1994) 68–72; for a different view see G. R. T. Ross (1906) 1: 'They [the *Parva naturalia*] are essays on psychological subjects of very various classes, and there is so much detail in the treatment that, if incorporated in the *De Anima*, they would have detracted considerably from the unity and the plan of that work. Consequent on the separateness of the subjects in the *Parva Naturalia*, the method of treatment is much more inductive than in the *De Anima*. There, on the whole, the author is working outwards from the general definition of soul to the various types and determinations of psychic existence, while here, not being hampered by a general plan which compels him to move continually from the universal to the particular, he takes up the different types of animate activity with an independence and objectivity which was impossible in his central work.' It is true that in the *Parva naturalia* Aristotle makes more (though still very selective) use of empirical data, but he goes out of his way to make them consistent with his general psychological theory (see ch. 6 in this volume). In spite of Aristotle's own characterisation of the scope of the *Parva naturalia* in the beginning of *On Sense Perception*, it is not easy to characterise the difference with regard to *On the Soul* in such a way as to account for the distribution of information over the various treatises. Even if one is prepared to regard *On the Soul* and *Parva naturalia* as a continuous discussion of what it basically means for a living being (an animal or a plant) to live and to realise its various vital functions, or to explain the relative lack of physiological detail in *On the Soul* as the result of a deliberate argumentative strategy, it remains strange that some very fundamental *formal* aspects of the various psychic functions are dealt with at places where one would hardly expect them (e.g. the discussion of the 'common sense' faculty in *On Sleeping and Waking*, the discussion of the relation between thought and imagination in *On Memory and Recollection*, etc.) and that so many seemingly crucial issues in Aristotle's psychology are left vague.

to a large extent, but the study of soul comprises both more and less than the study of living beings: 'more' in the sense that there seems to be at least one psychic function which does not involve bodily organs or processes (although it cannot function without bodily organs or processes being present or taking place and its functioning can be influenced, i.e. both improved and disturbed, by bodily factors); and 'less' in the sense that it only studies living things under a certain aspect (their being ensouled, i.e. alive), or perhaps not so much 'ensouled beings' as 'soul' itself, whereas biology also deals with characteristics of living things that seem to have hardly any, or even no 'psychic' aspect at all, for example differences in the shape of certain bodily organs, or characteristics that are at best very *indirectly* related to the psychic functions they are supposed to serve.

These considerations are of some importance when it comes to comparing the various accounts of psychic powers and activities we find in Aristotle's works. For these accounts sometimes show discrepancies or even divergences that cannot easily be reconciled. Any attempt at relating, or even uniting, Aristotle's statements on soul functions in *On the Soul*, the *Parva naturalia*, and the zoological writings (not to mention the *Ethics* and the *Rhetoric*) into a comprehensive picture should take into account the differences in scope, purpose, method and subject matter of the various works concerned in order to arrive at a correct assessment of what Aristotle may be up to in these contexts and of the kind of information we may reasonably expect there. For example, concerning a psychic function such as sense-perception, one might say that its treatment in *Hist. an.* 4.8–10 (together with voice, sleep and sex differentiation) is mainly determined by the question of its distribution over various kinds of animals, and so Aristotle is only interested in dealing with questions such as whether all animals have sense-perception, whether they all have all the special senses, whether they all partake in sleep, and so on. One might subsequently say that *Hist. an.* 7–9 and *Gen. an.* 5 discuss the *differences* that manifest themselves among different species of organisms with regard to, among other things, their perceptual apparatus, whereas in *On the Soul* and the *Parva naturalia* Aristotle focuses on what all living beings possessing sense-perception have *in common*. The discussion of the sense-organs in *Parts of Animals* may then be said to be determined by a 'moriologic' perspective in which the special sense-organs are considered with a view to their suitability for the exercise of their respective special sense-functions. And finally, Aristotle's reasons for dealing with particular aspects of sense-perception at one place rather than another may be quite trivial, for example when, in *Gen. an.* 5.7, he says that he has been discussing those aspects of voice that have not yet been dealt with in *On the Soul* and *On Sense Perception*.[15]

Yet not always can differences in Aristotle's treatment of a particular soul power at different places be so easily related to the principles or strategies underlying the arrangement of his biological works. To continue with the example of sense-perception, there is a discrepancy between his rather formal and abstract enunciations on visual perception in *De an.* 2.7 (the 'canonical' doctrine of sight being moved by the visible object through the medium of the transparent) and, on the other hand, his rather technical discussions of various forms and degrees of sharpness of sight (ὀξὺ ὁρᾶν) and seeing over a great distance in *Gen. an.* 5, and of observing certain cosmic phenomena such as haloes as a result of reflection (ἀνάκλασις) in *Meteorologica* 3, which seem to presuppose an emanatory view on visual perception consisting in visual 'rays' departing from the eye and reaching the object of sight (or failing to do so properly). Even if this 'emanatory' doctrine is not identical to the view that Aristotle seems to reject in *On Sense Perception* and *On the Soul*, it remains unclear how it is to be accommodated within the 'canonical' theory of visual perception expounded in those works.[16]

In general, one gets the impression that divergences like this[17] tend to occur when Aristotle is dealing with the more 'technical' or 'mechanical' aspects of how soul powers actually operate and how, in particular cases or circumstances, these operations may *deviate* from the normal procedure. In dealing with these deviations, Aristotle sometimes refers to physical or physiological mechanisms or entities in respect of which it is not quite clear how they fit in the general picture or what part, if any, they play in the *normal* procedure. Thus in the example of visual perception over great distances, Aristotle does not explain what atmospheric conditions are conducive to the process of the object setting the visual faculty in motion, resulting in successful seeing. Similarly with regard to the 'type' of the melancholics[18] – one of Aristotle's favourite examples of deviations in the area of action

---

[15] 788 a 34-b 2. As for the relationship between 'psychology' and 'biology' in Aristotle, it would be interesting to examine the relationship between *Gen. an.* 5 on the one hand and *On the Soul* and *On Sense Perception* on the other; the many references in the former to the latter (786 b 23ff.; 781 a 21; 779 b 22) should indicate that Aristotle is very much aware of possible differences in levels of explanation or in status of the psychic phenomena to be discussed in either of these works.

[16] On this problem see van der Eijk (1994) 183 and 189–91.

[17] Other examples are Aristotle's discussion of the central sense faculty in *De an.* 3.2, *Sens.* 6 and *Somn. vig.* 2, or his doctrine of the 'kindled soul' in *De iuv.* 469 b 16 and *Resp.* 474 b 13, or the problem of animal intelligence (see below and Coles (1997)).

[18] See ch. 5 in this volume.

and cognition – we are told that they suffer from certain disturbances in their recollective capacities because of the presence of moisture around their 'perceptual parts',[19] but we are not informed about the *normal* physiological conditions for a successful operation of the recollective faculty.

One reason for this may be that Aristotle believed his audience to be sufficiently aware of these physical or physiological processes, perhaps because they were part of a medico-physiological tradition which he took for granted,[20] or he may not have quite made up his mind on them himself; in both cases, lack of clarity in the texts[21] prevents us from seeing how all these brief references to physiological processes fit together and are to be accommodated within the more 'formal' account of *On the Soul*, in which the emphasis is, as I said, on what ensouled beings have *in common* and in which deviations are rarely considered (although they are occasionally taken into account in passing in that treatise as well, as in *De an.* 421 a 22ff., to be discussed below).

However, it would also seem that these discrepancies are, at least partly, the result of a fundamental tension in Aristotle's application of the concept of 'nature' (φύσις), that is, what it means for the psychic functions to operate 'naturally' (κατὰ φύσιν). On the one hand, there is what we might call his 'normative' (or perhaps 'idealistic') view of what it naturally means to be a living plant, animal or human being – an approach which dominates in *On the Soul* and in the *Ethics*. On the other hand, there is also a more 'technical' or perhaps 'relativistic' perspective, in which he is concerned with the mechanics of psychic processes and with a natural explanation of the *variations* that manifest themselves in the actual performance of psychic functions among different living beings (e.g. degrees of accuracy in sense-perception, degrees of intelligence, degrees of moral excellence). Thus from the one perspective he might say that every human being is intelligent by definition, but from the other that not all human beings are equally intelligent, or from the one perspective that all animals have sense-perception by definition, but from the other that not all animals possess all senses. Whilst some of these variations exist between different species (e.g. some species of animals have only one sense, touch, whereas others have more), others exist between individual members of one species or between different *types* within one species (thus Aristotle distinguishes, within the human species, types such as the melancholics, dwarfs, 'ecstatic' people,

---

[19] *Mem.* 453 a 19ff.
[20] This seems to be the case with his concept of the melancholics; see ch. 5 in this volume.
[21] On the general lack of clarity of physiological descriptions in the *Parva naturalia* see Lloyd (1978) 229.

'irritable' people, 'quick' and 'slow' people, very young, youthful and very old people, people with prominent veins, people with soft flesh vs. people with hard flesh, etc., all of which are invoked to account for variations in cognitive capacities and performances).[22] Some of the variations of this latter category are on the structural level of an animal's 'disposition' (ἕξις) or natural constitution (φύσις), in that they are, for example, determined by heritage, natural constitution, or dependent on age and gender, but others are incidental (i.e. dependent on particular transitory states of the body or particular transitory circumstances). And whilst, depending on their effects, these variable factors are mostly to be regarded as *disturbing* agents impeding the actualisation of the animal's capacities (or even, on the level of the 'first actuality', affecting the basic vital apparatus of the animal, in which case it counts as a 'deformation', πεπηρωμένον), they can also be *conducive* to a better and fuller development of these capacities.

Some of these variations are explained by Aristotle in an entirely 'mechanistic' way without reference to a higher purpose they are said to serve, because they merely represent residual phenomena to be accounted for (material which is typically suitable for works like the *Problemata*). However, there are also variations which are, or can be, explained teleologically. Thus also in the seemingly mechanical account of the various forms and degrees of sharpness of sight in *Gen. an.* 5.1 an underlying teleological motive can be discerned: Aristotle distinguishes two types of sharpness of sight—seeing over a great distance (πόρρωθεν ὁρᾶν) and sensitivity to differences (διαισθάνεσθαι τὰς διαφοράς);[23] and the fact that the latter manifests itself in humans[24] (whereas many other animals are better at seeing sharply over a great distance) can be related to the cognitive and epistemological importance of the discrimination of differences, which is (like its counterpart, the

---

[22] Little attention has been paid to this aspect of Aristotle's biology, and to its medical background. On constitution types in the Hippocratic Corpus see Dittmer (1940). On dwarfs (οἱ νάνοι) see below, p. 223; for the 'ecstatics' (οἱ ἐκστατικοί) see *Div. somn.* 464 a 24–5; *Eth. Nic.* 1145 b 8–14; 1146 a 16ff.; 1151 a 1; 1151 a 20ff.; *Mem.* 451 a 9, and the discussion in Croissant (1932) 41ff., and in van der Eijk (1994) 321ff. The 'irritable' (οἱ ὀξεῖς) are mentioned in *Eth. Nic.* 1150 b 25; for the quick and the slow (οἱ ταχεῖς, οἱ βραδεῖς) see *Mem.* 450 b 8, *Physiognomonica* (*Phgn.*) 813 b 7ff. and below, p. 228; for the 'very young' (οἱ πάμπαν νέοι), the young and the old see *Hist. an.* 581 b 2; 537 b 14ff.; *Mem.* 450 b 2; 453 b 4; *Insomn.* 461 a 12; 462 a 12; *Gen. an.* 779 a 12f.; 778 a 23ff.; *Somn. vig.* 457 a 3ff.; *Rh.* 2.12–14 and below p. 225; for people with prominent veins (said to influence their sleep behaviour) see *Somn. vig.* 457 a 26 (cf. *Hist. an.* 582 a 15; *Pr.* 863 a 23); for 'people with soft' or 'hard flesh' (οἱ μαλακόσαρκοι, οἱ σκληρόσαρκοι) see *De an.* 421 a 25, and below, pp. 226–7.
[23] *Gen. an.* 780 b 15ff.
[24] *Gen. an.* 781 b 20: 'the reason is that the sense organ is pure and least earthy or corporeal, and man by nature has for his size the most delicate skin of all animals' (αἴτιον δὲ ὅτι τὸ αἰσθητήριον καθαρὸν καὶ ἥκιστα γεῶδες καὶ σωματῶδες, καὶ φύσει λεπτοδερμότατον τῶν ζώων ὡς κατὰ μέγεθος ἄνθρωπός ἐστιν).

power to see resemblances, ἡ τῶν ὁμοιοτήτων θεωρία)[25] at the basis of rational understanding, which is characteristic of human cognition. Thus variations that seem to be merely necessary concomitants of other, purposive biological structures and processes – and thus seem to be 'natural' (κατὰ φύσιν) only in the mechanical sense – can sometimes be accounted for *indirectly* as being 'natural' (κατὰ φύσιν) in a teleological sense as well.

This coexistence of two approaches need not be problematic: Aristotle is very much aware of the difference between teleological and mechanical explanations and is convinced of their being, to a very large extent, complementary. One might also say that the principle of 'naturalness' (κατὰ φύσιν) is applied by Aristotle at different levels: he does not shrink from saying that even within the category of things happening 'contrary to nature' (παρὰ φύσιν), such as the occurrence of deviations, deformations and monstrosities, there is such a thing as 'the natural' (τὸ κατὰ φύσιν);[26] deviations from the natural procedure can nevertheless display regularity, such as, again, the melancholics, who are said to be *naturally* abnormal.[27] The difficulty that remains, however, is how explanations offered for these variations and deviations are to be related to explanations offered for the normal procedure. This difficulty is especially urgent with variations in intellectual capacities; for these are explained with a reference to differences in *bodily* conditions of the individuals concerned, which raises the question of what the bodily conditions for a 'normal' operating of the intellect are and how this is to be related to Aristotle's 'normative' view of thinking as an incorporeal process: is the influence of these bodily conditions in deviations to be regarded as 'interference' in a process which *normally* has no physical aspect whatsoever, or is there also such a thing as a 'normal' or 'healthy' bodily state which acts as a physical substrate to thinking?

A related difficulty presents itself in the ethical domain. On the one hand, Aristotle tries to connect his views on what is best for man with what he believes to be man's *natural* activity (κατὰ φύσιν).[28] On the other hand, he also notoriously tries to provide a biological foundation for his belief that not all human beings are equally capable of realising the moral and intellectual virtues,[29] which is at the basis of his views on political organisation (e.g. his views on the naturalness of the state, slavery, and

---

[25] On this principle see Lambert (1966) and van der Eijk (1994) 326 and 333.
[26] *Gen. an.* 770 b 10ff.   [27] *Eth. Nic.* 1154 b 11; *Pr.* 954 b 8ff.; 955 a 40.
[28] See *Eth. Nic.* 1097 b 25ff.
[29] See the condition of natural ability in *Eth. Nic.* 1099 b 17ff.: 'In this way, happiness is also common to many; for it is possible for it to be available through some sort of learning and practising to all those who are not disabled in respect of virtue' (εἴη δ᾽ ἂν καὶ πολύκοινον [sc. ἡ εὐδαιμονία]· δυνατὸν γὰρ ὑπάρξαι πᾶσι τοῖς μὴ πεπηρωμένοις πρὸς ἀρετὴν διά τινος μαθήσεως καὶ ἐπιμελείας).

the position of women, or on the natural disposition of the good citizen). Moreover, he also seems to recognise that natural dispositions, though being necessary conditions for the realisation of human moral and intellectual capacities, are not *sufficient* to provide human beings with virtue and with happiness, but need development, training, and education.[30] To be sure, he recognises the existence of 'natural virtues' (φυσικαὶ ἀρεταί),[31] but they are in need of regulative principles (such as 'prudence', φρόνησις) in order to develop in the right direction, and they are even potentially harmful without these regulative principles, as his discussion of 'shrewdness' (δεινότης) shows.[32] Thus in the sphere of such distinctly human things as virtue, he acknowledges that nature requires further elaboration and even correction by 'art' (τέχνη). There is a tension here between a 'biological' and an 'ethical', perhaps 'anthropocentric' approach to human activity which has been well expressed by Gigon in his discussion of Aristotle's treatment of the contribution of nature to human happiness in the first chapter of the *Eudemian Ethics*: 'In the background lurks the problem (which is nowhere explicitly discussed in the Corpus Aristotelicum as we have it) why nature, which arranges everything for the best, is not capable of securing happiness for all people right from the start.'[33]

To summarise this first section: a comprehensive study of Aristotle's views on the bodily structures and processes involved in the actualisation of the various psychic functions of organisms (nutrition, growth and decay, locomotion, sense-perception, desire, imagination, thinking) would be very desirable.[34] Such a study would be even more interesting if it could demonstrate to what extent these views are determined by a concern, on his part, to provide a physical foundation for his normative views on hierarchy in

---

[30] See the discussion in *Eth. Nic.* 2.1, esp. 1103 a 24: 'Therefore virtues occur neither naturally nor contrary to nature, rather they occur to us because we are naturally suited to receive them and to bring them to perfection by habituation' (οὔτ' ἄρα φύσει οὔτε παρὰ φύσιν ἐγγίνονται αἱ ἀρεταί, ἀλλὰ πεφυκόσι μὲν ἡμῖν δέξασθαι αὐτάς, τελειουμένους δὲ διὰ τοῦ ἔθους, and 10.9, esp. 1179 b 21ff.; cf. also *Eth. Eud.* 1.1.
[31] *Eth. Nic.* 1144 b 15–16 and b 35ff.
[32] *Eth. Nic.* 1144 a 24ff., b 3, 9.
[33] Gigon (1971) 108: 'Im Hintergrund lauert das Problem (das in unserem corpus Aristotelicum nirgends expressis verbis verhandelt wird), warum die φύσις, die doch alles κατὰ τὸ βέλτιστον einrichtet, nicht in der Lage ist, alle Menschen von vorneherein mit der Eudaimonie auszustatten.'
[34] This is not to deprecate the importance of, indeed my indebtedness to, existing scholarship on this topic. Extremely useful (and deserving to be taken into account much more thoroughly by students of Aristotle's psychology) are the contributions by Tracy (1969); and by Solmsen (1950), esp. 464ff., (1955), (1957), (1961a), and (1961b). Nor are some German contributions from the nineteenth century to be neglected, such as Bäumker (1877); Neuhäuser (1878a, b); Schmidt (1881); Kampe (1870); Schell (1873). Still useful are Beare (1906); Rüsche (1930); and Peck (1953). See further Manuli and Vegetti (1977); Webb (1982); G. Freudenthal (1995) and Sisko (1996) 138–57.

the animal kingdom, in particular for his philosophical anthropology, and to what extent the description of these bodily structures and processes is guided by teleological concerns. However, such a study would have to take into account the different levels of explanation on which Aristotle is at work in various contexts as well as the *types* of context in which Aristotle expresses himself on these issues. The following typology of contexts (which does not claim to be exhaustive) would seem helpful:

(1) First, there are contexts in which Aristotle explains the bodily structures with a view to their suitability (ἐπιτηδειότης, οἰκειότης) for the fulfilment of the psychic functions in which they are involved, for example, when he describes the structure of the human hand by reference to the purpose it is intended to serve,[35] or man's upright position with a view to man's rational nature.[36] This is because he believes that a purely material description of the bodily structures would be just as insufficient as a purely formal description of soul functions, because it ignores the suitability of these structures for the exercise of the powers for the sake of which they exist and with a view to which they are shaped. As G. E. R. Lloyd summarises: 'whenever he is dealing with an instrumental part that is directly concerned with one of the major faculties of the soul identified in the *De anima*, Aristotle cannot fail to bear in mind precisely that *that* is the function that the part serves, and he will indeed see the activities in question as the final causes of the parts'.[37] However, as Lloyd himself recognises, this is just one of several concerns Aristotle has in the zoological works, and it is not consistently implemented.

(2) Secondly, there are contexts in which the 'mechanics' of psychic processes are discussed in physiological terms. Thus in his explanations of memory, recollection, sleeping and dreaming, Aristotle goes into great (though not always clear) physiological detail to describe the bodily parts involved in these 'psychic' activities and the physical processes that accompany them (e.g. the discussion of the 'bodily imprints' in memory,[38] or of the 'reactivation' of sense-movements in sleep due to the withdrawal of the blood).[39] As I have tried to show elsewhere, these discussions deal with operations of the sensitive (and perhaps also the intellectual) part of the soul under rather special circumstances, but they also have important implications for the physiology of *normal* sense-perception (on which the relevant sections in *On the Soul* and *On Sense Perception* are rather uninformative).[40]

---

[35] *Part. an.* 687 b 6ff.   [36] *Part. an.* 686 a 27ff. (see below); cf. also *IA* 706 a 19.
[37] Lloyd (1992) 149.   [38] *Mem.* 450 a 27ff.   [39] *Insomn.* 459 b 7ff.; 461 b 11ff.
[40] See van der Eijk (1994) 75–87.

(3) Thirdly, there are contexts in which Aristotle is giving a physiological explanation of *variations* in the distribution of psychic capacities or in their performance among various species of animals or types within one species – variations which, as I said, can be either purposive or without a purpose.

Such a comprehensive analysis is clearly beyond the scope of the present study. Moreover, the anatomical and physiological aspects of nutrition and of visual perception have recently been dealt with by Althoff (1997) and Oser-Grote (1997). For these practical reasons, the second part of the chapter will attempt to apply these general considerations to the highest psychic function only, the notoriously tricky subject of thinking and intelligence.

2 THE BODILY ASPECTS OF THINKING

Aristotle's sketchy and intriguing remarks on νοῦς and its relation to the body in *De an.* 3.4–5 have attracted a lot of scholarly attention, and the discussion on the precise implications of Aristotle's statements concerning the incorporeality of the intellect is still continuing.[41] Rather than adding to the vast amount of secondary literature on that topic, I shall confine myself to a discussion of a number of passages, mostly from the zoological writings, but also from *On the Soul* itself, in which Aristotle deals with the physical aspects of human (and animal) thinking. In order to avoid misunderstanding, it is perhaps useful to say from the outset that I shall be concerned with the intellectual activity of organisms rather than with the (divine) intellect itself, that is, with operations of the intellect in human (and to some extent also animal) cognition.[42] However, this does not mean a restriction to concrete *acts* of thinking (which might be seen as instances of participation by embodied souls in an incorporeal principle), for some of the passages to be discussed deal with structures and dispositions rather than with instantaneous acts of thinking, that is to say, they also pertain to the level of the 'first actuality'. A second preliminary remark is that the focus will be on the *role* these physical factors play rather than on the factors themselves: a comprehensive and systematic account of all individual factors involved (e.g. the

---

[41] For two recent interpretations see Kahn (1992), especially 366ff., and Wedin (1994); see also Wedin (1989).

[42] Cf. the distinction between 'the principle or faculty of *nous* as such and its concrete activity in us, in human acts of thinking' made by Kahn (1992) 362 and 367. It should be said, however, that this distinction is less clear in Aristotle than Kahn suggests; nor is it clear why the distinction between the principle and its concrete activities does not apply just as well to sensation – and if it does, what remains of the unique status of *nous*. Cf. Frede (1992) 105–7.

role of heat, or *pneuma*, or blood) is beyond the scope of this chapter.[43] In particular, the question will be raised to what extent these roles can be subsumed under the rubric of 'the dependence of thought on appearances' (φαντάσματα); for this is a dependence Aristotle acknowledges[44] but which seems to open the door to a variety of serious bodily influences on the operation of the intellect and thus may present a challenge to his 'canonical' view that thinking is not a bodily process taking place in a particular bodily organ (a view that can be related to other parts of his philosophy, e.g. his epistemological and ethical views about man, man's being akin to the gods, man's highest activity consisting in contemplation, etc.).

First, there are a number of texts that describe thinking itself in seemingly physical terms. Thus a passage in *Ph*. 247 b 1ff. describes thinking as a state of 'rest' (ἠρέμησις) or 'coming to a standstill' (ἐφίστασθαι) following upon, indeed emerging from, a state of bodily motion or turbulence:

Nor are the states of the intellectual part qualitative changes ... nor is the original acquisition of knowledge a process of becoming or a modification. For it is through [discursive] reasoning (διάνοια) coming to a standstill that we are said to know and understand (ἐπίστασθαι καὶ φρονεῖν), and there is no process of becoming leading to the standstill, nor indeed to any kind of change ... Just as when someone changes from [a state of] drunkenness or sleep or disease into the opposite states we do not say that he has come to have knowledge again – although he *was* unable to realise the knowledge – so likewise when he originally acquires the state [of knowing] we should not say so [i.e. that he is 'coming to be' possessed of knowledge]. For it is by the soul (ψυχή) coming to a standstill from the natural turbulence that something becomes understanding (φρόνιμον) or knowing (ἐπιστῆμον) – and this is also why children cannot acquire knowledge (μανθάνειν) or pass judgements according to their senses as grown men can, for they are in a state of great turbulence and movement. It [i.e. the soul] is brought to a standstill and to rest, with regard to

---

[43] It would be very useful indeed to study the role of particular factors, especially heat and blood, in the various psychic powers and to see what part they play in the explanation of variations in psychic performances among different kinds of animals (for a thorough treatment of the role of the elementary qualities in Aristotle's biological writings see Althoff (1992a), whose *index locorum* will guide the reader to useful discussions of the relevant passages). This might also shed light on the difficult question of how the different 'parts' of the soul are interrelated and how, or rather, *whether* operations of 'lower' soul functions may be influenced by higher ones, e.g. whether human perception is *itself* different from animal perception because of the presence of the intellectual capacity. Thus in addition to speaking of 'sense informed by a noetic capacity' and saying that 'It is only in the case of *human* perception, enriched by the conceptual resources provided by its marriage with *nous*, that Aristotle can speak of us *perceiving a man*' (Kahn (1992) 369), one might also consider saying that according to Aristotle the human bodily structures and conditions for perception are better and more conducive to knowledge and understanding than in animals (e.g. because man has a better, purer blend of heat and cold).

[44] *Mem.* 449 b 31–450 a 1; *De an.* 403 a 9; 427 b 15; 431 a 17; 431 b 2; 432 a 3ff.

some things by nature itself, with regard to others by other factors, but in either case while certain qualitative changes take place in the body, just as with the use and the activity [of the intellect] when a man becomes sober or wakes from sleep. It is clear, then, from what has been said, that being changed and qualitative change occurs in the perceptible objects and in the perceptive part of the soul, but in no other [part], except incidentally (κατὰ συμβεβηκός).

The passage stands in the context of an argument in which Aristotle is trying to prove that dispositions of the soul (ἕξεις τῆς ψυχῆς) are not qualitative changes (ἀλλοιώσεις), and in the case of thinking he even goes further to deny that any activity of the intellectual part of the soul is a process of 'coming to be' (γένεσις), although it is accompanied by such processes taking place in the body, that is, in the perceptual part of the soul. In the passage quoted it is clearly stated that thinking, while carefully distinguished from bodily motions, is accompanied by, and is the result of, these bodily motions. The acquisition of knowledge is compared with the transition from having knowledge to using it which takes place when somebody wakes up from sleep or emerges from drunkenness, states which are said to impede the *use* of knowledge, namely the transition from 'first' to 'second actuality'.[45] This comparison, and the remark about children's inability to think and judge because of their physical constitution, clearly indicates that thinking, though not equated with physical movement, is very much dependent on bodily states and processes; it is said to result from 'the *soul* (ψυχή) coming to a rest' or even from '*reasoning* (διάνοια) coming to a standstill'. The use of these two terms may be significant: 'soul' apparently refers to the embodied nutritive and perceptual powers as a whole, and as for *dianoia*, there are indications in Aristotle's works that this is a wider concept covering a variety of cognitive actions in the border area between perceiving and thinking (see below).

The idea that thinking consists in 'rest' or 'standing still' is a traditional notion which also occurs elsewhere in Greek literature and which

[45] In his discussion of this and related passages, Tracy (1969) 274 comments: 'Now the very nature of thought and knowledge demands that the phantasm upon which they depend be undisturbed and tranquil. For, psychologically, thought and knowledge are not a movement but the *termination* of movement, a *settling down* or repose of the mind in the possession of its object, which depends upon a corresponding tranquillity in the sense power serving it... Thus the original acquisition and subsequent actualization of intellectual virtues like scientific knowledge or wisdom are brought about not by any movement in the intellect itself, but by "*something else* coming to be present" so that the intellect "rests" or "halts" upon it. From what we have seen of the intellect and its operation we may infer that Aristotle has in mind here the *phantasm*, which presents the *universal*, – the intelligible form – as embodied in *particular* sensible qualities... Thus the virtue of knowledge and its activation, being dependent upon the phantasm produced by the sense power, are impeded or rendered impossible by the physical disturbances accompanying drunkenness, sleep, disease and growth, as well as the dissolution of old age.'

is sometimes justified by means of the alleged etymological relation between ἐπιστήμη and ἐφίστασθαι,[46] and it occurs a number of times in Aristotle's works.[47] There is nothing to suggest that this should be understood in a metaphorical way; on the contrary, the reference to bodily motion and to children who because of their structural state of motion are not capable of thinking strongly suggests that Aristotle actually believes that thinking emerges from the 'coming to a standstill' of a bodily process. Where this coming to a standstill takes place (the heart?) and what bodily factors are involved (the blood?) are not explained in any of these texts.[48] Whether thoughts 'emerge' from the standing still of movements, or whether thought *brings about* the standing still of images (e.g. by abstraction) remains unclear.[49] The physiological picture to be drawn with the transition from having knowledge to using it, which is said to occur at the transition from drunkenness (or sleep) to sobriety (or waking), is also referred to in Aristotle's discussion of *akrasia* in *Eth. Nic.* 1147 b 6ff., where it is said: 'The explanation of how the ignorance (which caused the weak person's action) is dissipated (λύεται) and the weak person returns to a state of knowing is the same as concerning a drunk and a sleeping person, and it is not peculiar to this condition: it is to be obtained from the physiologists.' This physiological explanation is provided by scattered remarks in Aristotle's physical works and is conveniently summarised by Tracy: 'knowledge is acquired and activated only when the body, and the sensory system in particular, *calms down*, being freed from disturbance and brought to a state of stable equilibrium in all respects, that is, to a state of maturity, health, sobriety and moral excellence. Some of these may be produced by natural processes alone; others, like health and moral excellence, may require assistance from the physician and trainer, the moral guide and statesman.'[50] As emerges from *On Sleep and Waking* and *On Dreams*, one of these 'natural processes' is the restoration of the balance between warm and cold in the body which is brought about when the process of digestion (the material cause of sleep) has been completed; another, which accompanies this, is the process of separation of blood into a thinner, clearer part and a thicker, more troubled part;[51] and yet another (in the case of

---

[46] See Plato, *Phaedo* 96 b 8.
[47] See *De motu an.* 701 a 27; *An. post.* 100 a 1ff. and 15ff.; *Int.* 16 b 20; *De an.* 407 a 32–3. Cf. *Pr.* 956 b 39ff.; 916 b 7ff.
[48] Except in *Pr.* 916 b 7ff., where, perhaps significantly, a disturbance in intellectual activity (διάνοια, in this case reading) is attributed to the cooling effect of 'pneumatic movements' and melancholic humours; a few lines later on, however, the intellect (νοῦς) is localised in the head (916 b 16).
[49] Perhaps one should think of an act of viewing (θεωρεῖν) the relevant items in a confused whole; see *Insomn.* 461 a 8–25; *Div. somn.* 464 b 7–16 (cf. 463 b 15–22); *Mem.* 450 b 15ff.
[50] Tracy (1969) 276.
[51] On the physiological explanation of sleep in *Somn. vig.* see Wiesner (1978).

drunkenness) is the dissolution of movement and confusion (κίνησις καὶ ταραχή) brought about by *pneuma*.[52] How exactly these processes interact and influence cognitive processes, Aristotle does not make very clear; but it is evident that he believes that healthy bodily conditions (such as an empty stomach) may be conducive to a successful operation of the intellectual part of the soul.[53]

Another passage, however, suggests that movement (κίνησις) and even 'agility' (τὸ εὐκίνητον) are essential to thinking and that physical impediment to movement also affects thinking. At *Part. an.* 686 a 25ff. we are told that man's body is in an upright position in order to promote the performance of his 'divine' function, namely thinking and being intelligent (νοεῖν καὶ φρονεῖν).[54]

Man, instead of forelegs and forefeet, has arms and the so-called hands. For man is the only animal that stands upright, and this is because his nature and essence is divine. The activity of that which is most divine is to think and to be intelligent; but this is not easy when there is a great deal of the upper body weighing it down (τοῦτο δὲ οὐ ῥᾴδιον πολλοῦ τοῦ ἄνωθεν ἐπικειμένου σώματος), for weight hampers the motion of the intellect and of the common sense (τὸ γὰρ βάρος δυσκίνητον ποιεῖ τὴν διάνοιαν καὶ τὴν κοινὴν αἴσθησιν). Thus, when the weight and the corporeal condition (of the soul) become too great, the bodies themselves must lurch forward towards the ground; consequently, for the purpose of safety, nature provided quadrupeds with forefeet instead of arms and hands. All animals which walk must have two hind feet, and those I have just mentioned became quadrupeds because their soul could not sustain the weight bearing it down (οὐ δυναμένης φέρειν τὸ βάρος τῆς ψυχῆς). In fact, compared with man, all the other animals are dwarf-like... In humans, the size of the trunk is proportionate to the lower parts, and as they are brought to pefection (τελειουμένοις), it becomes much smaller in proportion. With young people, however, the contrary happens: the upper parts are large and the lower are small... In fact, all children are dwarfs. The genera of birds and fishes, as well as every animal with blood in it, as I have said, are dwarf-like. This is also the reason why all animals are less intelligent (ἀφρονέστερα) than man. Even among human beings children, for example, when compared to adults, and among those who are adults those who have a dwarf-like nature, though having some exceptional capacity,[55] are nevertheless inferior in their having intelligence (τῷ τὸν νοῦν ἔχειν ἐλλείπουσιν). The reason, as has already been said, is that in many of them the principle of the soul is sluggish and corporeal (ἡ τῆς ψυχῆς

---

[52] *Insomn.* 461 a 23–5.
[53] It is interesting to note that ancient commentators on *De an.* 403 a 16 were already worried about the implications of this belief for the doctrine of the separateness of the intellect (see Philoponus, *In Arist. De anima I comment.* p. 51, 10ff. Hayduck).
[54] Cf. *Part. an.* 653 a 30; cf. *Pol.* 1254 b 30 and the comments ad loc. by Saunders (1995). For a discussion of the various physiological factors mentioned in this passage (*Part. an.* 686 a 25ff.) see Coles (1997).
[55] For Aristotle's appreciation of τὸ περιττόν cf. *Rh.* 1390 b 27; see also *Pr.* 30.1, which exploits this notion for the explanation of the melancholics' exceptional performances.

ἀρχὴ πολλοῖς δὴ δυσκίνητός ἐστι καὶ σωματώδης).[56] If the heat which raises the organism up wanes still further and the earthly matter waxes,[57] then the animals' bodies wane, and they are many-footed; and finally they lose their feet and lie full length on the ground.

This passage clearly speaks of the 'movement' of thought and the common sense admitting of being impeded by the position of the body. Again the mention of 'intellect' (διάνοια) and of 'the principle of the soul' as being susceptible to bodily disturbances (even acquiring a 'body-like' state, σωματώδης) is significant.[58] The seemingly indiscriminate use of νοῦς, νοεῖν, διάνοια, φρονεῖν, and ἀφρονέστερος may suggest that Aristotle is not talking about a specific intellectual function but about thinking in general; however, it might also indicate that the *gradual* difference of intelligence between man and other animals (ἀφρονέστερος) amounts to a *principal* difference of having *nous* or not having it – although the expression τῷ τὸν νοῦν ἔχειν ἐλλείπουσιν occurs in a context where he is discussing differences *within* the human species, which suggests that the inferiority of dwarfs consists in their having a lower degree of intelligence rather than having no intelligence at all. This point is of relevance for the question whether Aristotle believed in lower or higher levels of thinking which are to a higher or lower extent susceptible to bodily influence, and for whether Aristotle believed in animal intelligence (see below).

It is further significant that, perhaps somewhat to our surprise, the passage states the *reason* why man is the most intelligent of all blooded animals – something which is usually simply postulated as a fact without argument by Aristotle in *On the Soul* and in the *Ethics* – by stating the *material* cause for man's being intelligent.[59] All blooded animals are less intelligent than man because of their dwarf-like nature (νανώδη), and also within the human species differences in intelligence are accounted for by the dwarf-like shape

---

[56] The text is uncertain here; πολλοῖς is A. L. Peck's emendation of the manuscript reading πολλῷ.

[57] A. L. Peck, in his Loeb translation, compares this to the Hippocratic *On Regimen* 1.35; on this see below, pp. 230–1. On 'earthiness' as an impeding factor cf. *Gen. an.* 781 b 20.

[58] The mention of the 'common sense', and 'the principle of the soul' suggest that a principle located in the heart is meant here (cf. *De iuv.* 469 a 5ff.; b 5–6; *Gen. an.* 743 b 26; *Somn. vig.* 456 b 1). For the difficulty of relating this passage to Aristotle's conception of the soul see Althoff (1992) 73 n. 146: 'Der Seele selbst die Eigenschaft des Körperhaften zuzusprechen ist nach der aristotelischen Seelenauffassung sehr problematisch. Es scheint vielmehr so zu sein, dass die mangelnde Beweglichkeit der Seele (und damit die mangelnde Intelligenz) zurückgeführt wird auf eine Druckeinwirkung, die der obere Teil des Körpers auf das Herz als den ersten Sitz der Seele ausübt.' However, also in *Part. an.* 672 b 16–17 Aristotle seems to allow the 'principle of the sensitive part of the soul' to be affected by the evaporation of food.

[59] Further below in the same chapter (686 a 7ff.) Aristotle also gives a teleological explanation for the difference in bodily shape between man and other animals with a view to man's being intelligent. There, however, the material explanation offered by Anaxagoras and rejected by Aristotle is different: it is not man's upright position, but his having hands which is at issue.

of the body. In this respect, it may be useful to note that dwarfs (νάνοι) represent a special human type[60] to which Aristotle refers a number of times and which is said to suffer from all sorts of structural cognitive weaknesses and disturbances. Thus at *Mem.* 453 a 31, dwarf-like people are said to have poorer memories (ἀμνημονέστεροι) than their opposites because of much weight on their perceptual faculty, which makes it difficult for them to retain the movements and which also makes it difficult for them to recollect – which is an *intellectual* process, as he has said in 453 a 10ff. – along a straight line.[61] At *Somn. vig.* 457 a 22ff., they are said to sleep much because of the great upward movement and evaporation (of hot moisture derived from food). Young children suffer from the same defects,[62] but in their case growth will bring them to perfection later in their lives.

It is not very clear how the idea of agility of thought and common sense is to be reconciled with the statement in the *Physics* passage that thinking consists in rest and stillness. It may be that Aristotle is talking about different stages of the process, *duskinēton* referring to a disturbance of the supply of appearances (φαντάσματα) that provide the intellect with material to think about and to halt upon (although it is hard to read this into the Greek); or it may be that he is speaking about different levels, or different *types* of movement, *duskinēton* referring to a more abstract, less physical type of movement – although, again, this is not expressed very clearly in the Greek. It may also be that *duskinētos*, as the opposite of *eukinētos*, should be understood as a disturbance of the balance between movement and stillness (cf. εὐκρασία vs. δυσκρασία), and that the ideal state consists in a mean between two extremes (cf. *Mem.* 450 b 1–11); however, the difficulty that remains is that this still presupposes some sort of movement, whereas the *Physics* passage seemed to say that thinking depends on the coming to a standstill of bodily motion. Anyway, the passage also seems to commit itself to a *location* of thinking at a relatively high part of the body.[63]

A number of passages briefly allude to incidental disturbances of the intellect by bodily conditions. Thus in his discussion of 'imagination' (φαντασία)

---

[60] As appears from *Gen. an.* 749 a 4, they are a deformation (πεπηρωμένον). On Aristotle's views on dwarfs (and their medical background) see Dasen (1993) 214–20.
[61] For the notion of εὐθυπορεῖν see 453 a 25; see also below, p. 229.
[62] Children are also mentioned in *Mem.* 453 b 4; 450 b 6; *Somn. vig.* 457 a 18ff.
[63] The question might be raised why, if the bodily structure of man is supposed to be subservient to the performance of his 'most divine' part, thinking is not located in the brain (as was Plato's argument in the *Timaeus* (90 a ff.), of which the present passage is clearly reminiscent). However, Aristotle may have had other reasons for not considering the brain as an ideal location (see Kullmann (1982) 233–4), and he may have been reluctant to express himself on *any* location of the intellect (see below, n. 65).

in *De an.* 3.3, Aristotle says that animals (ζῷα) perform many actions in accordance with imagination, some animals, such as the beasts (τὰ θηρία), because they have no intellect (i.e. they have nothing else to guide their actions except for imagination), others, such as humans, because thinking (νοῦς) is 'overshadowed' (ἐπικαλύπτεσθαι) by emotion, disease or sleep (*De an.* 429 a 5–8).[64] At *Part. an.* 653 b 5, mental disturbances (παράνοιαι) are said to occur as a result of the brain's failure to cool the bodily heat. In his discussion of the diaphragm in *Part. an.* 672 b 28ff., Aristotle remarks that reasoning and perception (διάνοια καὶ αἴσθησις) are 'evidently confused' (ἐπιδήλως ταράττει) by the presence of a warm, moist residual substance in the neighbourhood of the diaphragm:

> This is why it [i.e. the diaphragm] is called *phrenes*, as if it had some part in thinking (φρονεῖν). Yet it does not have any part [in thinking], but being close to [parts] that do have part [in thinking], it evidently causes a change of the intellect (μεταβολὴ τῆς διανοίας).

This is one of the very few places where Aristotle says something about the *place* where thinking – if it is anywhere – is located, or at least about bodily parts that partake in reason; the passage points, not surprisingly, to the heart, although this is not directly stated and there may be other candidates as well.[65]

In other passages, we are told that within the human species, age is a factor that influences an individual's intellectual capacities: very young people do not yet have the power to think, they are similar to animals (*Hist. an.* 588 a 31ff.; cf. *Part. an.* 686 b 23ff. discussed above); similarly, old age is accompanied by a decay of thinking (*Pol.* 1270 b 40 and, more hesitantly, *De an.* 408 b 19–31).[66] The influence of age and descent (εὐγένεια) on

---

[64] Physical factors as disturbing agents in the process of rational deliberation about the right way of action are also mentioned several times in Aristotle's discussion of ἀκρασία and pleasure in *Eth. Nic.* 7 (1147 a 13–14; 1147 b 7; 1152 a 15; 1154 b 10). What part they play in practical reasoning, i.e. to what extent Aristotle believes the actualisation of the right premises in a practical syllogism to be dependent on physiological conditions ('deliberations' (λογισμοί) being 'kicked away' (ἐκκρούεσθαι) by physical movement, cf. *Eth. Nic.* 1119 b 10; 1175 b 3ff.; *Eth. Eud.* 1224 b 24), deserves further examination (cf. Gosling 1993).

[65] It is striking indeed that although in later doxographical literature Aristotle is always credited with holding a cardiocentrist view on the seat of the intellect, there is surprisingly little in his works to confirm this interpretation (only *Pr.* 954 a 35 speaks of a νοερὸς τόπος, which is probably the heart; elsewhere in the *Problemata*, however, the intellect is located in the head, 916 b 16). Cf. Mansfeld (1990) [and ch. 4].

[66] A striking passage on the correlation between age and intelligence (νοῦς) is *Pr.* 30.5, where νοῦς is said to be the only intellectual activity which is present to us by nature, whereas the other forms of wisdom and skill (ἐπιστῆμαι καὶ τέχναι) are brought about by human effort (955 b 26–7; cf. *Eth. Nic.* 1143 b 7–9).

character (ἦθος)⁶⁷ is discussed in *Rh.* 2.12–15; and a passage in *Pol.* 7.6 on the best natural constitution (φύσις) for citizenship in the city-state suggests a correspondence between environment (τόποι) on the one hand and intelligence and courage (διάνοια καὶ θυμός) on the other (1327 b 20ff.): while the inhabitants of cold regions and of 'Europe' are courageous but defective in intelligence and skill (διανοίας δὲ ἐνδεέστερα καὶ τέχνης) and the inhabitants of Asia intelligent but lacking in spirit (διανοητικὰ μὲν καὶ τεχνικὰ τὴν ψυχήν, ἄθυμα δέ), the Greeks represent a mean both geographically and in virtue of their character as determined by their physical constitution (τὰ δὲ εὖ κέκραται πρὸς ἀμφοτέρας τὰς δυνάμεις ταύτας).⁶⁸

There are also the well-known passages on states of the blood that are of influence on thinking. At *Part. an.* 648 a 2ff. we are told that while thick and warm blood produce strength, thinness and coldness of the blood are conducive to sharper intellectual and perceptive capacities (αἰσθητικώτερον δὲ καὶ νοερώτερον τὸ λεπτότερον καὶ ψυχρότερον), and this also applies to the substance analogous to blood in bloodless animals: 'This is why bees and other similar animals are naturally more intelligent (φρονιμώτερα) than many blooded animals, and of the blooded animals, those with cold and thin blood are more intelligent than their counterparts.' The best combination of properties – in actual fact a sort of compromise – is blood that is warm, thin and pure, which makes the animal both intelligent and courageous. This indicates that thinness is apparently more important for intelligence than coldness, which is confirmed by *Part. an.* 650 b 19ff., where we are told that some animals have a more subtle intelligence (γλαφυρωτέραν τὴν διάνοιαν), 'not because of the coldness of the blood, but rather because of its being thin and pure' (διὰ τὴν λεπτότητα μᾶλλον καὶ διὰ τὸ καθαρὸν εἶναι); and he adds that more 'earthy' blood does not have these characteristics.⁶⁹ Thinness and purity of the bodily moisture (blood or its analogue) are also said to make sensation more *agile* (εὐκινητοτέραν), and this accounts for the fact that some bloodless animals (with a thin and pure moisture) have 'a more intelligent soul' (συνετωτέραν τὴν ψυχήν) than some blooded animals – an important remark indicating that not the blood itself, but its *state* is conducive of intelligence. The chapter proceeds with some remarks about the influence of blood on character (ἦθος) and concludes that blood is the cause of many things, in the sphere both of character

---

[67] I have discussed the 'ethopoietic' influence of bodily factors (such as the size of the heart, *Part. an.* 667 a 11ff.) in ch. 5 above.
[68] Cf. *Pr.* 14.15 and the Hippocratic *Airs, Waters, Places* 16 (2.62ff. L.).
[69] On 'earthiness' cf. *Part. an.* 686 b 28ff. discussed above (see n. 57), and see Althoff (1992) 73, 80.

and of perception, since it is the matter of the body, and its influence varies according to its being hot, cold, thin, thick, troubled or pure.

In these two passages, the influence of blood on intelligence is closely linked with its influence on perception, and this again suggests that what makes for greater intelligence is a better, that is, swifter, more accurate, supply of perceptions for the intellect to halt upon. Aristotle's remarks here seem to refer to *structural* differences existing between different species of animals, but there is no reason to doubt whether similar *incidental*, or individual, variations in the state of the blood may make for incidental, or individual, variations in intellectual performances.[70] Nor is there any reason to believe that Aristotle is only referring to animals and not to man: his remarks on the importance of the blood in the process of dreaming, for example, indicate that also in human cognition the quality of the blood is an important factor.[71] Again, this is of considerable importance to the question whether Aristotle believed in animal intelligence: there is nothing in these two passages to suggest that Aristotle is not referring to *really* intellectual activities of animals, but only to something analogous; on the contrary, there is every reason to believe that similar variations in the state of the blood affect human intelligence just as well as animal intellectual capacities.

The most remarkable passage in this respect is *De an.* 421 a 22ff., which suggests that there is a direct connection between degrees of softness of the flesh and degrees of intelligence in human beings.[72] Aristotle deals with the sense of smell, and he remarks that man has a very weak, unarticulated sense of smell in comparison with many other animals: he is only capable of labelling smells as pleasant or unpleasant. Similarly, he says, animals with hard eyes (σκληρόφθαλμα) do not have an accurate sense for seeing a variety of colours. The situation is slightly better with taste, he says, for man's sense of taste is more accurate than his sense of smell, because taste is a form of touch, and as regards touch man is the most accurate of all animals.[73] He then continues:

---

[70] See Kullmann (1982) 229: 'Es kommt freilich Aristoteles in 2.4 vor allem darauf an, die physiologische Bedeutung der beiden Bestandteile des Blutes hervorzuheben. Ihr jeweiliger Anteil ist nach seiner Meinung von Tierart zu Tierart (und wohl auch von Individuum zu Individuum) verschieden.'

[71] See *Insomn.* 461 a 25; b 11ff.

[72] The passage seems to be a sort of embarrassment to most interpreters, for it is hardly ever commented upon. Freeland (1992) 234 says that 'this should be taken with a grain of salt because Aristotle offers several alternative explanations for human "superior intelligence"'. However, Freeland does not consider how these 'alternative explanations' are interrelated in Aristotle's physiology, and of the instances she cites only *Part. an.* 4.10 is comparable to (and fully consistent with) the one here.

[73] Cf. *Hist. an.* 494 b 17; *Part. an.* 660 a 12.

This is also the reason why man is most intelligent of all animals (φρονιμώτατον). A sign of this is that also within the species of man it is in accordance with this sense organ that one is well or poorly endowed [with intelligence], but not in accordance with any other sense organ: for people with hard flesh are poorly endowed with intelligence, but people with soft flesh are well endowed with it (οἱ μὲν γὰρ σκληρόσαρκοι ἀφυεῖς τὴν διάνοιαν, οἱ δὲ μαλακόσαρκοι εὐφυεῖς).

Here Aristotle distinguishes not only between different species of animals, but also between different members (or types of members) within the human species. Man is more intelligent than other animals because of the accuracy of his sense of touch, and this is indicated also by the fact that within the human species individuals with soft flesh (which is obviously conducive to touch) are by nature more intelligent (εὐφυὴς τὴν διάνοιαν) than those with hard flesh. Thus variations in intellectual capacities are here directly related to variations in the quality of the skin. Just *how* they are related, does not emerge from the text. It is not inconceivable that the connection is teleological and that διό should be interpreted as 'therefore', or 'to that end', that is, to use his sense of touch in a sensible way, just as in *Part. an.* 4.10, where it is said that man is the only animal to have hands because he is the most intelligent and so best qualified to use them sensibly; the remark that man is inferior to other animals in so many other respects, but superior in his rationality and sense of touch (421 a 20–2) might be paralleled by a similar remark in *Part. an.* 4.10 (687 a 25ff.). However, there is nothing in the text of *De an.* 2.11 to suggest that this is what Aristotle has in mind here; the text rather points to a relation of efficient causality between touch and intelligence. This relation is not further spelled out by Aristotle: it may have something to do with the fact that touch is the fundamental sense which is closely connected with, if not identical to, the 'common sense faculty'[74] (also referred to at *Part. an.* 686 a 31), which is most closely related to intellectual activity; hence variations in the performance of this faculty might also bring about variations in intellectual performance. Another possibility is that delicacy of the skin is somehow conducive to thinness and agility of the blood, which in its turn, as we saw, is of influence on the degrees of intellectual activity.[75] Anyway, it is significant that again the word *dianoia* and the adjective *phronimos* are used, and again *degrees* of intelligence are at issue: man is compared with other animals in what seems to be a gradualist view of intelligence, and within the human species a typology is made on the basis of a physical criterion.

---

[74] *Somn. vig.* 455 a 23.   [75] I owe this suggestion to Jochen Althoff.

Several other passages further confirm the picture that has so far emerged from the texts. Thus we are told in *Gen. an.* 744 a 30 that in man the brain has more moisture and is greater than in other animals, because in man the heat in the heart is most pure (τὴν ἐν τῇ καρδίᾳ θερμότητα καθαρωτάτην). 'This good proportion is indicated by man's intelligence: for the most intelligent of all animals is man' (δηλοῖ δὲ τὴν εὐκρασίαν ἡ διάνοια· φρονιμώτατον γάρ ἐστι τῶν ζῴων ἄνθρωπος). Here man's intelligence is said to be a *sign* of the fine blend of warm and cold, which again suggests that there is a direct connection between the two. And two passages in *On Memory and Recollection* very well illustrate the influence of bodily conditions of cognitive activity. First, in 450 a 27ff., memory is said to take place 'in the soul, that is, in the part of the body that contains soul', as a kind of picture, just as the seal of a signet ring.

This is also the reason why no memory occurs in people who are in [a state of] great movement because of disease or age, just as if the movement and the seal were to fall into water; with other people, owing to the detrition of the [part] that receives the affection, no impression is made. This is why the very young and the very old have no memory: the first are in a state of flux because of growth, the others because of decay. Similarly, neither those who are excessively quick nor those who are excessively slow [of wit][76] appear to have a good memory: the former are moister than they should be, the latter dryer: with the former, the appearance does not remain in the soul, with the latter, it does not take hold.

It may be objected that this passage is about memory, and therefore not about an activity of the intellectual but of the sensitive part of the soul whose physical substrate is not at issue (although it is striking that Aristotle seems to present the soul as an extended entity *in* which things are going on and in which surfaces are present which should receive the impression of the phantasm; again, Aristotle only refers to these physical aspects when discussing variations or even deviations: what the 'normal' physical components of a successful act of memory are is not explained). However, it also refers to the physiological conditions of quick-witted and slow-minded people, excessive states that are related to an undue predominance of moisture or dryness. And the passage as a whole again speaks of typological differences in cognitive and intellectual behaviour within the human species that are caused by differences in physiological conditions.

Further on in *On Memory and Recollection* (453 a 14ff.), this connection becomes even clearer, when Aristotle is dealing with the difference between memory and recollection. One of the differences is that while

---

[76] That quickness and slowness of wit are meant is indicated by *Phgn.* 813 b 7ff.

memory also occurs with other animals, recollection is confined to man, because recollection is 'like inference' (οἷον συλλογισμός), because it clearly involves searching and deliberation. This, however, does not mean that it is an incorporeal process:

> That the affection [i.e. recollection] is something physical and that recollection is a search for an image in something of this [i.e. physical] kind, is indicated by the fact that some people are disturbed whenever they cannot recollect, even though they keep their attention fixed, and when they make no more effort, they recollect nonetheless [i.e. the recollective process keeps going on]. This occurs especially with the melancholics, for they are particularly moved by images. The reason why they have no control over their recollective activity is that just as people are unable to stop something they have thrown away, likewise the person who recollects and chases something sets something physical in motion, in which the affection takes place. This disturbance particularly occurs with those with whom there happens to be moisture around the perceptive place, for this [moisture] does not easily stop when set in motion, until the object sought turns up and the movement runs a straight course... Those who have large upper parts and those who are dwarfish are less good at memorising than their counterparts because they have much weight on their perceptual faculty, and their movements cannot remain in their original condition but are scattered; nor can they easily run a straight course in recollecting. The very young and the very old have poor memories because of the movement: the latter are in a state of decay, the former in rapid growth; and small children are also dwarfish until they have advanced in age.

Again, the thesis (that recollection is a physical process) is demonstrated with a reference to a *disturbance* in the act of recollection. The word διάνοια is used in a context which deals with mental concentration, and also the melancholics make their appearance; reference is made to moisture around the 'perceptive place'; and in the following section, which again deals with special groups, dwarfs, the very young and the very old are mentioned. So we have a rational process (although Aristotle, perhaps significantly, does not say that it is an affection of the intellectual part of the soul) which takes place in a bodily part and which is susceptible to influences and disturbances of bodily conditions. Again, it remains unclear what the normal physical conditions for a successful operation of recollection (searching 'along a straight course', εὐθυπορεῖν)[77] are.

The passages that I have discussed clearly suggest that, according to Aristotle, bodily conditions can be of influence on intellectual activities

---

[77] On this expression see above, n. 61. It is also used in *Gen. an.* 781 a 2 and b 12 to refer to the transmission of sense movement outside the body (from the perceptible object to the perceiving subject); cf. also *Pr.* 934 a 17.

(νοῦς, διάνοια, φρονεῖν).⁷⁸ Whether they always are, or only in abnormal cases, or whether the influence in abnormal cases is of a different kind rather than of a different degree compared with normal cases is hard to decide, for these bodily conditions are mostly referred to by Aristotle in the context of a discussion of *variations* in intellectual performances (type (3) distinguished above, p. 217). It is clear, however, that apart from incidental bodily states such as drunkenness or sleep (which may be characterised as disturbing agents, although the former is παρὰ φύσιν, the latter κατὰ φύσιν), there are also more structural conditions such as the quality of the blood, age, the overall balance between warm and cold in the body and the quality of the skin. Variations in these structural conditions account for variations in intellectual capacities. The variations exist among different species, but also among individual members of one species or types within a species, such as dwarfs or melancholics. For the most part, these types represent 'imperfect' (ἀτελεῖς) or 'deformed' (πεπηρωμένοι) groups of human beings with special characteristics due to their physical aberrations. However, some types (such as the μαλακόσαρκοι) seem to represent special classes of humans whose distinctive characteristics are not to be regarded as deformations, but as variations *within* one species that may be either conducive, or harmful, or just neutral to the exercise of certain psychic powers.

We hear very little about what the bodily conditions of a normal, successful operation of the intellectual powers are, but, as I have already said, there is good reason to assume that this is just because, in the writings that have survived, Aristotle simply does not have much reason to dwell on them. Our picture of Aristotle's psycho-physiology is likely to remain very incomplete – as is also indicated by the difficulties involved in piecing together his scattered remarks about physiological conditions such as *pneuma*, blood, and so forth. This has perhaps to do with his indebtedness to a medical tradition which supplied a lot of material which he could simply take for granted. As has already been demonstrated by Tracy – and is confirmed by more recent work on Aristotle's acquaintance with medical literature⁷⁹ – this indebtedness is probably much greater than the scanty references to medical authorities in Aristotle's works suggest. In this particular context, the Hippocratic work *On Regimen* comes to one's mind, which in chapters 35 and 36 has an extremely interesting discussion on variations in intellectual performance due to variations in the proportion between fire and water in

---

⁷⁸ Other, more peripheral evidence (dealing less explicitly with *intellectual* capacities) is discussed in ch. 5 above. See also Tracy (1969), *passim*.
⁷⁹ For further references to scholarly discussions of Aristotle's relation to medical literature see ch. 9; see also Longrigg (1995) and Oser-Grote (1997).

the body;[80] and there may be other medical influences as well,[81] especially of dietetics, for it was certainly one of the claims of dietetics in Aristotle's time to provide a physiologically founded doctrine of 'the good life'.[82] The Peripatetic school was very receptive to these medical views, as is shown, for example, by the *Problemata physica*, and Aristotle was almost certainly aware of them. Now it is certainly true that Aristotle's psychology is much richer and much more sophisticated than that of the medical literature, but it should not be overlooked that there is also a 'technical' side to Aristotle's psychology, an interest in the 'mechanics' of cognition and in modalities of thinking such as concentration, analytical powers, creativity, quickness (ταχυτής) of thinking and intuition (ἀγχίνοια, εὐστοχία),[83] habituation and repetition, and *degrees* in capacities to all these activities. It very rarely comes to the surface in *On the Soul*, but it figures more prominently in the *Parva naturalia* and in the zoological works, mostly when one species of animals is compared with another or when different members of one species are compared with one another, and mostly in contexts in which some sort of disturbance or aberration in cognitive behaviour is discussed. It is in these contexts that bodily factors are made responsible for these disturbances or aberrations; Aristotle does not explain what the *normal* bodily conditions for a normal functioning of thinking are, and they can only be deduced indirectly. However, it is very likely that the concept of 'the mean' plays an important part here.[84]

This situation provides a parallel (though not a solution) to another problem in Aristotle's theory of thinking – which has recently received much attention and which has already been alluded to above – namely the question of animal intelligence.[85] In many (although admittedly not all) of the passages in which Aristotle seems to credit animals with intellectual capacities he compares one species with another, and in this comparative perspective man is simply seen as the most intelligent (the use of comparatives such as φρονιμώτεροι or superlatives such as φρονιμώτατοι in these contexts is striking). Here, too, there seems to be a tension between a 'relativistic', biological view of man as a ζῷον at the end of a scale which

---

[80] For a discussion of these chapters see the commentary by Joly and Byl (1984). See also Jouanna (1966) and Hankinson (1991b) 200–6.
[81] The cognitive role of the blood reminds us, of course, of Empedocles (see Kullmann (1982) 230). The doctrine of *pneuma* may be inspired by Diocles of Carystus (see Longrigg (1995) 441).
[82] See Tracy (1969), *passim*. On the claims of dietetics, and its relation to philosophy in the fourth century see also G. Wöhrle (1990), chs. 4 and 5.
[83] Cf. *An. post.* 89 b 10ff.; *Eth. Nic.* 1142 b 3–6; *Rh.* 1362 b 24; 1412 a 13; *Top.* 151 b 19; *Div. somn.* 464 a 33.
[84] On this see the excellent discussion by Tracy (1969).
[85] For a survey of the recent discussion see Coles (1997).

may easily give rise to statements to the effect that he is *more* intelligent than other animals, and an 'idealistic', anthropocentric view which postulates a distinction of kind rather than degree between animals and men to the effect that man is the only intelligent living being and the other animals have no intelligence at all.

I should suggest that this difficulty is to be related to Aristotle's endeavours to account for variations in psychic capacities and their performance by reference to variable *bodily* (anatomical, physiological, pathological) factors – although it is not quite clear how these factors are to be accommodated within the 'canonical' doctrine of the incorporeality of the intellect and the changelessness of the soul. It is certainly to Aristotle's credit as a scientist that he recognises the existence of these variations, most of which are probably to be classified as belonging to the category of 'the more and the less' (διαφοραὶ καθ' ὑπεροχήν).[86] And just as, at the one end of the scale, he is prepared to account for disturbances in intellectual behaviour by reference to physical aberrations or disturbances, he also recognises the existence of exceptionally good performances of the intellectual part of the soul and tries to account for these by assuming that some people have extraordinary intuitive powers that enable them to think quickly, to perceive hidden resemblances, to invent good definitions and to create effective metaphors;[87] and he tries to explain these positive deviations too as the results of differences in bodily constitution, as we have seen in the case of the 'people with soft flesh' (μαλακόσαρκοι). Moreover, when it comes to physical defects, he also seems to apply a sort of principle of natural *compensation*, which manifests itself in his belief that nature (i.e. the natural, bodily constitution) provides even people with low intellectual capacities with a special endowment or ingenuity (εὐφυία),[88] which is at the basis of such marginal powers as the ability to foresee the future in sleep, the instinctive power to make the right choice (εὐτυχία, see ch. 8 below), the manifestations of 'the exceptional' (τὸ περιττόν), or 'natural virtues' (φυσικαὶ ἀρεταί) such as moral shrewdness (δεινότης) – capacities which seem to flourish when the reasoning faculties are impeded or absent and which are, of course, obviously inferior to the intellectual virtues such as 'prudence' (φρόνησις),

---

[86] Cf. *Part. an.* 645 b 24; 644 a 17; 692 b 3ff.; *Gen. an.* 737 b 4–7; 739 b 31–2.
[87] See the passages referred to above (n. 83) and, for metaphors, *Poet.* 1459 a 5–7, 1455 a 32, and *Rh.* 1405 a 8–10.
[88] The word εὐφυία, meaning 'natural suitability', seems to have acquired the special sense of 'natural cleverness', 'ingenuity' (with τὴν διάνοιαν to be understood), and οἱ εὐφυεῖς represent a special type of people with a particular cleverness (which, however, may easily change into insanity: *Rh.* 1390 b 28); see *Eth.Eud.* 1247 b 22, b 39; *Eth. Nic.* 1114 b 8; *Mag. mor.* 1203 b 1–2; *Phgn.* 807 b 12 and 808 a 37; *Poet.* 1459 a 7 and 1455 a 32; *Pr.* 954 a 32.

but whose existence, however marginal their importance may be, Aristotle recognises as interesting and in need of explanation[89] – an explanation which invokes the principle that even within the category of 'what is contrary to nature' (τὸ παρὰ φύσιν) there is such a thing as 'according to nature' (τὸ κατὰ φύσιν).

However much this may seem to be applauded, it remains unclear how these gradualist and compensatory explanations should be accommodated within the 'normative' theory of *De an.* 3.4–8, for in explaining all these variations by reference to bodily variables he seems to grant physical conditions a greater influence on intellectual activities than his 'canonical' view of the incorporeality of *nous* would seem to allow.

To be sure, it may be asked whether there is actually such a tension, for it might be argued that all instances of bodily influence on intellectual activity discussed above can be classified under the rubric of the 'dependence of the intellect on appearances'.[90] Yet even if this is true, we still have gained a much more detailed view on how this dependence may work out in particular cases, what may go wrong in the supply of images to the intellect and what range of bodily factors may actually influence this supply, and indeed not only the supply but also the quality of images, and even the act of thinking itself. Whether this affects the thesis of the incorporeality of the intellect, remains to be seen.[91] One way in which it would not do so, is to assume that the bodily influences only apply to *lower* levels of intellectual activity such as *doxa* ('opinion'), *hupolēpsis* ('supposition'), *dianoia* ('discursive thought'), not to *nous*, or to 'practical' not 'theoretical' intellect, or to 'passive' not 'active' intellect.[92] This is a problematic solution because, as is well known, it is not easy to see how the various terminological distinctions between intellectual powers that Aristotle makes are related to each other, and we have also seen that the passages on bodily influence do not seem to be very specific with regard to the precise intellectual power they are

---

[89] On all these phenomena, and their place in Aristotle's philosophy, see ch. 5 in this volume, pp. 164 ff.

[90] This seems to be the view taken by most interpreters who have dealt with (some of) the passages I have discussed; see, e.g., Kahn (1992) 366 n. 11 on *De an.* 408 b 9: 'In mentioning bodily change in connection with thinking, Aristotle must be referring to phantasms'; Tracy (1969) 272ff.; and Verbeke (1978) 201–2 with n. 55.

[91] See Aristotle's uneasiness about this in *De an.* 403 a 8–10.

[92] See Kahn (1992) 362–3: 'It is not the disembodied principle of *nous* that requires phantasms; it is our use of *nous*, the penetration of *nous* into our embodied activity as sentient animals, which must take place by means of the phantasms, that is, through the neurophysiological mechanism of sense and the mental imagery of conscious thought.' A distinction between διανοεῖσθαι and νοεῖν seems to be implied in *De an.* 408 b 24–5, although Aristotle is very tentative (cf. the use of ἴσως in b 29). On different modes of thinking see also Lowe (1983) 17–30.

said to act on (cf. the use of νοερός, σύνετος, γλάφυρος, φρόνιμος, νοεῖν, φρονεῖν, διάνοια, νοῦς). The only terminological point we can make is that a number of passages assign an important role to *dianoia*, and it may be that this is Aristotle's favourite term for intellectual activity on the borderlines between sense-perception and thinking; one sometimes gets the impression that it refers to a particular kind of thinking, a sort of attention, in any case a directed and concentrated intellectual activity (or the capacity to this).[93] In this connection, it may be worth referring to a dispute between two German students of Aristotle's psychology in the second half of the nineteenth century, namely Clemens Bäumker and Joseph Neuhäuser. Bäumker, in his monograph on Aristotle's physiology of sense perception, argued that Aristotle adopted a fourth 'part of the soul' in between perception and intellect (νοῦς), for which διάνοια was supposed to be the technical term;[94] and Bäumker did so on the strength of a number of passages I have also discussed above. Neuhäuser, however, rejected Bäumker's view by pointing to a number of passages in which the verb *dianoeisthai* seems to be used as a general, non-specific term for *any* intellectual activity, including that of *nous*.[95] Although there is no evidence that Aristotle really regarded 'lower' intellectual capacities as constituting a separate 'part' of the soul, it must be conceded that especially in passages where he adopts a gradualist point of view, *dianoia* seems to be the appropriate term, and it may be that Aristotle associates this term more closely with activities of the sensitive part of the soul, and thus with bodily influences, than other terms such as *logos, nous, sunesis, phronēsis, doxa* and *hupolēpsis*. There is, indeed, abundant evidence that in the border area between sense-perception and thinking, where elusive faculties such as 'incidental perception' (the perception that that white thing over there is the son of Diares), 'common sense' and imagination are at work, Aristotle is not always clear whether we are dealing with operations of the sensitive or the intellectual part of the soul.[96] The passage on recollection (an intellectual activity restricted to human beings but taking place in physical material) from *Mem.* 453 a 14ff. provided a good illustration of this point.

---

[93] Cf. *Div. somn.* 464 a 22, where a failure to exercise this capacity is described.
[94] Bäumker (1877) 7 with n. 2.
[95] Neuhäuser (1878a) 10ff. See also Neuhäuser's review of Bäumker's monograph (1878b).
[96] For incidental perception see Cashdollar (1973). The question whether the judgement of images is a sensitive or an intellectual activity presents itself very strongly in *On Dreams*, where sometimes one sense (sight) corrects the other (touch), as in 460 b 21–2, but sometimes also an intellectual faculty is at work (as in 460 b 18–19), and sometimes it is unclear which faculty is judging (461 b 3ff.; 461 b 25; 462 a 4, 6). For a discussion of this difficulty see van der Eijk (1994) 50ff.

Let us finally turn to the question of the *kind* of connection or correspondence between the bodily conditions referred to and the intellectual activities they are said to accompany or influence. Of course, Aristotle has appropriate language at his disposal: on a structural level (where bodily influences are related to constitution types such as the melancholic nature, to deformations such as dwarfs, or to natural conditions such as hardness of the flesh) he may say (as he often does in *Parts of Animals* and *Generation of Animals*) that form does not completely 'master' (κρατεῖν) matter, which results in deformed (πεπηρωμένα) or 'imperfect' (ἀτελῆ) structural capacities, or that material natural factors 'impede' (ἐμποδίζειν) the full realisation of the formal nature.[97] He may say that physical factors are responsible as additional causes, as in *De an.* 416 a 14, where he says that fire is a συναίτιον of the real αἰτία, the soul, or at *Part. an.* 652 b 10ff., where he says that of all bodily factors heat (τὸ θερμόν) is 'most serviceable to the activities of the soul' (τοῖς τῆς ψυχῆς ἔργοις ὑπηρετικώτατον τῶν σωμάτων τὸ θερμόν ἐστιν), although these passages relate especially to the nutritive activities of the soul which constitute, as Aristotle himself recognises, 'the most physical' (φυσικώτατον) of the psychic functions (*De an.* 415 a 26).[98] Passages (as discussed above) in which weight is said to 'make' (ποιεῖν) the soul slow, or disease or sleep are said to 'overshadow' the intellect, or certain material substances are said to 'confuse' and 'change' the intellect, indicate an *active* role of bodily factors in the operations of the intellect. Thus apart from saying that bodily changes 'correspond with' or 'accompany' psychic activities, which does not commit itself to a specific type of causal relationship,[99] we may go further and say that bodily states and processes *act* on psychic powers or activities just as well as psychic powers may be said to 'inform' bodily structures.

---

[97] See *Gen. an.* 766 a 15ff.; 767 b 10ff.; 772 b 30ff.; 737 a 25; 780 b 10. See the discussion by A. L. Peck in his Loeb edition of *Generation of Animals*, pp. xlv–xlvii.

[98] For a similar reason, the remark in *Part. an.* 667 a 11ff. that differences in the size and the structure of the heart 'also in a certain way extend to' character (τείνουσί πῃ καὶ πρὸς τὰ ἤθη) cannot be used as evidence of bodily influence on the *intellectual* part of the soul.

[99] Cf. *De motu an.* 701 b 17ff., in particular b 34: ἐξ ἀνάγκης δ' ἀκολουθεῖ τῇ νοήσει καὶ τῇ φαντασίᾳ αὐτῶν θερμότης καὶ ψύξις, on which see the useful comments by Kollesch (1985) 51–2. See also her comments on *De motu an.* 703 a 15 and *Gen. an.* 736 b 31ff. (ὡς δὲ διαφέρουσι τιμιότητι αἱ ψυχαὶ καὶ ἀτιμίᾳ ἀλλήλων, οὕτω καὶ ἡ τοιαύτη διαφέρει φύσις, sc. of the *pneuma*): 'Die Unterschiede, die das Pneuma aufweist, sind abhängig von der unterschiedlichen Wertigkeit der einzelnen Seelenvermögen, mit denen das Pneuma jeweils verbunden ist. Das heisst, einer höheren Seelentätigkeit, wie sie z.B. die Wahrnehmung gegenüber der Ernährung und Zeugung darstellt, entspricht auch eine höhere Qualität des Pneumas' (p. 60).

It is perhaps significant that passages like the ones discussed were used by writers such as the Peripatetic author of the *Physiognomonica* – who may well have been Aristotle himself – in support of their assumption of the fundamental correspondence between mental dispositions (διάνοιαι) and bodily states (ὅτι αἱ διάνοιαι ἕπονται τοῖς σώμασιν);[100] again, the word *dianoia* is used here, although it is very difficult to decide whether it refers to intellectual capacities alone or has a wider meaning of 'mental dispositions' (as the sequence of the passage in *Physiognomonica* shows, where the author refers to παθήματα τῆς ψυχῆς or just to ψυχή). To be sure, in the *Physiognomonica* intellectual capacities are rarely referred to,[101] and the author mainly deals with moral dispositions and characteristics. He refers to stock examples such as drunkenness and illness, and he also uses love, fear, pleasure and pain as examples of how emotional states may influence the condition of the body, thus indicating that there is a reciprocal relationship between body and soul.[102] In doing so, the author is in accordance with genuine Aristotelian doctrine, for example with what we read about the bodily aspects of emotion in *Movement of Animals*, where Aristotle says that heat and cold may be causative – in the sense of 'efficient causality' – of emotions, or accompaniments of emotions, but he also acknowledges that emotions in their turn may produce heat or cold in the body.[103]

Thus to dismiss works such as the *Physiognomonica* (and parts of the *Problemata*) as un-Aristotelian[104] on the strength of their alleged 'materialistic' doctrine of the soul and of the intellect in particular, ignores the presence of a number of passages in genuine Aristotelian works in which very similar views are being expressed.[105] The purpose of the present chapter has been to draw attention to these passages and to encourage students of Aristotle's psychology and 'philosophy of mind' to take them into more serious consideration. In particular, it should be asked to what extent these passages present a challenge to the doctrine of the

---

[100] *Phgn.* 805 a 1ff.; cf. the ancient commentaries on *De an.* 403 a 16 referred to above (n. 53). On physiognomics see Barton (1994), ch. 2 (with abundant bibliography).
[101] 813 a 29; 813 b 7ff. Cf. 808 b 10.   [102] 805 a 3ff.
[103] *De motu an.* 701 b 17ff.; 702 a 3ff.
[104] I have occasionally referred to passages in the *Problemata* in the footnotes to show how certain tenets vaguely alluded to in Aristotle's genuine works are elaborated there, although I am aware that this work is of a later date; the question of to what extent *Problemata* can be used to reconstruct Aristotelian views on which the authentic works provide only fragmentary information deserves further examination.
[105] See Solmsen (1950) 463–4, who uses the word 'materialistic' in connection with the passages in *Part. an.* 648 a 2ff. and 650 b 19ff. about the cognitive role of the blood.

changelessness of the soul and the incorporeality of the intellect; for it seems that the variety of psychic performances, including the intellectual ones, which the animal kingdom displays makes Aristotle acknowledge that there is a material aspect to thinking as well, which he, in the 'canonical' theory of *nous* in *De an.* 3.4–8, is conspicuously reluctant to recognise.

CHAPTER 8

Divine movement and human nature in Eudemian Ethics 8.2

In *Eudemian Ethics* (*Eth. Eud.*) 8.2 Aristotle is searching for an explanation of *eutuchia* (εὐτυχία), which might be defined as 'good fortune' – sheer luck in matters in which the lucky man does not have any rational or technical competence, befalling the same man so frequently that it cannot be a matter of coincidence.[1] Textual problems, extreme brevity and looseness of expression as well as the enormous span of the argument make it difficult to follow Aristotle's reasoning in detail. Yet there seems to be a consensus among modern interpreters concerning the conclusion of the chapter. The principal question was whether *eutuchia* is caused by nature or not (1247 a 2), and Aristotle's answer to this question, briefly summarised in 1248 b 3–7, is as follows. There are two forms of *eutuchia*, the first of which is both 'divine' (*theia*) and 'by nature' (*phusei*),[2] and the second of which is caused by 'chance' (*tuchē*); both forms are 'irrational' (*alogoi*), but the first form is 'continuous' (*sunechēs*), whereas the latter is not. The first form is the one which Aristotle has been trying to explain from the beginning; the existence of the second form he was compelled to recognise in the course of his argument.

It appears that this first form of *eutuchia* is based on a kind of interaction between a principal divine movement (1248 a 25ff.) and a human natural constitution (1248 a 30–1; 39–41). Thus the explanation of *eutuchia* involves a rather specific conjunction of two factors, nature (*phusis*) and God (*ho theos*), which at an earlier stage of the argument (1247 a 23–31) – and also in the first chapter of the *Eudemian Ethics* (1214 a 16–24) – were distinguished among others as two different possible causes of *eutuchia*. This conjunction

---

This chapter was first published in *Hermes* 117 (1989) 24–42.

[1] Actually Aristotle nowhere explicitly defines *eutuchia*, since the explanation of the phenomenon consists for a substantial part in trying to attain such a definition. For an analysis of Aristotle's argument see Woods (1982) 176ff.; and Mills (1981) and (1983).

[2] Spengel's conjecture in 1248 b 4 (ἡ δὲ φύσει), adopted by Susemihl (1884), is no longer accepted by modern interpreters. On 'chance' (τύχη) as the cause of the second form see Dirlmeier (1962a) 492; Gigon (1969) 211.

is in accordance with an assertion in *Nicomachean Ethics* (*Eth. Nic.* 1179 b 21–3); the part played by 'nature' (*phusis*) as a possible cause of 'excellence' (*aretē*), Aristotle says there, is 'not within our control, but is present in those who are truly fortunate (*eutuchesin*) through certain sorts of divine causes'.[3]

The problem to be discussed in this chapter concerns the discrepancy between these two stages (1247 a 23ff. and 1248 a 25ff.) of the argument in *Eth. Eud.* 8.2. In 1247 a 23ff. Aristotle suggests as a possible explanation of *eutuchia* that it is caused not by nature (*phusis*) but by a god or demon:

or because they [i.e. these 'fortunate' people] are loved, as people say, by a god, and the cause of their success is something external: just as a ship that has been built badly often sails better not because of itself, but because it has a good navigator, likewise the fortunate person has a good navigator.[4]

But this explanation is immediately ruled out by the following objection:

but it is paradoxical that a god or demon should love such a person rather than the best or the wisest. (1247 a 28–9)[5]

It is obvious that Aristotle is thinking here of the popular concept of a personal guardian deity or demon.[6] It is evident that his rejection of this conception as a possible explanation of *eutuchia* is not inconsistent with his own final conclusion that *eutuchia* is 'divine' (*theia*) and happens 'through God' (*dia theon*).[7] But the problem is that it is far from evident in what way this final conclusion is proof against the objection stated in 1247 a 28–9 about the distribution of the phenomenon among different groups of people ('but it is paradoxical...', ἀλλ' ἄτοπον κτλ.), for in his final conclusion Aristotle explicitly asserts that God is 'moving more strongly' in people who are 'without reason' (*alogoi*) than in those who practise reason, intellect and rational deliberation (*logos, nous, bouleusis*, 1248 a 32–4; 40–1).[8]

---

[3] τὸ μὲν οὖν τῆς φύσεως δῆλον ὡς οὐκ ἐφ' ἡμῖν ὑπάρχει, ἀλλὰ διά τινας θείας αἰτίας τοῖς ὡς ἀληθῶς εὐτυχέσιν ὑπάρχει.

[4] ἢ τῷ φιλεῖσθαι, ὥσπερ φασίν, ὑπὸ θεοῦ, καὶ ἔξωθέν τι εἶναι τὸ κατορθοῦν, οἷον πλοῖον κακῶς νεναυπηγημένον ἄμεινον πολλάκις πλεῖ, ἀλλ' οὐ δι' αὑτό, ἀλλ' ὅτι ἔχει κυβερνήτην ἀγαθόν, οὕτως εὐτυχὴς τὸν δαίμον' ἔχει κυβερνήτην ἀγαθόν.

[5] ἀλλ' ἄτοπον θεὸν ἢ δαίμονα φιλεῖν τὸν τοιοῦτον, ἀλλὰ μὴ τὸν βέλτιστον καὶ φρονιμώτατον.

[6] On this popular conception see Détienne (1963) 129–30 and Hanse (1939) 8–12.

[7] See von Fragstein (1974) 375; Mills (1982) 206; von Arnim (1929) 12; and von Arnim (1927) 130, who argues that there is an inconsistency between 1247 a 23–31 and 1248 a 32ff. and accounts for this inconsistency by arguing that these passages represent different stages in the development of Aristotle's ideas.

[8] See Bodéüs (1981) 55 n. 44: 'La principale difficulté vient peut-être moins d'une conception selon laquelle Dieu pourrait intervenir dans les affaires humaines (ce dont la doctrine du *nous* dans la *Mét.* XII ne semble pas envisager les modalités) que de l'idée selon laquelle pareille intervention serait, contre toute logique, en faveur des faibles d'esprit exclusivement.'

This problem, then, concerns the consistency of the argument within this chapter of the *Eudemian Ethics*. That it is a genuine problem is further shown by the fact that the same objection as that raised in 1247 a 28–9 concerning the distribution of the phenomenon ascribed to divine dispensation (and which I shall henceforth refer to as the 'distribution argument') is found in two other Aristotelian writings which are closely parallel to *Eth. Eud.* 8.2, but there, contrary to *Eth. Eud.* 8.2, it is sufficient to reject *any* explanation which ascribes *eutuchia* (or a comparable phenomenon) to a god. The passages in question are the parallel discussion of *eutuchia* in chapter 2.8 of the so-called *Great Ethics* (*Magna moralia*, *Mag. mor.*) and the treatment of prophetic dreams in the *On Divination in Sleep* (*De divinatione per somnum*, *Div. somn.*).

Thus at a certain point of the discussion in *Mag. mor.* 1207 a 6ff., as in *Eth. Eud.* 1247 a 23ff., it is tentatively suggested that *eutuchia* might be explained as a form of divine dispensation:

But is *eutuchia* a kind of dispensation of the gods? Or would it appear to be not that?[9]

But this suggestion is rejected on the strength of the following argument:

We hold that God, who is in supreme control of such things [i.e. external goods], distributes both good and evil to those who deserve it, whereas chance and the results of chance truly happen as chance would have it. And if we attribute such a thing to God, we shall make him a poor judge, or at least not a just one; and that is not befitting for God. (1207 a 7–12)[10]

In line 15, this conclusion is repeated:

Surely, neither the concern nor the benevolence of God would seem to be *eutuchia*, because it [i.e. *eutuchia*] also occurs among the wicked; and it is unlikely that God would care for the wicked.[11]

The conclusion of the discussion of *eutuchia* in *Mag. mor.* 2.8 is that *eutuchia* is caused by an 'irrational nature' (*alogos phusis*), more specifically by irrational 'impulses' or instinctive drives (*hormai*) (1207 a 35ff.). These 'impulses' also play an important part in the explanation in *Eth. Eud.* 8.2 (1247 b 18ff.), but the major difference between *Eth. Eud.* 8.2 and *Mag.*

---

[9] ἀλλ' ἆρά γε ἡ εὐτυχία ἐστὶν ὡς ἐπιμέλειά τις θεῶν; ἢ τοῦτ' οὐκ ἂν δόξειεν;
[10] τὸν γὰρ θεὸν ἀξιοῦμεν κύριον ὄντα τῶν τοιούτων τοῖς ἀξίοις ἀπονέμειν καὶ τἀγαθὰ καὶ τὰ κακά, ἡ δὲ τύχη καὶ τὰ ἀπὸ τύχης ὡς ἀληθῶς ὡς ἂν τύχῃ γίνεται. εἰ δέ γε τῷ θεῷ τὸ τοιοῦτον ἀπονέμομεν, φαῦλον αὐτὸν κριτὴν ποιήσομεν ἢ οὐ δίκαιον· τοῦτο δ' οὐ προσῆκον ἐστι θεῷ.
[11] ἀλλὰ μὴν οὐδ' ἡ ἐπιμέλεια καὶ ἡ εὔνοια παρὰ τοῦ θεοῦ δόξειεν ἂν εἶναι εὐτυχία διὰ τὸ καὶ ἐν τοῖς φαύλοις ἐγγίγνεσθαι· τὸν δὲ θεὸν τῶν φαύλων οὐκ εἰκὸς ἐπιμελεῖσθαι.

mor. 2.8 is that in the latter chapter Aristotle (or the Peripatetic author of the *Magna moralia*) seems to be satisfied with these impulses as the cause of *eutuchia*, whereas in *Eth. Eud.* 8.2 Aristotle proceeds to a search for the cause of these impulses themselves.[12]

In his discussion of divination in *On Divination in Sleep*, Aristotle uses the distribution argument three times in order to combat the traditional view that dreams are sent by a god:[13] in each case the wording is strikingly similar to *Eth. Eud.* 1247 a 28–9:

462b 20–2: For that the sender [of such prophetic dreams] were a god is irrational in many respects, and it is particularly paradoxical that he sends them not to the best and the most intelligent of people but to ordinary people.[14]

463 b 15–18: For it is quite simple-minded people that tend to foresee the future and to have clear dream images, which suggests that it is not a god that sends them but rather that all those people whose nature is, so to speak, melancholic and garrulous see all kinds of dream visions.[15]

464a 19–20: And for this reason, this experience [i.e. foreseeing the future in sleep] occurs in ordinary people and not the most intelligent. For it would happen during the daytime and in intelligent people, if it were a god who sent it.[16]

Moreover, it is remarkable that in 463 b 18 'the melancholics' are mentioned as an example of the fact that 'quite simple-minded people tend to foresee the future and have clear dreams' (προορατικοὶ καὶ εὐθυόνειροι), which is for Aristotle a sign that dreams cannot be sent by a god. This is barely, if at all, compatible with *Eth. Eud.* 1248 a 39–40, where he says that 'this is why the melancholics have clear dream images' (διὸ οἱ μελαγχολικοὶ καί εὐθυόνειροι), and where the causal connection marked by 'this is why' (διὸ) is with the assertion that God (ὁ θεός) foresees the future, and that God

---

[12] See Dirlmeier (1958) 421. I am aware that the authorship of the *Magna moralia* still is, and probably always will be, a matter of dispute, but the arguments in favour of an Aristotelian origin of much of the philosophical contents, at least, are so strong that I have thought it desirable to include *Mag. mor.* 2.8 in my discussion (see ch. 5 above, n. 42). I have refrained from an explanation of the discrepancy between *Eth. Eud.* 8.2 and *Mag. mor.* 2.8 concerning the cause of the 'impulses', and from a discussion of the implications of this discrepancy, should it be an inconsistency, for the dating and authorship of this part of the *Magna moralia*.
[13] 463 b 13: θεόπεμπτα οὐκ ἂν εἴη τὰ ἐνύπνια. On the wider context of these three passages see ch. 6 above.
[14] τό τε γὰρ θεὸν εἶναι τὸν πέμποντα, πρὸς τῇ ἄλλῃ ἀλογίᾳ, καὶ τὸ μὴ τοῖς βελτίστοις καὶ φρονιμωτάτοις ἀλλὰ τοῖς τυχοῦσι πέμπειν ἄτοπον.
[15] πάνυ γὰρ εὐτελεῖς ἄνθρωποι προορατικοί εἰσι καὶ εὐθυόνειροι, ὡς οὐ θεοῦ πέμποντος, ἀλλ' ὅσων ὥσπερ ἂν εἰ λάλος ἡ φύσις ἐστὶ καὶ μελαγχολικὴ παντοδαπὰς ὄψεις ὁρῶσιν.
[16] καὶ διὰ ταῦτα συμβαίνει τὸ πάθος τοῦτο τοῖς τυχοῦσι καὶ οὐ τοῖς φρονιμωτάτοις. μεθ' ἡμέραν τε γὰρ ἐγίνετ' ἂν καὶ τοῖς σοφοῖς, εἰ θεὸς ἦν ὁ πέμπων.

also works in those people 'whose reasoning is disengaged' (ὧν ὁ λόγος ἀπολυόμενος), as is the case with the melancholics.[17]

The problem, then, might also be put as follows. At first sight there seems to be a discrepancy between, on the one hand, the conclusion of *Eth. Eud.* 8.2 that *eutuchia* is 'divine' and happens 'through God', and, on the other hand, the statements in *On Divination in Sleep*, which repeatedly reject the attribution of divination in sleep[18] to a god.[19] Yet the argument which Aristotle uses in *On Divination in Sleep* (as in *Mag. mor.* 2.8) against this attribution is the same distribution argument as that used in *Eth. Eud.* 8.2: in the latter chapter, it is at first sufficient to reject the popular conception of divine guidance or dispensation, but later it no longer forms an impediment to the conclusion that *eutuchia* is divine (*theia*). On any interpretation it is clear that developmental arguments, such as those used

---

[17] See also the discussion in ch. 5 above. On this contrast see Dirlmeier (1962a) 490 and 492; Flashar (1966) 60 n. 2. Effe (1970, 84–5), argues that the sentence 1248 a 39–40 is a parenthesis: 'Die Träume der Melancholiker werden jedoch nicht in dem Sinn verglichen, daß auch sie auf Gott zurückgeführt werden, sondern nur insofern, als sie – wie die irrationale Mantik – ohne Verwendung des rationalen Elements das Richtige treffen.' But Effe fails to appreciate the force of διό ('this is why'), which connects the sentence with 38–9: 'he well sees both the future and the present, also in those people in whom this reasoning faculty is disengaged' (τοῦτο καὶ εὖ ὁρᾷ καὶ τὸ μέλλον καὶ τὸ ὄν, καὶ ὧν ἀπολύεται ὁ λόγος οὗτος), and which establishes a causal connection between the clear dreams of the melancholics and the divine movement, which is stronger in those whose reasoning faculty is disengaged. It is not correct, therefore, to speak of a *comparison*: the melancholics are an *example*. Moreover, given that the clear dreams of the melancholics are mentioned in this particular context, what other cause is there to account for them than God?

[18] Divination (μαντική) is closely connected with *eutuchia*, as is shown by the mention of μαντική in 1248 a 35 and of the 'clear dreams' (εὐθυονειρίαι) of the melancholics in 1248 a 39. See Woods (1982) 183: 'The power of prophecy is relevant because of the close connection between the right choice and foreknowledge of the future.'

[19] This discrepancy has been noted by many interpreters, e.g. by Huby (1979) 54–5, 57, 59; Natali (1974) 175–7; Dirlmeier (1962a) 483, 490, and 492; Effe (1970) 84–5; Bodéüs (1981) 52–3, 55. On the place of *Eth. Eud.* 8.2 in Aristotle's theology see also Pépin (1971) 220–2 and 272–6; Aubenque (1963) 71–5; and von Arnim (1928) 17ff. Out of all these interpreters, Effe is the only one who tries to account for the discrepancy on the strength of non-developmental arguments. According to him, the form of divination described in *Eth. Eud.* 8.2, which he calls 'enthusiastic divination', is not what is spoken of in *On Divination in Sleep*: 'Aristoteles erkennt also die enthusiastische Mantik, bei der Gott direkt durch den Menschen spricht, an. Das steht nicht in Widerspruch zu *De div. p. somn.*, denn dort wird nur die Zurückführung der Träume auf Gott abgelehnt; die enthusiastische Mantik ist nicht thematisiert.' Apart from being forced, in order to sustain this interpretation, to regard 1248 a 39–40 as a parenthesis (on which see n. 17 above), Effe fails to appreciate that the argument which Aristotle here uses to reject the attribution of prophetic dreams to a god, is the same distribution argument as that used in 1247 a 28–9 to reject the attribution of *eutuchia* to a god. Effe does not make it clear why this argument is no impediment to Aristotle's conclusion of a θεία εὐτυχία in *Eth. Eud.* 1248 a 32ff. (which he conceives as 'enthusiastic divination'), whereas it actually is an impediment to the theory of 'god-sent dreams' (θεόπεμπτα ἐνύπνια) in *On Divination in Sleep*. Moreover, I do not think that what Aristotle has in mind in *Eth. Eud.* 8.2 is the 'enthusiastic divination' ('in which God speaks directly through human beings'; cf. Effe's typology of divination on p. 79): on this see below, especially n. 28.

Aristotle on divine movement and human nature 243

by Dirlmeier,[20] are insufficient to account for this discrepancy, for the problem can be regarded as a problem of consistency both within *Eth. Eud.* 8.2 and between *Eudemian Ethics* and *On Divination in Sleep*. It is therefore necessary to study the part played by the distribution argument in both contexts.

Aristotle's assertion that it is 'paradoxical' (*atopon*) that a god should send gifts to foolish people and not to the best and the wisest, may be understood in the light of a passage in *Eth. Nic.* 1179 a 21ff. There it is argued that if there is such a thing as a divine concern (*theia epimeleia*) with human affairs, this will be directed to those people who cultivate intelligence (*nous*), the thing in which they are most akin to the gods and in which the gods take pleasure. These people are the wise (*sophoi*), who act rightly and nobly, and therefore they are the most beloved by the gods.

Although it is by no means certain that Aristotle himself accepted the existence of such a 'divine concern',[21] it is clear in his view that *if* there is such a thing it will be concerned with the best and wisest, for they are most beloved by the gods just because they cultivate their intelligence. The same, hypothetical frame of argument is to be found in *Div. somn.* 462 b 20–2: if the gods really sent dreams to people – an idea which in itself is 'irrational on other grounds as well' – then it would be 'paradoxical'[22] that they should send them to simple and foolish people, not to the best and wisest. Thus the degree to which a person is 'loved by the gods' (*theophilēs*) depends on the extent to which someone actualises 'excellence' (*aretē*, both intellectual and

---

[20] From Dirlmeier's remarks in his commentary (1962a) it can be concluded that he has not noticed the problem. At 1247 a 28–9 he refers to *On Divination in Sleep*: 'Gegen eine von Gott verursachte Traummantik erhebt Ar. denselben Einwand: es sei paradox, daß Gott der Sender sei, das Wahrsehen aber nicht den βέλτιστοι καὶ φρονιμώτατοι senden sollte, sondern den gewöhnlichen Leuten' (p. 483). On 1248 a 15 he remarks: 'er hat bezüglich der Gottgesandtheit der Träume seine Ansicht (man darf wohl sagen: später) modifiziert' (p. 490). On 1248 a 34 he says: 'In der Richtigkeit von Träumen hat Ar. später keine Gottesgunst mehr gesehen. Ich beschränke mich, auf den Traktat De divinatione per somnum zu verweisen ... und bezüglich der "Melancholiker" auf *Probl.* 953 a 10–955a 4' (p. 492).

[21] This question has been hotly disputed, as has the question whether Aristotle really believed in the existence of these 'gods'. It is to be noted that in *Eth. Nic.* 1179 a 23ff., as well as in 1099 b 10ff., Aristotle neither accepts nor rejects the conception of 'divine concern' (θεία ἐπιμέλεια) and of 'divine dispensation' (θεία μοῖρα); it seems that he did not want to go so far as to draw the conclusion, which in the light of his theology in its strictest form was perhaps inescapable, that there is no room for such divine concern. See on this Verdenius (1960) 60; Pötscher (1970) 69–71; Bodéüs (1975) 28.

[22] It should be noted that both in *Eth. Eud.* 1247 a 28 and in *Div. somn.* 462 b 22 the word ἄτοπον is used, which connotes both 'out of place' and 'paradoxical': it expresses an element of surprise, either in respect to what can be, generally speaking, thought real and reasonable, or in respect to the context in which the ἄτοπον element stands; as such it is often used by Aristotle to point his finger to inconsistencies in the theories of others; cf. *Ph.* 196 b 1; *Eth. Eud.* 1239 a 1–6; *Metaph.* 1079 a 25; *Eth. Nic.* 1178 b 14.

moral), and thus the degree of excellence found in the people among whom *eutuchia*, or divination in sleep, or any other phenomenon commonly attributed to divine dispensation, occurs, actually becomes for Aristotle a criterion by which he judges whether this attribution is correct. Just as the fact that 'happiness' (*eudaimonia*) is found with the 'wise' (the *sophoi*), who are 'most beloved by the gods' (*theophilestatoi*), supports the idea that it is granted by the gods, likewise the fact that *eutuchia* occurs with people who are not 'wise' and do not possess excellence furnishes an argument against the idea that *eutuchia* is given by the gods. This is consistent with Aristotle's remark (*Div. somn.* 464 a 20; see above) that if foresight of the future were given by the gods, they would give it 'during the daytime' (*meth' hēmeran*), not at night; for at night the faculty in virtue of which good people can be distinguished from bad people is inactive.[23]

This whole complex of thought on the relationship between a 'divine concern' (*theia epimeleia*) and human moral qualification – irrespective of whether there is such a thing as divine concern at all – is firmly rooted in Aristotle's ethics, as is shown by the passages cited above (to which might be added *Eth. Eud.* 8.3, 1249 b 3–23).[24] It is clear, therefore, that the distribution argument is not simply an occasional, or even (as was claimed by Dirlmeier) an un-Aristotelian argument,[25] and it is all the more surprising that this argument does not pose an impediment to Aristotle's conclusion that *eutuchia* is 'divine' (*theia*) in 1248 b 4.

The first part of the solution to this problem is in that the 'movement' of God in the fortunate men (the εὐτυχεῖς who succeed without reasoning, ἄλογοι ὄντες κατορθοῦσι), as described in 1248 a 25ff., is not regarded by Aristotle as a form of 'divine concern' (θεία ἐπιμέλεια). The idea which is labelled as 'paradoxical' (ἄτοπον) in 1247 a 28–9 is that a god or demon 'loves' (φιλεῖν) a man who does not possess reason (λόγος): the emphasis is on 'loving' no less than on 'a god or demon' (θεὸν ἢ δαίμονα). But in his

---

[23] Cf. *Eth. Nic.* 1102 b 3–11; *Eth. Eud.* 1219 b 19ff.; *Mag. mor.* 1185 a 9ff.
[24] See especially 1249 b 16ff.: the man who makes such a choice of the 'natural goods' (φύσει ἀγαθά) that they advance the contemplation of God possesses the best standard for the practical life; this is 'the wise man' (ὁ σοφός). I follow the interpretation of this passage offered by Verdenius (1971) 292: 'When God has revealed himself through the channel of contemplation, his influence gets the character of a directive power. This directive power is turned towards practical action through the intermediary of φρόνησις.' The fact that this standard (ὅρος) consists in 'paying as little attention as possible to the irrational part of the soul' (τὸ ἥκιστα αἰσθάνεσθαι τοῦ ἀλόγου (or: ἄλλου) μέρους τῆς ψυχῆς) is in marked contrast with 1248 a 40: 'It seems that this starting-point is more powerful when reason has been disengaged' (ἔοικε γὰρ ἡ ἀρκὴ ἀπολυομένου τοῦ λόγου ἰσχύειν μᾶλλον).
[25] Dirlmeier (1935) 60–1 'Sie gehört noch dem suchenden Aristoteles an, ja sie ist gar nicht aristotelisch, sondern platonisch.' But Dirlmeier also labels *Eth. Nic.* 1162 a 5 and 1179 a 23ff. as 'un-Aristotelian'. See also Vidal (1959) 179.

own explanation in 1248 a 25ff. Aristotle speaks of 'God' (ὁ θεός) as 'principle of movement in the soul' (ἀρχὴ τῆς κινήσεως ἐν τῇ ψυχῇ) who 'sees both the future and the present' (ὁρᾷ καὶ τὸ μέλλον καὶ τὸ ὄν, 38) and who 'moves more powerfully' (ἰσχύει μᾶλλον) (40–1). For the rest, this 'God' is in the main passive: he is the object of 'having' (ἔχειν, 32) and of 'using' (χρῆσθαι, 38),[26] and it is worth noting that verbs like 'give' (διδόναι) or 'be concerned' (ἐπιμελεῖσθαι, cf. πέμπειν in *On Divination in Sleep* and ἀπονέμειν in *Magna moralia*) are absent here.[27] The idea of a divine movement which Aristotle here expounds does not, as has often been claimed, amount to an incidental and momentaneous inspiration or possession by a god comparable, for instance, with Plato's description of divine frenzy in the *Ion* and the *Phaedrus* (as the word ἐνθουσιασμός might suggest).[28] It

[26] Χρῆσθαι is mostly translated here as 'use', probably because it is supposed that the god (θεός) of whom Aristotle here speaks is an immanent principle, some sort of psychic faculty. Apart from the question of whether this is correct (see below), χρῆσθαι in the context of divination has the meaning 'consult'; it is thus often connected with θεῷ ('god', Herodotus 1.47; Aeschines 3.124), with μάντεσι ('sooth-sayers', Aristophanes, *Birds* 724; Plato, *Laws* 686 a) and with μαντείᾳ ('divination', Plato, *Timaeus* 71 d). This use of χρῆσθαι is, according to Redard (1953) 44, derived from the principal meaning 'seek the use of something', which is an 'essentially human' activity ('rechercher l'utilisation de quelque chose. C'est un verbe essentiellement humain. Le procès exprimé est restreint à la sphère du sujet qui fait un recours occasionel à l'objet'), in which the object remains passive ('Le rapport sujet–objet se définit comme un rapport d'appropriation occasionelle').

[27] The question of divine activity in this chapter is connected, of course, with the question of how this 'god' (θεός) should be conceived. The analogy in 1248 a 26, 'as it is a god (or, God) that moves the universe, so it is in the soul' (ὥσπερ ἐν τῷ ὅλῳ θεὸς κἂν ἐκείνῳ) seems to exclude the possibility that it is an immanent principle. In any case this 'god' is not identical with 'the divine element in us' (τὸ ἐν ἡμῖν θεῖον, line 27), for this is the 'intellect' (νοῦς), whereas 'God' is 'superior to intellect' (κρεῖττον τοῦ νοῦ). This is why I prefer the MSS reading θεῷ over Spengel's conjecture θείῳ in line 38. If the Unmoved Mover is referred to, then the wording 'principle of movement' (ἀρχὴ τῆς κινήσεως), which is usually set aside for efficient causality, is awkward, since the Unmoved Mover moves as a final cause (but see Pötscher (1970) 57). But it is questionable whether the theology of *Metaphysics* Λ should serve as a guiding principle here: passages such as *Pol.* 1362 a 32, *On Coming to Be and Passing Away* (*Gen. corr.*) 336 b 27, *On the Heavens* (*Cael.*) 271 a 33 and *Metaph.* 1074 b 3 show a greater resemblance to the theology of *Eth. Eud.* 8.2. The same applies to 1248 a 38: 'he sees well both the future and the present' (τοῦτο καὶ εὖ ὁρᾷ καὶ τὸ μέλλον καὶ τὸ ὄν), which seems inconsistent with God's activity of 'thinking of thinking' (νοήσεως νόησις) in *Metaph.* 1074 b 34–5 and also with *Eth. Eud.* 1245 b 17 ('he is too good to think of anything other than himself', βέλτιον ἢ ὥστε ἄλλο τι νοεῖν παρ'αὑτὸς αὑτόν), but which might be connected with *Metaph.* 983 a 5–10, where it is stated that God knows the 'principles and causes' (ἀρχαί and αἴτια) of all things (see Owens (1979) 227). On these matters see Huby (1979) 57.

[28] The idea expressed by 'using God' (χρῆσθαι θεῷ, see n. 26 above) is in contrast with the concept of enthusiastic divination in Plato's *Ion*: 'this is why God takes out the mind of these people and uses them as his servants, as well as the sooth-sayers and godly diviners' (διὰ ταῦτα δὲ ὁ θεὸς ἐξαιρούμενος τούτων τὸν νοῦν τούτοις χρῆται ὑπηρέταις καὶ τοῖς χρησμῳδοῖς καὶ τοῖς μάντεσι τοῖς θείοις, 534 c 7–d 1), where 'God' (ὁ θεός) is the subject of 'use' (χρῆσθαι) and man the object. This contrast supports the view that Aristotle here does not, as Effe (1970) argues (cf. my note 29), have in mind Plato's notion of divine madness (μανία). The presence of the word ἐνθουσιασμός ('divine inspiration') here in Aristotle's text does not alter this view, for this is used by Aristotle elsewhere to denote an affection (a πάθος) of the human soul (cf. *Pol.* 1342 a 6; *Eth. Eud.* 1225 a 25) and here seems to be used in a somewhat metaphorical way. See also Croissant (1932) 30 n. 2: 'Le mot ἐνθουσιασμός

should rather be conceived as a psycho-physiological mechanism: in virtue of their particular natural constitution (their *phusis*) the 'irrational people' (ἄλογοι) are more open to the divine movement (which turns the 'impulses' in the right direction so that the fortunate people make the right choice)[29] than are people who use reason and deliberation (λόγος and βούλευσις). The conclusion that *eutuchia* is found among simple-minded people is therefore not incompatible with the statement that *eutuchia* is 'divine' (θεία): the psycho-physiological process that Aristotle here has in mind does not presuppose an active and purposive divine choice (ἐπιμέλεια or φιλία) – whereas the theory rejected in 1247 a 28–9 does presuppose such a choice, as the verb 'love' (φιλέω) shows – but is based on a general physical divine movement which works more strongly with those people whose reasoning faculty is disengaged. The process seems similar to the workings of the 'superhuman nature' (δαιμονία φύσις), to which Aristotle ascribes the phenomenon of prophetic dreams in *On Divination in Sleep* (463 b 14); there the susceptibility of simple-minded people to foresight and clear dream images, as well as the absence of this susceptibility in intelligent people, is accounted for by the absence (or, in the case of the intelligent people, the presence) of rational activity: 'for the mind of such [i.e. simple-minded] people is not inclined to much thinking, but is, as it were, vacant and devoid of everything, and once set in motion it moves along with the agent of motion' (ἡ γὰρ διάνοια τῶν τοιούτων [= τῶν τυχόντων] οὐ φροντιστική, ἀλλ' ὥσπερ ἔρημος καὶ κενὴ πάντων, καὶ κινηθεῖσα κατὰ τὸ κινοῦν ἄγεται (464 a 21–2). By contrast, in intelligent people the presence of 'their own proper movements' (οἰκεῖαι κινήσεις) prevents this susceptibility.[30] Like *eutuchia*, divination in sleep is for Aristotle not a

---

ne me paraît pas devoir être compris, d'accord avec cette interprétation, comme le résultat d'une influence directe de la divinité suprême. Il faut plutôt rapprocher ce passage des dialogues de Platon où l'on voit cités les mêmes phénomènes psychiques et notamment de Ménon.' Cf. Gigon (1969) 211: 'Man wird allerdings auch zugestehen müssen, daß der Einschub über den Enthusiasmus verwirrend wirkt: denn in ihm liegt eine göttliche Einwirkung vor, die ihrer besonderen Art nach kaum συνεχής genannt werden kann.' I agree with Croissant's conclusion that 'ni la chance, ni la divination par les songes ne sont le fait d'une inspiration divine et elles sont conditionnées par des facteurs qui n'ont rien de noble, mais elles découlent cependant en droite ligne de ce que l'homme possède de plus divin' (1932, 30), and with her statement that 'Ainsi la θεία μοῖρα reste bien une θεία φύσις', although here I would prefer to refer to the 'superhuman nature' (δαιμονία φύσις) of *Div. somn.* 463 b 14 (see below).

[29] This seems to be the working of God in the soul. Cf. von Fragstein (1974) 375, *contra* Woods (1982) 183 and Dirlmeier (1962a) 490.

[30] It seems best to interpret δαιμονία φύσις in *Div. somn.* 463 b 14 as applying not to nature in general (for on this view, it is difficult to see why Aristotle stipulates that nature is 'superhuman, though not divine', ἡ γὰρ φύσις δαιμονία, ἀλλ' οὐ θεία) but as *human* nature, and not as human nature in general, but as the particular natural constitution of a human individual, as is shown by the example of the 'garrulous and melancholic nature' (λάλος καὶ μελαγχολικὴ φύσις) in the sequel. This is called

form of 'divine concern' (θεία ἐπιμέλεια), but the theory of others that a god 'sends' (πέμπει) dreams to people does suppose divination in sleep to be such, for 'sending' presupposes an active and purposive divine choice, whereas such a choice is for Aristotle, as we have seen, incompatible with the fact that prophetic dreams are found among simple people and not among the best and wisest. For this reason he uses three times the same distribution argument as that in *Eth. Eud.* 1247 a 28–9.

The second part of the solution is in that the movement of God is, in principle, not limited to the class of the 'irrational' (ἄλογοι) people, but extends to the 'wise and intelligent' (σοφοὶ καὶ φρόνιμοι) as well. What Aristotle has in mind here is a general and universal divine causality. To demonstrate this I shall first summarise my interpretation of the passage 1248 a 15ff.; then I shall give a detailed account of this interpretation and of my treatment of the various textual problems.

Having established that *eutuchia* proceeds from natural desire (ὁρμαί and ἐπιθυμίαι), Aristotle asks in turn for the starting-point of this desire, probably because it is not yet clear why this natural desire should be aimed in the right direction. He considers that this starting-point will also be the origin of rational activity (νοῦς and βούλευσις), and having disposed of 'chance' (τύχη) as an evidently unsatisfactory candidate for this function he argues that the starting-point wanted is in fact the starting-point of movement in the soul; then it is clear that this starting-point is God. Thus God is the starting-point of all psychic activity, both of reasoning (νοῆσαι) and of the irrational impulses (ὁρμαί) on which *eutuchia* is based. God is even more powerful than the divine principle in man, the intellect (νοῦς), and it is for this reason that people who are devoid of rational activity, too, can make the right choice: they succeed without reasoning because they still have God, although the wise people also have God and use his movement in their calculation of the future, either by experience or by habit: thus there is a more rational form of divination as well. Both irrational and rational divination, then, 'use' God (who sees the future as well as the present), but God moves more strongly in those people whose reasoning faculty is disengaged. Thus God's movement is present both in the irrational people

daimonia because it is beyond human control, as is indicated by the use of the word δαιμόνιος in *Somn. vig.* 453 b 23, where τὸ δαιμόνιον is presented as the opposite of what is done by human agency and is subdivided into things that happen 'naturally' (φύσει) and things that happen 'spontaneously' (ἀπὸ ταὐτομάτου). The individual human nature is further called *daimonia* because it works more strongly when reason is inactive, and because it plays the part of intermediary between God and man, which Greek tradition assigned to demons. For this interpretation see van der Eijk (1994) 292–6, and ch. 6 above.

and in the intelligent ones, but it is stronger in the irrational ones: in the latter it is an immediate movement, whereas in the intelligent people God works through the intermediary of 'the divine in us' (τὸ ἐν ἡμῖν θεῖον), the intellect. This is an obvious reference to the distribution argument in 1247 a 28–9, where it was stated that it is 'paradoxical' that a god or demon should love simple people, not the best and wisest (μὴ τὸν βέλτιστον καὶ φρονιμώτατον); evidently Aristotle remains aware of the distribution argument and anticipates it by means of a careful presentation of his own explanation.

I will now support this interpretation with a detailed analysis of the text. For the purpose of clarity I will print first a text and a translation of each section and then add comments on the section in question. The text of the manuscript tradition will be followed as closely as possible; any deviations from it will be accounted for from line to line.[31]

1248 a 16–26:

16 τοῦτο μέντ' ἂν ἀπορήσειέ τις, ἆρ' αὐτοῦ τούτου τύχη αἰτία,
17 τοῦ ἐπιθυμῆσαι οὗ δεῖ καὶ ὅτε δεῖ; ἢ οὕτως γε πάντων ἔσται;
18 καὶ γὰρ τοῦ νοῆσαι καὶ βουλεύσασθαι· οὐ γὰρ δὴ ἐβουλεύσατο
19 βουλευσάμενος καὶ τοῦτ' ἐβουλεύσατο,[32] ἀλλ' ἔστιν
20 ἀρχή τις, οὐδ' ἐνόησε νοήσας πρότερον ἢ[33] νοῆσαι, καὶ τοῦτο
21 εἰς ἄπειρον. οὐκ ἄρα τοῦ νοῆσαι ὁ νοῦς[34] ἀρχή, οὐδὲ τοῦ
22 βουλεύσασθαι βουλή. τί οὖν ἄλλο πλὴν τύχη; ὥστ' ἀπὸ τύχης

---

[31] In the light of the harassed transmission of the text it may seem rather naive to keep as closely as possible to the MS tradition, but I have done so for methodological reasons. It seems to me that the numerous problems of interpretation in this chapter are due at least as much to Aristotle's concise and often frankly clumsy way of writing as to possible corruptions in the text. Therefore the interpreter should maintain a fundamental distinction between hypotheses concerning the original text which Aristotle wrote down, and hypotheses concerning what he intended to say. This distinction seems to have often been ignored, and apparently interpreters have, with an appeal to the abysmal state of the text, proposed many conjectures with a view to making the text comply with interpretations mainly prompted by theological assertions in other Aristotelian writings. The unfortunate consequence of this process is that there is no generally accepted text on which to base a debate concerning the tenability of a particular interpretation: in order to scrutinise it, one has to be willing to accept, for the sake of argument, the readings proposed by the interpreter, while these readings were actually chosen to support the interpretation. An interpretation open to falsification must necessarily keep as closely as possible to the, admittedly narrow, basis of the MS tradition, and should propose conjectures only where this is absolutely necessary, and render an account of every conjecture. This account should be based principally on the immediate context and only secondarily on statements on the subject in other Aristotelian writings.

[32] The MS tradition καὶ τοῦτ' ἐβουλεύσατο is emended by Dirlmeier (1962a) and Woods (1982) into πρότερον ἢ βουλεύσασθαι, analogously to πρότερον (ἢ) νοῆσαι in line 20, but this is unnecessary, as von Fragstein (1974, 375) points out, for the articulation οὗ δεῖ καὶ ὅτε δεῖ is also present here.

[33] The MS tradition is πρότερον νοῆσαι; I follow Spengel in inserting ἢ.

[34] The MS tradition is τοῦ νοῆσαι συνοῦσα ἀρχή, which does not make sense and which can easily be emended into τοῦ νοῆσαι ὁ νοῦς ἀρχή analogously to τοῦ βουλεύσασθαι ἀρχή.

Aristotle on divine movement and human nature   249

23 ἅπαντα ἔσται· ἢ[35] ἔστι τις ἀρχὴ ἧς οὐκ ἔστιν ἄλλη ἔξω, αὕτη
24 δὲ διὰ τὸ τοιαύτη εἶναι τοιοῦτο δύναται ποιεῖν;[36] τὸ δὲ
25 ζητούμενον τοῦτ' ἔστι, τίς ἡ τῆς κινήσεως ἀρχὴ ἐν τῇ ψυχῇ; δῆλον
26 δὴ ὥσπερ ἐν τῷ ὅλῳ θεὸς κἂν ἐκείνῳ.[37]

'However, one might raise the question whether good fortune is the cause of this very fact, that we desire the right thing at the right moment. Or will good fortune be in that way the cause of everything? For then it will also be the cause of thinking and deliberation. For we did not deliberate at a particular moment concerning a particular thing after having deliberated – no, there is a certain starting-point, nor did we think after having already thought before thinking, and so on to infinity. Intelligence, therefore, is not the starting-point of thinking nor is counsel the starting-point of deliberation. So what else if not good fortune? Thus everything will be caused by chance. Or is there some starting-point beyond which there is no other, and is this starting-point such as to be able to produce such an effect? What we are looking for is this: what is the starting-point of the movement in the soul? It is now evident that, as it is a god that moves the universe, so it is in the soul.'

Comments: So far the text provides few interpretative difficulties. It is of vital importance to notice that the 'starting-point' (ἀρχή) Aristotle is seeking is the starting-point of all movement in the soul, both of 'thinking' (νοῆσαι) and of 'desiring' (ἐπιθυμῆσαι, ὁρμαί). Thus God is also the 'principle of movement' in the souls of those people who actualise 'intellect and deliberation' (νοῦς, βούλευσις).[38]

---

[35] The MS tradition is ἔσται εἰ ἔστι, which does not make sense, since the sentence obviously marks a disjunction (cf. the Latin tradition *aut est aliquod principium*, etc.).

[36] The MS tradition is αὕτη δὲ διὰ τι τοιαύτη τὸ εἶναι τὸ τοῦτο δύνασθαι ποιεῖν. I follow Jackson (1913) 197 and Mills (1983) 289 n. 13 in reading: αὕτη δὲ διὰ τ: τοιαύτη εἶναι τοιοῦτο δύναται ποιεῖν, which accounts for the corruption better than Dirlmeier's αὕτη δὲ ὅτι τοιαύτη κατὰ τὸ εἶναι τὸ τοιοῦτο δύναται ποιεῖν (1962a).

[37] The MS tradition is καὶ πᾶν ἐκείνῳ which, if translated as 'also everything is moved by him (i.e. God)', yields a tautology with ὥσπερ ἐν τῷ ὅλῳ (sc. ἀρχὴ τῆς κινήσεως). W. J. Verdenius (private correspondence) suggested to me as a translation of the whole sentence: 'It is clear that this starting-point is analogous to the part which God plays in the universe, where he moves everything' (reading καὶ πᾶν ἐκείνῳ and taking καί as specifying ὥσπερ ἐν τῷ ὅλῳ). However, the connection with the following then becomes difficult, for the ἀρχή sought is not τὸ ἐν ἡμῖν θεῖον (which is the νοῦς) but ὁ θεός (who is κρεῖττον τοῦ νοῦ). The analogy which Aristotle wants to express is best achieved when we read κἂν ἐκείνῳ, where ἐκείνῳ refers to ψυχή (as so often in this chapter a neuter pronoun refers to a masculine or feminine noun; for this reason Wood's conjecture κἂν ἐκείνη can be left aside). Dirlmeier reads καὶ πᾶν ἐκεῖνο and translates: 'so bewegt er auch alles jene (in der Seele)', but this is awkward as Greek.

[38] See Gigon (1969) 211.

1248 a 26–9:
26 κινεῖ γάρ
27 πως πάντα τὸ ἐν ἡμῖν θεῖον· λόγου δ' ἀρχὴ οὐ λόγος.
28 ἀλλά τι κρεῖττον· τί οὖν ἂν κρεῖττον καὶ ἐπιστήμης εἴη
29 πλὴν θεός;[39] ἡ γὰρ ἀρετὴ τοῦ νοῦ ὄργανον.

'For in a certain way the divine element in us moves everything; but the starting-point of reasoning is not reasoning, but something stronger. Well, what then could be even stronger than knowledge, other than God? (Not virtue) for virtue is an instrument of intelligence.'

Comments: I regard 'the divine element in us' (τὸ ἐν ἡμῖν θεῖον) as an equivalent of 'the intellect' (νοῦς, λόγος), in accordance with *Eth. Nic.* 1177 a 13–17, 1177 b 27–31 and 1179 a 27–8.[40] The point of this sentence is that it makes explicit another possible answer to Aristotle's question, to the effect that it is the intellect (νοῦς) which is the principle of movement in the soul: for after all, the intellect is 'the divine element in us'. Aristotle anticipates this idea by arguing that, admittedly, this is true in a certain way (πως), but the intellect itself has got its movement from something which is 'superior' (κρεῖττον, cf. 1248 a 18–20 above). (It is not necessary to alter the MS reading κινεῖ γάρ πως πάντα τὸ ἐν ἡμῖν θεῖον.[41] The sentence ἡ γὰρ ἀρετὴ τοῦ νοῦ ὄργανον anticipates a possible objection to the effect that the ἀρχή sought for is ἀρετή).[42]

---

[39] The MS tradition is τί οὖν ἂν κρεῖττον καὶ ἐπιστήμης εἴποι πλὴν θεός; The emendation of εἴποι into εἴη as well as the addition of καὶ νοῦ, which are generally accepted by modern interpreters, are based on the Latin tradition: *quid igitur utique erit melius et scientia et intellectu nisi deus*, but the addition καὶ νοῦ is probably prompted by the mention of νοῦς in the following sentence and by line 32 κρεῖττον τοῦ νοῦ καὶ τῆς βουλεύσεως; ἐπιστήμη seems equivalent in this context to νοῦς and λόγος.

[40] Following Dirlmeier (1962a) 490, and von Arnim (1928) 21, contra Woods (1982) 182, who argues that in *Eth. Nic.* 1177 a 13–17 'the divine element is tentatively identified with the intelligence (*nous*), whereas here the divine element is distinguished from intelligence'. Cf. Wagner (1970) 105–8, who wrongly follows Dirlmeier (1962a) 108 in concluding that 'this divine element moves the processes in the soul' ('dieses θεῖον bewegt die Vorgänge in der Seele'), which is incompatible with Wagner's own conclusion that τὸ ἐν ἡμῖν θεῖον is equivalent to ὁ νοῦς which is distinguished from ὁ θεός: if Wagner reads θεῷ in 1248a 38, how can he conclude that not ὁ θεός but τὸ θεῖον is the ἀρχὴ τῆς κινήσεως ἐν τῇ ψυχῇ?

[41] Mills (1983, 289 n. 13) reads κινεῖ γάρ πως πάντα τὰ ἐν ἡμῖν θεός, but this change is not necessary, and it makes the following sentence (lines 27–9) redundant. I do not understand Mills' objection to the MS tradition, 'for how could the λόγος in us move πάντα?', for this seems consistent with Aristotle's ideas on the subject in general (cf. *De motu an.* 700 b 18ff.) and, besides, Aristotle qualifies this statement by πως ('in a way which it is not relevant now to explain').

[42] The objection is probably Socratic, and ἀρετή should be regarded here as moral virtue. Woods (1982, 182) and Dirlmeier (1962a, 490) refer to 1246 b 10–12: ἀλλὰ μὴν οὐδ' ἀρετή· χρῆται γὰρ αὐτῇ· ἡ γὰρ τοῦ ἄρχοντος ἀρετὴ τῇ τοῦ ἀρχομένου χρῆται (on which see Moraux (1971) 264–5).

Aristotle on divine movement and human nature   251

1248 a 29–34:
29   καὶ διὰ τοῦτο,
30   ὃ⁴³ οἱ πάλαι ἔλεγον, εὐτυχεῖς καλοῦνται οἳ ἂν ὁρμήσωσι
31   κατορθοῦσιν⁴⁴ ἄλογοι ὄντες, καὶ βουλεύεσθαι οὐ συμφέρει
     αὐτοῖς.
32   ἔχουσι γὰρ ἀρχὴν τοιαύτην ἣ κρεῖττον⁴⁵ τοῦ νοῦ καὶ τῆς
     βουλεύσεως
33   (οἳ δὲ τὸν λόγον· τοῦτο δ' οὐκ ἔχουσι) καὶ ἐνθουσιασμόν.⁴⁶
     τοῦτο
34   δ' οὐ δύνανται· ἄλογοι γὰρ ὄντες ἐπιτυγχάνουσι.⁴⁷

'And for this reason, as people spoke of old, those people are called fortunate people who, when they make a start, succeed though lacking reasoning, and it is not profitable for them to deliberate. For they have such a starting-point which is stronger than intelligence and deliberation (others have reasoning; this the lucky people do not possess) and they have divine inspiration,⁴⁸ but they are not capable of intelligence and deliberation: they hit the mark without reasoning.'

Comments: The question about the cause of the lucky people's success is now answered: they succeed owing to 'the starting-point which is stronger than intelligence and deliberation'. The adjunct 'though lacking reasoning' (ἄλογοι ὄντες) again stresses what has already been noted in the beginning of the chapter (1247 a 4; 13), that their success is not due to reason or intelligence; the sentence 'it is not profitable for them to deliberate' refers to 1247 b 29–37, where Aristotle says that in the case of *eutuchia* the natural impulse (ὁρμή) is contrary to reasoning and that reasoning is idle (ὁ δὲ λογισμὸς ἦν ἠλίθιος, 35). The anticipation in lines 26–9 now turns out to be very appropriate: having discussed the part played by the intellect (νοῦς being on a par in this context with λόγος and βούλευσις) in human action, Aristotle stipulates that there is a starting-point which is even more powerful than this, and that this starting-point is the cause of the lucky people's success.

---

⁴³ The MS tradition is τοῦτο οἱ πάλαι, with ὃ omitted, having dropped out (cf. the Latin tradition: *propter hoc quod olim dicebatur*).
⁴⁴ The MS tradition is κατορθοῦν, but a finite verb is obviously appropriate here.
⁴⁵ For the neuter κρεῖττον (cf. line 28) see n. 37 above.
⁴⁶ The MS tradition is ἐνθουσιασμοί.
⁴⁷ The MS tradition is ἀποτυγχάνουσι, but this is completely out of place here, since the subject must be the εὐτυχεῖς (see below).
⁴⁸ On the word ἐνθουσιασμός see n. 28 above.

Lines 33–4 contain many difficulties. οἳ δέ ('others') are the people who actually owe their sucess to reasoning (λόγος). But it is improbable that these οἳ δέ should be the subject of ἔχουσι ('they have') and that τοῦτο ('this') should refer to ἀρχή, since it is hardly credible that these people do *not* have this starting-point (ἀρχή), for this starting-point was said to be the origin of all movement in the soul, including intellect, reason and deliberation. Various solutions to this problem might be suggested:

(1) The subject of ἔχουσι ('they have') is not οἳ δέ, but the 'irrational people' (the ἄλογοι); and τοῦτο ('this') refers to λόγος ('reason'). It might be objected to this possible solution that the sentence τοῦτο δ' οὐ δύναται ('they are not capable . . . ') is then redundant, since this second τοῦτο refers to νοῦς and βούλευσις. But this objection can be countered in two ways: either (i) the sentence οἳ δὲ τὸν λόγον· τοῦτο δ' οὐκ ἔχουσι ('others have reasoning; this the lucky people do not possess') can be taken as a parenthesis (as does Susemihl, who puts it between brackets): in this case the redundancy is not unacceptable; or (ii) there is a new change of subject: the second τοῦτο ('this') refers to ἐνθουσιασμόν ('divine inspiration') and the subject of δύνανται ('they are capable') is οἳ δέ, the people with reason (λόγος). But this seems to be going too far, since in the next sentence the 'irrational people' (ἄλογοι) are again the subject; moreover, δύνασθαι ἐνθουσιασμόν is linguistically an awkward combination.

(2) The subject of ἔχουσι ('they have') is οἳ δέ ('the other people'); Aristotle is thinking here of a specific form of divine movement (as the word ἐνθουσιασμός suggests); this movement (some sort of inspiration) does not affect those who have λόγος. There is a shift in the argument from a general divine causality of *all* psychic movement to a *specific* divine causality.[49] But the problem is that this shift is nowhere marked explicitly in the text; moreover the conjunction with the following sentence now becomes problematic.

(3) von Fragstein (1974) 376 reads: οἳ δὲ τὸν λόγον (sc. ἔχουσιν) τοῦτο δ' οὐκ ἔχουσιν, οὐδὲ ἐνθουσιασμόν· τοῦτο δ' οὐ δύνανται· ἄλογοι γὰρ ὄντες ἀποτυγχάνουσι: 'Die Andern aber haben die Fähigkeit logischen Durchdringens; dieses aber, den Anstoß von der Gottheit her, haben sie nicht, auch nicht die göttliche Begeisterung; das können sie nicht. Wenn nämlich ihr Denken einmal versagt, gehen sie in die Irre.' Against this it must be objected that τοῦτο δ' οὐ δύνανται is redundant after τοῦτο δ'

---

[49] See Woods (1982) 183: 'although the previous section apparently introduced the divine element in the soul as the source of all psychic activities, it is clear that in this section a divine causation of a rather special kind is in question; instead of initiating a fallible train of reasoning from the desired end to the conclusion, the divine element produces action of the appropriate kind in a manner superior to rational calculation'.

οὐκ ἔχουσιν and that the sentence ἄλογοι γὰρ ὄντες ἀποτυγχάνουσιν (which is, in fact, the MS reading) is completely out of place in this context: the translation of ἄλογοι ὄντες as 'Wenn nämlich ihr Denken einmal versagt' is certainly incorrect (cf. the same phrase in line 31), and Aristotle's argument does not seem to leave any room for the possibility that those people should fail who have λόγος but do not use it (at a certain moment) and follow their ὁρμαί.[50]

Since the second and the third solution yield insurmountable difficulties, the first solution seems the most acceptable; this requires that we allow argument (i) to count as a sufficient justification of the redundancy of τοῦτο δ' οὐ δύνανται.

1248 a 34–41:
34 καὶ τού-
35 των φρονίμων καὶ σοφῶν ταχεῖαν εἶναι τὴν μαντικήν, καὶ
36 μόνον οὐ τὴν ἀπὸ τοῦ λόγου δεῖ ἀπολαβεῖν, ἀλλ' οἱ μὲν δι'
37 ἐμπειρίαν οἱ δὲ διὰ συνήθειάν τε ἐν τῷ σκοπεῖν χρῆσθαι.
38 τῷ θεῷ δὲ αὗται· τοῦτο καὶ εὖ ὁρᾷ καὶ τὸ μέλλον καὶ
39 τὸ ὄν, καὶ ὧν ἀπολύεται ὁ λόγος οὗτος·[51] διὸ οἱ μελαγ-
40 χολικοὶ καὶ εὐθυόνειροι. ἔοικε γὰρ ἡ ἀρχὴ ἀπολυομένου τοῦ
41 λόγου[52] ἰσχύειν μᾶλλον.

'The divination of those who are intelligent and wise, too, is swift, and it may almost be said that we must distinguish the form of divination founded on reason, but in any case some people use this by experience, others by habituation in observation. These forms make use of God: he well sees both the future and the present, also in those people in whom this reasoning faculty is disengaged. This is why melancholics have clear dreams too. For the starting-point appears to be stronger when reason is disengaged.'

Comments: This passage is bristling with difficulties. In lines 34–5 it is not clear what the infinitive construction depends on, but it is unnecessary to assume a lacuna before καί, as is done by Dirlmeier (1962a) and Woods (1982), following Spengel:[53] the sentence can be understood as equivalent

---

[50] Unless this possibility should be provided for in 1248 a 7–8; but the meaning of this section is extremely obscure; cf. Dirlmeier (1962a) 489, and Mills (1983) 294.
[51] I follow the MS tradition in reading οὗτος, which has been emended by most interpreters into οὕτως; see on this n. 63 below.
[52] The MS tradition is ἀπολυομένους τοὺς λόγους, where the plural accusative is obviously wrong (cf. line 39).
[53] Dirlmeier (1962a) reads: ⟨δῆλον δὲ⟩ καὶ τὸ τῶν φρονίμων καὶ σοφῶν ταχεῖαν εἶναι τὴν μαντικήν καὶ μόνην οὐ τὴν ἀπὸ τοῦ λόγου δεῖ ἀπολαβεῖν, ἀλλ' οἱ μὲν δι' ἐμπειρίαν οἱ δὲ διὰ συνήθειαν (δοκοῦσι) [τε ἐν] τῷ σκοπεῖν χρῆσθαι – τῷ θεῷ δ' ⟨αὐτῷ⟩ αὗτη.

το καὶ τούτων φρονίμων καὶ σοφῶν ταχεῖα ἐστι ἡ μαντική, or it can be connected zeugmatically with ἀπολαβεῖν ('distinguish'),[54] which has often, though unnecessarily, been changed into ὑπολαβεῖν ('suppose'); in that case the infinitive χρῆσθαι ('use') also depends on ἀπολαβεῖν.

Who are 'those who are intelligent and wise' (τούτων φρονίμων καὶ σοφῶν)? Several interpreters (Woods (1982); Décarie (1978); Düring (1966)) suppose that the 'irrational people' (the ἄλογοι) are meant, that is, the fortunate people (εὐτυχεῖς) who were the subject of ἐπιτυγχάνουσι ('they hit the mark without reasoning') in line 34.[55] But it is very unlikely that Aristotle should call these people 'intelligent and wise' (φρόνιμοι καὶ σοφοί). It seems better (with Dirlmeier (1962a) and von Fragstein (1974)) to identify these 'intelligent and wise' people with οἳ δέ in line 33, the people who possess reason. Aristotle asserts that these people too, just like the irrational people, have a prophetic capacity which is swift, but in them it actually *is* due to reason.[56]

The next sentence is taken by nearly all interpreters[57] as if it read οὐ μόνον, 'not only', but μόνον οὐ means 'very nearly', 'almost': the construction μόνον οὐ *p* ἀλλὰ *q* expresses that we may almost say *p* but in any case *q*.[58] Aristotle does not want to go so far as to say that there exists such a thing as rational divination founded on reason, but he does recognise the fact that some people, by means of experience or habit, perform divination,[59] and that this kind of divination is different from the irrational process by which the lucky people foresee the future. Given this interpretation, Dirlmeier's (1962a) emendation of μόνον into μόνην can be discarded. τε is deleted by all interpreters, but it might be connected with διὰ συνήθειαν: 'others also by habit'. In any case ἐν should certainly be retained, for the object of χρῆσθαι ('use') is not τῷ σκοπεῖν ('observation'), which is linguistically an awkward combination, but μαντική ('divination'; cf. τὴν ἀπὸ τοῦ λόγου sc. μαντικήν): 'they use divination by habituation in observing'.

---

[54] I do not see how Dirlmeier can translate ἀπολαβεῖν as 'als abgesonderte (einfach) abtun', for ἀπολαμβάνειν means 'to take apart, to distinguish' (see LSJ s.v.).

[55] See Woods (1982) 43, 183; Décarie (1978) 215; Düring (1966) 453.

[56] See Dirlmeier (1962a) 481; Effe (1970) 84; von Fragstein (1974) 376–7. The distinction between rational and irrational divination is made by Plato, *Phaedrus* 244 a–d; rational divination is referred to by Aristotle in *Mem.* 449 b 10 and in *Pol.* 1274 a 28.

[57] Except Jackson (1913) 198–9, who translates: 'and it may almost be said that they should put a check upon the divination which depends on reason. The fact is that some by experience, and others by habit, have this power.' However, Jackson's translation of ἀπολαβεῖν as 'put a check upon' is certainly incorrect (see n. 54 above).

[58] For this use of μόνον οὐ... ἀλλὰ cf. Aristophanes, *Wasps* 515–17: καταγελώμενος μὲν οὖν οὐκ ἐπαΐεις ὑπ᾽ ἀνδρῶν, οὓς σὺ μόνον οὐ προσκυνεῖς ἀλλὰ δουλεύων λέληθας.

[59] Cf. Aristotle's cautious reference to the idea, expressed by others, that divination is an ἐπιστήμη ἐλπιστική (*Mem.* 449 b 12: εἴη δ᾽ ἂν καὶ ἐπιστήμη τις ἐλπιστική, καθάπερ τινές φασι τὴν μαντικήν).

This interpretation may seem over-subtle, but the interpretations in which μόνον... οὐ is taken as 'not only... but' involve the difficulty that the structure of the sentence (καὶ μόνον οὐ... ἀλλ' οἳ μέν, οἳ δέ) would mark a contrast between the two forms of divination to be distinguished, whereas such a contrast is lacking in the actual contents of the sentence: for both experience (ἐμπειρία) and habituation (συνήθεια) seem to belong to the rational form of divination, a capacity based on some sort of inductive process of repeated observation and registration. To this it could be objected that perhaps they do not really belong there, and (1) we might have to classify experience and habituation under the irrational form of the divination: then we would have the contrast, marked by ἀλλά, with τὴν ἀπὸ τοῦ λόγου (sc. μαντικήν). However, on that interpretation (i) the connection with the previous sentence, marked by καί, remains awkward, and (ii) it is hard to imagine how ἐμπειρία and συνήθεια can be regarded as irrational activities, for they result in τέχνη ('technical skill') whereas *eutuchia* is not founded on technical skill but on natural talent (φύσις) and on irrational impulses (ὁρμαί). Alternatively, one might consider (2) that ἐμπειρία is the rational form, συνήθεια the irrational form of divination; but objection (i) would remain, and the word σκοπεῖν seems peculiar to rational divination; moreover it seems impossible to regard irrational *eutuchia*, based on natural impulses, as identical or comparable with μαντικὴ διὰ συνήθειαν.[60]

The interpretation of μόνον οὐ as 'almost' and of ἐμπειρία and συνήθεια as forms of rational divination is at any rate consistent with the following sentence. In τῷ θεῷ δὲ αὗται we must understand a form of χρῆσθαι, and τῷ θεῷ is the ἀρχή of line 32 (and of 23, 25 and 27). It is unnecessary to emend this to τῷ θείῳ, as Verdenius (1971), following Spengel, proposes.[61] αὗται refers to the two types of divination[62] or to the two sub-types of rational divination, ἐμπειρία and συνήθεια; the first alternative seems

---

[60] Habit is explicitly distinguished from nature by Aristotle in what is plainly a reference to εὐτυχία at *Eth. Nic.* 1179b 21ff.: γίνεσθαι δ' ἀγαθοὺς οἴονται οἱ μὲν φύσει οἱ δὲ ἔθει οἱ δὲ διδαχῇ. τὸ μὲν οὖν τῆς φύσεως δῆλον ὡς οὐκ ἐφ' ἡμῖν ὑπάρχει, ἀλλὰ διά τινας θείας αἰτίας τοῖς ὡς ἀληθῶς εὐτυχέσιν ὑπάρχει. ὁ δὲ λόγος καὶ ἡ διδαχὴ μὴ ποτ' οὐκ ἐν ἅπασιν ἰσχύει, ἀλλὰ δεῖ προδιειργάσθαι τοῖς ἔθεσι τὴν τοῦ ἀκροατοῦ ψυχὴν πρὸς τὸ καλῶς χαίρειν καὶ μισεῖν, ὥσπερ γῆν τὴν θρέψουσαν τὸ σπέρμα (cf. *Eth. Nic.* 1148 a 30, 1152 a 29; *Eth. Eud.* 1214 a 16–21). Moreover, as ἕξις is implicitly rejected as a possible cause of εὐτυχία in 1247 a 7–13, it is unlikely that συνήθεια, which is closely connected with ἕξις (cf. *Rh.* 1354a 7: διὰ συνήθειαν ἀπὸ ἕξεως), is identical with the psycho-physiological mechanism on which εὐτυχία is based (see on ἕξις Dirlmeier (1962a) 480 and Mills (1981) 253–6). Finally, it appears from *Eth. Nic.* 1181 a 10ff. that ἐμπειρία and συνήθεια cannot be regarded as opposites: οὐ μὴν μικρόν γε ἔοικεν ἡ ἐμπειρία συμβάλλεσθαι. οὐδὲ γὰρ ἐγίνοντ' ἂν διὰ τῆς πολιτικῆς συνηθείας πολιτικοί.
[61] For the ἀρχή is not τὸ ἐν ἡμῖν θεῖον, but ὁ θεός. Cf. Huby (1979) 57 and Dirlmeier (1962a) 491–2, contra Verdenius (1971) 291 n. 14. For the neuter τοῦτο cf. my note 37.
[62] See von Fragstein (1974) 377.

preferable in view of the bipartition which runs through this whole section of the text. In any case, both irrational and rational divination are caused by ὁ θεός; also the φρόνιμοι καὶ σοφοί use the divine movement, and this conclusion can, as we have seen above, be read as a plain reference to the distribution argument of 1247 a 28–9. Only then can it be understood that Aristotle says that God moves *also* (καί) in those whose λόγος is disengaged, and that he moves *more strongly* (ἰσχύειν μᾶλλον)[63] in those: he does *not* say that God does not move in the φρόνιμοι καὶ σοφοί.[64]

The rest of the chapter does not contain any further problems of interpretation as distinct from textual difficulties.[65]

To sum up, we may say that there are two reasons why the distribution argument actually poses an impediment to the attribution of *eutuchia* to a god in 1247 a 23–9, but does not do so in 1248 b 4. First, in 1247 a 28–9 Aristotle speaks of 'being loved' (φιλεῖν) by the gods; *eutuchia* is,

---

[63] The words ἰσχύειν and ἀπολύεσθαι seem to form a contrast here, but it remains obscure what exactly Aristotle means when he says that 'reason is disengaged' (λόγος ἀπολυόμενος), and through what cause it is supposed to be so. The example of the blind in 1248 b 1–2 points to a physical defect, but perhaps we should not press the analogy too far (see my note 65 below). In view of this obscurity it is questionable whether the traditional reading οὗτος should be emended into οὕτως, for this vague reference can only be to the way in which the εὐτυχεῖς succeed ἄλογοι ὄντες.

[64] Dirlmeier's (1962a) remark that, if rational divination too consulted God, 'die ganze Argumentation sinnlos würde', cannot be approved. On the contrary, if rational divination did not consult God, many elements in the text (lines 26–9 and 34–8) would be out of place.

[65] In 1248b 1–2 the MS tradition is καὶ ὥσπερ οἱ τυφλοὶ μνημονεύουσι μᾶλλον ἀπολυθέντες τοῦ πρὸς τοῖς εἰρημένοις εἶναι τὸ μνημονεῦον. The difficulty is ἀπολυθέντες τοῦ πρὸς τοῖς εἰρημένοις εἶναι τὸ μνημονεῦον, for which many emendations have been proposed, none of which are free from difficulties. The simplest solution is that suggested by von Fragstein (1974) 377: ἀπολυθέντες τῷ πρὸς τοῖς εἰρημένοις εἶναι τὸ μνημονεῦον; but how can the blind be called ἀπολυθέντες without further qualification (although the aorist participle, after ἀπολυομένου, is striking?) Dirlmeier (1962a) and Woods (1982) propose τῷ ἀπολυθέντος τοῦ πρὸς τοῖς ὁρωμένοις [sc. εἶναι] σπουδαιότερον εἶναι τὸ μνημονεῦον, but this is based on the Latin tradition *amissis hiis quae ad visibilia virtuosius esse quod memoratur*. It is safer, though not free from difficulties either, to read ἀπολυθέντος τοῦ πρὸς τοῖς ὁρωμένοις εἶναι τὸ μνημονεῦον. Anyhow, the point must be, as Woods (1982, 219) puts it, that 'just as the blind man has better powers of memory as a result of lack of preoccupation with the visible, the power of divination is improved when reason is in abeyance'. Then the text runs as printed by Susemihl, who emends φανερὸν into φανερὸν δή, but for Spengel's conjecture in 1248 b 4 (ἡ δὲ φύσει) which is certainly wrong (see n. 2 above): 'It is clear, then, that there are two forms of good fortune, the former of which is divine. For this reason the fortunate man seems to owe his success to a god. He is the one who succeeds in accordance with impulse, the other succeeds contrary to impulse; but both are irrational. It is the first form, rather, which is continuous; the second is not continuous.' The second form is the one caused by τύχη referred to in the section 1247 b 38–1248 a 15, as Dirlmeier (1962a, 492) rightly observes. But his contra-predestinarian remark 'Weiterdenken darf man hier nicht, also nicht fragen, warum Gott in solchen Seelen nicht tätig wird', is certainly out of place, for God is moving in all souls: the second form also occurs with people who have the first form, but in them its cause is different. For συνεχής meaning 'continuous' cf. *Eth. Nic.* 1150b 34: ἡ μὲν γὰρ συνεχὴς ἡ δ' οὐ συνεχὴς πονηρία, and *Insomn.* 461 a 10.

in the theory criticised there, a specific form of divine dispensation (θεία μοῖρα), whereas in 1248 a 32ff. Aristotle is thinking of a process which does not consist in such a divine dispensation but in people making use of a universal divine causality. Secondly, the theory criticised by Aristotle in 1247 a 23ff. presupposes that divine dispensation regards only the 'irrational' (ἄλογοι) people, whereas in 1248 a 32ff. not only these ἄλογοι but also the 'wise and clever' (φρόνιμοι καὶ σοφοί) use the divine movement; the difference between these two classes of people in their susceptibility to the divine movement is one of degree rather than kind, and it is based not on deliberate divine choice but on human nature (φύσις).

If this interpretation is convincing, then the discrepancy between *Eth. Eud.* 8.2 and *Div. somn.* has disappeared as well. What Aristotle has in mind in *Eth. Eud.* 1248 a 32ff. is the same process of interaction between a divine movement and a human natural constitution as what he refers to as the 'superhuman nature' in *Div. somn.* 463 b 14 (δαιμονία φύσις). The only difference is that the *Eudemian Ethics* explicitly mentions 'God' (ὁ θεός) as the starting-point (ἀρχή) of the process, whereas in *On Divination in Sleep* Aristotle seems to reject any divine influence whatsoever. But the reason for this is that in *On Divination in Sleep* he combats a theory which is comparable with the view, rejected in *Eth. Eud.* 1247a 23–9, that prophetic dreams are caused by deliberate divine dispensation (θεόπεμπτα). The reason why he does not explicitly mention the divine aspect of the process of interaction is that the subtleties of *Eth. Eud.* 8.2 would certainly undermine his own purpose in *On Divination in Sleep*, which is to reject this popular attribution of prophetic dreams to a god. In the *Eudemian Ethics*, however, the argument does not breathe the polemical atmosphere of *On Divination in Sleep*. It seems that Aristotle is arguing here positively in defence of a view which is unlikely to be accepted by an audience who, in accordance with the main tenets of Aristotle's ethical theory, tend to reject any possible cause of human success which is not within human control (ἐφ' ἡμῖν) and who will cling to a rational way to success based on λόγος and φρόνησις.[66] In the face of such an audience, 'God' (ὁ θεός) is a far more satisfactory candidate as 'principle of movement in the soul' (ἀρχὴ τῆς κινήσεως ἐν τῇ ψυχῇ) than 'chance' (τύχη), the rejection of which remains implicit because of its obvious unsuitability (1248 a 22: ὥστ' ἀπὸ τύχης ἅπαντ' ἔσται); and it is now easy to understand why Aristotle concludes that God is the starting-point of *eutuchia* only after a long and tentative and often aporetic argument.

---

[66] See, e.g., *Eth. Eud.* 1215 a 12–20; cf. *Eth. Nic.* 1099 b 10ff. and 1179 b 21ff.

In the light of this argumentative situation in *Eth. Eud.* 8.2 it can be understood, on the one hand, why Aristotle repeatedly makes concessions to the champions of a rational way to human success; for this reason he pays much attention to the part played by 'intellect' (νοῦς, τὸ ἐν ἡμῖν θεῖον) in lines 26–9; he asserts that intellect, reasoning and deliberation (νοῦς, λόγος and βούλευσις), too, go back to God (18–21; 27); and he admits that rational divination, too, 'uses' God (34–7). On the other hand, it has now become clear why Aristotle repeatedly stresses the existence of an *eutuchia* which is based neither on reason nor on chance (a 32, 34, 39, b 4), and why he explains that it is not profitable for the 'irrationally lucky' people to use deliberation (βούλευσις) – on the contrary, they owe their success to the very fact that their reasoning faculty is disengaged (ἀπολυόμενος).

In this chapter, then, I have tried to solve a problem of textual consistency both within *Eth. Eud.* 8.2 and between *Eth. Eud.* 8.2 and *On Divination in Sleep*. As a result of this interpretation, the concept of *eutuchia* has become much less isolated from Aristotle's ethical and theological ideas in general than used to be assumed. However, a discussion of the implications of the theory of *Eth. Eud.* 8.2 for a possible development in Aristotle's theology is beyond the scope of this chapter.[67]

Postscript
Since the original publication of this chapter, the Oxford Classical Text of the *Eudemian Ethics* edited by Walzer and Mingay has come out (1991) and has been incorporated in Woods' (1992) revision of his (1982) commentary (with discussion of textual problems on 196–8). Other discussions of this chapter can be found in Bodéüs (1992); Verbeke (1985); Kenny (1992); and Johnson (1997). None of these publications, however, have led me to change my interpretation of the text of *Eth. Eud.* 8.2 or my overall views on what Aristotle argues in this chapter.

[67] [See Bodéüs (1992) 242–57.]

CHAPTER 9

On Sterility ('Hist. an. 10'), a medical work by Aristotle?

Whether its title, ὑπὲρ τοῦ μὴ γεννᾶν ('On Sterility', 'On Failure to Produce Offspring'), is authentic or not, the work transmitted as 'Book 10' of Aristotle's *History of Animals* (*Hist. an.*) deals with a wide range of possible causes for failure to conceive and generate offspring. It sets out by saying that these causes may lie in both partners or in either of them, but in the sequel the author devotes most of his attention to problems of the female body. Thus he discusses the state of the uterus, the occurrence and modalities of menstruation, the condition and position of the mouth of the uterus, the emission of fluid during sleep (when the woman dreams that she is having intercourse with a man), physical weakness or vigour on awakening after this nocturnal emission, the occurrence of flatulence in the uterus and the ability to discharge this, moistness or dryness of the uterus, wind-pregnancy, and spasms in the uterus. Then he briefly considers the possibility that the cause of infertility lies with the male, but this is disposed of in one sentence: if you want to find out whether the man is to blame, the author says, just let him have intercourse with another woman and see whether that produces a satisfactory result.[1] The writer also acknowledges that the problem may lie in a failure of two otherwise healthy partners to match sexually, or as he puts it, to 'run at the same pace' (ἰσοδρομῆσαι) during intercourse, but he does not go into this possibility at great length,[2] and he proceeds to discuss further particulars on the female side. There is some discussion of animal sexual behaviour in chapter 6, but compared to the rest of *History of Animals*, the scope of the work is anthropocentric, and the lengthy discussion of the phenomenon of *mola uteri* with which the work concludes is also human-orientated.

This chapter was first published in *The Classical Quarterly* 49 (1999) 490–502.
[1] 636 b 11–13; see also 637 b 23–4.   [2] 636 b 15–23.

Among the relatively few scholars who have occupied themselves with this work (on which the last monograph dates from 1911),³ it has been the source of continuous disagreement. Apart from numerous difficulties of textual transmission and interpretation of particular passages, the main issues are (1) whether the work is by Aristotle and, if so, (2) whether it is part of *History of Animals* as it was originally intended by Aristotle or not,⁴ or, if not, (3) what the original status of the work was and how it came to be added to *History of Animals* in the later tradition. From the eighteenth century onwards the view that the work is spurious seems to have been dominant,⁵ with alleged doctrinal differences between '*Hist. an.* 10' and other writings of Aristotle, especially *Generation of Animals* (*Gen. an.*), constituting the main obstacles to accepting the text as genuine. These concerned issues such as the idea that the female contributes seed of her own to produce offspring, the idea that *pneuma* draws in the mixture of male and female seed into the uterus, the idea that heat is responsible for the formation of moles, and the idea that multiple offspring from one single pregnancy is to be explained by reference to different places of the uterus receiving different portions of the seed – views seemingly advocated in '*Hist. an.* 10' but explicitly rejected in *Generation of Animals*. In addition, arguments concerning style (or rather, lack of style), syntax and vocabulary, as well as the observation of a striking number of similarities with some of the Hippocratic writings, have been adduced to demonstrate that this work could not possibly be by Aristotle and was more likely to have been written by a medical author.

This view has in recent times been challenged by at least two distinguished Aristotelian scholars. J. Tricot conceded that there were differences of doctrine, but argued that '*Hist. an.* 10' represents an earlier stage of Aristotle's thinking on the matter which he later abandoned and critically reviewed in *Generation of Animals*.⁶ More recently, David Balme has argued that the accounts in *Generation of Animals* and '*Hist. an.* 10' do not contradict each other and that there is no reason to assume that the latter work is not by Aristotle – indeed, Balme claimed that our interpretation

---

³ Rudberg (1911). For some briefer discussions see Aubert and Wimmer (1868) 6; Dittmeyer (1907) v; Gigon (1983) 502–3; Louis (1964–9) vol. I, xxxi–xxxii and vol. III, 147–55; Peck (1965) lvi–lviii; Poschenrieder (1887) 33; Rose (1854) 172ff.; Spengel (1842); Zeller (1879) 408ff.
⁴ It should be noted that the question of 'belonging to *History of Animals*' does not necessarily depend on the book's Aristotelian authorship being settled, if one is prepared to consider the possibility (once popular in scholarship but currently out of fashion) that *History of Animals* was, from the start, a work of multiple authorship.
⁵ For a survey of older scholarship see Balme (1985) 191–206.
⁶ Tricot (1957) 17.

of *Generation of Animals* would benefit from accepting '*Hist. an.* 10' as Aristotelian, since Aristotle's silence, in *Generation of Animals*, on the rival (Platonic) view that the uterus changes its place in the female body would be explained by the fact that he had already refuted this view in '*Hist. an.* 10'.[7] According to Balme, the work known as '*Hist. an.* 10' is by Aristotle but does not belong to *History of Animals*,[8] because it makes use of causal explanation whereas the rest of *History of Animals* deliberately refrains from this.[9] Thus in Balme's view the relation of *Generation of Animals* to '*Hist. an.* 10' is the reverse of that between *Generation of Animals* and the rest of *History of Animals*, which Balme believes to be not the preliminary data-collection which it was always held to be, and on which the explanatory biological works (*Generation of Animals* (*Gen. an.*), *Parts of Animals* (*Part. an.*), *Movement of Animals* (*De motu an.*), *Progression of Animals* (*IA*)) were believed to be based, but a later summary based on these explanatory works.[10] In the case of '*Hist. an.* 10', however, Balme claims that we are dealing with a preliminary study of the role of the female in reproduction which is later 'refined' – but not contradicted – in the more mature *Generation of Animals*.

Yet the issue is by no means definitively settled. Quite recently, Sabine Föllinger, in her monograph on theories of sexual differentiation in ancient thought, once again advocated scepticism with regard to the question of authenticity.[11] Apart from pointing out a number of serious difficulties in Balme's argumentation, her main argument against Aristotelian authorship is that the author does not speak of the process of reproduction in the characteristically Aristotelian terms of form (εἶδος) and matter (ὕλη).

It seems to me that many of Föllinger's objections to Balme's analysis are justified and that her cautious attitude to the question of authenticity is prudent, because in the present state of scholarship (i.e. in the absence of a proper commentary on '*Hist. an.* 10') truly decisive arguments in favour of or against Aristotelian authorship are very difficult to find, and any judgement is likely to remain, to a considerable extent, subjective. However, this does not necessarily mean that scepticism is the only acceptable position. It is one thing to establish divergences of opinion between two works, but quite another to say that these divergences cannot coexist in the mind of one thinker, or at different stages in the development of his thought. Indeed, there are other, notorious and perhaps much more serious divergences of

---

[7] Balme (1985); see also Balme's introductory remarks in his (1991) 26–30, and his notes to the text and translation (476–539).
[8] For the ancient evidence that it was added later to *History of Animals*, see below.
[9] See also Louis (1969) 148.   [10] Balme (1991) 21–6.   [11] Föllinger (1996) 143–56.

doctrine between works whose Aristotelian authorship is beyond dispute, or even within one and the same work (see below), so the question is whether the divergences between '*Hist. an.* 10' and *Generation of Animals* are such that they cannot conceivably be derived from Aristotle's own mind.

In this chapter, however, I will approach this question from a rather different angle by drawing attention to the special nature of '*Hist. an.* 10'. I will argue that the divergences of doctrine between '*Hist. an.* 10' and other Aristotelian works need not exclusively be interpreted as evidence of different authorship, or indeed of a development in Aristotle's thought, but may be better appreciated when we relate them to differences in scientific status and methodology between these works. To put it briefly, '*Hist. an.* 10' is a 'practical', that is, medical work, unsystematic and limited in scope, intended to provide diagnostic clues as to the possible causes of failure to conceive, or in other words, pursuing knowledge that is useful for practical application.[12] Thus it is very different in nature from a thoroughly theoretical, systematic, and comprehensive work such as *Generation of Animals*. From this perspective, it becomes understandable that '*Hist. an.* 10' mainly discusses additional factors that are supplementary to the account of *Generation of Animals*, and on the other hand does not mention a number of factors which play such a crucial role in *Generation of Animals*. It also explains the book's anthropocentric approach, the fact that it deals almost exclusively with problems on the female side and why it so persistently considers aspects of failure to conceive in relation to whether they require, or allow of, 'treatment' (θεραπεία).

The assumption that Aristotle wrote medical works at all (and that '*Hist. an.* 10' was one of them) may need some elaboration. As is well known, Aristotle makes a clear distinction between practical and theoretical sciences[13] and is well aware of its implications for the way in which a particular topic is discussed within the context of one kind of science rather than the other[14] – such implications pertaining, among other things, to the degree of exactitude with which the topic is to be discussed, the kind of questions to be asked and the amount of technical detail to be covered (a good example of such differences in treatment is the discussion of the soul and its various parts in the *Ethics* and in *On the Soul*). As far as medicine is concerned, Aristotle expresses a similar view on the differences between

---

[12] The possibility that '*Hist. an.* 10' is different in style and doctrine from other Aristotelian works because it is practical in nature and addresses a wider readership is suggested by Gigon (1983) 503, but he does not elaborate on this, and he also seems to think that the work was revised and updated by a later Peripatetic in the light of new evidence.
[13] See, e.g., *Metaph.* 1025 b 25; 993 b 21; *Top.* 145 a 16.
[14] See, e.g., *Eth. Nic.* 1094 b 1ff.; 1098 a 21ff.; 1102 a 5ff.

the theoretical 'study of nature' (φυσικὴ φιλοσοφία) and the practical[15] art of 'medicine' (ἰατρική). This becomes clear from three well-known passages in the *Parva naturalia*,[16] where Aristotle not only speaks approvingly of doctors who build their medical doctrines on 'starting-points' (ἀρχαί) derived from the study of nature, but also of 'the most refined students of nature' (τῶν περὶ φύσεως πραγματευθέντων οἱ χαριέστατοι), who deal with the principles of health and disease; the latter is what Aristotle himself apparently did, or intended to do, in his work *On Health and Disease* (Περὶ ὑγιείας καὶ νόσου), which is not extant.[17] To be sure, in the third of these passages (*On Respiration* (*Resp.*) 480 b 22ff.) Aristotle stresses that although medicine and the study of nature are, up to a point, coterminous, they are different in method as well as in subject matter; hence, scholars have concluded that any discussion of medical topics by Aristotle was (or would have been) fundamentally different from works such as those contained in the Hippocratic Corpus.[18] However, this conclusion seems to ignore the fact that Aristotle's remarks here in the *Parva naturalia* apply to his project of 'the study of nature' (to which also *On Health and Disease* would have belonged), and it fails to take account of the possibility that Aristotle, within another, more specialised and technical framework, may have gone into far greater medical detail.

That such an 'other framework' actually existed is suggested by the references, both in Aristotle's own works and in the indirect tradition, to more specialised medical studies. Thus Aristotle himself refers on numerous occasions to a work called Ἀνατομαί.[19] In his catalogue of Aristotle's writings (5.25), Diogenes Laertius lists a work called Ἰατρικά in two books, a title that suggests that this was possibly a collection of medical problems not dissimilar to the first book of the extant – but presumably post-Aristotelian – *Problemata*.[20] Interestingly, the same catalogue also lists a work ὑπὲρ

[15] Strictly speaking, medicine is a 'productive' art for Aristotle, since its purpose, health, is distinct from its activity (cf. *Eth. Nic.* 1140 a 1–23; *Pol.* 1254 a 2; *Mag. mor.* 1197 a 3); but this distinction is irrelevant for the contrast 'theoretical' vs. 'practical'.
[16] *Sens.* 436 a 17–b 2; *Div. somn.* 463 a 4–5; *Resp.* 480 b 22–31. See also *Long. et brev. vitae* 464 b 32ff.; *Part. an.* 653 a 8ff. For a discussion of these passages see ch. 6 above, pp. 192–5.
[17] On this work, and its reputation in the later tradition, see Strohmaier (1983) 186–9.
[18] E.g. Flashar (1962) 318: 'Aristoteles sagt von sich selbst, er sei kein Fachmann in der Medizin und betrachte medizinische Fragen nur unter philosophischem oder naturwissenschaftlichem Blickpunkt.' For a more positive attitude to the possibility that Aristotle wrote on medicine see Marenghi (1961) 141–61.
[19] The references can easily be found with the aid of Bonitz's *Index Aristotelicus* or Gigon's collection of fragments (see n. 3 above), frs. 295–324. For a recent discussion of this (lost) work see Kollesch (1997) 370; see also Kullmann (1998) 130–1.
[20] The Aristotelian authorship of this section of the *Problemata* was defended by Marenghi (1966), and later by Louis (1991–4) vol. 1. Flashar (1962) 385, is more cautious. [See ch. 5 n. 168.]

τοῦ μὴ γεννᾶν in one book. Furthermore, Caelius Aurelianus quotes literally from a medical work *De adiutoriis* ('On Remedies', in Greek probably Περὶ βοηθημάτων) by Aristotle.[21] There is also evidence that Aristotle wrote a doxographical work on the causes of diseases, which served as a basis for the literary activities of the so-called Anonymus Londiniensis.[22] These medical works are lost (unless ὑπὲρ τοῦ μὴ γεννᾶν survives in the form of '*Hist. an.* 10'), but there is no reason to believe that they were not written by Aristotle – who was, after all, the son of a doctor and in whose works medical analogies and metaphors are prominent.[23] The situation seems similar to that of the more specialised works on harmonics, acoustics, mechanics, optics, and so forth attributed to Aristotle in the catalogues and the indirect transmission:[24] here, as in the case of the medical works, there is no *a priori* reason to believe that Aristotle did not write them. The burden of proof lies on those who wish to deny the authenticity of these works, and since the works are lost, the only basis for questioning their authenticity seems to have been a tacit distinction between 'philosophy' and 'science' and the assumption that these writings were too 'specialised' and 'unphilosophical' for the mind of Aristotle, who would have left it to his pupils (such as Theophrastus, Meno and Eudemus) to deal with the technical details. There is, however, little evidence for this assumption, which has every appearance of a prejudice and does not do justice to the fact that Aristotle's 'philosophical' writings themselves contain a large amount of 'technical' detail.[25]

If we assume that *On Sterility*, rather than being book 10 of *History of Animals*, is one of these medical works – indeed, perhaps, the work ὑπὲρ τοῦ μὴ γεννᾶν mentioned in two catalogues of Aristotle's writings, which incidentally also list *History of Animals* as containing nine books[26] – we need not be surprised to see divergences between it and a thoroughly theoretical, comprehensive and systematic work such as *Generation of Animals*.

---

[21] *Acute Affections* 2.13.87: *Hanc definiens primo De adiutoriis libro Aristoteles sic tradendam credidit: 'Pleuritis', inquit, 'est liquidae materiae coitio siue densatio'*.

[22] Anon. Lond. V 37 and VI 42. The Aristotelian authorship of the work of which Anon. Lond. is an adaptation is taken seriously by Manetti (1994) 47–58, and by Gigon (1983) 511. Other scholars, basing themselves on a passage in Galen's *Commentary on Hippocrates' On the Nature of Man* 1.25–6 (pp. 15–16 Mewaldt; 15.25 K.), assume that this work was in fact written by Aristotle's pupil Meno.

[23] This is, of course, not to say that these analogies and metaphors *prove* that Aristotle had medical interests. But the frequency of these analogies is remarkable and may be significant. For a discussion of the role of medicine in Aristotle's thought and a bibliography on the subject see ch. 6. Little attention has been paid to the lengthy discussion of animal diseases in *Hist. an.* 602 b 12–605 b 21.

[24] See frs. 113–16 and 123 Gigon.

[25] A good example of such 'technical' aspects is Aristotle's discussion of various aspects of sense-perception in *Gen. an.* 5.

[26] For further details see Balme (1985) 191.

Aristotle On Sterility

For we can then appreciate that '*Hist. an.* 10' does not intend to give a comprehensive, theoretically satisfactory account of reproduction, and we can see why it discusses a number of factors that are supplementary to, and hence not envisaged in, the account of *Generation of Animals*.

This brings us to a further methodological point. Even if one is reluctant to believe that Aristotle wrote medical works, the special nature of '*Hist. an.* 10' makes it pertinent to ask what sort of thing we can reasonably expect the author to say. For the doctrinal divergences it shows are related to a *pattern* that can be perceived in Aristotle's works as a whole.[27] When Aristotle is dealing with *deviations*, irregularities, exceptions to the rule, deformations, errors or disturbances of certain vital functions, or variations in the degree of perfection with which these vital functions are performed – in short, aspects of a subject which are typically suitable to be dealt with in an appendix, or in a collection such as the *Problemata*[28] – he often makes use of explanatory factors in respect of which it is not easy to see how and where they are to be accommodated within his account of the *standard* procedure.[29] Often when Aristotle focuses on such special, 'technical' aspects of a topic which he has first discussed in general outline and without qualification, apparent discrepancies of doctrine tend to occur, even within one and the same treatise. For example, in *Generation of Animals* itself,[30] generation *without qualification* is explained in books 1–2 as the male seed acting as the form and the female menstrual blood as the matter, but in book 4 attention is given to what the offspring will be like, whether it will be male or female, whether it will resemble the father or the mother, or the grandfather or grandmother from the father's side or the mother's side, and so on. In the explanation of these variations a number of additional factors are brought into the picture, some of which point to a much more active role of the female part than the sheer passivity the first two books seemed to suggest (e.g., different degrees

---

[27] On this pattern, see ch. 7 above, pp. 211 ff.

[28] It may not be a coincidence that there are more cases of scientific writing in antiquity where the final book or part of a work seems rather different in nature and subject matter from the rest (cf. book 4 of the *Meteorologica*; book 9 of Theophrastus' *Historia plantarum*; and the final parts of Hippocratic works such as *On the Sacred Disease, On Fleshes, On Ancient Medicine*). However, if '*Hist. an.* 10' does not belong to *History of Animals*, as I am claiming, this is irrelevant to the present argument. On the *Problemata* see below.

[29] Two examples may suffice. Aristotle's remarks (in *On the Heavens* and the *Meteorologica*) about atmospheric conditions influencing keenness of sight apparently presuppose an emanatory theory of vision which is difficult to accommodate within his 'canonical' view of normal visual perception as expounded in *De an*. 2.5. And his remarks about various bodily factors being responsible for different degrees of human intelligence seem difficult to reconcile with his 'orthodox' view that thinking is a non-corporeal process. For a more elaborate discussion of these problems see ch. 7 above.

[30] On this well-known problem see Lesky (1951) 1358–79; Düring (1966) 533; Föllinger (1996) 171–9. For a recent discussion see Bien (1998) 3–17.

of συμμετρία, 'right proportion', between the hotness of the seed and the coldness of the menstrual blood). Indeed, in the course of this discussion, we are told by Aristotle that συμμετρία also determines whether there is going to be any offspring at all – which raises the question why Aristotle has not mentioned it earlier.[31]

Now the topic of '*Hist. an.* 10' is precisely such a disturbance of a vital function: the power to generate offspring. As the first sentence says, the purpose of the treatise is to identify whether the causes of this disturbance lie in both partners or in one of them, so that on the basis of this an appropriate treatment can be determined: 'The cause of a man and a woman's failure to generate when they have intercourse with each other, when their age advances, lies sometimes with both, sometimes only in either of them. Now first one should consider in the female the state of things that concern the uterus, so that it may receive treatment if the cause lies in it, but if the cause does not lie in it attention may be given to another one of the causes.'[32] It is true that in what follows the author frequently refers to the normal, healthy state of the relevant bodily parts, but this is because his procedure consists in eliminating potential causes in order to facilitate a diagnosis of the actual cause of the disturbance: if something functions normally, it can be ruled out as a cause of the disturbance. This procedure is very clearly expressed in 636 b 6–10: 'But where none of these impediments is present but the uterus is in the state that we have described, if it is not the case that the husband is the cause of the childlessness or that both are able to have children but are not matched to each other in simultaneous emission but are very discordant, they will have children.'[33] It is as if the author has in mind a routine medical examination, in which one would

---

[31] *Gen. an.* 767 a 25. (I owe this observation to Sophia Elliott, who has dealt with this tension in Aristotle's thought in her Cambridge PhD dissertation.) To be sure, Aristotle had briefly alluded to the principle of συμμετρία in 723 a 29–33, but this is in a polemical context and it is not elaborated. It is interesting to note that in '*Hist. an.* 10' the principle of συμμετρία is applied to generation without qualification (636 b 9), whereas in *Generation of Animals* it is introduced when the question of what the offspring will be like is at stake (767 a 24), although in the sequel it is also brought to bear on the issue of fertility.

[32] προϊούσης δὲ τῆς ἡλικίας ἀνδρὶ καὶ γυναικὶ τοῦ μὴ γεννᾶν ἀλλήλοις συνόντας τὸ αἴτιον ὁτὲ μὲν ἐν ἀμφοῖν ἐστὶν ὁτὲ δ' ἐν θατέρῳ μόνον. πρῶτον μὲν οὖν ἐπὶ τοῦ θηλέος δεῖ θεωρεῖν τὰ περὶ τὰς ὑστέρας ὅπως ἔχει, ἵν' εἰ μὲν ἐν ταύταις τὸ αἴτιον αὗται τυγχάνωσι θεραπείας, εἰ δὲ μὴ ἐν ταύταις περὶ ἕτερόν τι τῶν αἰτίων ποιῶνται τὴν ἐπιμέλειαν (633 b 12–17) (tr. Balme, slightly modified).

[33] ὅσαις δὲ τούτων μηδὲν ἐμπόδιον ᾖ, ἀλλ' ἔχουσιν ὃν τρόπον δεῖν εἴρηται ἔχειν, ἂν μὴ ὁ ἀνὴρ αἴτιος ᾖ τῆς ἀτεκνίας, ἀμφότεροι μὲν δύνανται τεκνοῦσθαι... (tr. Balme). See also 635 a 31–2: 'Concerning the mouth of the uterus, then, those are the grounds from which to consider whether it is in the required state or not' (περὶ μὲν οὖν τὸ στόμα τῶν ὑστέρων ἐκ τούτων ἡ σκέψις ἐστίν, εἰ ἔχει ὡς δεῖ ἢ μή, tr. Balme).

go through a questionnaire: is the womb healthy? Does the woman secrete fluid normally? Is the mouth of the uterus dry after intercourse, and so on? All these points are presented as indicators for the observer: they serve as clues to an answer to the original question, whether sterility is due to a defect in the female or in the male.

This 'diagnostic' character is underscored by the frequency of expressions such as 'on touching, this will appear . . .', or 'whether you touch this or not . . .'.[34] It is as if he is giving instructions as to how one can determine the situation by touching various parts of the female body. Furthermore, the author shows a great interest in 'signs': he very frequently uses expressions such as 'this indicates . . .', 'you can infer from this . . .', 'this is not difficult to judge . . .'.[35] In fact, he seems more interested in the significance of certain symptoms or conditions than in how they are causally related to the disorder. A third point which is relevant in this respect is his frequently recurring observation that a particular condition 'is in need of treatment' (θεραπείας δεόμενον), or 'does not require treatment', or 'does not admit of treatment'.[36] To be sure, he does not indicate what sort of treatment should be applied, but he does seem to find it important to comment, in the case of each condition, on the curability, the need for cure, or the absence of this need.

These characteristics, in combination with the above-mentioned resemblances to the Hippocratic writings, suggest that we are not dealing with a biological but with a predominantly medical work, intended to provide instructions on how to deal with an important practical problem. For, in the context of early Greek medicine, to establish whether a certain bodily affection *required* treatment, and whether it *admitted* of treatment, was

---

[34] μηδὲν ἀναισθητοτέρας εἶναι θιγγανομένας. τοῦτο δὲ κρίνειν οὐ χαλεπόν (634 a 4–5); λέγω δὲ τὸ καλῶς τοιοῦτον ὅπως ὅταν ἄρχηται τὰ γυναικεῖα, θιγγανόμενον ἔσται τὸ στόμα μαλακώτερον ἢ πρότερον καὶ μὴ διεστομωμένον φανερῶς (635 a 7–10); φανερῶς ἔσται ἀνεστομωμένη ἄνευ ἀλγήματος, κἂν θιγγάνῃ κἂν μὴ θιγγάνῃ (635 a 12–13); ἔτι δὲ θιγγανομένης τὰ ἐπὶ δεξιὰ καὶ τὰ ἐπ' ἀριστερὰ ὁμαλὰ αὐτῆς εἶναι (635 b 15–16); ἔστι δ' οὐ χαλεπὸν γνῶναι, ἂν μύλη ᾖ, θιγγάνοντα τῆς ὑστέρας (638 b 30–1; but the text is uncertain here).

[35] σημαίνειν (*passim*, e.g. 634 a 14, 26, 635 a 11, 12, 17, 23, etc.); τοῦτο δὲ κρίνειν (or γνῶναι) οὐ χαλεπόν (634 a 5; 636 b 3); φανερόν (634 a 5); ἐπίδηλον γίνεται (634 a 29); περὶ μὲν οὖν τὸ στόμα τῶν ὑστέρων ἐκ τούτων ἡ σκέψις ἐστίν, εἰ ἔχει ὡς δεῖ ἢ μή (635 a 31–2); διασημαίνει (634 a 37); δηλοῖ (634 b 12); εἰδέναι . . . σημεῖα λαβεῖν φαίνοιτο (636 b 11–12). In themselves, these expressions are not peculiar to this treatise, but the high frequency and the emphasis the author puts on indicators are significant.

[36] θεραπείας δεόμενον (634 a 12, 21, 34; 634 b 7, 10–11, 31; 635 a 36, b 27; 637 b 29); οὐ μέντοι νόσος ἀλλὰ τοιοῦτόν τι πάθος οἷον καθίστασθαι καὶ ἄνευ θεραπείας (634 a 39–41); οὐθὲν αὐταὶ δέονται θεραπείας (634 b 7); ἐὰν μὲν οὖν ἰσχυρῶς τῇ φύσει οὕτως ἔχωσιν ἢ ὑπὸ νόσου, ἀνίατον τὸ πάθος (635 a 2–4); ὃ ἔστι θεραπευτόν (636 a 25); καὶ ἰατὸν καὶ ἀνίατον (636 b 3). In the short discussion of sterility in *Gen. an.* 746 b 16–25 Aristotle also distinguishes forms of sterility that can be cured and those that cannot.

of the highest possible significance: several Hippocratic writings reflect uncertainty and hesitation as to whether doctors should engage in treatment of certain afflictions.[37]

This reading of '*Hist. an.* 10' is rather different from David Balme's analysis of the purpose and the structure of the text. Balme clearly wishes to play down the medical character of the work: 'the book is not iatric and its "medical" content has been overstated... its subject-matter is not the sterile or diseased condition but the normal fertile condition'.[38] According to Balme, the book's 'central thesis' is that the female contributes seed to generation, and the discussion of the normal, healthy state and actions of the uterus 'are set out in order to elicit the female's contribution; incorrect conditions are mentioned only to show the contrast, and are dismissed as "needing treatment" without further discussion'.[39] This is a forced and hardly defensible reading of the text,[40] and Balme seems to be aware of this when he says that 'To follow the argument, which is swift and economical, one must dismiss the preconception that it concerns sterility.' The fact that this 'preconception' is actually inspired by the first sentence of the text (quoted above) is dismissed by Balme as being a case of 'Aristotle's normal dialectical manner', and places where Balme concedes that there is a 'lack of connecting argument' for what he sees as 'the purpose of the whole argument' (viz. that the female contributes seed) are dismissed as instances of Aristotle's 'uncompromising presentation'.[41]

Now, this study is not primarily intended to criticise Balme – indeed, it is difficult to see why it would be in the interest of Balme's main thesis (i.e. that the work is by Aristotle) to play down its medical character. A number of discrepancies between '*Hist. an.* 10' and other works of Aristotle can better be accounted for on the assumption that this is a practical, not a theoretical work: its predominantly human orientation, the fact that it only discusses animal behaviour in so far as this casts light on the human situation, the fact that the work mainly considers defects on the female side, and the fact that the possibility that the male is to blame is dealt with so superficially, all point in this practical direction. The author does not pursue the issue of male sterility and does not offer any guidelines as to what causes might be identified if his practical test (referred to above) were to suggest that there was something wrong with the male contribution. This is again different from the much shorter, but at the same time more

---

[37] See the discussion by von Staden (1990).   [38] Balme (1985) 194.   [39] Balme (1985) 195.
[40] Apart from the considerations already mentioned above, there is also the frequent use of δεῖ in relation to the normal state: 'it should be like this...' (e.g. 634 a 1).
[41] Balme (1985) 196.

wide-ranging account of sterility in *Generation of Animals* (746 b 16ff.), where we do find a discussion of weakness of the male seed and of various means of ascertaining this.

What Balme seems to mean when he denies the 'iatric' nature of the work is that it is not written by a practising doctor and that it is not intended for a medical readership, for example midwives or doctors. However, Balme seems to make this claim on the basis of the alleged absence of what he calls 'the typical Hippocratic discussion of diseases and remedies'. As Föllinger has pointed out, this concept of Hippocratic medicine is too simplistic.[42] There is no such thing as 'typical Hippocratic' medicine or 'Hippocratic doctrine'. The Hippocratic Corpus is the work of a great variety of authors from different periods and possibly different medical schools; as a consequence, the collection displays a great variety of doctrines, styles and methods. There are several works in the Hippocratic Corpus which certainly intend a wider readership than just doctors and which explore in great detail the 'normal', 'natural' state of affairs (e.g. the embryological *Nature of the Child*); and in the case of some works in the collection (e.g. *On the Art of Medicine*, *On Breaths*) it has even been questioned whether they were really written by a doctor with practical experience. This indicates that the distance between the Hippocratic writers and Aristotle was not so great and that we must assume a whole spectrum of varying degrees of 'specialism' or 'expertise': we need not assume that Aristotle was a practising doctor himself in order to allow for a vivid interest, on his part, in medical details, nor need we assume that in '*Hist. an.* 10' he was addressing an audience of doctors or midwives (although this is an interesting possibility). In this respect, the fact that '*Hist. an.* 10' does not go into therapeutic details (see above) may be significant; it simply says that a condition is 'in need of treatment', but it does not say what the proper treatment consists of.[43] But it is clear from the treatise that the author has been listening carefully to what such medical experts had to say.[44]

Nor is there any reason, from this point of view, to be worried about resemblances to the Hippocratic writings. As recent research has shown, Aristotle's awareness of Hippocratic views seems to have been much greater than used to be assumed,[45] and several Hippocratic works were at least

---

[42] Föllinger (1996) 147–8.
[43] The only statement to this effect is in 635 b 28, where the treatment the uterus is said to require is compared with the mouth's need to spit (ὥσπερ καὶ τὸ στόμα πτύσεως sc. δεῖται).
[44] Indeed he is critical of 'many doctors' (638 b 15) who misidentified cases of dropsy as cases of *mola uteri*.
[45] See, e.g., Oser-Grote (1997) 333–49, and her forthcoming book *Aristoteles und das Corpus Hippocraticum*. See also the literature quoted in ch. 6 above.

known in the Lyceum, as is shown by the abundant use made of them in the first books of the extant *Problemata physica*. The fact that '*Hist. an.* 10' shows greater receptivity to medical doctrine than other Aristotelian works may be related to the fact that, as Balme has observed, '*Hist. an.* 10' does display certain characteristics of *Problemata*-literature, and the text may well be identical to, or a version of, what Aristotle refers to (in *Gen. an.* 775 b 36–7) as a section of 'the *Problems*' where a more elaborate discussion of the cause of *mola uteri* is said to have taken place. It could be seen as an elaborate answer to the question 'why is it that women often do not conceive after intercourse?' – a question which has indeed made its way into later doxographical literature[46] – although its length is rather excessive compared with most other *Problemata* chapters.

What is there to be said, in the light of these considerations, about the objections to Aristotelian authorship raised by earlier scholars? Leaving aside arguments about style and indebtedness to Hippocratic doctrines, which are inconclusive,[47] the main difficulties are the view that the female contributes 'seed' to generation and the view that air (*pneuma*) is needed to draw the seed into the uterus. With regard to the first difficulty, Balme and Föllinger have pointed out that also in *Generation of Animals* Aristotle frequently calls the female contribution 'seed', or 'seed-like' (σπερματικός),[48] which is understandable when one considers that for Aristotle both the menstrual discharge and the sperm have the same material origin. In fact, Aristotle seems to waver on the precise formulation, and the view which he is really keen to dismiss in *Generation of Animals* is that the female seed is of *exactly the same nature* as the male[49] – a view which he attributes to other thinkers but which is not expressed, at least not explicitly, in '*Hist. an.* 10'. The fact that in '*Hist. an.* 10' this female contribution remains an unspecified fluid, whereas it is identified as menstrual blood in *Generation of Animals*, which Balme regards as a later 'refinement', need not be a serious problem as long as one accepts that '*Hist. an.* 10' does not intend to give a full, accurate account of normal, successful reproduction. This would explain

---

[46] See, e.g., Aëtius 5.9 and 5.14 (Diels, *Dox. Graec.*, pp. 421 and 424). For the relation between *Problemata* and doxography see Mansfeld (1993) 311–82.

[47] See the discussion of the linguistic evidence by Louis (1964–9) vol. III, 151–2; Balme (1985) 193–4; and Föllinger (1996) 146–7.

[48] E.g. in 727 b 7; 746 b 28; 771 b 22–3; 774 a 22. To the passages already quoted by Balme and Föllinger, *Gen. an.* 747 a 13ff. should be added, where the mechanism of a certain type of fertility test applied to women (rubbing colours on to their eyes and then seeing whether they colour the saliva) is explained by Aristotle by reference to the fact that the area around the eyes is the most 'seedlike' (σπερματικώτατος).

[49] 727 b 7.

why menstrual blood *is* mentioned in '*Hist. an.* 10', but only in the context of irregularities in menstruation, which are to be taken as signs pointing to a certain cause of failure to conceive.[50] In fact, throughout '*Hist. an.* 10' it remains unclear what exactly the female contribution consists of. To be sure, there is frequent mention of an emission, by the female, of fluid,[51] indeed of seed (σπέρμα);[52] but on two occasions (636 b 15–16 and 637 b 19) the female is said to 'contribute *to* the seed' (συμβάλλεσθαι εἰς τὸ σπέρμα).[53] And in the only apparently unambiguous statement to this effect, in 637 b 30–1 (φανερὸν ὅτι παρ' ἀμφοῖν γίνεται πρόεσις σπέρματος εἰ μέλλει γόνιμον ἔσεσθαι), the text does not make clear what actually happens at the moment of conception. Interpreters have usually assumed that the author believes that both male and female seed *mix* in the mouth of the uterus and that this mixture is subsequently drawn into the uterus with the aid of *pneuma*. Now, if this was his position, it would be tantamount to the view which Aristotle vigorously combats in *Gen. an.* 727 b 7 (οὐδὲ μεμιγμένων ἀμφοῖν γίνεται, ὥσπερ τινές φασιν),[54] and we would have a serious inconsistency. Yet on looking closer at the actual evidence for this, it is by no means certain that this is what the author has in mind. The statement in 637 b 30–1 quoted above can also be taken to mean that female ejaculation brings about a favourable condition – but does not necessarily constitute the material agent – for fertility, which would explain why it is so often mentioned as an indicator:[55] the fact that she ejaculates (also in sleep), indicates that she is ready to receive the male seed and draw it into the uterus, because it shows that the uterus is positioned in the right direction.[56] This does not contradict Aristotle's statement in *Gen. an.* 739 a 21 that the fluid women discharge during intercourse does not represent the female material contribution to conception, nor his insistence that the fact that women also discharge this fluid while having erotic dreams is no sign of it actually contributing to conception. To be sure, *Hist. an.* 638 a 8 and a 20ff. speak of a mixture ('Why do not the females generate by themselves, since it is granted that the uterus draws in the male emission too when it

---

[50] 634 a 12ff.
[51] 634 b 29, 37; 635 a 21; 635 b 37; 636 a 6, 10ff.; 636 b 4–5, 37; 637 a 2–3; 637 a 15; 637 a 37; 637 b 12; 637 b 19; 637 b 31; 638 a 1.
[52] 634 a 37; 635 b 37; 636 a 11–12; 637 b 31.
[53] Cf. the use of συμβάλλεσθαι εἰς τὸ κύημα in *Gen. an.* 739 a 21 and συμβάλλεσθαι εἰς τὴν γένεσιν in *Gen. an.* 729 a 21f.
[54] See also *Gen. an.* 739 b 16ff.   [55] 634 b 30ff.; 635 b 2; 635 b 22ff.; 637 b 25–32.
[56] See 635 b 2: πάντα γὰρ ταῦτα σημαίνει δεκτικὴν τὴν ὑστέραν εἶναι τοῦ διδομένου, καὶ προσπαστικὰς τὰς κοτυληδόνας καὶ καθεκτικὰς ὧν λαμβάνουσι καὶ ἀκούσας ἀφιείσας. Cf. *Gen. an.* 739 a 35.

has been mixed... if the emission from both has not been mixed'),[57] but this is in a rather special context (the discussion of the *mola uteri*) and again it does not specify what the contribution of each partner consists in. On two other occasions, however, it is said that the woman draws in 'what she has been given' (τὸ διδόμενον, τὸ δοθέν),[58] which does not really suggest that what is drawn in is a mixture of two contributions from both sides.

It seems that '*Hist. an.* 10' contains no statement that really contradicts the orthodox Aristotelian view that conception takes place when male seed and female menstrual blood meet. To be sure, this view is nowhere expressed or even suggested in '*Hist. an.* 10'; but, as mentioned above, '*Hist. an.* 10' does not offer, and probably does not intend to offer, a complete, profound, philosophically satisfactory account of animal reproduction; this is why it does not discuss the reproductive role of menstrual blood, why it does not say what exactly happens when male and female contribution meet, and why it does not speak in terms of 'form' and 'matter'. And to say emphatically – as the author of '*Hist. an.* 10' does – that the female also contributes to generation, is not inconsistent with this orthodox view from *Generation of Animals*.

Yet one may object that even if it is not a problem that the author of '*Hist. an.* 10' calls the female contribution 'seed', the fact remains that he seems to say that the female contribution is ejaculated in a moment of sexual excitement, which is not what Aristotle says about menstrual blood in *Generation of Animals*.[59] This makes it very hard to believe that the female contribution, as depicted in '*Hist. an.* 10', would have to be identified after all with menstrual blood.[60] Yet perhaps this depends on what one means by 'contribution': even in *Generation of Animals* Aristotle concedes that the female ejaculation during intercourse facilitates conception in that it causes the mouth of the uterus to open.[61] So although the fluid itself does

---

[57] (διὰ τί οὐ γεννᾷ αὐτὰ καθ' αὑτὰ τὰ θήλεα, ἐπείπερ καὶ μιχθὲν ἕλκει τὸ τοῦ ἄρρενος... ἐὰν μὴ μεμιγμένον ἐστὶ [*sic*] τὸ ἀπ' ἀμφοῖν) (tr. Balme).

[58] 635 b 2; 637 a 2.

[59] Even though, as Balme notes (1985, 198), 739 a 28 allows that some of the menstrual blood may already be outside the uterus when conception takes place; and Aristotle sometimes uses the verb 'ejaculate' (προίεσθαι) for menstrual discharge (*Gen. an.* 748 a 21). See also *Hist. an.* 9 (7) 582 b 12ff. on the various possible positions of menstrual blood at conception.

[60] Related to this is the difficulty that in *Gen. an.* 727 b 7–11, Aristotle seems to think that the sexual act does not influence fertility, whereas the author of '*Hist. an.* 10', as we have seen, regards 'keeping the same pace' (ἰσοδρομεῖν) as a very important, indeed a crucial factor for conception (636 b 15–23). However, it seems that the author of '*Hist. an.* 10' does envisage the situation referred to in *Gen. an.* 727 b 9–11, for ἰσοδρομεῖν becomes relevant only after the other conditions for male and female fertility have been met. Nor does the author of '*Hist. an.* 10' assume that ejaculation is necessarily accompanied by pleasure.

[61] *Gen. an.* 739 a 32ff.

not constitute the female contribution in a material sense, the mechanism of its emission does contribute, though perhaps indirectly, to the female's ability to receive the male seed. It might be objected to this interpretation that it is questionable whether the fluid would then still qualify as 'seed'. I see no immediate answer to this question, except that it is the kind of difficulty that, one could imagine, might cause Aristotle, in *Generation of Animals*, to be more specific and to conclude explicitly that the female emission during intercourse does not constitute the female contribution in the material sense.

As far as the role of *pneuma* is concerned, the view criticised in *Gen. an.* 737 b 28–32[62] is that *pneuma* is involved in the *emission* of seed by the male,[63] not that it is involved in the seed's being drawn into the uterus, which is what '*Hist. an.* 10' claims (634 b 34; 636 a 6; 637 a 17). As the use of terms such as ἀπόκρισις, ἐξόδους, συνεκκρίνειν and ἐκκρίνεσθαι in this *Generation of Animals* passage shows, Aristotle is not discussing copulation but the transport of seed from various sections within the body of the discharging agent to the genital organ (the οἰκεῖος τόπος) where it is discharged.[64]

As for the explanation of *mola uteri* in terms of heat, which seems to contradict *Gen. an.* 776 a 2, where Aristotle insists that this is not due to heat but to a deficiency of heat (καὶ οὐ διὰ θερμότητα, ὥσπερ τινές φασιν, ἀλλὰ μᾶλλον δι' ἀσθένειαν θερμότητος), it should be said that the author of '*Hist. an.* 10' seems to toy with the idea rather than actually commit himself to heat as a cause. At 638 a 19f. he asks whether it is through heat that this phenomenon occurs (πότερον δὲ διὰ θερμότητα γίνεται τὸ πάθος τοῦτο...), but in the course of his answer he gets sidetracked; at 638 b 1 he addresses himself again to this possibility, but again fails to make up his mind as to the actual cause: 'But is heat the cause of the affection, as we said, or is it rather because of fluid – something that in fact constitutes the fullness of pregnancy – that it closes its mouth as it were? Or is it when the uterus is not cold enough to discharge it nor hot enough to concoct it?'[65] There is no clear answer, and this is again typical *Problemata*-style, stating various alternative explanations that must have

---

[62] Cf. 739 a 3.
[63] A view which is incidentally advocated in *Hist. an.* 9 (7) 586 a 15.
[64] That this is the subject matter of this passage is also indicated by the fact that in the sequel Aristotle is discussing how the female residue reaches the uterus (which is also called οἰκεῖος τόπος in 739 a 3–5) in order to be discharged.
[65] πότερον δ' ὥσπερ εἴρηται, διὰ θερμότητα γίνεται τὸ πάθος ἢ μᾶλλον δι' ὑγρότητα (ὅτι καὶ ἔστι τὸ πλήρωμα) οἷον μύει, ἢ ὅταν μὴ οὕτως ἢ ψυχρὰ ἡ ὑστέρα ὥστε ἀφεῖναι, μηδ' οὕτω θερμὴ ὥστε πέψαι; (tr. Balme).

been in the air. Contrary to Föllinger,[66] I find it not at all difficult to imagine that in *Generation of Animals* Aristotle would refer to one of such possible explanations by means of ὥσπερ τινές φασιν, even if he himself had considered it on another, possibly earlier occasion.

The only problem concerning a divergence of doctrine for which I fail to see an immediate solution is the explanation of multiple offspring from one pregnancy in *Hist. an.* 637 a 8ff. to the effect that different places in the uterus each receive a different portion of the seed. This seems to be the very theory which Aristotle rejects in *Gen. an.* 771 b 27ff. Balme comments in a footnote *ad loc.* that *Generation of Animals* 'corrects and further develops' the view expounded in '*Hist. an.* 10', but this is a very gentle way of putting it. However, it is not very clear what the author is up to in 637 a 8ff., and there are several textual problems that make it difficult to fathom the meaning of this passage.

Clearly, then, not all difficulties have disappeared.[67] To sort all this out, a probing analytical commentary on '*Hist. an.* 10' is needed, which would examine the alleged inconsistencies with *Generation of Animals* on the basis of close consideration of each individual context in which a relevant statement is made, and which would also examine in much closer detail the relationship with the Hippocratic writings (where the differences may be just as significant as the similarities). However, such a commentary would at least have to take account of the difference in status, method and purpose between '*Hist. an.* 10' and *Generation of Animals* – which seems undeniable – and consider the consequences of this for the kind of thing we can reasonably expect the author to say.

So although Balme's analysis of the text is open to serious question and many of Föllinger's objections to his arguments are justified, Balme's conclusions have some plausibility, although they would be better presented in the form of a hypothesis in need of further investigation; '*Hist. an.* 10' is by Aristotle – at least there is no reason to believe it is not – but it is to be disconnected from the other books of *History of Animals* and regarded as a separate work. It is possibly identical with the work entitled ὑπὲρ τοῦ

---

[66] Föllinger (1996) 150.
[67] As stated above (pp. 268–9), the discussion of sterility (ἀγονία) in *Gen. an.* 746 b 16ff. displays several differences with regard to '*Hist. an.* 10', although there are no genuine inconsistencies. The *Generation of Animals* passage distinguishes various kinds of sterility with various causes but these are stated in very general terms, and the cases '*Hist. an.* 10' mentions could well be accommodated within this typology: they are all instances of infertility that arises when man and woman get older (προιούσης δὲ τῆς ἡλικίας), and they are due either to physical defects (πηρώματα) or to disease (νόσος); some are curable, others incurable.

μὴ γεννᾶν which is mentioned in the same ancient catalogues that also list *History of Animals* as having nine books – a detail that need not carry much weight but fits the argument nicely. How the work came to be added to *History of Animals* in the later tradition is not difficult to imagine, seeing that it provides a more or less smooth continuation of the subject matter of book 9 (7). The work known as '*History of Animals* book 10' constitutes one of the several 'medical' works attributed to Aristotle in the indirect tradition. Thanks to its erroneous inclusion in *History of Animals* in the later transmission, it is the only one of these works to have survived.

Postscript
Since the original publication of this chapter, vol. 1 of Balme's critical edition of the *Historia animalium* has come out (Cambridge, 2002), which also contains a new text of 'Book 10'. A commentary on 'Book 10' is in preparation by Lesley Dean-Jones and Jim Hankinson.

PART III

Late antiquity

CHAPTER 10

Galen's use of the concept of 'qualified experience' in his dietetic and pharmacological works

I INTRODUCTION

It is well known that Galen, in the epistemological debate (as he saw it) between the so-called Dogmatists and the Empiricists, adopted a position which might be defined both as an attempt at maintaining his cherished ideal of intellectual independence and as an endeavour to preserve the valuable insights that the different strands of tradition provided. The latter resulted in his conviction that medical knowledge is arrived at by means of a rather special conjunction of, on the one hand, reason (*logos*), that is, a set of theoretical and logical concepts, definitions, axioms, arguments, and ideas referring both to observable and unobservable entities, and, on the other hand, experience (*peira*), that is, a more or less systematic collection of data derived from sense-perception.[1] What makes his position more complicated is that according to Galen both reason and experience should be used or applied *in a correct way*, in a correct order, interrelation and/or proportion. This requirement may have different consequences for different areas within medical science. Moreover, it is precisely in this respect that Galen explicitly distances himself from the other medical schools, who, as he believes, either failed to take into account empirical data which would seem to him to be inconsistent with their theoretical assumptions, deductions, inferences or analogies, or who formulated unqualified generalising claims on the *exclusive* basis of empirical data.

As far as dietetics and pharmacology are concerned,[2] Galen similarly stipulates on various occasions that both reason and experience are

---

This chapter was first published in A. Debru (ed.), *Galen on Pharmacology. Philosophy, History and Medicine* (Leiden, 1997) 35–57.
[1] See Frede (1987c) 279–98 and (1985) xx–xxxiv.
[2] These more or less overlap, given Galen's views on the relative distinction between foodstuffs and drugs (see below).

indispensable instruments for the acquisition of knowledge and understanding.[3] To be sure, he sometimes says that experience merely has to confirm or check what reason has already expected (ἐλπίζειν) or guessed (στοχάζειν).[4] At the same time, he repeatedly stresses the relative predominance of experience over reasoning: experience, he says, is the 'teacher' (διδάσκαλος) of this subject matter;[5] it is the primary source of knowledge and the ultimate judge.[6] Yet he also frequently insists that experience should be used correctly, that is, with proper qualification. This applies in particular to one of the central questions the dietician/pharmacologist has to face: the quest for the 'powers' (δυνάμεις) of foodstuffs or drugs – their powers to bring about certain effects in the body of the organism to which they are administered. Galen's point seems to be that when trying to *discover* what the power of a particular foodstuff or drug is when it is administered to a patient, or when making a statement about the power a foodstuff or drug is supposed to have, the pharmacologist should not just rely on a small number of isolated empirical data related to the substance in question, collected at random without any underlying principle guiding his search. Moreover, when it comes to *judging* or *refuting* a theory or general statement about the supposed power of a particular foodstuff, the pharmacologist should not, according to Galen, believe that one random counter-example is sufficient to discard the theory or statement in question. Both for heuristic and for critical purposes, Galen stresses, the pharmacologist's use of experience should not be ἀδιορίστως, that is, 'unqualified', 'without distinctions', or 'without proper definition'.[7] It is here that Galen's concept of 'qualified experience' (διωρισμένη πεῖρα) enters the discussion.

---

[3] See, for example, *On the Method of Healing* (*De methodo medendi, De meth. med.*) 3.1 (10.159 K.); 14.5 (10.962 K.); *On the Composition of Drugs according to Places* (*De compositione medicamentorum secundum locus, De comp. med. sec. loc.*) 8.6 (13.188 K.); *On the Mixtures and Powers of Simple Drugs* (*De simplicium medicamentorum temperamentis ac facultatibus, De simpl. med. fac.*) 9.2 (12.192–3 K.). See also Jacques (1997).

[4] See for example *On The Composition of Drugs according to Kinds* (*De compositione medicamentorum per genera, De comp. med. per gen.*) 6.7 (13.887 K.); *De meth. med.* 5.1 (10.306 K.). An interesting example of theoretical reasoning about the powers of foodstuffs or drugs is found in *De simpl. med. fac.* 1.13 (11.401ff. K.); for fallacies in pharmacology cf. 1.25 (11.424–45 K.).

[5] *On the Powers of Foodstuffs* (*De alimentorum facultatibus, De alim. facult.*) 1.1.7 (*CMG* v 4, 2, p. 204.3–5 Helmreich, 6.457 K.); see also *De simpl. med. fac.* 1.37 (11.449 K.); 2.1 (11.459–62 K.); *De comp. med. sec. gen.* 4.5 (13.706f. K.); 6.7 (13.886ff. K.); 6.8 (13.891f. K.). See also Harig (1974) 78–83; Fabricius (1972) 36ff.

[6] See Frede (1987c) 295, who refers, among others, to *De simpl. med. fac.* 2.2 (11.462 K.); 1.40 (11.456 K.); *De meth. med.* 2.6 (10.123 K.); 13.16 (10.916 K.); *On Mixtures* (*De temperamentis, De temper.*) 1.5 (p. 16 Helmreich, 1.534 K.); *De alim. facult.* 1.1.3 (*CMG* v 4, 2, p. 202.14ff. Helmreich, 6.454 K.); *De comp. med. sec. gen.* 1.4 (13.376 K.); *On Antidotes* (*De antidotis*) 1.2 (14.12 K.).

[7] Cf. *De simpl. med. fac.* 1.3 (11.385 K.); 1.4 (11.388 K.); 1.34 (11.441 K.); 6.1 (11.803 K.); *De alim. facult.* 1.1.33 (*CMG* v 4, 2, p. 212.3 Helmreich, 6.472 K.); 3.29 (*CMG* v 4, 2, p. 370.5 Helmreich, 6.723 K.). I am indebted to Heinrich von Staden for pointing out that Galen's use of the concept of *diorismos*

Galen on qualified experience 281

It seems that this concept has not received the attention it deserves.[8] In fact it is a genuinely Galenic technical term which is used a number of times, especially in his dietetic and pharmacological works,[9] and which is of interest for a variety of reasons. First, it has a bearing on the

---

is not restricted to pharmacological experience, but adopted as a general principle of sophistication and accuracy in order to reduce the possibility of error; see von Staden (1997) and his references to *De comp. med. sec. loc.* 2.1 (12.498 K.); 7.6 (13.107–8 K.); 9.1 (13.229 K.); *De comp. med. per gen.* 4.5 (13.681–2 K.); *De simpl. med. fac.* 2.23 (11.523–5 K.). Thus Galen frequently stresses the urgency of *diorismos* with regard to the writings of other physicians, whose statements (λόγοι) are said to suffer from incorrectness or inaccuracy, ἀδιορίστως being used on a par with συγκεχυμένως ('confused'), ἁπλῶς ('without specification') or ἀδιαρθρώτως ('unarticulated'), as in *Commentary on Hippocrates' Prognostic* (*In Hippocratis Prognosticon librum commentaria, In Hipp. Progn. comment.*) 1.30 (*CMG* v 9, 2, p. 248.5–6 Heeg, 18b.93 K.), *De simpl. med. fac.* 1.18 (11.412 K.), and *De comp. med. per gen.* 1.14 (13.426 K.). Cf. *De meth. med.* 6.4 (10.420 K.): 'Some of the things written by him [i.e. Hippocrates] can be found to be lacking in qualification, or deficient or unclear' (καὶ γὰρ ἀδιόριστά τινα τῶν ὑπ' αὐτοῦ [sc. Ἱπποκράτους] γεγραμμένων ἐστιν εὑρεῖν καὶ ἐλλιπῆ καὶ ἀσαφῆ); 6.5 (10.425 K.); *De simpl. med. fac.* 2.12 (11.490 K.); 6.1 (11.805 K.); *De comp. med. sec. loc.* 2.1 (12.526, 529, and 532 K.); 3.1 (12.619 K.): 'Many others have in the same manner and for many parts and affections (of the body) described drugs without further qualification, not knowing what great power qualification (*diorismos*) has for the establishment of the art (of medicine)' (γέγραπται δὲ καὶ ἄλλοις πολλοῖς τὸν αὐτὸν τρόπον ἐπὶ πολλῶν μορίων τε καὶ παθῶν ἀδιόριστα φάρμακα, μὴ γινώσκουσιν ὅσην ὁ διορισμὸς ἔχει δύναμιν εἰς τέχνης σύστασιν). Galen occasionally also uses ἀορίστως (e.g. in *De simpl. med. fac.* 1.18 (11.412 K.)), ἀπεριορίστως (*On the Sects* (*De sectis*) 5, p. 9.21 Helmreich, 1.75 K.), ἀφορίζειν (*De simpl. med. fac.* 1.31 (11.435 K.)) and ὁρίζειν (e.g. *De simpl. med. fac.* 1.27 (11.429 K.)) to express the same idea. On the Aristotelian origins of the concept of *diorismos* see below.

[8] Although much has been written on Galen's attitude towards experience, the concept of διωρισμένη πεῖρα has not, to the best of my knowledge, been studied or even recognised before as a technical term. Harig (1974, 77ff.) provides some important remarks without actually mentioning the term (see esp. p. 85: 'Denn ein Pharmakon, das einen eukratischen Gesunden erwärmt, braucht keineswegs bei einer kalten Dyskrasie und noch viel weniger bei einer kalten Krankheit wärmend zu wirken, so dass eine zuverlässige Aussage über seine wärmende Eigenschaft nur durch den Vergleich seiner Wirkung unter verschiedenen Ausgangsbedingungen gewonnen werden kann'); cf. Frede (1987c) 295–6: 'Proposed theorems arrived at by experience tend to lack the proper qualifications... Though experience puts one into a position to deal with familiar situations, it is not as resourceful as the rational method when it comes to dealing with qualitatively new cases'; Grmek and Gourevitch (1985) 24–5: 'Le raisonnement seul peut déterminer le rapport entre les qualités d'un médicament et leurs degrés d'une part et les effets pharmacologiques d'autre part; le raisonnement seul peut prendre en considération la nature du malade, le stade de la maladie, la puissance du remède et le moment propice à son administration pour arriver ainsi à la découverte du traitement dont la valeur sera confirmée par l'épreuve clinique... La découverte des médicaments composés est, selon Galien, une affaire très complexe, où le raisonnement joue un rôle important en guidant le travail du médecin sans éliminer pour autant la nécessité de la confirmation expérimentale.' For general studies on Galen's views on experience see Debru (1991) and (1994) (with abundant bibliography), esp. 1750ff.; Fabricius (1972) 36–51; Tieleman (1995) 32–4.

[9] The expression ἡ διωρισμένη πεῖρα occurs in *De alim. facult.* 1.1.45 and 46 (*CMG* v 4, 2, p. 216.5 and 14 Helmreich, 6.479 K.); 1.12.1 (*CMG* v 4, 2, p. 233.2–3 Helmreich, 6.508 K.); *De meth. med.* 3.7 (10.204 K.); *De simpl. med. fac.* 3.13 (11.573 K.); 4.19 (11.685 K.); 4.23 (11.703 K.); 6.1 (11.800 K.); 7.10 (12.38 K.). Slightly different formulations of the same idea (e.g. that πεῖρα should not be executed without διορισμός) can be found in *De alim. facult.* 1.1.7–8 (*CMG* v 4, 2, p. 204.3–5 and 15 Helmreich, 6.457–8 K.); 1.1.43 (*CMG* v 4, 2, p. 215.18–20 Helmreich, 6.478 K.); 2.59 (*CMG* v 4, 2, p. 323.8–9 Helmreich, 6.648 K.); *De meth. med.* 3.3 (10.181 K.); 3.7 (10.204 K.); *De simpl. med. fac.* 3.6 (11.552 K.); 10.1 (12.246 K.). For occurrences of the notion in non-pharmacological contexts see *On Critical Days* (*De diebus decretoriis, De diebus decr.*) 2.2 (9.842–3 K.); 2.6 (9.872 K.); *On Diagnosis of Pulses* (*De dignotione pulsuum, De dign. puls.*) 2.2 (8.848–52 K.).

hotly debated question of the presence, or absence, of pharmacological 'experiments' in Galen's works or – as I would rather put it – on Galen's theory of experimentation, namely his ideas on the requirements for a correct use of, and sufficiently specific search for, the relevant empirical data – indeed, for a correct *identification* of the relevant empirical data. Secondly, the concept of 'qualified experience' is of interest for an assessment of the originality of Galen's position, in particular with respect to the medical sect to which his pharmacological work is probably most indebted, the Empiricists. For, on the one hand, Galen uses the notion to articulate his own refined and sophisticated use of experience as against its allegedly unqualified application by the Empiricists;[10] on the other hand, as we shall see, he clearly distinguishes it from 'rational' methods of discovery as well, such as 'indication' (ἔνδειξις) on the basis of the 'essence' (οὐσία) or the 'nature' (φύσις) of the substance, various other forms of inferential thinking (συλλογίζειν, τεκμαίρεσθαι, ἀναλογίζεσθαι, etc.) as well as his own systematic 'method' (μέθοδος) of treatment as expounded in *On the Method of Healing*. This raises the question of to what extent the concept represents a successful attempt at combining reason and experience. Finally, the concept raises some fascinating problems about the philosophical conceptualisation of what seems to be a rather straightforward commonsensical idea, namely that a foodstuff or drug does not produce the same effect in all cases (which had been recognised by Greek dietetic writers from the Hippocratic author of *On Ancient Medicine* onwards), or to be more precise – and perhaps less commonsensical – that one and the same substance may act either as a foodstuff (τροφή) or as a drug (φάρμακον) or even as a poison (δηλητήριον) depending on the manner and the circumstances under which it is applied.

2 GALEN ON DIORISMOS

Galen's notion of 'qualified experience' should not be confused with his more straightforward, much more frequently expressed belief that something – a statement or claim, an issue, idea or notion – may be in need of qualification *by means of* experience. Thus in *De simpl. med. fac.* 2.7 (11.483 K.), in an obvious lash at the Empiricists, he says that the question

---

[10] See *De alim. facult.* 1.1.4 (*CMG* v 4, 2, p. 202.23–5 Helmreich, 6.455 K.); *De meth. med.* 3.3 (10.181 K.); cf. *De comp. med. sec. loc.* 1.7 (12.469 K.): 'This is what Archigenes has written, making his teaching not only empirical but also without qualification' (ταῦτα μὲν ὁ Ἀρχιγένης ἔγραψεν, οὐ μόνον ἐμπειρικὴν ποιησάμενος τὴν διδασκαλίαν, ἀλλὰ καὶ ἀδιόριστον).

Galen on qualified experience 283

whether all olive oil is irritating to the eyes should be decided on the basis of experience rather than by improvisation.[11] Here, as elsewhere, he uses the expression διορίζειν (or διορίσασθαι) πείρα, which obviously means that a statement or belief about the nature, characteristics or power of a substance has to be checked against, or qualified and sophisticated *by means of* the results of empirical research. Here πεῖρα is the *instrument* by which such a qualification is achieved; as its co-occurrences with words such as βασανίζειν and δοκιμάζειν ('test') in these contexts indicate,[12] it is here adopted as a critical, testing instrument rather than as a heuristic device aiming at discovering new data.

However, we also find the expression that some issues can, or have to be settled – discovered, found out, investigated, tested – on the strength of the διωρισμένη πεῖρα, experience which has *itself* been the object of qualification,[13] and statements to the effect that πεῖρα, 'experience', should

---

[11] 'The solutions to all such difficulties are very problematic if one raises them as physical problems, but if one considers them in relation to the practical execution of the art, all they require is much experience, and [only] some reasonings that are accurate and qualified, though not many. For, to begin with, as to the question whether olive oil is irritating to the eyes or not, it is better to determine this by means of experience, rather than to try it either way, just as rhetoricians do by way of exercise' (εἰσὶ δὲ τῶν τοιούτων ἀπασῶν ἀποριῶν αἱ λύσεις, εἰ μὲν ὡς φυσικὰ προβλήματα προβάλλοιντο, παγχάλεποί τινες, εἰ δ᾽ ὡς πρὸς τὴν χρείαν τῆς τέχνης ἀναφέροιντο, πείρας μὲν πολλῆς, ἐπιλογισμῶν δὲ οὐ πολλῶν μέν, ἀκριβῶν δὲ καὶ διωρισμένων δεόμεναι. πρῶτον μὲν γάρ, εἰ πᾶν ἔλαιον τοῖς ὀφθαλμοὺς δακνῶδές ἐστιν ἢ μή, **τῇ πείρᾳ διορίσασθαι** βέλτιον, οὐκ αὐτοσχεδιάζειν, ὥσπερ ῥήτορας ἐπιχειροῦντας εἰς ἑκάτερον). See also *De dign. puls.* 1.7 (8.803 K.); *De comp. med. per gen.* 2.5 (13.502 K.); *Commentary on Hippocrates' Regimen in Acute Diseases* (*In Hippocratis De victu acutorum commentarium, In Hipp. Acut. comment*). 1.15 (*CMG* v 9, 1, p. 129.33–130.3 Helmreich, 15.444 K.).

[12] Cf. *De comp. med. per gen.* 2.5 (13.502 K.); *De comp. med. sec. loc.* 5.5 (12.884 K.); *De temper.* 3.5 (p. 113.20ff. Helmreich; 1.691 K.); *De simpl. med. fac.* 1.40 (11.456 K.); 4.7 (11.642 K.).

[13] See the instances listed in n. 9 above. Although with διορίζειν in the sense of 'distinguish', 'discriminate', when used in the aorist and the perfect, Greek authors seem to prefer middle rather than active verb forms (see LSJ s.v., who quote Demosthenes 24.192: ἃ χρὴ ποιεῖν διωρισμέθα [and Arist. *Part. an.* 644 b 2–3]), it is obvious that the participle διωρισμένος should be interpreted as passive: 'experience that has been discriminated/qualified', i.e. has *undergone* discrimination or qualification [cf. Arist. *Eth. Nic.* 1138 b 33], not 'experience that has performed discrimination' (which would come very close to the use of πεῖρα as an instrument of qualification discussed in the previous sentence). This distinction is confused in Beintker and Kahlenberg's translation (1948) of the term in *De alim. facult.* 1.1.45 (*CMG* v 4, 2, p. 216.4–6 Helmreich, 6.479 K.): they translate ἡ γνῶσις δ᾽ αὐτῶν ἐν χρόνῳ πολλῷ κατορθοῦται μόλις ἔκ τε τῆς διωρισμένης πείρας καὶ τῆς τῶν ἀτμῶν τε καὶ χυμῶν φύσεως as 'Eine sichere Kenntnis derselben erwirbt man sich nur mit Mühe und in langer Zeit, und zwar auf Grund einer durch scharfe Unterscheidung gewonnenen Erfahrung, der Beschaffenheit der Ausdünstungen und der Säfte' (which suggests that ἡ διωρισμένη πεῖρα is not an *instrument* of research but rather the attitude or the state that results from empirical research, the experience or expertise (ἐμπειρία) constituted by the cumulative body of empirical knowledge one has built up during a process of trial and error and further refining); however, at 1.1.46 (*CMG* v 4, 2, p. 216.16 Helmreich, 6.479 K.) they translate ἐὰν τῇ διωρισμένῃ πείρᾳ κρίνῃς as 'wenn man es nicht mit einer genau unterscheidenden Erfahrung beurteilt' (the Latin translation printed by Kühn has 'ex certa definitaque experientia' and 'si experientia definita ipsa exploraris'). Nor is

be executed with due consideration of, or at least not without, certain διορισμοί – 'qualifications', 'distinctions', or 'specifications'.[14] Thus at *De simpl. med. fac.* 3.13 (11.573 K.) Galen says that he will endeavour to give an account of drugs in a systematic order in accordance with the range of their powers, and that he will adopt as an infallible criterion for determining what these powers are 'not plausible (theoretical) accounts but qualified experience' (οὐ λόγοις πιθανοῖς ἐπιτρέψοντες αὐτῶν τὴν κρίσιν, ἀλλὰ τῇ διωρισμένῃ πείρᾳ). This high degree of exactness and reliability of qualified experience is also referred to at *De simpl. med. fac.* 4.23 (11.703 K.).[15] Qualified experience is said to be an important instrument for testing (δοκιμάζειν) the power of a drug;[16] it is sometimes presented as superior

ἡ διωρισμένη πεῖρα equivalent to the 'trained perception' referred to in *De comp. med. per gen.* 3.2 (13.570 K.), on which see Harig (1974) 82. For the use of the active perfect forms διώρικα in Galen see *On the Affected Parts (De locis affectis, De loc. aff.)* 2.8 (8.108 K.): διὰ τοῦτο συγκεχυμένως τε καὶ ἀδιορίστως ὑπὲρ αὐτῶν ἔγραψεν, ὡς ἂν μηδὲ τὰς αἰτίας τῶν διαθέσεων ἀμφοτέρων ἀκριβῶς που **διωρικώς**, and *De comp. med. per gen.* 7.4 (13.961 K.): ἐμοῦ δὲ ἐπὶ τῶν ἀρίστων καθ' ἕκαστον εἶδός τε καὶ γένος ἀποφηναμένου τὴν δύναμιν, ἐὰν ἐπὶ τοῦ χειρίστου ποιήσηταί τις τήνδε διὰ τῆς πείρας ἐξέτασιν, ποιήσεται μὲν ψευδῶς, οὐ **διώρικε** δέ τὰς τῆς δυνάμεως αὐτῶν τάξεις.

[14] See the instances listed in n. 9 above. The basic meaning of διορίζειν is 'to discriminate', 'to discern', 'to distinguish'; Galen frequently uses the noun διορισμός in combination with the preposition ἀπό, thus approximating our notion of 'criterion', e.g. the διορισμὸς ἀπὸ τῶν ἐθῶν ('criterion based on habits') adopted by the Empiricists (cf. *De meth. med* 3.7, 10.207 K.) or the διορισμὸς ἀπὸ τοῦ μετρίου τε καὶ σφοδροῦ τῆς ὀδύνης ('criterion based on moderateness or excessiveness of the pain') adopted by Archigenes (*De comp. med. sec. loc.* 3.1 (12.620 K.)). On the antecedents of this use of διορισμός see below; on the meaning see Manetti and Roselli (1994) 1601, who translate the term as 'una specificazione della verità' (e.g. of a statement by Hippocrates); Beintker and Kahlenberg (1948) translate 'begriffliche Unterscheidung'.

[15] 'Therefore, if it is possible on this basis to make inferences about the power of drugs, the best addition to the theory, as has been said many times, is to discover them on the basis of qualified experience. For you won't go wrong in this, even though before detecting the power by experience, taste provides most indications, with smell, as I have said, providing some additional evidence' (ὥστ' εἴ τι κἀντεῦθεν ἐγχωρεῖ περὶ φαρμάκων δυνάμεως τεκμαίρεσθαι, προσκείσθω τῷ λόγῳ κάλλιστον μέν, ὡς εἴρηταί τε καὶ λέλεκται πολλάκις, ἐκ **τῆς διωρισμένης πείρας** ἐξευρίσκειν τὰς δυνάμεις. οὐ γὰρ ἂν σφαλείης οὐδὲ ἐν τῇδε, πρὶν μέντοι τῇ πείρᾳ διαγνῶναι τὴν δύναμιν, ἡ γεῦσις ἐκδείκνυται τὰ πολλά, συνεπιμαρτυρούσης, ὡς εἴρηται, βραχέα καὶ τῆς ὀσμῆς).

[16] *De simpl. med. fac.* 7.10 (12.38 K.): 'This is why in our previous discussions, when we held that one must test the power of each drug by means of qualified experience, we advised to select an affection that is as simple as possible' (διὰ τοῦθ' ἡμεῖς ἐν τοῖς ἔμπροσθεν λόγοις, ὁπότε **τῇ διωρισμένη πείρᾳ δοκιμάζειν** ἑκάστου τῶν φαρμάκων τὴν δύναμιν ἠξιοῦμεν, ἁπλοῦν ὡς ἔνι μάλιστα τὸ πάθος ἐκλέγεσθαι συνεβουλεύομεν). See also *De simpl. med. fac.* 6.1 (11.800 K.), which conveys a good impression of what such a 'qualified' test consists of: 'Surely when performing the test accurately by means of qualified experience, which we have discussed many times before, we will discover the medicinal power [sc. of wormwood] from its mixture itself. For if one crushes the foliage together with the flowers (for the rest of the fruit is useless) and applies it to a clean wound, it turns out to be pungent and irritating, but if you want to soak it in olive oil and pour it over the head or down the stomach, it will be found to be intensely heating' (οὐ μὴν ἀλλὰ καὶ **τῇ διωρισμένῃ πείρᾳ**, περὶ ἧς ἔμπροσθεν εἴρηται πολλάκις, ἀκριβῶς βασανίσαντες ἐκ τῆς αὐτῆς εὕρομεν τὸ φάρμακον τοῦτο κράσεως. εἴτε γὰρ κόψας τὴν κόμην ἅμα τοῖς ἄνθεσιν, ἄχρηστον γὰρ αὐτοῦ τὸ λοιπὸν κάρφος, ἐπιτάττοις ἕλκει καθαρῷ, δακνῶδές τε καὶ ἐρεθιστικὸν φαίνεται, εἴτε ἀποβρέξας ἐν ἐλαίῳ καταντλεῖν ἐθελήσαις ἤτοι κεφαλὴν ἢ γαστέρα, θερμαῖνον σφοδρῶς εὑρεθήσεται).

Galen on qualified experience 285

to, but occasionally also as supplementary to, inference (τεκμαίρεσθαι) by reason.[17] What does Galen mean by this, and what kind of 'qualifications' are there to be considered? And how is this concept related to reason and experience?

At some places where he uses the term διωρισμένη πεῖρα, Galen says that he has explained the notion in greater detail elsewhere, but none of these references turned out on checking to point to a really systematic or exhaustive treatment of the concept.[18] The most instructive textual elucidation is provided by the first chapter of *On the Powers of Foodstuffs* and the third book of *On Mixtures*, the latter being a sort of short treatise on elementary pharmacology which, as Galen does not grow tired of stressing repeatedly,[19] is an indispensable prerequisite for a correct understanding of all his pharmacological works – a typically Galenic schoolmasterly recommendation to students of his pharmacological works to do their homework properly.

In the long introductory chapter of *On the Powers of Foodstuffs*, which precedes his actual discussion of the powers of the various foodstuffs, Galen points out that an exclusively empirical approach to the subject of the

[17] See *De simpl. med. fac.* 4.19 (11.685 K.): 'That all bitter humours have not only a hot but also a dry mixture is shown first of all by qualified experience, which I have discussed many times, and in addition to experience the same result is also found if one examines it rationally' (ὅτι δ' οὐδὲ θερμὸς μόνον, ἀλλὰ καὶ ξηρὸς ἐστι τὴν κρᾶσιν ὁ πικρὸς ἅπας χυμός, ἥ τε διωρισμένη πεῖρα πρώτως καὶ μάλιστα διδάσκει, περὶ ἧς ἔμπροσθεν εἴρηταί μοι πολλάκις, ἔτι τε πρὸς τῇ πείρᾳ τῷ λόγῳ σκοπουμένοις ὡσαύτως συμβαίνει). *De alim. facult.* 1.12.1 (*CMG* v 4, 2, p. 233.2–3 Helmreich, 6.508 K.): '(On maza.) As to the power of each food, even before subjecting it to qualified experience, you can infer this from its nature. For to any intelligent man the fine, white flour free from any bran-like material would indicate etc.' (Περὶ μάζης. τὴν δύναμιν ἑκάστου τῶν ἐδεσμάτων ἔνεστί σοι καὶ πρὸ τῆς διωρισμένης πείρας ἐκ τῆς φύσεως αὐτῶν τεκμήρασθαι. τίνι γὰρ ἀνδρὶ συνετῷ τὸ μὲν ἀκριβῶς λεπτὸν καὶ λευκὸν καὶ καθαρὸν ἁπάσης πιτυρώδους οὐσίας ἄλευρον ἐνδείξαιτο κτλ.). Cf. *De alim. facult.* 2.59 (*CMG* v 4, 2, p. 323.8–10 Helmreich, 6.647–8 K.), where qualified experience is presented as supplementary to 'indication from the structure of the plant' (ἔνδειξις ἀπὸ τῆς συστάσεως τοῦ φυτοῦ), and *De simpl. med. fac.* 10.1 (12.246 K.): 'We have shown that the general power is clearly indicated by one experiential trial, and not any random trial, but one that has been carried out with the qualifications mentioned' (ἐδείχθη δὲ καὶ ὡς ἡ καθόλου δύναμις ἐκ πείρας μιᾶς ἐνδεικτικῶς εὑρίσκοιτο, καὶ οὐ τῆς τυχούσης πείρας, ἀλλὰ μετὰ τῶν εἰρημένων διορισμῶν γιγνομένης). On Galen's use of ἔνδειξις see Kudlien (1991) 103–11.

[18] Thus in *De alim. facult.* 1.1.7 (*CMG* v 4, 2, p. 204.3–5 Helmreich, 6.457 K.) he refers to *On the Mixtures and Powers of Simple Drugs* and to the third book of *On Mixtures*; Helmreich in his apparatus does not specify the first reference, but the second is taken to refer to pp. 109–15 of his edition of *On Mixtures*. In *De simpl. med. fac.* 3.13 (11.573 K.), Galen says that he has explained the urgency of deciding pharmacological issues on the basis of qualified experience 'quite often throughout the preceding sections of the work' (καθότι καὶ τοῦτο πολλάκις εἴρηται διὰ τῶν ἔμπροσθεν), which may be no more than an overstatement; similarly vague references are given in 4.19 (11.685 K.); 4.23 (11.703 K.); 6.1 (11.800 K.); and 7.10 (12.38 K.).

[19] E.g. in *De simpl. med. fac.* 1.1 (11.381 K.); 1.3 (11.385 K.); 1.11 (11.400 K.).

'powers' (δυνάμεις) is likely to bring many errors with it.[20] For a generalising statement about the supposed dietetic or pharmacological power of a substance may in many particular cases turn out to be completely false when it lacks important qualifications (διορισμοί) concerning the particular bodily constitution of the patient and the circumstances under which it is to be administered.[21] This error may be due to the fact that the empirical evidence adduced in favour of the statement has not been properly interpreted, for instance because it has been torn out of context or incorrectly extrapolated or generalised.[22] Galen illustrates this by means of examples concerning the digestibility or laxativeness of certain foodstuffs such as honey-drink (μελίκρατον) and 'rock fish' (πετραῖοι ἰχθύες).[23] Thus a foodstuff which is said to be easily digestible may in certain cases be quite difficult to digest because of an incidental or structural predominance of yellow bile in the intestines due to a bad temperament (δυσκρασία) or a peculiarity of the bodily condition of the patient (κατασκευῆς ἰδιότης).[24] A general statement about the power of this particular foodstuff should take this kind of complicating, variable factors into account.

[20] 1.1.7 (*CMG* v 4, 2, p. 204.6–7 Helmreich, 6.457 K.). On the connection between error and lack of qualification see n. 7 above and von Staden (1997). As becomes clear from the sequel of Galen's argument, his criticism is especially directed towards too rash generalisations and overconfident causal explanations; cf. *De simpl. med. fac.* 1.34 (11.441 K.): 'Neither of the two statements is true when put simply and without qualification, neither when people say that all astringent substances cause a wound to close, nor when they say that all [wounds] that are closed are closed because of astringent substances' (οὐδέτερος οὖν ἀληθὴς λόγος ἁπλῶς καὶ ἀδιορίστως λεχθείς, οὔθ᾽ ὅταν ἅπαντα φάσκωσι τὰ στύφοντα κολλᾶν ἕλκος, οὔθ᾽ ὅταν πάντα τὰ κολλώμενα διὰ τῶν στυφόντων κολλᾶσθαι), and 2.3 (11.466 f. K.). This Galenic criticism stands in a long tradition already attested in the Hippocratic Corpus and in Diocles: see ch. 2 in this volume.
[21] The term διορισμός occurs a number of times in this chapter: see p. 210.14–16 (6.469 K., a criticism of Diocles' failure to distinguish between the notions of 'foodstuff' and 'drug'), p. 212.3 and 7 (6.472 K.), p. 215.19 (6.478 K.), p. 216.5 and 14 Helmreich (6.479 K.).
[22] On undue generalisations see also *De alim. facult.* 1.1.43 (*CMG* v 4, 2, p. 215.18–20 Helmreich, 6.478 K.): 'I said "not few", being very careful not to say "all", for here, too, qualifications are needed according to which the conditions of people with chronic diarrhoea will be discovered' (οὐκ ὀλίγοις δ᾽ εἶπον, ἅπασι φυλαξάμενος εἰπεῖν, ὅτι κἀνταῦθα διορισμῶν ἐστι χρεία, καθ᾽ οὓς αἱ διαθέσεις εὑρεθήσονται τῶν διαρροϊζομένων χρονίως).
[23] Thus at 1.1.8 (*CMG* v 4, 2, p. 204.17 Helmreich, 6.458 K.) he refers to Erasistratus (fr. 117 Garofalo) for having pointed out that 'neither does honey-wine cause the stomach to flow in all cases, nor do lentils check it in all cases; rather is it the case that some people, in addition to experiencing neither of these, are affected by the opposite, to the effect that their stomachs are checked by honey-wine, but are caused to flow by lentils; and some people have been found to digest beef more easily than rock fish' (μήτε τὸ μελίκρατον ὑπάγειν τὴν γαστέρα πάντων μήτε τὴν φακῆν ἐπέχειν, ἀλλ᾽ εἶναί τινας, οἳ πρὸς τῷ μηδέτερον πάσχειν ἔτι καὶ τοῖς ἐναντίοις περιπίπτουσιν, ὡς ἵστασθαι μὲν ἐπὶ τῷ μελικράτῳ τὴν γαστέρα, λαπάττεσθαι δ᾽ ἐπὶ τῇ φακῇ, καί τινας εὑρίσκεσθαι τὰ βόεια κρέα ῥᾷον πέττοντας ἢ τοὺς πετραίους ἰχθύας).
[24] 1.1.9–10 (*CMG* v 4, 2, p. 205.5ff. Helmreich, 6.459 K.).

In the rest of the chapter, Galen further lists a number of διορισμοί that are relevant to the question of the powers of foodstuffs, such as:

- the amount of time spent on the preparation of the substance, as well as the manner of preparation, which may influence its power;[25]
- the particular condition (both natural and acquired) of the bowels and the stomach, which determines which constituents of the substance are activated in the process of digestion;[26]
- season, geographical area, age, sex, way of life (the list of factors familiar from the Hippocratic Corpus), each of which may influence the actual outcome of an empirical test;[27]
- variations in the intensity of the substance's effect;[28]
- degrees of mixture with other substances, which may significantly influence the substance's power;[29]
- different parts of the body, which may react differently to one and the same substance.[30]

The general thrust of the argument is that the actual effect a substance may produce not only depends on the 'mixture' (κρᾶσις) of the substance, but also on the mixture of the body;[31] variations on either side bring complications with them. When testing the substance's power, and when prescribing the substance in particular cases, it is the task of the dietician to take all those variations into account.

On the matter of 'mixtures' (κράσεις), *On Mixtures* book 3 presents a more systematic discussion of the διορισμοί to be taken into account when describing the effects of a particular foodstuff or drug. After explaining a number of notions that are very fundamental to the study of pharmacology, such as δύναμις and ἐνέργεια (to which I shall turn later), Galen enumerates a long list of factors which determine the possible effects of a foodstuff or drug:

- some drugs immediately bring about warmth when brought into contact with a human body, but others have to be cut into smaller pieces before actually bringing about the effect;[32]

---

[25] 1.1.12–15 (*CMG* v 4, 2, pp. 205.23–206.28 Helmreich, 6.460–2 K.).
[26] 1.1.16–17 (*CMG* v 4, 2, p. 207.1–18 Helmreich, 6.462 K.).
[27] 1.1.30–2 (*CMG* v 4, 2, p. 211.9–30 Helmreich, 6.470–1 K.). Cf. *De simpl. med. fac.* 3.12 (11.570 K.).
[28] 1.1.26–8 (*CMG* v 4, 2, pp. 208.8–209.3 Helmreich, 6.468–70 K.). Cf. *De simpl. med. fac.* 1.27 (11.428–9). Harig (1974), 117ff.
[29] 1.1.40–1 (*CMG* v 4, 2, p. 214.4–22 Helmreich, 6.475–6 K.).
[30] 1.1.42–3 (*CMG* v 4, 2, p. 214.2–9 Helmreich, 6.477 K.).
[31] 1.1.34 (*CMG* v 4, 2, p. 212.12–13 Helmreich, 6.472 K.).
[32] *De temper.* 3.1 (p. 89.15ff. Helmreich, 1.651ff. K.); cf. *De simpl. med. fac.* 1.11 (11.400 K.).

some drugs work 'in virtue of their whole essence' (καθ'ὅλην τὴν οὐσίαν), others in virtue of one, or several particular qualities (warm, cold, dry or wet); and some drugs admit of both possibilities depending on the circumstances;[33]

the effect of a drug depends on the way of consumption: it makes all the difference whether a substance (for example, mustard) is brought onto the skin or taken in via the mouth;[34]

a very fundamental distinction is whether a particular power such as hotness is present in the foodstuff 'primarily and by itself' (πρώτως καὶ καθ' ἑαυτό) or 'accidentally' (κατὰ συμβεβηκός): thus water is by itself cold (i.e. cooling), but it may be accidentally warm (i.e. warming), because it has acquired its warmth (ἐπίκτητος vs. σύμφυτος θερμασία). [35]

Further distinctions mentioned are:

whether a certain substance acts as a foodstuff (which just preserves the state of the body), or as a drug (which changes the state of the body in a beneficial way), or a poison (which harms the state of the body);[36]

the distinction between the power a substance has 'in itself' versus the power 'it is said to have in relation to something' (πρὸς ὃ λέγεται), and, within that latter category, the distinction between the power it has 'with regard to us', namely humans (πρὸς ἡμᾶς), versus the power it has when brought into contact with other organic or inorganic substances or entities, such as fire;[37]

bodily state (διάθεσις) and time (χρόνος), that is, whether the state of the body is simple or complex, and whether the drug works immediately or after an elapse of some time;[38]

---

[33] *De temper.* 3.1 (p. 91.6ff. Helmreich, 1.654 K.); cf. *De simpl. med. fac.* 1.3 (11.385 K.). On this notion see Harig (1974) 108ff., who refers to *De simpl. med. fac.* 5.1 (11.705 K.); 4.9 (11.650 K.); 5.17 (11.760 K.); 5.18 (11.761–4 K.).

[34] *De temper.* 3.3 (p. 95.26ff. Helmreich, 1.661ff. K.).

[35] *De temper.* 3.3 (p. 98.17ff. Helmreich, 1.666 K.); 3.4 (p. 102.15–16 Helmreich, 1.672 K.); cf. *De comp. med. per gen.* 1.6 (13.401 K.); *De simpl. med. fac.* 1.2 (11.382 K.); 1.31 (11.435 K.); 3.4 (11.545 K.).

[36] *De temper.* 3.1 (p. 91.15 Helmreich, 1.655 K.); 3.2 (p. 91.19 Helmreich, 1.655 K.); 3.4 (p. 100.22–4 Helmreich, 1.670 K.); cf. *De alim. facult.* 1.1.24–29 (*CMG* v 4, 2, pp. 209.16–211.3 Helmreich, 6.467–70 K.); *De simpl. med. fac.* 1.1 (11.380 K.); 1.3 (11.385 K.); 3.3 (11.545 K.); 5.1 (11.705 K.). On this distinction, and on the physiological factors determining whether a substance acts as a foodstuff, or a drug, or a poison, see Harig (1974) 87–95.

[37] *De temper.* 3.5 (p. 109.14ff. Helmreich, 1.684 K.); cf. *De simpl. med. fac.* 1.2 (11.382 K.). On this distinction see Harig (1974), p. 84 nn. 26–7, who refers to *De simpl. med. fac.* 1.40 (11.455f. K.); 2.3 (11.467 K.); 2.20 (11.518 K.); 3.6 (11.552 K.); 3.9 (11.557 K.).

[38] *De temper.* 3.5 (p. 111.24ff. Helmreich, 1.688 K.).

Galen on qualified experience 289

variations in the quantity and the proportion in which a substance (or a combination of various substances) is administered.³⁹

Additional types of relevant qualifications can easily be found in *On the Mixtures and Powers of Simple Drugs*:

it makes all the difference whether a substance consists of fine particles (λεπτομερές) or of thick ones (παχυμερές);⁴⁰

it makes all the difference whether a substance is applied to a healthy body (ἀμέμπτως ὑγιαῖνον) with a good temperament (εὔκρατον), a body which naturally has a bad temperament (φύσει δύσκρατον), or a body which is ill or accidentally badly tempered (νοσοῦν, δύσκρατον κατὰ πάθος);⁴¹

if a substance's power is tested by applying it to an ill body, it is important to apply it to a body suffering from a 'simple disease' (ἁπλοῦν νόσημα) rather than from a 'complex disease' (σύνθετον νόσημα), because in the latter case there may be all kinds of complicating variables;⁴²

within one genus of substance, one should take into account that different species (e.g. of water) may have different powers;⁴³

the *cause* of the state to be dispelled by the drug may vary: thus a thirst-quenching substance may not be efficacious in a particular case because the body suffers from a special kind of thirst which is different from normal thirst.⁴⁴

Thus what Galen seems to mean when he says that a pharmacological question or issue should be decided on the basis of 'qualified experience' (ἡ διωρισμένη πεῖρα) is an empirical test of a substance's dietetic or pharmacological power which takes into account the conditions that have to be fulfilled in order to make the test have an evidential value and provide sufficiently specific information. Though the passages discussed are by no means exhaustive, it turns out that Galen recognises a fairly comprehensive list of *diorismoi*, 'qualifications' or 'distinctions' that serve as requirements for a correct use of, or search for, empirical data, and thus for a truly informative execution of experience (πεῖρα). His primary concern, to which

---

³⁹ *De temper.* 3.5 (p. 113.20ff. Helmreich, 1.691 K.). For further elaborations of these *diorismoi* in pharmacology see *De comp. med. sec. loc.* 5.1 (12.805ff. K.) and 7.2 (13.14ff. K.).
⁴⁰ 1.3 (11.385 K.). On the topic of λεπτομέρεια see Debru (1997).
⁴¹ 1.4 (11.386 K.); 1.21 (11.416 K.); 1.33 (11.438 K.); 2.9 (11.485 K.); 2.21 (11.518 K.); 3.13 (11.572–3 K.). Cf. Grmek and Gourevitch (1985) 25; Harig (1974) 84 n. 32.
⁴² See the example of erysipelas in *De simpl. med. fac.* 7.10 (12.39f. K.), and of κόπος in 2.10 (11.485ff. K.). Cf. Harig (1974) 85 nn. 33–4, who refers to *De simpl. med. fac.* 2.21 (11.518 K.); 4.7 (11.641 K.); 6 proem (11.791 K.).
⁴³ *De simpl. med. fac.* 1.18 (11.413 K.).   ⁴⁴ *De simpl. med. fac.* 1.32 (11.437 K.).

most of the qualifications can be reduced, is to distinguish essential (καθ' αὑτό) from accidental (κατὰ συμβεβηκός) factors. Some distinctions concern variations between different substances, but several may apply to one and the same substance, or occur with different species of one and the same substance.

Hence we may say that there is a keen awareness, on Galen's part, of the fact that the outcome of an empirical test of a certain substance's effect depends to a very high degree on the conditions under which it is applied. In a number of cases we can see Galen actually defining these conditions on the basis of a set of *diorismoi*, qualifications or distinctions that are to be taken into account, and on the basis of a knowledge of which conditions are relevant and which are not. Only by taking the relevant qualifications into account can one arrive at a correct general *statement* (λόγος) about the power of a particular substance.[45]

As for the relation of 'qualified experience' to reason and experience, it is interesting to note that Galen, as already stated, presents the notion in opposition both to 'reason' (λόγος)[46] and to 'experience without reason'.[47] This can be well understood when considering the qualifications that I have just enumerated. Some of these *diorismoi* can be accepted as observable: for example, we can simply *observe* that in summer the effects of a given drug are different from those brought about when it is administered in winter, or that a certain drug is beneficial to younger people but harmful to older people, and we may conclude from this that these distinctions are the relevant determining factors (although it may be objected that their actually having a causative influence is, strictly speaking, not observable). Yet there are also determining factors which do not admit of being observed, at least not in a straightforward sense. This is especially the case with physiological states and processes of the kind referred to in the chapter of On the Powers of Foodstuffs (such as a δυσκρασία, a 'bad mixture' of humours, a particular state of the bowels or the stomach, etc.). The existence or occurrence of these, *and their actually being a conditioning factor,* is – as Galen himself acknowledges without any misgivings[48] – to be theoretically postulated, or to be inferred on the basis of symptoms, such as the occurrence of a

---

[45] For examples of such statements see n. 65 below. [46] See n. 17 above.
[47] De alim. facult. 1.1.7 (CMG v 4, 2, p. 204.6–9 Helmreich, 6.458 K.); see also next note.
[48] De alim. facult. 1.1.44 (CMG v 4, 2, p. 215.21–3 Helmreich, 6.478 K.): 'For in general it is not possible to test anything properly by experience without first discovering accurately by means of reason the condition of the body to which the food or drug that is being tested is applied' (ὅλως γὰρ οὐδὲν οἷόν τ' ἐστὶ τῇ πείρᾳ βασανίσαι προσηκόντως ἄνευ τοῦ **τῷ λόγῳ** πρότερον εὑρεῖν ἀκριβῶς τὴν διάθεσιν (sc. τοῦ σώματος), ᾗ προσφέρεται τὸ βασανιζόμενον ἤτοι σιτίον ἢ φάρμακον).

particular kind of pain (this raises the question of the empirical basis of Galen's physiology).[49]

3 THE ORIGINALITY OF GALEN'S POSITION

We have seen that Galen is aware that knowledge of the relevant διορισμοί to be considered by the pharmacologist is, at least partly, of a theoretical nature: an empirical test of a substance's power or a search for the relevant empirical data that is *not* guided by an *a priori* expectation founded on reason is likely to be fruitless or even misleading. In this respect a major difference manifests itself between Galen's set of διορισμοί and those of the Empiricists, who also frequently used the term (although we are told that they preferred the term διαστολή in order to avoid confusion with the Dogmatists' notion of διορισμός),[50] and who also allowed *epilogismos*, a kind of common sense reasoning, to play a part in the acquisition of medical knowledge.[51] To be sure, it would be grossly unfair to suggest – as Galen occasionally does[52] – that the Empiricists had an unqualified concept of experience. Yet none of the various types of *peira* they distinguished (περιπτωτική πεῖρα, αὐτοσχεδιαστική πεῖρα and μιμητική πεῖρα)[53] seem to approximate Galen's concept of διωρισμένη πεῖρα; and as for their notion of 'practised experience' (τριβική πεῖρα), which would at first sight seem to be a promising equivalent, the scanty information on this, derived exclusively from Galen's own reports in *Outline of Empiricism*

---

[49] *De alim. facult.* 1.1.9 (*CMG* v 4, 2, p. 205.3–5 Helmreich, 6.459 K.).
[50] See Galen, *Outline of Empiricism* (*Subfiguratio empirica, Subf. emp.*) 6–7 (pp. 54–65 Deichgräber); the distinction between διορισμός and διαστολή occurs at p. 59.2 Deichgräber and p. 62.12–13 Deichgräber; cf. also *In Hipp. Acut. comment.* 1.17 (*CMG* v 9, 1, p. 134.13–15 Helmreich, 15.454 K.). On the Empiricists' notion of διορισμός see Deichgräber (1965), 305f.
[51] On this see Frede (1985) xxiii, and (1987c) 248; see also his (1988). See *De simpl. med. fac.* 2.7 (quoted above, n. 11), where Galen says that we need not many ἐπιλογισμοί, but accurate ones.
[52] For example in *De meth. med.* 3.3 (10.181 K.); cf. *De sectis* 5 (p. 9.21–2 Helmreich, 1.75 K.). A much more nuanced characterisation of the Empiricists is found in *Subf. emp.* 7 (p. 64.22ff. Deichgräber): 'If, then, they had discovered each of the things they have written about before they wrote about them, so that the empiricist who uses qualification could discover these, at least all things would be true exactly in the way they have described, yet since some of them have relied on unqualified experience, and since some have not observed many times what they describe, while others have followed theoretical conjectures and have written things not according to truth, for these reasons ...'
(*'si itaque ita inuenissent prius singula eorum que scripserunt antequam scriberent, ut inuenire posset ea empericus qui utitur determinatione* (ὁ τῷ διορισμῷ χρώμενος ἐμπειρικός), *omnia essent uera utique que scribuntur ab eis, sed quia quidam quippe indeterminate experientie credentes* (τινὲς μὲν δὴ τῇ ἀδιορίστῳ πείρα πιστεύοντες), *quidam uero quia non uiderunt multotiens ea que scripserunt, quidam uero logicas suspitiones secuti non scripserunt secundum ueritatem quedam, propter ea ...'*).
[53] Galen, *De sectis* 2 (p. 3.1ff. Helmreich, 1.67 K.); *Subf. emp.* 2 (p. 44.13ff. Deichgräber).

and *On the Sects*, rather points in a different direction.[54] The fundamental difference between Galen and the Empiricists concerns the *kind* of *diorismoi* considered to be relevant: the Empiricists apparently allowed only observable entities such as age, sex, hardness or softness of the flesh, and the 'distinction made on the basis of the habits of the patient' (διορισμὸς ἀπὸ τῶν ἐθῶν) to play a part as criteria in order to describe the individual condition of each patient and to decide what medicaments should be prescribed in a particular case.[55] This use of *peira* must have inevitably appeared insufficiently specific to Galen,[56] just as the Empiricists' exclusive reliance on chance and analogy for the discovery of the powers of drugs must have looked too haphazard and unsystematic to be taken seriously as sources for scientific knowledge and understanding.[57] Moreover, Galen's use of διωρισμένη πεῖρα, 'qualified experience', also provides him with an answer to the criticism raised by Asclepiades against the Empiricists concerning the non-reproducibility of their applications of *peira*.[58] According to this criticism, one never knows for certain, at least not within the concept of knowledge adopted by the Empiricists, whether two empirical tests are precisely the same. Galen echoes this criticism by repeatedly insisting that experiments should be reproducible; but in order for them to be reproducible one has to know exactly under what conditions and circumstances they were carried out and which conditions and circumstances are relevant and which are not. Galen firmly believes that the set of *diorismoi* he has at his disposal, and the knowledge of the particular role they play in a certain

[54] *De sectis* 2 (p. 4.12 Helmreich, 1.68 K.); *Subf. emp.* 2 (p. 45.18 Deichgräber). On the *trivica experientia* of the Empiricists see von Staden (1975) 191. Even less is known about the notion of ἐπιλογιστικὴ πεῖρα with which the Empiricist Theodas is credited (Galen, *Subf. emp.* 4, p. 50.3 Deichgräber, on which see Frede (1988) 95), but this, like the τριβικὴ πεῖρα, seems to be related to the principle of 'transition to the similar' on the basis of generally accepted empirical knowledge (see, however, Menodotus' use of τρίβαξ and τρίβων as attested in *Subf. emp.* 7, p. 65.8ff. Deichgräber).

[55] See *Subf. emp.* 7 (p. 62.18ff. Deichgräber); *De meth. med.* 3.7 (10.207 K.); *De loc. aff.* 3.3 (8.142 K.).

[56] The difference in approach appears most clearly in *De simpl. med. fac.* 1.16 (11.412 K.), *De meth. med.* 3.3 (10.181 K.), and 3.7 (10.204 K.), where it is stated that the Empiricists never arrive at a really scientific and solid (ἐπιστημονικὴ καὶ βέβαια) knowledge of the individual patient's bodily state (ἰδιοσυγκρασία). See also *De simpl. med. fac.* 5.2 (11.712–13 K.), and *On the Doctrines of Hippocrates and Plato* (*De plac. Hipp. et Plat.*) 9.6.20 (*CMG* V 4, 1, 2, p. 576.24–5 De Lacy, 5.767–8 K.).

[57] *De comp. med. per gen.* 1.1 (13.366 K.). The provisional nature of these remarks on Galen's attitude towards (and indebtedness to) Empiricist pharmacology cannot be overstated. An enormous amount of work still needs to be done here (just as on his attitude towards the Pneumatists, esp. Archigenes). For the fragments and testimonies on Empiricist pharmacology see Deichgräber (1965) 146–62; for a discussion of his excerpts from, among others, Empiricist pharmacological writings, see the monograph by Fabricius (1972). See also the general remarks by Harig (1974) 135–6, who refers for Galen's criticism of the Empiricist method of discovery to *De comp. med. per gen.* 1.4 (13.366 K.), 2.1 (13.463 K.), 3.2 (13.594 K.), 6.8 (13.892 K.), *De simpl. med. fac.* 2.7 (11.482 K.) and *De comp. med. sec. loc.* 2.1 (12.524 K.), a passage which very well illustrates the difference between Galen's method of 'indication' (ἔνδειξις) and the Empiricists' use of 'transition to the similar' (ἡ ὁμοία μετάβασις).

[58] *De sectis* 5 (p. 9.9–13 Helmreich, 1.75 K.); cf. *De exper. med.* 1 (pp. 85f. Walzer).

set of conditions and circumstances, actually enables the pharmacologist to carry out reproducible experiments.[59]

Rather than looking for the origin of Galen's notion of qualified experience in medical Empiricism (that the Empiricists preferred διαστολή over διορισμός seemingly indicates that they modified an already existent concept), one might argue that his insistence on adequate qualification, or specification, of empirical statements once more testifies to his indebtedness to Aristotelian philosophy. As in so many other respects, Aristotelian methodology and terminological sophistication also provides the basic constituents of Galen's scientific instrumentarium in pharmacology (e.g. the use of the distinctions between καθ' αὐτό and κατὰ συμβεβηκός and between δύναμις and ἐνέργεια).[60] The need for appropriate specification of scientific statements is one of the cornerstones of Aristotle's philosophy of science, in which an 'unqualified premise' is defined as 'a statement which applies or does not apply without reference to universality or particularity',[61] and in which it is clearly stated that premises that are 'unqualified' (ἀδιόριστος) are not suitable for syllogisms.[62] Aristotle's classical example of the difference between experience (ἐμπειρία) and 'art' (τέχνη), derived from therapeutics, aptly illustrates the principle of qualification.[63]

4 THE CONCEPTUALISATION OF POWER AND EFFECT

We have seen so far that Galen's notion of qualified experience serves as an appropriate instrument for dealing with the fact that a certain substance does not always produce the same results in all cases. Even the very

---

[59] On the requirement of reproducibility see, e.g., *De simpl. med. fac.* 11.1 (12.350 K.), and *De plac. Hipp. et Plat.* 7.3.13 (*CMG* v 4, 1, 2, p. 442.13–18 De Lacy, 5.604 K.).

[60] On Aristotelian elements in Galen's pharmacology see Harig (1974) 87, 93f., 99–105, 156–8, 166. On Galen's use of Aristotle's philosophy of science see Tieleman (1996), ch. 4.

[61] *An. pr.* 24 a 20: ἀδιόριστον δὲ τὸ ὑπάρχειν ἢ μὴ ὑπάρχειν ἄνευ τοῦ καθόλου ἢ κατὰ μέρος, οἷον τὸ τῶν ἐναντίων εἶναι τὴν αὐτὴν ἐπιστήμην ἢ τὸ τὴν ἡδονὴν μὴ εἶναι ἀγαθόν (the usual translation of ἀδιόριστον in Aristotle is 'indeterminate'). This is exactly the point raised by Galen with regard to statements about the powers of foodstuffs and drugs (see nn. 20, 22 and 23 above).

[62] Arist., *An. pr.* 29 a 7–10; cf. *An. pr.* 26 b 23 and *Top.* 131 b 5–19, and the insistence on qualification in the discussion of the law of contradiction in *Metaph.* 4.3ff. (e.g. 1005 b 21, 28–9).

[63] *Metaph.* 981 a 7–12: 'For to have a judgement that when Callias was suffering from this particular disease, this particular treatment benefited him, and similarly with Socrates and other individual cases, is a matter of experience; but to have a judgement that all people of a certain type, defined as one specific kind, who suffer from this particular disease benefit from this treatment, e.g. phlegmatic or bilious people or people suffering from burning fever, is a matter of skill' (τὸ μὲν γὰρ ἔχειν ὑπόληψιν ὅτι Καλλίᾳ κάμνοντι τηνδὶ τὴν νόσον τοδὶ συνήνεγκε καὶ Σωκράτει καὶ καθ' ἕκαστον οὕτω πολλοῖς, ἐμπειρίας ἐστίν. τὸ δ' ὅτι πᾶσι τοῖς τοιοῖσδε κατ' εἶδος ἓν **ἀφορισθεῖσι**, κάμνουσι τηνδὶ τὴν νόσον, συνήνεγκεν, οἷον τοῖς φλεγματώδεσιν ἢ χολώδεσιν [ἢ] πυρέττουσι καύσῳ, τέχνης). For a discussion of the meaning of this example, and of the textual difficulties involved, see Spoerri (1996).

distinction Galen makes between foodstuff, drug and poison depends on this very issue, for this is a *functional* distinction depending on whether a substance just preserves the body in the state it already has, or whether it brings about a change in the state of the body.[64] Thus the whole corpus of dietetic and pharmacological knowledge would consist of a systematic set of statements (λόγοι) defining precisely what a *certain* substance, under *certain* circumstances, when applied to a *certain* kind of patients and in the case of a *certain* kind of bodily affection may bring about, thus covering and explaining all effects a substance may bring about in various types of cases.[65]

However, this does raise a problem concerning the philosophical conceptualisation of what is going on in these different cases. Since the primary question the pharmacologist has to face is that of the power (δύναμις) a particular substance has, one might ask how the power of a substance producing different results under different circumstances is to be defined: should we speak of *one* power present in the substance but not always being realised, that, is of *one* power whose realisation is impeded or disturbed by interfering circumstances? Or should we rather speak of *several different*, even *opposed* powers in one and the same substance, that is, different

---

[64] See Harig (1974) 92: 'In Abhängigkeit von der Eigentümlichkeit der verschiedenen Physeis kann darum jede eingenommene Substanz entweder die Eigenschaft des Pharmakons oder die der Nahrung oder die von beiden haben.' As Harig points out (pp. 93–4), there is, again, heavy Aristotelian (or at least Peripatetic) influence to be recorded here (he refers to Ps.-Arist. *Plant.* 820 b 5f.; *Pr.* 864 a 26–30; b 8–11; 865 a 6f.; 9–18; *Oec.* 1344 b 10f.).

[65] For an example of such statements see *De simpl. med. fac.* 1.4 (11.388 K.), where we can actually follow Galen tentatively formulating a statement with a growing degree of exactness, using the verb προστιθέναι to denote the addition of important specifications: 'But if we do not at some point in one's statement add the word "fresh", but simply say "in so far as water is cold in itself", one should not be pedantic and criticise us for having made a statement that is deficient or lacking qualification' (εἰ δὲ καὶ μὴ **προσθείη** μέν ποτε ἐν τῷ λόγῳ τὸ πότιμον, ἀλλ' **ἁπλῶς** εἴποιμεν ὅσον ἐφ' ἑαυτὸ ψυχρὸν εἶναι τὸ ὕδωρ, οὐ χρὴ συκοφαντεῖν ὡς **ἐλλιπῶς** ἢ **ἀδιορίστως** εἰρηκότας). For another example see *De alim. facult.* 1.1.33 (*CMG* v 4, 2, p. 212.2–11 Helmreich, 6.472 K.): 'One cannot forgive doctors who leave many of their most useful theoretical points without qualification. For they should not state without qualification that rock fish are easily digestible for most people although some people are found to digest beef more easily, but one should qualify both groups, just as with honey one should not make statements without qualification, but with the addition to which age-groups and which natural constitutions it is beneficial or harmful, and in which seasons or places or modes of life. For example, one would have to say that it is most damaging to dry and hot people, and most beneficial to those who are moist and cold, whether they have such a temperament through age, or natural constitution, or place, or season, or mode of life, etc.' (τοῖς δ' ἰατροῖς οὐκ ἄν τις συγγνοίη παραλιποῦσιν **ἀδιόριστα** πολλὰ τῶν χρησιμωτάτων θεωρημάτων. οὐ γὰρ **ἁπλῶς** προσήκει λέγειν αὐτούς, εὐπέπτους μὲν εἶναι **τοῖς πλείστοις** τοὺς πετραίους ἰχθύας, εὑρίσκεσθαι δέ **τινας**, οἳ τὰ βόεια κρέα ῥᾷον πέττουσιν, ἀλλ' ἑκατέρους **διορίζεσθαι**, καθάπερ γε καὶ περὶ μέλιτος οὐχ **ἁπλῶς** εἰπεῖν, ἀλλὰ μετὰ τοῦ **προσθεῖναι**, τίσιν ἡλικίαις τε καὶ φύσεσιν ὥραις τε καὶ χώραις καὶ βίοις ἐστὶν ὠφέλιμον ἢ βλαβερόν· οἷον ὅτι τοῖς μὲν ξηροῖς καὶ θερμοῖς ἐναντιώτατον, ὠφελιμώτατον δὲ τοῖς ὑγροῖς τε καὶ ψυχροῖς, εἴτε δι' ἡλικίαν ἢ διὰ φύσιν ἢ χώραν ἢ ὥραν ἢ ἐπιτηδεύματα τοιοῦτοι τὴν κρᾶσιν εἶεν). Cf. *De comp. med. sec. loc.* 5.1 (12.807 K.).

potential or virtual states present in the substance whose actualisation is dependent on the circumstances, for example the nature of the particular triggering factors?[66]

It is not completely clear, at least not to me, which of these options Galen preferred. In book 3 of *On Mixtures*, he repeatedly mentions the condition that 'no external agent should interfere with or impede' (μηδενὸς τῶν ἔξωθεν ἐμπόδων αὐτῷ γενομένου) the process of a δύναμις ('power' or 'potentiality') developing into an ἐνέργεια ('actuality');[67] and in *On the Mixtures and Powers of Simple Drugs* he stresses the connotations of stability and regularity which he apparently considers to be inherent in the notion of δύναμις (τὸ διὰ παντὸς ἕν τι ποιεῖν).[68] But there is also some evidence, albeit of a rather indirect nature, in favour of the second option.[69] A third possibility would be to include the διορισμοί in the definition of the δύναμις, for example by saying that the power of honey-wine is 'being laxative under such and such conditions'.[70]

At the core of this problem lies a certain ambiguity in the word δύναμις which also occurs in earlier Greek medical thinking[71] and which, if I am permitted to venture a rather speculative statement, might be seen as a not completely successful attempt at applying the Aristotelian distinction between δύναμις and ἐνέργεια to the area of dietetics and pharmacology. For it makes a great difference whether this distinction is applied to a situation in which something has the power *to become* something else (to change in a passive sense, i.e. to undergo change or be changed) or to a situation in which something has the power *to cause something to undergo change or be*

---

[66] Cf. *De temper.* 3.1 (p. 89.1–14 Helmreich, 1.651 K.); *De simpl. med. fac.* 3.20 (11.602f.K.).
[67] *De temper.* 3.1 (p. 86.14–15 Helmreich, 1.647 K.); 3.1 (p. 87.5–6 Helmreich, 1.647 K.).
[68] *De simpl. med. fac.* 1.2–3 (11.384 K.).
[69] See *De simpl. med. fac.* 1.3 (11.384 K.): 'And perhaps on some occasion you will say that water not only has the power of cooling, but also of heating. For on some occasions it is evidently cooling in all circumstances, whenever we come into contact with it, but on many other occasions it has effected a heating reaction. One should therefore not leave these things without qualification for any drug that is being examined, as I have said in On Mixtures' (καὶ ἴσως δέ ποτε καὶ τὸ ψυχρὸν ὕδωρ οὐ ψυχρὸν μόνον ἐρεῖς τὴν δύναμιν, ἀλλὰ καὶ θερμόν. ὅτε μὲν ψῦχον φαίνεται, διὰ παντός, ἔστ' ἂν ἡμῖν πλησιάζῃ, ψυχρόν, ὅτε δὲ πολλάκις ἐπανάκλησιν θερμότητος ἤνεγκεν θερμόν. οὔκουν χρὴ ταῦτα παραλιπεῖν ἀδιόριστα καὶ τῶν κρινομένων ἕκαστον φαρμάκων, ὡς κἂν τοῖς περὶ κράσεων ἐλέγετο). A clearer example is *De simpl. med. fac.* 7.10 (12.36 K.): 'Coriander consists of opposite powers: it has much bitterness, which was shown to reside in its fine and earthy texture, but it also has the power to produce quite a bit of watery, fatty moisture, and it also has something astringent' (σύγκειται γάρ [τὸ κορίανον] ἐξ ἐναντίων δυνάμεων πολὺ μὲν ἔχουσα πικρᾶς οὐσίας, ἥτις ἐδείκνυτο λεπτομερὴς ὑπάρχειν καὶ γεῶδες, οὐκ ὀλίγον δὲ καὶ ὑδατώδους ὑγρότητος χλιαρᾶς κατὰ δύναμιν, ἔχει δέ τι καὶ στύψεως ὀλίγης). See also *De alim. facult.* 1.1.11 (*CMG* v 4, 2, p. 205.16–23 Helmreich, 6.460 K.).
[70] See the passage from *De alim. facult.* 1.1 quoted in n. 65 above
[71] It can also be detected in the Hippocratic Corpus and in Diocles; see ch. 2 in this volume, pp. 79 ff.

changed into something else. While the physiological description of these processes of change in terms of qualities acting on, or competing with, each other may not be very different in either type of situation,[72] the formal description in terms of a power, or powers, being realised does present a difficulty. There seems to be an awareness of this difficulty on Galen's part. On the one hand, his definition of the concept of δύναμις in *On Mixtures* book 3 contains the same normative and teleological elements as Aristotle's notion of potentiality:[73] it certainly is Nature's intention that the δύναμις will actually be realised, as Galen's use of μέλλειν, μήπω, ἤδη, ἐπιτήδειος and ἀτελές indicates,[74] and this seems to be the normal, natural way of affairs; the possibility implied in the condition 'nothing external occurring as an impediment' (μηδενὸς τῶν ἔξωθεν ἐμποδὼν αὐτῷ γενομένου), also derived from Aristotle's analysis of change,[75] seems to rule out only *exceptional* cases (such as monstrosities). On the other hand, when it comes to the power *to bring about* change, Galen, in his discussion of the powers of foodstuffs and drugs, uses a slightly different concept of δύναμις, which is defined in the first chapter of *On the Mixtures and Powers of Simple Drugs* as an αἰτία δραστική,[76] an 'active cause', and which in its turn allows of a distinction between two stages: a stage of 'being about to' (ἐν τῷ μέλλειν) and an actual stage (κατ' ἐνέργειαν).[77] Thus the power of hotness (i.e. of *causing something else to become* hot) is 'actually' present in fire, but 'about to be' present in a flint. Now, with this concept of δύναμις, the normative or teleological connotation is more difficult to maintain, and the condition 'nothing external occurring as an impediment' (μηδενὸς τῶν ἔξωθεν

---

[72] This would be along the lines that Aristotle draws in *On Coming to Be and Passing Away* and the fourth book of the *Meteorologica* and that Galen himself applies in *On Mixtures*, on which see Harig (1974) 105ff. Galen refers to Aristotle in *De temper.* 3.3 (p. 98.23 Helmreich, 1.666 K.) and 3.4 (p. 102.16 Helmreich, 1.672 K.)

[73] *De temper.* 3.1 (p. 86.9–15 Helmreich, 1.646–7 K.): 'For we say that what is not yet such as it is said to be, but has the nature to become like that, is present potentially ... In all cases that which each of these things is about to become, if no external factor gets in the way, this we say is already present... Potentially in the strictest sense we call only those things where nature itself brings about the completion (of the process), if no external factor gets in the way' (ὃ γὰρ ἂν ὑπάρχῃ μὲν μήπω τοιοῦτον, οἷον λέγεται, πέφυκε δὲ γενέσθαι, δυνάμει φαμὲν ὑπάρχειν αὐτό ... ὅπερ ἔσεσθαι πάντως ἕκαστον αὐτῶν μέλλει μηδενὸς τῶν ἔξωθεν ἐμποδὼν αὐτῷ γενομένου, τοῦθ᾽ ὡς ὂν ἤδη λέγοντες ... κυριώτατα μὲν οὖν ἐκεῖνα μόνα δυνάμει λέγομεν, ἐφ᾽ ὧν ἡ φύσις αὐτὴ πρὸς τὸ τέλειον ἀφικνεῖται μηδενὸς τῶν ἔξωθεν ἐμποδὼν αὐτῇ γενομένου). Cf. *De temper.* 1.9 (p. 32.17–19 Helmreich, 1.560 K.); 2.2 (p. 51.21–22 Helmreich, 1.590 K.).

[74] *De temper.* 3.1 (p. 86.18–19 Helmreich, 1.647 K.): 'What is potentially is incomplete and still about to be and as it were suited to become (what it is to be), but it is not yet (what it is to be)' (τὸ δυνάμει δ᾽ ἀτελές τι καὶ μέλλον ἔτι καὶ οἷον ἐπιτήδειον μὲν εἰς τὸ γενέσθαι, μήπω δ᾽ ὑπάρχον ὃ λέγεται).

[75] Arist., *Phys.* 199 a 11; b 18, 26; 215 a 21; 255 b 7. Cf. *Rh.* 1392 b 20 and *Pol.* 1288 b 24.

[76] Cf. *De simpl. med. fac.* 1.1 (11.380 K.); cf. *On the Seed (De semine)* 1.1 (*CMG* v 3, 1, p. 64.5 De Lacy, 4.512 K.).

[77] *De simpl. med fac.* 1.1 (11.380 K.).

ἐμποδών αὐτῷ γενομένου), if applicable, would refer *not* just to a few exceptional cases in which something has gone wrong, but to quite a considerable number of different types of situation in which the power of a substance is not realised or the process is turned in another direction. For as Galen's list of διορισμοί indicates, there may be quite a lot of possibly interfering or even impeding factors changing the course of the process, and as a consequence it may be difficult to distinguish between effects brought about 'by the substance itself' (καθ' αὐτό) and effects produced 'accidentally' (κατὰ συμβεβηκός).

Although Galen was apparently aware of this difficulty, the possibility that a dietetic or pharmacological power may be prevented from being actualised by interfering factors is apparently *not* taken into account by him when it comes to refuting generalising statements about the power of a foodstuff or drug. Galen's refutation of such statements usually follows the pattern of deducing the power (or the absence of it) from the effect.[78] Thus 'A has the power to bring about X' is refuted by pointing out that in a certain case A does not bring about X but Y; but to conclude from this that A does not possess the *power* to bring about X ignores the possibility that A *may* have this power but does not realise it in this particular case, and may therefore be false. Thus Galen fails to apply the concept of διωρισμένη πεῖρα consistently to his own critical scrutiny of other pharmacologists' statements.

5 CONSEQUENCES FOR THE QUESTION OF EXPERIMENT IN GALEN'S PHARMACOLOGY

To sum up: what does the concept of qualified experience have to say on the question of pharmacological 'experiment' in Galen's works? As is well known and has already been alluded to above, there has been a long-standing dispute as to whether we are actually justified in speaking of experiment in ancient science (and, as a consequence, of ancient *science* at all). It has often been argued that this word is too evocative of modern connotations of a deliberate and systematical examination of what happens when, in a determined set of circumstances, a definite change is brought about;[79] and it

---

[78] See Harig (1974) 104: 'die Feststellung der potentiellen Wirkung eines Pharmakons... erst retrospektiv aus der eingetretenen aktuellen Wirkung erkannt werden kann'. For an example of Galen falsifying statements by means of counter-examples see *De simpl. med. fac.* 1.34 (11.440ff. K.).

[79] For a definition of experiment see von Staden (1975) 180. See also the discussions by Grmek and Gourevitch (1985) 3–4; Debru (1994) 1718–21; Tieleman (1995) 32 (all with abundant references to secondary literature) and Lloyd (1964) 50–72.

may suggest the idea of a systematical elimination of all the other incidental variables that may interfere with the process of change and determine the actual outcome. Related to this problem is the disagreement as to whether πεῖρα should be translated as 'experience' rather than as 'experiment' – an issue which is closely connected with the question whether πεῖρα is used as a heuristic instrument for the discovery of hitherto unknown facts, or as a critical instrument in order to check whether an *already existent* view or claim about the effect of a foodstuff or drug is correct.

It is impossible, within the scope of this chapter, to go into the details of all these questions – although it should be said that there are certainly passages in Galen's pharmacological works where we see him actually describing what one may call without hesitation an attempt at experimentation in the modern sense.[80] In any case Galen's insistence on a *qualified* use of experience strongly suggests that he is, at least *theoretically*, rather close to the modern concept of experiment. The texts discussed above have shown that qualified experience is used both for judging whether a particular, already existent view on the power of a foodstuff or drug is true and for making new discoveries.[81] This may now be well understood: to refute a view in a correct way presupposes the same knowledge of determining circumstances as interpreting the result of an empirical test as a new and significant discovery. A scientist using a counter-example in order to falsify an hypothesis should ensure that the counter-example is actually a good example. That Galen himself does not always live up to this latter requirement in actual practice, is another story.

[80] See, e.g., *De simpl. med. fac.* 1.21 (11.418 K.).
[81] Heuristic: *De alim. facult.* 1.12.1; *De simpl. med. fac.* 4.19; 4.23; 6.1; critical: *De alim. facult.* 1.1.46; *De simpl. med. fac.* 3.13; 7.10.

CHAPTER II

The Methodism of Caelius Aurelianus: some epistemological issues

Caelius Aurelianus' Methodism is often taken for granted. Yet the question may be asked how profoundly, pervasively and consistently Methodist doctrine and methodology is applied in Caelius' work. In this chapter I will attempt to answer this question with regard to some epistemological principles of Methodism as they are known to us from Soranus and from Caelius himself;[1] and I will consider whether the difficulties that arise here are just apparent or amount to genuine inconsistencies, and, if the latter, whether these are to be explained as the result of a development in Methodism after Soranus or as tensions inherent in Methodist medicine as such. In so doing, I will treat Caelius Aurelianus (not Soranus) as the author of *Acute Affections* (*Acut.*) and *Chronic Affections* (*Chron.*). This is not to deny Caelius' dependence on Soranus – a dependence which is probably great, but in the absence of most of Soranus' work impossible to assess – but should leave room, at least theoretically, for Caelius' own contribution, whether that merely consisted of translating and partially rearranging Soranic material or of substantial revision with additions and omissions of his own.[2]

This chapter was first published in P. Mudry (ed.), *Le traité des Maladies aiguës et des Maladies chroniques de Caelius Aurelianus: nouvelles approches* (Nantes, 1999) 47–83.

[1] I will deal with external sources on Methodism such as Celsus, Galen and Sextus Empiricus only in so far as they confirm what is found in Soranus and Caelius; I will not go into the question of to what extent their reports distort Methodist doctrines (as they undoubtedly do in the case of Galen, but perhaps less so in the case of Celsus).

[2] Scholarly controversy continues to exist about the precise relationship of Caelius' work to that of Soranus, and about what exactly Caelius *claims* this relationship to be (on this latter point see Vázquez Buján (1999)). For other discussions of this relationship see Pigeaud (1982); Lloyd (1983) 186 n. 258; Vallance (1990) 5 n. 7; Rubinstein (1985) 155 n. 3; Kollesch (1990) 5; Hanson and Green (1994) 979; Vázquez Buján (1991) 87–97 [and van der Eijk (1999c) 415–28]. A passage which deserves closer attention in this respect is *Acut.* 3.14.105, where Soranus seems to be just one of the authorities (apart from Artorius and Eudemus) to whom Caelius appeals (although here, again, it is possible that Caelius bases himself on a text by Soranus in which Soranus juxtaposes his own observations with remarks made by Artorius and Eudemus); another passage is the proem of *Chronic Affections*, where Soranus seems to be treated on a par with other authorities such as Themison and Thessalus.

To be sure, there is no question about Caelius' actually belonging to the Methodist school, to which he frequently refers as 'our sect' and whose doctrines he often presents as the standard for his therapeutic instructions.[3] Nor is there any doubt about Caelius' commitment to Soranus, whom he often mentions as the point of reference for his own work and with whom he never expresses disagreement.[4] Yet the unprejudiced reader of *Acute Affections* has to wait until chapter 11 of the first book (a good twenty pages in Bendz and Pape's edition) for the first reference to the 'Method';[5] and it is no earlier than in book 2, chapter 1 that he is told that what he is presented with there is a Latin version of Soranus.[6]

To this it could be responded that this is just a matter of presentation, that Caelius did not write for unprejudiced readers and that he must have assumed his audience[7] to be sufficiently aware of his intellectual background[8] and his indebtedness to the *Methodicorum princeps*.[9] Yet in the absence of any certainty about the setting and readership of Caelius' works one has to be careful with such presuppositions. Moreover, there is the fact that, as far as other Methodists such as Themison, Thessalus, or more generally 'the older Methodists' are concerned, Caelius frequently castigates them for

---

[3] E.g. *Acut.* 3.4.47; 2.33.179; *Chron.* 2.1.16.

[4] The entry 'Soranus' in the (otherwise invaluable) *index nominum* to Bendz and Pape's edition prepared by J. Kollesch and D. Nickel should be used with caution, for it also lists (with some exceptions such as *Chron.* 2.1.60 (p. 580,1) and *Chron.* 4.9.134 (p. 850,17)) occurrences of the authorial *ego* and *nos* as referring to Soranus (this is based on their view that Caelius' work is in the main a faithful translation of Soranus, for which see n. 2 above).

[5] *Acut.* 1.11.99: 'This is the treatment of the affection phrenitis according to the Method' (*Haec est secundum methodon curatio phreniticae passionis*).

[6] *Acut.* 2.1.8: 'But Soranus, whose [views] these are, which we have undertaken to present in Latin' (*Soranus uero, cuius haec sunt, quae latinizanda suscepimus*). Cf. *Acut.* 2.10.65 (where, however, the word *Soranus* is an editorial addition); 2.28.147; 2.31.163. For this observation – that the first reference to Soranus occurs not earlier than here and that neither in the preface of *Acute Affections* nor in that of *Chronic Affections* does Caelius give any indication that he is offering a translation of Soranus – and for a discussion of the other passages where Caelius defines his work as a Latinisation of Soranus (which actually represent only a small minority of all the references to Soranus) see Hanson and Green (1994) 979, who rightly make the point that this does not really support the hypothesis that Caelius' work is a *translation* of Soranus (but their own translation of *cuius haec sunt* in *Acut.* 2.1.8 and 2.10.65 as 'his works' is unnecessarily specific: Caelius may just mean Soranus' views). They also rightly stress that the relationship between Soranus' *Gynaecia* and Caelius' version of it need not be the same as that between Soranus' work on acute and chronic diseases and that of Caelius (contra Kollesch 1990).

[7] Little can be said with any certainty about Caelius' intended audience. Nothing is known of the Bellicus addressed in the proem to *Acute Affections*, but the fact that he is addressed as 'best pupil' (*discipule summe*) suggests at least some familiarity of the audience with Methodism.

[8] This might be inferred from the occurrence of several Methodist terms in the pages preceding *Acut.* 1.11.99, e.g. the use of *accessio* in *Acut.* 1.4.42 and 1.5.47, and of *strictura* and *solutio* in *Acut.* 1.9.58 and 1.9.60.

[9] For this characterisation of Soranus see *Chron.* 1.1.50.

their erroneous beliefs and their 'looseness' of doctrine.[10] Whether these criticisms in Caelius' work simply reproduce similar criticisms found in Soranus (who did not shy away from taking his fellow Methodists to task either, as we can see from his *Gynaecia*)[11] we do not know, but they do indicate that there was a development in Methodism, that there was room for disagreement and further refinement of doctrine, and that authority and orthodoxy played a less prominent role here than in other medical sects.[12]

It is therefore an interesting and legitimate question to ask whether this development continued after Soranus, or was brought to a halt by the 'rigour' which Soranus is said to have instituted,[13] or to put it differently, whether Caelius (the first Methodist author after Soranus whose works have survived) faithfully followed the footsteps of his great example or had the boldness to go beyond Soranus in matters of doctrine and methodology – and if the latter is the case, whether this is to be seen as an expression of intellectual independence by a writer with a strong personality, or as a sign of susceptibility to influences from outside the Methodist sect. Theoretically, such a development is by no means inconceivable or improbable. For if the tentative dating of Caelius Aurelianus in the early fifth century CE is correct,[14] there is a time-span of at least three centuries separating him from Soranus. What the historical setting of Caelius' works was and what the Methodist sect looked like in the early fifth century we do not know, but it is difficult to believe that when Caelius wrote his works the school had ceased to exist or had come to a complete intellectual standstill.[15]

---

[10] For criticism of Themison see, e.g., *Acut.* 1.16.155–65 (where, however, at the beginning (p. 108, 11–13 Bendz) and at the end (p. 114, 9–10 Bendz) he is said to have done the Methodist school much good at a later stage of his development); *Chron.* 1.1.50. For criticism of the older Methodists in general see, e.g., *Acut.* 3.4.47; *Chron.* 2.7.96. An interesting passage is *Chron.* 5.2.51, where Themison is said to have discussed the treatment of arthritis and podagra, 'discussing some things as a Methodist, others as if he were not a Methodist' (*aliqua ut Methodicus, aliqua ut non Methodicus decurrens*), and where Thessalus is said to have given therapeutic instructions 'not quite perfectly, but in accordance with Methodist principles' (*imperfecte quidem, sed consequenter Methodicis intentionibus*). For criticism of Thessalus see, e.g., *Acut.* 3.17.172 (where he is reported to have said 'some things as a Methodist, others in a way that deserves censure', *alia quidem ut Methodicus, alia culpabiliter*); *Chron.* 2.7.112 (where also Themison is mentioned); 2.1.60–1 (where the criticism is said to be derived from Soranus); 3.8.155.

[11] For criticism of other Methodists by Soranus see *Gynaecia* 3.24; 3.42; 4.39; 1.29.

[12] This point has also been made by Lloyd (1983) 188 and 198, and (1991a) 400–1; see also von Staden (1982) 83–5; Pigeaud (1991) 36.

[13] On this rigour see *Chron.* 2.7.109; *Chron.* 3.4.65. Cf. *Acut.* 2.9.46; *Chron.* 3.8.98.

[14] This is mainly based on linguistic and stylistic evidence such as similarities with Cassius Felix. A renewed examination of this question would be very desirable.

[15] On the interest taken in Methodism in the early fifth century see Hanson and Green (1994) 1043.

To be sure, Caelius does not mention any Methodist, or indeed any other medical writer, known to be later than Soranus[16] (surprisingly, he does not even mention Galen)[17] – which might suggest that at least in the area of doxography he had nothing to add to Soranus, but for which there may be other reasons as well[18] – and he nowhere explicitly disagrees with Soranus. Yet we cannot rule out that Methodist doctrine developed further and, by the time of Caelius, had, perhaps unintentionally, evolved beyond the strict boundaries of Soranus' teaching.[19] There are indeed indications that this happened. Thus P. H. Schrijvers, in his commentary on Caelius' rejection of homosexuality in *Chron.* 4.9, has pointed out that Caelius' use of a theological and indeed teleological argument about the natural purpose of the bodily organs is incompatible with Soranus' often expressed anti-teleological views on nature, and is perhaps to be understood against the later background of Christian or Stoic intolerance towards homosexual behaviour.[20] To this it may be objected that *Chron.* 4.9 is a rather exceptional chapter and cannot be regarded as representative of the whole work;[21] but, as I will show here, there are more signs to suggest that Caelius took a line which is not always easy to accommodate within what we know – both

---

[16] It should be stressed that of some authorities the date and identity are not known, e.g. Valens physicus (*Acut.* 3.1.2) and Leonides Episyntheticus (*Acut.* 2.1.6).

[17] As Mirko Grmek pointed out during the discussion of the original version of this paper, in the light of the subject matter of the *Acute* and *Chronic Affections*, the absence of any reference to Aretaeus of Cappadocia (first century CE) is perhaps even more surprising; also one would expect a more prominent place for Archigenes of Apamea, who seems to have been in close contact with the Methodist school (cf. Waszink (1947a) 25) but who is only mentioned twice (*Acut.* 2.10.58 and 61). For Caelius' references to earlier authorities see van der Eijk (1998) and (1999c); see also von Staden (1999a).

[18] Alternatively, it may suggest an earlier date for Caelius himself (see n. 14 above); however, Caelius' silence on intermediary authorities is not without parallel: Galen's *On the Doctrines of Hippocrates and Plato* does not discuss authorities later than Posidonius either (for this observation see Vegetti (1999)). For the observation that Caelius does not mention medical authors later than Soranus see Hanson and Green (1994) 980; however, I fail to see the point of their remark that 'Particularly important for the suggestion that Caelius Aurelianus draws his doxographic accounts from Soranus is the impression the text gives of having appended onto an existing framework opinions from Asclepiades, Themison (e.g. Cel. Pass. I xiv 105–xvi 165; II xxxix 225–xl 234), and sometimes Thessalus (e.g. Tard. Pass. II i.55–62).' I do not see how the text should give this impression or why the 'appending' should have been done by Caelius rather than by Soranus (who may have updated the doxography of Alexander Philalethes, as Hanson and Green suggest on p. 980 n. 33). – The fact that in Caelius' *Gynaecia* doxographic passages are far less frequent than in Soranus' original, whereas such passages abound in Caelius' *Acute* and *Chronic Affections*, suggests that in this respect there is an important difference between the relationship between Soranus' and Caelius' gynaecological works and that between Caelius' and Soranus' works on acute and chronic diseases (see also n. 2 above).

[19] A similar case would be Plotinus, whose philosophical system represents a major development in Platonic doctrine but who claimed to do nothing else than interpret Plato.

[20] Schrijvers (1985) 22–5.

[21] Caelius' own contribution in this chapter also becomes clear in the Latin hexametric translation of Parmenides. The chapter is also exceptional in that there is no section on therapeutics.

from Soranus and from external evidence provided by Galen, Celsus and Sextus Empiricus – about Methodism.

I should not exaggerate. Certainly, Caelius provides abundant evidence of 'orthodox' Methodist teaching. In his works we do find frequent mentions of the three 'common states' or 'generalities', to which he even refers by their Greek name *coenotetes*;[22] we also find the characteristic Methodist therapy intended to restore these pathological conditions to their normal state.[23] Again, we can perceive the characteristic Methodist indifference to which part of the body is affected by the disease,[24] and, more generally, their reluctance to attach any importance to questions which cannot be answered with certainty and whose outcome is at best 'plausible' (*existimabile*).[25] We also find confirmation in Caelius for Galen's testimony[26] about the Methodists' refusal to pay any attention, as far as diagnosis is concerned, to such variables as the patient's age, sex, constitution, way of life, the climate, the season, and so forth[27] – factors which from Hippocratic medicine onwards were believed to affect the bodily condition of the individual patient and to be relevant for the therapeutic decision about which course of treatment was to be followed. And to mention a final example, we find abundant confirmation in Caelius for Galen's and Celsus' testimony about the Methodists' disregard for so-called 'antecedent causes'.[28]

Yet, even with regard to these examples of clear Methodist tenets in Caelius Aurelianus, closer examination of the way in which they are implemented in various contexts does raise some problems. Thus the doctrine of the *coenotetes* is not so prominent as one would expect in a systematic work on acute and chronic diseases:[29] in a number of cases, the general heading under which a particular disease should be classified is not discussed at all[30] or is only given in passing, and at any rate it does not seem to have been among the *primary* concerns of Caelius as they appear in the questionnaire which he, whether more or less systematically, follows in the discussion of all diseases.[31] Also the concept of *indicatio* (ἔνδειξις) is

---

[22] E.g. *Chron.* 2.12.145ff.; 3.1.12; *Acut.* 3.16.136.
[23] E.g. *Chron.* 1.1.21ff. (esp. pp. 440,20 and 442,12 Bendz); 1.4.97.
[24] E.g. *Acut.* 1.8.53–6; 2.6.26; 2.28.147; 2.34.183.
[25] E.g. *Acut.* 2.5.23; 2.28.147; 2.35.185; *Chron.* 4.1.5; cf. Soranus, *Gyn.* 1.45.
[26] Galen, *De sectis* 6 (p. 12 Helmreich, 1.79 K.). See also Frede (1987a) 268–9, who rightly stresses that in therapy the Methodists did take differentiating features into account; one may also point to Sor., *Gyn.* 1.22 (about differentiating factors with regard to menstruation).
[27] E.g. *Acut.* 1.3.41; 1.12.103; 2.20.125.   [28] See section 2 below.
[29] On this see Rubinstein (1985) 129.
[30] E.g. lethargy (*Acut.* 2.1–9), defluxio (*Acut.* 3.22.220–2), cephalaea (*Chron.* 1.1), scotomatica (*Chron.* 1.2), incubo (*Chron.* 1.3), melancholia (*Chron.* 1.6), hydropes (*Chron.* 3.8) and ischias (*Chron.* 5.1).
[31] On this questionnaire see van der Eijk (1998) 346.

remarkably under-represented;[32] and, as John Vallance has pointed out,[33] the Methodists' indifference to the question of the affected parts seems difficult to square with Caelius' statements – sometimes in the same context – that some parts suffer more than others.[34]

These doctrinal difficulties deserve closer examination,[35] but for practical reasons I cannot go into them here. Instead, I shall concentrate on what seem to be some paradoxical elements in what may be called the epistemology, or methodology, of Caelius Aurelianus – paradoxical in the sense that they seem to fit in less well with Methodism as we know it, not only from the sources just mentioned (which may have distorted Methodist doctrine) but also from Soranus and from Caelius' own references to Methodism. Four issues can be distinguished here:

(1) Caelius' attitude to the 'manifest' and the unobservable;
(2) his attitude to, and use of, causal explanations;
(3) his attitude to, and use of, definitions;
(4) his evaluation of reason and experience as sources of knowledge.

These issues are interrelated, but each of the paradoxes they present may require an explanation of its own and no option should be ruled out beforehand. Some may only be apparent and turn out to be soluble on closer examination; others may represent undeniable tensions in Methodism itself (an explanation which would be more plausible if it could be shown that such tensions also occur in Soranus);[36] and yet others may give the impression of being peculiarities of Caelius' own version of Methodism, or at any rate of a later stage in the history of the school. Yet, however tempting the explanatory scenario of a continuing development in Methodism may be – especially to those scholars who appreciate the originality of Caelius Aurelianus[37] – we should be careful here, for there is hardly any evidence on which to build such a developmental hypothesis. Of course one could

---

[32] E.g. *Acut.* 2.3.13; *Acut.* 1.15.121; *Chron.* 2.12.146. On *indicatio* as the Latin translation for ἔνδειξις see Durling (1991) 112–13.
[33] Vallance (1990) 140 n. 52; see also Gourevitch (1991) 66.
[34] E.g. *Acut.* 1.8.55. Cf. *Acut.* 2.28.147, where, however, Soranus is reported to have stipulated that the view that some parts suffer more than others is 'a matter of conjecture and not to be accepted as trustworthy' (*aestimatum et non ad expressam fidem accipiendum*). Another interesting passage is *Acut.* 3.14.117 (on the affected part in the case of hydrophobia), where Caelius makes three points: (1) the question of the affected part is of no relevance to the doctor; (2) the stomach suffers more than other parts; (3) treatment is applied locally 'wherever we find the disease to be situated' (*ubi passionem inuenerimus*).
[35] For a discussion of Caelius' use of Methodist concepts such as generalities see Pigeaud (1991) 41.
[36] A thorough and systematic comparison between Soranus and Caelius Aurelianus on all of these issues would lead into great detail and is therefore beyond the scope of this chapter. However, parallels in Soranus are occasionally mentioned in the footnotes where this seems relevant.
[37] See n. 2 above (especially Pigeaud, more moderately Vallance, and Hanson and Green).

try to compare Caelius Aurelianus with Soranus (or with the fragments of other Methodists),[38] but this comparison is complicated by the different status of the extant works; for Soranus' *Gynaecia*, his only major surviving work, is a very specialised treatise, and a very practical one at that, whereas Caelius' *Acute* and *Chronic Affections* deal with what may be called the central concern of Methodism, namely the diagnosis and treatment of diseases.[39] Now we know, for example, from a passage in Caelius Aurelianus[40] that the Methodists were keen to distinguish between different specialised areas within medicine, such as surgery, pharmacology and dietetics, and to assign the discussion of a particular aspect of a particular disease to one area rather than another. This strong sense of compartmentalisation is a potential source of discrepancies, and hence of apparent inconsistencies, between the ways a certain subject is dealt with in different contexts.

Yet also the possible explanation of tensions inherent in Methodism itself should be used with some caution. On the one hand, historians of ancient medicine have recently stressed that Methodism is not a philosophy but a way of doing medicine, and a thoroughly practical way of doing medicine at that – though admittedly not without relation to philosophy – and this should make us careful not to approach Methodism as if it were an applied form of Scepticism.[41] After all, practicability was not the major concern, or indeed the major strength, of Scepticism. On the other hand, we should demand from Caelius a reasonable degree of consistency and systematicity (although we may have to allow for some flexibility in the extent to which this is implemented or for potential divergences between theory and practice). The point is that doctrinal and methodological tensions may, in the case of Methodism, find their origin in the fact that the primary concern of Methodism is the successful diagnosis and treatment of diseases, and in the Methodists' belief that all issues that are not necessarily related to this (such as the question of what the cause of a disease is, or what its correct definition is, or which part of the body is affected by the disease, etc.) are considered to be irrelevant or inappropriate. The important consequence of this is that the Methodists might have been perfectly well aware of some

---

[38] See now Moog (1994) [and Tecusan (2004)].
[39] Incidentally, one might conclude from this that, other things being equal, for the reconstruction of mainstream Methodist doctrine we are in a much better position with Caelius Aurelianus than with Soranus (contra Lloyd (1983) 185–6: 'For our purposes the extant original Greek of the *Gynaecology* is both more reliable and more interesting than the paraphrastic Latin versions of his *Acute* and *Chronic Diseases* that we have from Caelius Aurelianus').
[40] *Chron.* 2.12.146. Cf. Sor., *Gyn.* 1.4.
[41] This point has been made by Gourevitch (1991) 67–8 against Edelstein (1967b) 173–91. See also Lloyd (1983) 183.

of these tensions, but simply could not be bothered with them because they did not matter for their purposes. It seems that *relevance* both to diagnosis and to treatment – rather than some sort of epistemological reluctance – is the crucial criterion for the Methodists not only to decide whether, in a particular case, to go into such a question or not but also, if one has to go into it, to decide to what degree of accuracy, detail and profoundness one has to go into it.

1 THE (UN)OBSERVABLE

We are told that the Methodists as a matter of principle based themselves only on what is 'manifest' and refused to commit themselves to the existence, and the identification, of hidden, unobservable entities, and that they did not speculate about hidden entities because of the uncertainty this would involve.[42] This receives confirmation from Caelius Aurelianus himself, for example in the following passages:[43]

(1) iudicare enim[44] est incertum, utrum passio post accessionem primam inesse corpori an soluta uideatur, siquidem ex occulta ueniat apprehensione causarum, et oportet Methodicum sine ulla falsitate regulas intendere curationum. (*Chron.* 1.4.83)

For one cannot judge with certainty whether the affection appears to be still present in the body after the first attack or to have been overcome, as this would be based on an obscure apprehension of causes, and a Methodist ought to adhere to the rules of treatment without any falsity.

(2) his enim, qui forsitan ob eius [sc. Heraclidis] defensionem dixerint eum praecauere, rursum ne febres irruant, respondemus hoc esse occultum et non oportere Methodicum esse suspicionibus incertis occupatum, et uere. (*Acut.* 3.21.219)

For to these people, who in his [i.e. Heraclides'] defence might say that he is taking precautions against a new attack of fever, we reply that this is an obscure matter, and a Methodist ought not to concern himself with uncertain suspicions, and rightly so.

(3) erat igitur melius, ut manifestis et consequentibus uerbis intelligendam traderet [sc. Asclepiades] passionem et non per occultam atque dissonantem obtrusionem et quae fortasse neque esse probetur, sicut libris, quos Contra Sectos sumus scripturi, docebimus. (*Acut.* 1.1.9)

---

[42] Sor. *Gyn.* 1.45 and 1.52; Celsus, *De medicina* 1, proem, 57; Galen, *De sectis* 6 (pp. 13–14 Helmreich, 1.79–80 K.).
[43] Unless otherwise indicated, all translations of Caelius are my own; however, I am happy to acknowledge my great indebtedness to the translations by I. E. Drabkin and by I. Pape.
[44] *etiam*, Drabkin.

It would have been better if he [i.e. Asclepiades] had described the disease in clear and consistent terms and not with reference to an obscure stoppage which results in inconsistency and which, perhaps, could be shown not even to be present at all, as we shall point out in the books we will write Against the Sects.[45]

At the same time, we frequently find Caelius referring to hidden entities without any reservation. These passages fall into three categories:

(i) reference to entities of which it may seem difficult to non-experts to accept that they are observable, but which Methodists may claim to be observable to the expert's eye, such as the generalities or common conditions,[46] as in the following passage:

(4) interiorum uero eruptionum diuisuras urgente solutionis coenoteta[m] ipsam magis cogimur iudicare, siquidem prior oculis occurrat solutio. (*Chron.* 2.12.147)

Yet as for the wounds that occur as a result of haemorrhage in the inner parts, since the generality of looseness prevails, we must judge it rather as just that, as it presents itself first to the eyes as a looseness.

(ii) reference to entities of which it is unclear whether the Methodists regard them as observable or not, such as *spiritus* (or *pneuma*), in, for example:

(5) cordis enim motus tarditate quadam defecti spiritu<s> motu torpescit, ut post factum saltum ad semet ex residuo corpore praerogatum spiritum trahat, difficulter alium faciat saltum, siquidem non possit spiritus usque ad articulorum finem uel omnium membrorum peruenire summitatem. (*Acut.* 1.11.87)

For the motion of the heart is paralysed by the movement of the pneuma which, as a result of a slowness, is not present in sufficient measure, so that after making a beat it draws to itself from the rest of the body the pneuma that had previously been distributed; then it makes another beat with difficulty, as the pneuma cannot reach the end of the limbs or the extremities of any of the parts.

There are about a dozen references to this *pneuma* in Caelius,[47] and although in some of these cases he is clearly just thinking of the air that is inhaled or exhaled via respiration,[48] the majority of these passages show that he believes

---

[45] See also *Acut.* 1.15.121; 2.1.8; *Chron.* 1.4.129; 5.10.103.
[46] Although there may also be generalities that are hidden, even to the expert's eye, as *Chron.* 3.2.19 shows: 'but if the loose state is hidden, which the Greeks call *adelos*, or if the signs are perceived by the mind, which the Greeks call *logotheoretos*...' (*sin uero occulta fuerit solutio, quam Graeci adelon appellant, aut mente sensa signa uideantur, quae Graeci logotheoreta uocauerunt*...) On this passage see below.
[47] E.g. *Acut.* 1.14.113; 1.15.119; 1.15.124; 1.15.127; 1.15.150; 2.9.48; 2.14.93; 2.34.180; 3.17.138; *Chron.* 1.1.30; 1.1.33; 1.4.84; 1.4.101; 2.1.32; 2.1.39; 3.4.65. The concept of *pneuma* also occurs in Soranus, e.g. *Gyn.* 1.34; 1.38; 2.11.
[48] E.g. *Chron.* 1.1.33; 2.1.39.

the *pneuma* to reside and to originate in the body and to play a major part in physiological processes such as digestion and muscular movement.

From some passages it appears that this *pneuma* is to be regarded as an inheritance of Asclepiadean physiology:

(6) neque ullam digestionem in nobis esse [sc. dicit Asclepiades], sed solutionem ciborum in uentre fieri crudam et per singulas particulas corporis ire, ut per omnes tenuis uias penetrare uideatur, quod appellauit leptomeres, sed nos intelligimus spiritum; et neque inquit feruentis qualitatis neque frigidae esse nimiae suae tenuitatis causa neque alium quemlibet sensum tactus habere, sed per uias receptaculorum nutrimenti nunc arteriam, nunc neruum uel uenam uel carnem fieri. (*Acut.* 1.14.113)

And [Asclepiades says that] there is no digestion in us, but a crude dissolution of foods takes place in the stomach, and it moves through each individual part of the body, so that it looks as if it penetrates through all narrow passages; this he calls *leptomeres* ('of fine parts'), which is what we mean by *pneuma*; this (he says) has neither the quality of hot nor that of cold because of its extreme thinness, nor does it have any other tangible quality, but as it passes through the passages of the parts that receive nourishment, it becomes now artery, now sinew, now vein, now flesh.

(7) Item aliqui Asclepiadis sectatores gestationes et lauacra et uaporationes cataplasmatum atque malagmatum excluserunt in iecorosis suspicantes tenuissimorum corpusculorum fore consensum, hoc est spiritus, quem leptomerian eorum princeps appellauit, atque in egestorum constrictione falsitate causarum adiutoria magna recusantes. (*Chron.* 3.4.65)

Again, some followers of Asclepiades have excluded passive exercise, bathing, and fomentations by means of poultices and emollient plasters in the case of people suffering from disease of the liver, because they suspected that there would be a sympathetic affection of the finest particles, that is, of *pneuma*, which their master called *leptomereia*, and in a situation of congestion of matter they refuse to employ important remedies because of their false assumptions about causes.

From these passages it emerges that *spiritus* is the Methodist term for Asclepiades' notion of the *leptomeres*.[49] However, it is not clear that this is true in all cases, and even if it is, whether this is a satisfactory solution to our paradox. For passage (7) shows that the Methodists were not only critical of Asclepiades' therapeutics, but also of the physiological justification he offered for it. This raises the question why certain parts of Asclepiades' physiology were acceptable to Methodists while certain others met with

---

[49] For a discussion of this notion in Asclepiades, see Vallance (1990) 50–79.

vehement criticism.⁵⁰ This problem presents itself even more clearly when we get to a third category,

(iii) passages in which Caelius refers to parts of the body, or processes within the body, of which he explicitly states that they are invisible, such as the following:

(8) in quibusdam etiam sine sudore uires soluuntur et naturalis uigor *disiectione occulta, quam Graeci ἄδηλον διαφόρησιν uocant*, exstinguitur, cum omnis corporis habitudo laxior atque dimissa et friabilis fuerit facta. (*Acut.* 2.32.172)

In some people their physical strength simply dissolves without sweating and their natural vigour is destroyed because of an invisible dissolution, which the Greeks call *adēlos diaphorēsis*, which happens when the whole normal state of the body has become flabby and dissolved and fallen into decay.

(9) at si omnes partes fuerint solutione laxatae, similiter haec omnibus sunt adhibenda, in illis etiam, *quae occulta diaphoresi contabescunt*. differentia etenim accidentium mutata uidetur, genus autem passionis idem manet. (*Acut.* 2.37.217)

But if all parts are relaxed because of a state of looseness, these [measures] have to be applied similarly to all [parts of the body], also to those that decay as a result of an invisible dissolution. For although there seems to have occurred a difference in concomitant characteristics, the kind of the disease remains the same.

(10) plena igitur de his [sc. uomicis] tradenda est ratio. haec enim sunt, *quae in occultis natae collectiones nuncupantur*, ut in splanchnis ac membrana, quae latera cingit, uel in pulmone aut discrimine thoracis ac uentris, quod Graeci diaphragma uocant, item stomacho uel uentre, iecore, liene, intestinis, renibus, uesica aut mictuali uia uel matrice aut peritoneo... usum chirurgiae non exigunt, *siquidem sint occultis in locis et plurimis superpositis membris*. (*Chron.* 5.10.91–2)

We must give a full account of these [i.e. abscesses]. For these are the gatherings that are said to originate in invisible parts, for example in the intestines and in the membrane that surrounds the sides or in the lung or in the membrane that divides the chest and the abdomen, which the Greeks call the diaphragm, and also in the oesophagus or the stomach, the liver, the spleen, the intestines, the kidneys, the bladder or urinary passage, or the uterus or the peritoneum... [These] do not require the use of surgical measures, as they are located in invisible places and have many structures lying on top of them.

(11) Interiorum uero eruptionum diuisuras urgente solutionis coenoteta[m] ipsam magis cogimur iudicare, siquidem prior oculis occurrat solutio ac deinde diuisura *ratione atque intellectu mentis apprehendi uideatur*. (*Chron.* 2.12.147, partly quoted before as no. 4)

---

⁵⁰ This question is ignored in discussions of Asclepiades' influence on Methodism by Vallance (1990) 131ff., and Frede (1987a) 272f.

Yet as for the wounds that occur as a result of haemorrhage in the inner parts, since the generality of looseness prevails, we must judge it rather as just that, as it presents itself first to the eyes as a looseness, and after that it seems to be apprehended as a wound by reason and by an understanding of the mind.

Categories (i) and (ii) seem to present a problem which applies to Soranus no less than to Caelius Aurelianus. The question whether the Methodists believed that the generalities are observable with the senses, or at least to the expert's eye, has been discussed by other scholars[51] and is apparently to be answered affirmatively, though perhaps with the reservation that they are not *always* observable but *may* also, in some cases, be unobservable.[52] And Temkin has drawn attention to the fact that in Soranus' *Gynaecia*, too, we find Soranus on at least two occasions engaging in 'downright physiology' by referring to 'ducts' which are only visible to the mind.[53] These instances of speculative physiology have been explained as the result of the continuing influence of Asclepiadean doctrine on Methodism. Yet this explanation is not entirely satisfactory in the light of the severe criticism Asclepiades receives in Soranus and even more fiercely in Caelius Aurelianus. Moreover, there is evidence in Caelius himself (*Acut.* 3.19.189) that some Methodists, apparently unhappy with certain aspects of Asclepiades' physiology, modified the definition Asclepiades gave of cholera by replacing *concursus corpusculorum* by *raritas uiarum* (although this still involves a commitment to an unobservable entity).[54] This leaves us with the question why the Methodists, while rejecting so many aspects of Asclepiades' teaching, did not abolish Asclepiadean physiology altogether, if they really believed it to be unacceptable, or inconsistent with other parts of their system.

The answer I wish to suggest is that the Methodists, or at least Caelius, did not think that physiological speculation was unacceptable altogether, but that it was allowed under certain well-defined circumstances: as long as it does not affect treatment, there is nothing wrong with it (although it is

---

[51] Frede (1987a) 269–70; Pigeaud (1991) 23–8; Lloyd (1983) 196.
[52] As *Chron.* 3.2.19 shows, a generality may also be hidden and be intellectually inferred: *sin uero occulta fuerit solutio, quam Graeci adelon appellant, aut mente sensa signa uideantur, quae Graeci logotheoreta uocauerunt etc.* (for a translation see n. 46 above).
[53] 2.46 and 1.35 (Temkin (1956) xxxiii–xxxiv, nn. 31 and 32; see also Lloyd (1983) 192–3). It should be said that of these passages 2.46 is not quite conclusive, because Soranus is engaged there in a discussion of Asclepiades' views and may just be arguing *ex hypothesi*. The other passage, however, leaves little room for doubt. For references to Soranus' *pneuma* see n. 47 above.
[54] 'Again, some of our own people have handed down the same definition [sc. as that given by Asclepiades for the affection of cholera], removing [from it] only the gathering of particles and adding the widening of passages' (*item aliqui nostrorum tradiderunt eandem diffinitionem [sc. cholericae passionis ab Asclepiade datam] solum concursum corpusculorum detrahentes atque uiarum raritatem adicientes*).

irrelevant and hence useless to debate). But if it does affect treatment, one has to ensure the greatest possible accuracy and factual correctness.[55] And there are cases in which reference to invisible entities is simply unavoidable because of the nature of the disease, as in the example of haemorrhage (*sanguinis fluor*), which I shall discuss below.

2 CAUSAL EXPLANATION

We are told that Methodism rejected speculation about hidden causes (because they are hidden) and that, as far as *visible* causes were concerned, they took the view that although in some cases it may very well be possible to list the antecedent causes of a disease, this is irrelevant to its treatment.[56] We also hear of a work by Soranus on the causes of diseases, in which he is said to have given a comprehensive attack on the causal explanations proposed by other schools.[57] Again, there is abundant evidence in Caelius to confirm these reports about the Methodists' attitude towards causal explanation, for example:

(12) quod etiamsi lateret in partibus, periculum <nullum> Methodicis afferebat, qui generaliter congruas passionibus posuerunt curationes, etiam quibus particulariter latentia curentur. sciendum igitur, quia haec passio [sc. oppressio] ex iisdem causis antecedentibus fiet, quibus aliae quoque passiones efficiuntur, indigestione, uinolentia, carnali cibo et horum similibus rebus. <Soranus> cuius haec sunt, quae nostra mediocritas latinizanda existimauit, se uidisse plurimos memorat ex intemporali cibo uel plurimo puerorum ista oppressos passione. sed non inquit necessarium praecedentium causarum differentiam in curationibus praeuidere, siquidem praesentia sint a Methodicis intuenda. (*Acut.* 2.10.65)

---

[55] In this respect I diverge from Frede (1987a) 271: 'Soranus thought that there is nothing wrong with having theoretical views, as long as one keeps in mind that they are purely speculative, and as long as one does not base one's treatment on these views.' Later on, Frede does acknowledge that the Methodists accepted 'a more positive connection between medical theory and the art practiced by the doctor', but this turns out to be rather meagre ('Speculation did help us to focus our attention in the right direction... the theory... does provide some understanding and makes sense of our medical knowledge', p. 273) and I find no confirmation for this connection in the texts.

[56] Celsus, 1, proem 54; cf. Soranus, *Gyn.* 1.4; 3.17.

[57] *Chron.* 1.3.55: 'For that neither a god nor a semigod nor Eros is the cause of this disease has been explained by Soranus most comprehensively in his books on causes, which he called "Theories about Causes"' (*nam quod neque deus neque semideus neque Cupido sit, libris causarum, quos Aitiologumenos Soranus appellauit, plenissime explicauit*). It is possible that this work is identical to the work referred to as *De passionum causis* ('On the Causes of Affections') at *Acut.* 1.1.11, where it is suggested that this work contained an interesting discussion about the logical status of causes, and at *Acut.* 1.8.54, although there Caelius does not attribute it to Soranus but presents it as a work he himself is going to write (for the problem of the identification of the authorial *ego* and *nos* see n. 4 above). See also Soranus, *Gyn.* 3.17 and the discussion by Lloyd (1983) 193.

And even if this were hidden in the parts, this would pose no problem for the Methodists, who have proposed general treatments appropriate to diseases, even medicaments with which particularly the hidden parts are to be treated. One should know, then, that this disease [sc. catalepsy] originates from the same antecedent causes by which the other diseases are brought about, indigestion, drunkenness, the eating of meat and things similar to these. <Soranus>, whose views are expounded here, which we have humbly intended to put into Latin, tells that he has seen many young children being laid low by this disease as a result of untimely or excessive eating. Yet he says that it is not necessary to take account of a difference in preceding causes for the treatment, as it is the present Methodists ought to observe.

(13) nos autem superfluum fuisse causas passionis dicere iudicamus, cum sit necessarium id, quod ex causis conficitur, edocere. multo autem ac magis superfluum dicimus etiam causas antecedentes diffinitionibus adiungi. (*Acut.* 3.19.190)

We however judge that it was superfluous to state the causes of a disease, when it is necessary to set forth what is brought about by [these] causes. Yet even much more superfluous we consider the inclusion of preceding causes in the definitions.

(14) una est enim atque eadem passio ex qualibet veniens causa, quae una atque eadem indigeat curatione. (*Acut.* 2.13.87)

For the disease is one and the same, from whatever cause it comes, and it calls for one and the same treatment.

(15) sed non secundum has differentias erit efficacia curationis mutanda, siquidem antecedentes causae, quamquam diuersae, unam facere passionem uideantur. (*Chron.* 2.14.196)

But the effectiveness of the treatment ought not to be changed in accordance with these differences, as preceding causes, diverse though they are, seem to bring about one [and the same] disease.

(16) sunt autem passionis [sc. sanguinis fluoris] antecedentes causae, ut saepe approbatum est, percussio uel casus . . . sed non erit secundum has differentias curationis regula commutanda. (*Chron.* 2.9.118)

The preceding causes of this disease [sc. haemorrhage] are, as has often been established, a blow, a fall . . . but the mode of treatment ought not to be changed according to these differences.

All these passages (and there are several more in Caelius' work making the same point)[58] are in unison and confirm the disregard for causal explanations of diseases which seems so characteristic of Methodism.

However, we frequently find Caelius engaged in the causal explanation of a disease without any explicit reservation, usually in the *significatio* of the disease, where he lists the antecedent causes of the disease (in the majority

---

[58] E.g. *Acut.* 1.1.23; 3.6.64; 3.22.221.

of cases these are visible causes) without in any way restricting the relevance of these causal accounts.[59] He sometimes refers to hidden, or unknown, causes;[60] and in some cases we see him actually allowing that the cause of a disease *is* relevant to its treatment and including this cause in the definition of the disease, because it constitutes one of the relevant differentiae for the treatment.

Some clear illustrations of these attitudes are provided by the following passages:

(17) antecedentes causae, quibus haec sufficitur passio [sc. synanche], aliquae sunt *occultae*, aliquae *manifestae* atque ceteris quoque communes passionibus, maxime tamen conabiles atque laboriosi uomitus, plus etiam, si post cibum iam corruptum, item uinolentia uel niuis potatio aut exclamatio uehemens atque eodem modo perseuerans, quam Graeci monotonon uocant, item catarrhus et acriores cibi praeter consuetudinem accepti, item feruentia atque ignita medicamina pota uel purgatio per helleborum prouocata, quibusdam etiam feminis menstrualis retentio purgationis. afficiuntur autem hac passione magis uiri quam mulieres, quorum plus aetatis mediae et iuuenes quam pueri atque senes . . . nos uero iuxta Sorani sententiam synanchen dicimus difficultatem transuorandi atque praefocationem acutam *ob uehementiam tumoris faucium siue in locis, quibus nutrimenta transuora[ui]mus.* (*Acut.* 3.1.4–6)

As for the preceding causes through which this disease [sc. synanche] is brought about, some are invisible, others are manifest and identical to those of other diseases, in particular difficult and laboured vomiting, especially if this is done after the consumption of food that has gone off, drunkenness, the drinking of snow, ecstatic shouting which persists at the same tone, which the Greeks call *monotonos*, catarrh, acrid foods which one is not accustomed to, burning and fiery medicinal drinks or a purge provoked by hellebore, and with some women also the retention of the monthly discharge. This disease occurs more with men than women, and of these, with those who have reached middle age, and with young men rather than children and elderly people [. . .] We however, in accordance with Soranus' statement, say that synanche is a difficulty in swallowing and an acute choking caused by severe swelling of the throat or in the places in which we swallow nourishment.[61]

---

[59] E.g. *Acut.* 3.6.62: 'But the antecedent causes of the affections mentioned above are the following: a blow on the larger sinews, which the Greeks call *tenontes*, or lying upon them for a long time in the same position with something hard underneath' (*sed antecedentes causae supradictarum passionum sunt hae: percussus maiorum neruorum, quos tenontas appellant, uel supra ipsos iacendi iugis positio duris incumbens suppositis*). Cf. Soranus, *Gyn.* 4.35 and the very interesting chapters 4.1–6 where Soranus reports Demetrius of Apamea's account of the causes of difficult labour, which he seems to endorse.

[60] Examples follow below. For an example in Soranus see *Gyn.* 4.36 (paralysis of the uterus due to 'an unknown cause').

[61] This final sentence also indicates that the cause is relevant to the *definition* of the disease; on this see below.

(18) antecedens autem causa passionis [sc. hydrophobiae] est canis rabidi morsus uel, ut quidam memorant, ceterorum quoque animalium... est praeterea possibile *sine manifesta causa* hanc passionem corporibus innasci, cum talis fuerit strictio sponte generata, quali<s> a ueneno. (*Acut.* 3.9.99)

The preceding cause of this disease [i.e. hydrophobia] is the bite of a mad dog or, as some people record, of other animals... It is also possible that this disease originates in the body without a visible cause, when a constricted state similar to that produced by a poison occurs spontaneously.

(19) Nos autem iuxta Sorani iudicium hac quaestione nullis commodis curationes adiuuari probamus, sed dicimus tres esse differentias fluoris sanguinis, hoc est eruptionis, uulnerationis et putredinis siue lacerationis ex tussicula uenientis, sicut operantium manus iugi fricatione lacessiti uulnerantur; item sudationis sine uulnere siue ex raritate uiarum effectus fluor osculationis differentiam tenet siue expressionis uel cuiuslibet alterius causae. (*Chron.* 2.10.125)

We, however, in accordance with Soranus' judgement, believe that the treatment is in no way advanced by this dispute [sc. about various kinds of haemorrhage]; instead, we say that there are three different kinds of haemorrhage, namely eruption, wound and decomposition or abrasion caused by coughing, just as the hands of workmen are injured by constant rubbing; and a flow which involves a sweating without a wound or which is caused by a narrowness of channels can be distinguished as [flow caused by] anastomosis, or diffusion, or another cause.

How are these seemingly conflicting attitudes to be explained? Once again, it seems that the relevance of causal explanations to diagnosis and treatment varies from one disease to another. In the majority of cases, Caelius believes, the causal explanation of a disease, whether by reference to hidden or to observable causes, is not necessary: in many cases it is irrelevant and thus to be avoided, as it may even lead to errors in treatment.[62] It is irrelevant because it does not affect the present nature of the disease and thus does not affect the way the disease is treated, as was stated in passage (14) quoted above.[63] The present nature of the disease is different from the causes which brought it about;[64] causes may differ from case to case, but the nature of

---

[62] E.g. *Acut.* 3.4.45: 'Furthermore, it is ridiculous that he says that those who have got the affection synanche as a result of a cold should not be venesected; [in doing so], he does not pay attention to present things but inquires after the causes of things that are past' (*denique ridendum est etiam quod eos qui ex prefrictione synanchici fuerint effecti phlebotomandos negat [sc. Heraclides] non aduertens praesentia et inquirens factorum causas*) and *Acut.* 3.17.154: '[Hippocrates is led here] by a suspicion of the causes: for he thinks, or rather it is his firm belief, that the affection is caused by a burning heat of the upper parts and a chilling of the lower parts' (*suspicione causarum sollicitatus [sc. Hippocrates]: existimat enim uel constituit fieri passionem incendio superiorum et frigore inferiorum*).

[63] See also Soranus, *Gyn.* 1.52.

[64] *Acut.* 3.6.64–5: 'But against all these one common answer should be given: the cause of an affection is very different from the affection itself. One therefore has to state not what the cause of tetanus is, but

the disease is always the same; and conversely the same causes may lead to different diseases, as is stated in the following passage:

(20) sciendum igitur, quia haec passio ex iisdem causis antecedentibus fiet, quibus aliae quoque passiones efficiuntur, indigestione, uinolentia, carnali cibo et horum similibus rebus. (*Acut.* 2.10.65, more fully quoted under no. 12 above)

One should know, then, that this disease [sc. catalepsy] originates from the same preceding causes by which the other diseases are brought about, indigestion, drunkenness, the eating of meat and things similar to these.[65]

This does not come as a surprise, for the lists of antecedent causes of various diseases that Caelius offers, are always roughly the same: the taking of certain foods or drinks, drunkenness, a cold, indigestion, and suchlike. Hence in the majority of cases, the relevance of antecedent causes is very limited (because they are not peculiar to the disease), and the reason why Caelius discusses them altogether may be that they have the same status as signs:[66] they *may* constitute information that is relevant for the diagnosis and thus for the identification of a disease – and as such indirectly for the treatment[67] – but in the majority of cases this is not so.

However, as we have seen, there are cases in which a reference to the cause (or causes) is relevant, and in these cases it is perfectly all right to engage in causal explanations, for example in cases where the causes constitute the relevant criteria or differentiae for treatment as, again, in the case of haemorrhage, and it does not come as a surprise that in such cases they appear also in the definition of the disease.

3 DEFINITIONS

Closely related to the subject of causal explanation is the role of definitions. Again, a similar pattern may be detected. We are told that the Methodists refused to give definitions or to make use of other epistemological or logical tools derived from 'Dogmatist' dialectic, such as arguments based on demonstration, analogy or inferences.[68] The reason for this is assumed to be that the use of such Dogmatist logical tools would commit them to assumptions about the essence of diseases, whereas, for the reasons mentioned

---

what tetanus is' (*Sed his omnibus [sc. Asclepiadis sectatoribus... aliis... aliis nostrae sectae] communiter respondendum est, quomodo causa a passione plurimum differt. dicendum est igitur, non quae causa sit distentionis, sed quae sit distentio*).
[65] Cf. *Acut.* 1.1.23.   [66] This is suggested by *Chron.* 1.4.105.
[67] For the requirement of completeness in the symptomatology of the disease see *Acut.* 1.1.22.
[68] Galen, *De meth. med.* 1.1 (10.5 K.); 1.3 (10.30 K.); 2.5 (10.109 K.); see Frede (1987a) 276.

above (and their affiliation with Scepticism in particular), they were reluctant to do so.[69]

At first sight, Caelius seems to confirm this, for he repeatedly says that the Methodists, in particular Soranus, refused to give definitions.[70] On the other hand, we frequently see him (and Soranus) give concise statements of what a disease is in a form which there is no reason not to call a definition in the proper sense.[71] This apparent inconsistency has been noted by previous scholars. Thus Michael Frede has suggested that although the Methodists seem to give definitions, they are in fact giving descriptions, which do not claim to be uniquely appropriate;[72] and Danielle Gourevitch has drawn attention to the fact that what appear to be definitions are in fact accounts of the symptoms.[73] This receives confirmation from a passage in *Acut.* 2.10.64, where Caelius mentions *uera significatio* as the only relevant criterion for the identification, or recognition (*intelligentia*), of the disease.[74] This is a plausible solution, but it does not work for all the definitions we encounter in Caelius. For we sometimes see him giving definitions of a more 'Dogmatist' type consisting of genus and differentia specifica. Moreover, we see Caelius using concepts such as *genus, species, differentia* and *accidens*, which, on the above account, his Methodist background would strictly speaking not allow him to use.

---

[69] Frede (1987a) 274ff.

[70] *Acut.* 2.26.142: 'In accordance with Soranus, the Methodists refuse to give definitions' (*Diffinire Methodici iuxta Soranum iudicium declinant*). 2.31.163: 'Soranus refused to give definitions' (*Definitiones enim Soranus dicere declinauit*).

[71] Examples follow below. Caelius even uses the word *diffinitio* (*Acut.* 1.1.21: *intelligentiam siue diffinitionem passionis trademus dicentes*...). Cf. *Acut.* 2.1.8, where a Soranic definition is quoted ('Soranus... says that lethargy is a rapid or acute form of stupor accompanied by acute fevers and a pulse that is large, slow and hollow': *Soranus uero... pressuram inquit celerem esse uel acutam cum acutis febribus et pulsu magno ac tardo atque inani*), although the term *diffinitio* is not used here.

[72] Frede (1987a) 274.   [73] Gourevitch (1991) 67.

[74] See also *Acut.* 1.3.34: 'Our understanding of phrenitis is based on the whole gathering of symptoms' (*intelligimus phrenitim ex toto signorum concursu*). Cf. *Acut.* 2.3.13. From *Acut.* 1.1.21 we learn that this *intelligentia* ('understanding', 'identification') is actually the required activity, although here it is actually referred to by Caelius by means of the word *diffinitio*: 'We shall therefore present clearly and briefly, in so far as matters allow, the understanding or definition of the affection by saying that phrenitis is an acute derangement of the mind, accompanied by acute fever and futile groping of the hands, as if the patient is trying to grasp something with the fingers, which the Greeks call *krokodismos* or *karphologia*, and accompanied by a small, fast pulse' (*Nos igitur manifeste atque breuiter, quantum res patiuntur, intelligentiam siue diffinitionem passionis trademus dicentes phrenitim esse alienationem mentis celerem cum febri acuta atque manuum uano errore, ut aliquid suis digitis attrectare uideantur, quod Graeci crocodismon siue carphologiam uocant, et paruo pulsu et denso*). See also *Acut.* 2.31.163: 'For Soranus refused to give definitions. Therefore the recognition or understanding of this affection as handed down by Artemidorus of Sidon, a follower of Erasistratus, is as follows...' (*Definitiones enim Soranus dicere declinauit. cognitio igitur siue intelligentia eius passionis ab Artemidoro Sidensi Erasistrati sectatoris tradita est hoc modo...*).

The following passage provides a good example:

(21a) secundum nos igitur distentio est siue extentio, quam, ut supra diximus, tetanon Graeci uocauerunt, inuoluntaria tensio, recto atque inflexibili porrecta cremento collorum ob uehementem stricturam siue tumorem. (*Acut.* 3.6.65)

But according to us the stiffening or stretching, which, as we said above, the Greeks call tetanos, is an involuntary straining of the neck and its rigid prolongation straight upward, caused by a severe constriction or swelling.

This definition is not even a remotely complete description of the symptoms of this disease; nor does it claim to be one, for in fact such a description follows in the next section.[75] Moreover, this definition makes reference to the cause of the disease (*ob uehementem stricturam siue tumorem*), which is not what one would expect from an account of the symptoms.

Another example of such a type of definition is

(22a) est agnitio hydrophobiae appetentia uehemens atque timor potus sine ulla ratione atque ob quandam in corpore passionem. (*Acut.* 3.10.101)

The distinctive characteristic of hydrophobia is a powerful appetite and fear of water without any reason and because of some affection in the body.

What is interesting is that in the sequel to both passages Caelius proceeds to explain why the definition consists of its particular components. In the first passage, after having distinguished three types of spasm, he goes on to say:

(21b) sed inuoluntaria haec dicta sunt ad discretionem eorum, qui uoluntate sua colla hoc schemate componunt; ob tumorem autem siue stricturam ad discretionem <eorum>, qui ligationibus tormentuosis organi eas partes positas habent. (*Acut.* 3.6.66)

But these have been called 'involuntary' in order to distinguish them from those people who deliberately hold their neck in this position; and [it has been said to be] 'because of a swelling or a constricted state' in order to distinguish it from those people whose relevant bodily parts are put on torturing instruments.

And similarly in the second case:

(22b) adiectum est autem sine ulla ratione atque ob quandam in corpore passionem, quod alii timeant potum ut ueneni admixti suspicione uel arte prouidentes, quia, si intemporaliter sumpserint, periclitabuntur; neque ilico hi ratione timentes hydrophobi esse uel dici possunt. (*Acut.* 3.10.101)

---

[75] 3.6.66: 'Those who are about to lapse into these affections get the following symptoms: difficulty in moving the neck, frequent gaping, etc.' (*tentantibus igitur in has passiones deuenire haec obueniunt: difficilis cervicis motus, iugis oscitatio etc.*).

The addition 'without any reason and because of some affection in the body' is made because other people fear drinking out of a suspicion that it may be mixed with poison, or they are deliberately careful because, if they drink at the wrong time, they may be in danger; and people who are afraid for these reasons cannot immediately be called hydrophobes.

In both cases the definition is stated in such a form as to distinguish the disease from other phenomena that present themselves in a similar way but are due to a different cause.[76]

Not only do these passages appear difficult to accommodate within the supposedly categorical rejection by the Methodists of definitions; they also seem to go against the more specific ban on the inclusion of the *cause* in the definition, which Caelius expresses in the following passage:

(23) Nos autem superfluum fuisse causas passionis dicere iudicamus, cum sit necessarium id, quod ex causis conficitur, edocere. multo autem ac magis superfluum dicimus etiam *causas antecedentes diffinitionibus adiungi*, quippe cum nec sola cholerica passio ex indigestione fiat neque sola indigestio hanc faciat passionem, sed etiam aliae speciales atque contraria<e> virtutis, quarum nihil ex ista diffinitione monstratur, dehinc quod rheumatismus siue humoris fluor non solum uentris atque intestinorum sit, sed etiam stomachi. Quapropter, ut Soranus ait, cholerica passio est solutio stomachi ac uentris et intestinorum cum celerrimo periculo. sed antecedentes causas eius passionis dicimus... *quorum sane intellectus aptus rationi est ob causarum scientiam, inutilis uero ac <non> necessarius curationi uel naturae.* (*Acut.* 3.19.190, partly quoted under no. 13 above)

We, however, judge that it was superfluous to state the causes of the disease, when it is necessary to set forth what is brought about by (these) causes. Even much more superfluous we hold to be the inclusion of antecedent causes in the definitions, for neither is cholera the only disease caused by indigestion nor is indigestion the only thing to bring about this disease, but there are other special (causes) of diverse kinds, none of which become clear from this definition. Moreover, it is superfluous because the rheumatism or a flux of humour is not only of the belly and the intestines but also of the oesophagus. For this reason, as Soranus says, the choleric disease is a loose state of the oesophagus and the belly and the intestines with acute danger. The antecedent causes, however, we state to be the following... Yet while the understanding of these is certainly appropriate to the theoretical knowledge of the causes, it is useless and not necessary for the treatment or for the nature of the disease.

---

[76] For similar explanations of the components of the definition by reference to distinction from other similar phenomena see *Acut.* 3.1.5 (quoted above under no. 17), where, again, the cause of the disease (in this case, synanche) is referred to in the definition; see also Soranus, *Gyn.* 1.12; 1.19; 1.36.

This ban is also expressed in the following passage:

(24) sed superfluum est *causas adicere, cum passionem diffinimus*, quibus fuerit confecta defluxio. item alii defluxionem esse dixerunt uentris turbationem celerem uel acutam, quae fit ex corruptione ciborum. sed etiam nunc habet quaedam *superflua diffinitio*; dehinc etiam sine corruptione ciborum aut simili causa posse defluxionem fieri praeuide[a]mus. (*Acut.* 3.22.221)

But it is useless, when we are giving a definition of the disease, to add the causes through which diarrhoea is brought about. Others have said that diarrhoea is a rapid or acute disturbance of the belly taking place as a result of food that has gone off. Yet even now the definition contains superfluous elements; moreover, we can perceive that diarrhoea also occurs without corruption of food or a similar case.

These very interesting passages show the compatibility of the various Methodist attitudes towards definitions and causal explanations that we find in Caelius. The reason why the definitions Caelius rejects here (definitions of cholera and of diarrhoea given by Asclepiades and other anonymous people) are unsatisfactory is that in their references to causes they are misleading (because the cause stated does not necessarily lead to the disease in question), incomplete (because there may be other causes as well) and factually inaccurate. The reason is not the alleged general reason why Methodists refuse to give definitions, namely that a definition would commit them to views about the essence of diseases, essential and accidental characteristics, and suchlike – which would amount to the kind of commitment they do not wish to make – this also being the reason for their reluctance to use other instruments of Dogmatist dialectic such as *genus, species, accidens*, and so on. On the contrary, passage (23) shows, first, that Caelius (and Soranus) have no difficulty with giving a definition, provided that it is a proper definition – in this case, a concise statement of the generality (*coenotes*), of the affected parts, and of the acuteness of the disease – where properness is determined not only by factual correctness but also by the relevance of the components of the definition to diagnosis and treatment.[77] Secondly, the passage indicates that Caelius has no qualms about speaking about the nature or essence of the disease (*id, quod ex causis conficitur*, or *natura*, or *quae sit distentio*, also referred to as the *genus passionis* or just *passio*). Indeed, we also see Caelius at a number of occasions using concepts such as *genus, species* and *accidens*, as in:

(25) at si omnes partes fuerint solutione laxatae, similiter haec omnibus sunt adhibenda, in illis etiam, quae occulta diaphoresi contabescunt. differentia etenim accidentium mutata uidetur, genus autem passionis idem manet. (*Acut.* 2.37.217)

---

[77] Cf. *Acut.* 2.1.5 for criticism of the definition of lethargy as given by Alexander of Laodicea.

Yet if all parts were loosened by a state of looseness, these (medicaments) should similarly be applied to all parts, even to those that are consumed by an invisible decay. For the difference seems to be one of concomitant symptoms, but the kind of the diseases remains the same.

(26) Conicienda sunt eius praeterea accidentia, quae Graeci symptomata uocant, cum generali congrua curatione. (*Chron.* 3.5.71)

Moreover, one should consider the concomitant characteristics of the diseases, which the Greeks call symptoms, in connection with the treatment that is appropriate to the kind of disease.[78]

(27) Sed haec utraque Soranus excludit; nam primo dicto respondens ait aliud esse signum, aliud accidens. nam signum neque recedit et semper significato coniunctum est, accidens autem, quod Graeci symptoma uocant, nunc aduenit, nunc recedit, ex quibus esse intelligimus singula, quae febricitantium accidentia dixerunt, ut corporis difficilem motum, grauedinem, tensionem praecordiorum. (*Acut.* 2.33.176)

But Soranus rejects both of these, for against the first statement he argues that a sign is something different from a concomitant characteristic. For a sign does not disappear and is always connected with what is signified, but a concomitant characteristic, which the Greeks call a symptom, now appears, now disappears, from which points we understand that there are individual phenomena, which they say are the concomitant characteristics of people who have fever, such as difficulty with moving, heaviness, and a distention of the praecordium.

(28) declinante passione omnia supradicta minuentur, quae Graeci symptomata uocauerunt, nos accidentia passionis. (*Acut.* 3.18.177)

When the disease declines, all the above mentioned phenomena will decrease, which the Greeks call symptoms, but which we call concomitant characteristics.

(29) ac si passionibus fuerint appendicia, quae saepe generandorum animalium fuerunt causae, erunt congrua iisdem passionibus adhibenda. (*Chron.* 4.8.118)

But if they are consequences of diseases, which have often been the causes of the generation of these animals, measures have to be taken that are appropriate to the same diseases.

Thus as far as definitions as such are concerned, it seems that when Caelius – apparently bluntly – says that he, or Soranus, refuses to give definitions, he means that he and Soranus object to the uncritical, automatic procedure of trying to catch the essence of a disease in a definition. This can perhaps be understood against the background of a certain keenness on definitions

---

[78] Cf. *Acut.* 2.6.30: 'One should also attend the other concomitant signs of the disease, which the Greeks call *symptomata*' (*attendenda etiam cetera passionum accidentia, quae symptomata Graeci uocauerunt*).

as attested particularly in Soranus' contemporaries, the Pneumatists, who seem to have used definitions as a means of codifying knowledge about a disease in a form which easily facilitates memory and thus transmission (which is related to the role of definitions in doxographic traditions).[79] The Methodists object to this because in many cases a disease is too complicated a phenomenon to be caught in such a short verbal statement: some definitions suffer from inaccuracy, others from incompleteness; and yet others are criticised for containing irrelevant elements, such as references to antecedent causes (which are not peculiar to the disease in question). It seems that Caelius and Soranus are not against definitions as such, but against too automatic and uncritical an application of them, and to the misleading expectations this use raises. They do, however, engage in definitions themselves from time to time, and even include the cause in the definition if this is relevant to its treatment or to the distinction of various species of the disease.

What strikes one here is the flexibility with which Caelius uses these logical tools. There is no unqualified rejection of them, no dogmatic refusal to use them because they are Dogmatist and thus to be dismissed. In each particular case it must be considered whether they are relevant or not, and, if they are, what shape they should take. This flexibility is comparable to Caelius' attitude to nomenclature: in some cases he says that the name of a disease is totally arbitrary and it is useless to quarrel about why the disease acquired its particular name;[80] but in other cases, where its name *is* significant, Caelius does not fail to draw this to his readers' attention.[81]

4 RATIO AND EXPERIMENTUM

The distinction between reason and experience played a crucial role in the debates between the medical sects of later antiquity. In these debates, the Methodists are usually represented as having taken the following position: they relied primarily on what is manifest to the senses and were hostile to *a priori* reasoning,[82] although on the other hand their Asclepiadean heritage and terminology (not to mention their therapy and pharmacology) would distinguish them from the Empiricists. Thus Methodism may be said to have steered a kind of middle course between two extremes by reacting critically to both the Empiricists and the Dogmatists, while at the same time

---

[79] Cf. *Acut.* 3.19.189. Also, according to *Acut.* 1.1.20, Asclepiades wrote a book entitled *Diffinitiones*.
[80] E.g. *Chron.* 5.2.28.   [81] E.g. *Chron.* 3.1.1–2.
[82] E.g. Sextus Empiricus, *Outline of Pyrrhonism* 1.236ff.; Galen, *De sectis* 6 (p. 12 Helmreich, 1.79 K.).

combining accurate observation of a patient's symptoms with a moderately strong theoretical apparatus.[83]

Yet here, too, the picture is more complicated. First, the question arises of in what way the Methodist attitude to experience was different from that of the Empiricists; for we find Caelius, perhaps somewhat surprisingly, on several occasions speaking very scornfully about *experimentum*, experience, as it was used by the Empiricists. It is also unclear to what extent the Methodists nevertheless allowed for a selective use of theoretical reasoning;[84] for we often see Caelius appealing to reason (*ratio*) not only in polemical contexts (where he criticises the therapies proposed by other people or schools for their 'lack of reason') but also when he sets forth his own course of treatment.

As for *ratio*, however, it is important to specify in what sense this word is used:

(i) One category of usages are polemical contexts, where Caelius wishes to reveal the absurdities and irrationalities of the therapeutic ideas of other physicians, as in the following passages:

(30) dehinc sine ratione ad dierum numerum cibum dandum putat [sc. Diocles]. (*Acut.* 2.29.155)

Then without reason he [i.e. Diocles] holds that food should be given in accordance with the number of days.

(31) quae omnia, ut ratio demonstrat, sunt acria et propterea tumori contraria. (*Acut.* 2.29.156)

All these measures, as reason proves, are sharp and therefore opposed to the swelling.

In both passages, Caelius is criticising Diocles – a 'Rationalist' authority – for lack of rationality in his therapeutic instructions. There are several other passages in which other Dogmatists are criticised on the same grounds: their therapeutic, in particular their pharmacological recommendations are dismissed by Caelius for being *sine ratione*,[85] or *nullius rationis*,[86] or *contra*

---

[83] For a characterisation of the difference between Methodists and Empiricists see Frede (1987a) 270.
[84] On the Methodists' use of reason, i.e. their acceptance of 'truths of reason', see Frede (1987a) 265ff; for their use of reason as an instrument of refutation see Lloyd (1983) 190; for a critical reaction see Gourevitch (1991) 69. I should stress that my discussion of reason and experience in Caelius Aurelianus lays no claim to comprehensiveness; a much more thorough investigation of all the relevant passages is very desirable.
[85] E.g. *Acut.* 2.19.121; 1.16.165 (against Themison); cf. 2.9.49 (against Themison); 3.8.97 (against the Empiricists); *Chron.* 5.2.48.
[86] E.g. *Acut.* 1.16.157; cf. Soranus, *Gyn.* 1.46.

manifestam rationem,⁸⁷ or *praua ratione aestimatum*,⁸⁸ or *ratione commoti uera quidem, sed deficienti*.⁸⁹ *Ratio* refers here to a reasonable account, a rational justification.⁹⁰ This might suggest that Caelius is just fighting them with their own weapons without necessarily endorsing the premises of the argument (although this criticism is not restricted to Dogmatist doctors, but also directed against Themison and Heraclides).

Yet *ratio* is also used in non-polemical contexts. These usages can be divided into two further categories.

(ii) *ratio* is referred to as a source or criterion of knowledge, mostly concerning treatment (primarily pharmacological, but also dietetic and surgical), as in the following passage:

(32a) dabimus ea, quae non satis aliena sint ab his, quae rationi conueniunt, ut olus aut ptisana. (*Acut.* 1.11.81)

We will give things that are not very different from those that are in accordance with reason, such as vegetables and barley-gruel.

where the 'reason' is stated in dietetic terms:

(32b) dabit enim quiddam laxamenti atque indulgentiae asperitatibus animorum concupita oblatio, et non omnino sine cibo atque nutrimento perseuerabunt.

For giving the patients what they wish will give some relaxation and alleviation of the diseased state of their minds, and also they will not have to carry on without any food and nourishment at all.

A similar *ratio curationis* is referred to in the following passages:

(33) cataplasma laxatiuum et, si ratio coegerit, phlebotomia. (*Chron.* 4.8.119)

A loosening plaster and, if reason calls for it, venesection.

(34) ... sicut ratio probat atque Democriti dilatae mortis exemplum fama uulgatum. (*Acut.* 2.37.206)

...as is proved by reason and the famous example of the delayed death of Democritus.

It seems that *ratio* here refers to a reasoning (no doubt partly based on experience, but probably also partly of a theoretical kind) as to the best

---

⁸⁷ E.g. *Chron.* 2.2.64. ⁸⁸ E.g. *Chron.* 5.11.140. ⁸⁹ E.g. *Acut.* 3.14.116.
⁹⁰ See also *Acut.* 2.38.219: 'For that venesection differs in no way from killing is shown by reason, since it brings about what the affection itself aims for, namely the disruption of the body, etc.' (*etenim phlebotomiam nihil iugulatione differre ratio testatur, quippe cum haec faciat, quae ipsa nititur passio, meatum disicere et corpus*...), and *Acut.* 3.15.122: 'Reason evidently shows this' (*ratio quoque hoc ostendere uidetur*). Related to this is the usage of *ratio* in the context of Caelius' attack on superstition (e.g. *Acut.* 3.16.137); see Mudry (1998).

way of treatment based on a consideration of the state of the patient and the powers of the medicament.[91] This is confirmed by *Chron.* 2.14.202, where Caelius refers to a 'theory of remedies, which is called pharmacology' (*medicaminum ratio, quam pharmacian appellant*), where clearly a corpus of pharmacological knowledge is referred to, which he accepts.

It may not be a coincidence that the criticism of experience (*experimentum*) occurs precisely in these therapeutic contexts. It seems that especially in this area, *ratio* is considered to be a more reliable guide than *experimentum* – predominantly[92] experience as it was relied upon by the Empiricists, who are criticised for their 'vain' attempts, that is, treating their patients by trial and error, as in the following passage:

(35) et est haec experimenti tentatio, quam Graeci schediasticen piran uocant, quae non destinata passionibus adhibeat adiutoria, sed probanda. (*Chron.* 5.2.46)

And this method is one of trying by means of improvisation, which the Greeks call *schediastice peira*, which makes use of remedies that are not directed at the diseases themselves but which (as yet) have to be tested.[93]

The wording of this passage suggests that what Caelius criticises is the lack of a suitable orientation (*destinata*) and the failure to make use of relevant information about the state of the patient and the powers of the medicament – and for this orientation and consideration of relevant information, reason is an indispensable guide.[94] To be sure, this criticism applies, to some extent, to *all* non-Methodist treatment,[95] since Caelius believes also

---

[91] For other examples see *Acut.* 3.8.97; 3.16.137; *Chron.* 1.4.87. Cf. Gourevitch (1991) 69: 'Le méthodisme, donc, nous l'avons déjà dit, est un dogmatisme; comme tout dogmatisme il va au traitement par un raisonnement.' In some cases, e.g. *Chron.* 1.5.175, Caelius' appeal to *ratio* is ironical, because it refers to the erroneous therapeutic reasoning of other medical schools (cf. Drabkin's note ad loc.).

[92] Though not exclusively, as is shown by the criticism of Praxagoras in *Chron.* 1.4.135 (see n. 95 below), and of Asclepiades in *Acut.* 2.9.43.

[93] For other criticisms of *experimentum* see, e.g., *Acut.* 1.15.127; 1.17.170; 3.4.45; 3.8.97; 3.16.137; *Chron.* 1.4.129; 1.5.178; 5.2.46. For *ratio* in criticism of Empiricist therapy cf. *Acut.* 2.29.160.

[94] Another illuminating passage is *Acut.* 3.4.45: 'But it is clear that this is all a matter of experimenting and trial and based on obscure speculations. For the Empiricist looks only at observation, which they call *teresis*, and believes that in this case only full-blooded people should be venesected, not realising that because of the severity of the stricture all those who suffer from synanche should be venesected, as long as their strength permits' (*sed hoc omne experimentum siue tentatio promptissime ex occultis suspicionibus uidetur esse prouisa. etenim Empiricus solam seruationem intuens, quam teresin uocant, sanguinosos nunc phlebotomandos existimat* **non aduertens, quia omnes synanchicos ob stricturae uehementiam oportet phlebotomari permittentibus uiribus**). Cf. also *Acut.* 3.8.97: 'Frog soup may be called an experiment and it is offensive, as of itself it has no advantage which reason proves' (*iuscellum autem ranarum experimentum esse dicitur et est odiosum, in semet nihil habens commodi, quod ratio probet*).

[95] See *Chron.* 1.4.135: 'All these measures are tested neither by reason nor by diet, but by trying them out' (*haec omnia [sc. remedia Praxagorae] experta neque ratione neque regula, sed tentatione probantur*). Cf. *Acut.* 3.8.97 (criticism of Asclepiades) and *Chron.* 1.5.178 (criticism of the leaders of the other sects).

the Dogmatists' views on the treatment of diseases to be pathetically and dangerously erroneous; but it is the Empiricists' claim to be basing themselves on experience which, so to speak, invites them to be singled out for Caelius' most vehement castigation.[96]

However, Caelius' acceptance of reason as a source of knowledge is not restricted to therapeutics (where it may seem to amount to a sort of practical reasoning based on experience, common sense and perhaps some specialised knowledge about medicaments):

(iii) *Ratio* may also be used as an instrument of theoretical knowledge about internal states of the body. Once again, the chapter on haemorrhage (*sanguinis fluor*) is important:

(36) Interiorum uero eruptionum diuisuras urgente solutionis coenoteta[m] ipsam magis cogimur iudicare, siquidem prior oculis occurrat solutio ac deinde diuisura *ratione atque intellectu mentis apprehendi* uideatur. (*Chron.* 2.12.147, quoted earlier under nos. 4 and 11)

Yet as for the wounds that occur as a result of haemorrhage in the inner parts, since the generality of looseness prevails, we must judge it rather as just that, since it presents itself first to the eyes as a looseness, and after that it seems to be apprehended as a wound by reason and by an understanding of the mind.[97]

This passage stands in a very complicated argument about the generality to which haemorrhage is to be assigned, and the chapter is of great importance for the Methodist doctrine of the generalities (for it suggests that there are actually more than three generalities – *ulcus, ruptio, emissio* also seem to be among them – and that the question of generalities is different in surgery from in dietetics and pharmacology).[98] The argument is further complicated by a polemic against Thessalus and by a division of medicine into treatment by surgery, on the one hand, and treatment by diet and drugs, on the other. The question which Caelius addresses is whether haemorrhage should be regarded as a wound (*incisura* or *diuisura*) or as a loose state (*solutio*), and Thessalus is presented by Caelius as arguing that, since a bleeding at the surface of the body is clearly a wound, and since differences in location do not affect the question of generality, internal bleeding must also be regarded as a wound. To this Caelius replies, first, that haemorrhage

---

[96] Cf. *Acut.* 3.4.45.
[97] For another example of the use of *ratio* as an instrument of mental apprehension see *Chron.* 2.1.14: 'It is theoretically plausible that the other individual inner parts are also affected by paralysis, such as the lungs... but the death of the patient prevents us from recognising this. These facts often escape our notice, since there are no signs peculiar to them that indicate them' (*Est autem ratione credibile ceterorum quoque interiorum singula paralysi uitiari, ut pulmonem... <sed> praeueniri apprehensione<m> morte[m] patientis; quae saepe latent facta, cum non propria possint apprehensione signari*).
[98] This is confirmed by Galen, *De optima secta* 32 (1.192–3 K.).

is treated by diet and drugs rather than by surgical measures, which would suggest that it is a loose state rather than a wound; secondly, he gives the argument quoted here: its state of looseness presents itself clearly to the eyes, whereas to label it as a wound, though not false, requires a mental activity.

In this surprisingly revealing passage, we read, first of all, an explicit statement to the effect that the generality, in this case a loose state, presents itself to the eyes: one can clearly see that haemorrhage is a *solutio*. But we also read that apprehension by the mind – *ratio atque intellectus mentis* – is a means of knowing that it is an internal wound. Caelius commits himself here to the existence of a state which can only be apprehended by reason – the principle of *logotheōrētos* which is familiar from Erasistratus and especially Asclepiades. Indeed, another passage states this principle explicitly:

(37) Sin uero occulta fuerit solutio, quam Graeci adelon appellant, aut mente sensa signa uideantur, quae Graeci logotheoreta uocauerunt, sequitur debilitas pulsus aegrotantis... (*Chron.* 3.2.19)

But if the state of looseness is invisible, which the Greeks call *adelos*, or if signs [of it] seem to be perceived by the mind, signs which the Greeks call *logotheoreta*, it is followed by a weakness of the pulse of the patient...

These passages clearly indicate that Caelius does not regard physiological speculation as wholly unacceptable, and that he believes that mental apprehension can lead to knowledge about internal states that can be relied upon for treatment. Thus it is simply not true that the Methodists do not wish to commit themselves to the existence, or the occurrence, of unobservable entities or processes, and there is no indication that they believe that knowledge about the invisible is *impossible*. It is rather that they prefer not to build their therapy on such speculations or commitments; but this is a matter of *preference*, based on the criterion of relevance,[99] rather than a matter of unqualified rejection based on the belief that such commitments would necessarily be uncertain. For the most part, the Methodists will claim that as long as it is not necessary to build one's therapy on such commitments, one should do without them. However, in cases in which reference to unobservable entities is unavoidable or even desirable, for example because such reference provides relevant distinctions (as in the case

---

[99] See *Chron.* 5.10.105, where Caelius comments on the dispute about 'passages in the body that are "rational, irrational or hidden"' (*rationales... irrationales... latentes uiae*): 'But one should not argue too much about these, for it is sufficient for the purpose of giving an account of the symptoms to consider only what is manifest' (*sed non oportet de his plurimum disputare, sufficit enim ad disciplinam significationis faciundae manifesta comprobare*).

of internal bleedings), there is no impediment to it, and it *is* possible to proceed on the basis of a sufficient degree of certainty about these entities.

5 CONCLUSION

To the best of my knowledge, passages like those just quoted are without parallel in Soranus, and it is tempting to believe that they represent a further development in Methodism. Yet bearing in mind what was said earlier about the difficulties involved in comparing Soranus with Caelius, we should be careful here not to overstate the case. Moreover, especially in the case of definitions, and to a lesser extent also in the case of causal explanations, we see Caelius actually appealing to Soranus for support and quoting Soranic definitions and statements about causes. Hence in these cases the explanatory scenario of 'tensions inherent in Methodism as such' would seem to present itself as more plausible; it may remain a matter of opinion whether these tensions are real or can be solved, mitigated or at least appreciated, along the lines of what I have called the criterion of relevance.

Against this, one might still argue that these appeals to Soranus concern Soranus as he appears in Caelius Aurelianus, who may have created his own image of his great precursor to make it suit his own version of Methodism (comparable to the way in which Galen created his image of Hippocrates for his own purposes); and it would certainly be worth examining in what types of context Soranus is quoted, and what (rhetorical) reasons underly Caelius' practice of quoting him (and other authorities).[100] Yet for the present it seems preferable to refrain from such developmental speculations: *neque ualde nobis de hoc certandum est, ne in occulta quaestione uersemur.*[101]

[100] On this question, see van der Eijk (1999c).   [101] *Acut.* 2.34.183.

Bibliography

Abel, K. (1958), 'Die Lehre vom Blutkreislauf im Corpus Hippocraticum', *Hermes* 86, 192–219 (reprinted with a 'retractatio' in Flashar (ed.) (1971) 121–64)
Ackerknecht, E. H. (1968), *A Short History of Medicine*, 2nd edn, Baltimore and London
 (1973), *Therapeutics from the Primitives to the Twentieth Century*, London and New York
 (1982), 'Diathesis: the word and the concept in medical history', *Bulletin of the History of Medicine* 56, 317–25
Ackrill, J. L. (1963), *Aristotle. Categories and De Interpretatione*, Oxford
 (1972–3), 'Aristotle's definitions of psuchê', *Proceedings of the Aristotelian Society* 73, 119–33 (reprinted in Barnes, Schofield and Sorabji (eds.), vol. IV (1979) 65–75)
Alexanderson, B. (1963), *Die hippokratische Schrift 'Prognosticon'. Überlieferung und Text*, Stockholm
Althoff, J. (1992a), *Warm, kalt, flüssig und fest bei Aristoteles. Die Elementarqualitäten in den zoologischen Schriften*, Stuttgart
 (1992b), 'Das Konzept der generativen Wärme bei Aristoteles', *Hermes* 120, 181–93
 (1993), 'Formen der Wissensvermittlung in der frühgriechischen Medizin', in Kullmann and Althoff (eds.) (1993) 211–23
 (1995), 'Von der Lehrdichtung zur Prosa. Zu den Formen und Gattungen frühgriechischer wissenschaftlicher Literatur', Freiburg (unpublished Habilitationsarbeit)
 (1997), 'Aristoteles' Vorstellung von der Ernährung der Lebewesen', in W. Kullmann and S. Föllinger (eds.), *Aristotelische Biologie. Intentionen, Methoden, Ergebnisse*, Stuttgart, 351–64
 (1998), 'Die aphoristisch stilisierten Schriften des Corpus Hippocraticum', in Kullmann, Althoff and Asper (eds.) (1998) 37–64
 (1999), 'Aristoteles als Medizindoxograph', in van der Eijk (ed.) (1999a) 33–56
Aly, W. (1929), *Formprobleme der frühgriechischen Prosa* (Philologus, Suppl. 21, no. 3), Leipzig
Amigües, S. (1988, 1989, 1993), *Théophraste. Recherches sur les plantes*, Books I–II, III–IV and V–VI, Paris

Amouretti, M. C. and Comet, G. (1995), *La transmission des connaissances techniques* (Cahier d'Histoire des Techniques 3, Publications de l'Université de Provence), Aix-en-Provence
Amundsen, D. W. and Diers, C. J. (1969), 'The age of *menarche* in Classical Greece and Rome', *Human Biology* 41, 125–32
André, J. (1981), *L'alimentation et la cuisine à Rome*, Paris
  (1985), *Les noms de plantes dans la Rome antique*, Paris
  (1991), *Le vocabulaire latin de l'anatomie*, Paris
Angelino, C. and Salvaneschi, E. 1982, *La 'melanconia' dell' uomo di genio*, Genova
Annas, J. (1986), 'Aristotle on memory and the self', *Oxford Studies in Ancient Philosophy* 4, 99–117
  (1992), *Hellenistic Philosophy of Mind*, Berkeley
Anton, J. and Kustas, G. (eds.) (1971), *Essays in Ancient Greek Philosophy*, Albany, New York
Arnim, H. von (1927), 'Die Echtheit der *Großen Ethik* des Aristoteles', *Rheinisches Museum* 76, 113–37 and 225–53
  (1928), *Eudemische Ethik und Metaphysik* (Sitzungsberichte der Akademie der Wissenschaften Wien 207.5), Vienna
  (1929), *Der neueste Versuch, die Magna Moralia als unecht zu erweisen* (Sitzungsberichte der Akademie der Wissenschaften Wien 211.2), Vienna
Artelt, W. (1937), *Studien zur Geschichte der Begriffe 'Heilmittel' und 'Gift'*, Leipzig
Asper, M. (1998), 'Zur Struktur eisagogischer Schriften', in Kullmann, Althoff and Asper (eds.) (1998) 309–40
Aubenque, P. (1963), *La prudence chez Aristote*, Paris
  (1979), *Etudes sur la Métaphysique d'Aristote*, Paris
Aubert, H. and Wimmer, F. (1868), *Aristoteles. Thierkunde*, vol. 1, Leipzig
Aubert, J.-J. (1989), 'Threatened wombs: aspects of ancient uterine magic', *Greek, Roman and Byzantine Studies* 30, 421–49
Aune, D. E. (1983), *Prophecy in Early Christianity and the Ancient Mediterranean World*, Grand Rapids
Babut, D. (1974), *La religion des philosophes grecs*, Paris
Balme, D. M. (1985), 'Aristotle *Historia Animalium* Book Ten', in J. Wiesner (ed.), *Aristoteles. Werk und Wirkung*, vol. 1, Berlin, 191–206
  (1987), 'The place of biology in Aristotle's philosophy', in Gotthelf and Lennox (eds.) (1987) 9–20
  (1991), *Aristotle, History of Animals VII–X*, Cambridge, Mass. and London
  (2002), *Aristotle. Historia Animalium*, vol 1: *Books I–X, Text*, Cambridge
Balss, H. (1936), 'Die Zeugungslehre und Embryologie in der Antike', *Quellen und Studien zur Geschichte der Naturwissenschaften und der Medizin* 5.2–3, 1–82
Bardong, K. (1954), 'Praxagoras', *RE* XII.2, 1735–43
Barker, A. (1981), 'Aristotle on perception and ratios', *Phronesis* 26, 248–66
Barnes, J. (1971–2), 'Aristotle's concept of mind', *Proceedings of the Aristotelian Society* 72, 101–14 (reprinted in Barnes, Schofield and Sorabji (eds.), vol. IV (1979) 32–41)

(1983), 'Ancient Scepticism and causation', in M. Burnyeat (ed.), *The Skeptical Tradition*, Berkeley, 190–1

(ed.) (1984), *The Complete Works of Aristotle. The Revised Oxford Translation*, 2 vols., Princeton

Barnes, J., Schofield, M. and Sorabji, R. (eds.) (1975–9), *Articles on Aristotle*, 4 vols. (I: *Science*; II: *Ethics and Politics*; III: *Metaphysics*; IV: *Psychology and Aesthetics*), London

Barra, G. (1957), 'Δαιμονία φύσις', *Rendiconti della Academia di Archeologia, Lettere e Belle Arti di Napoli*, N.S. 32, 75–84

Barton, T. (1994), *Power and Knowledge. Astrology, Physiognomics, and Medicine under the Roman Empire*, Ann Arbor

Baumann, E. D. (1925), 'Die heilige Krankheit', *Janus* 29, 7–32

Bäumker, C. (1877), *Des Aristoteles' Lehre von den äussern und innern Sinnesvermögen*, Leipzig

Beard, M. (1986), 'Cicero and divination', *Journal of Roman Studies* 76, 33–46

Beare, J. I. (1906), *Greek Theories of Elementary Cognition from Alcmaeon to Aristotle*, Oxford

Beare, J. I. and Ross, G. R. T. (1908), *The Parva Naturalia*, Oxford (reprinted in W. D. Ross (ed.), *The Works of Aristotle Translated into English*, vol. III, Oxford, 1931)

Beck, H. and Spät, F. (1896), *Auszüge eines Unbekannten aus Aristoteles–Menons Handbuch der Medizin und aus Werken anderer älterer Ärzte*, Berlin

Beintker, E. and Kahlenberg, W. (1948–52), *Galenos. Die Kräfte der Nahrungsmittel* (Die Werke des Galenos, vols. III–IV), Stuttgart

Bekker, I. (1831), *Aristotelis opera*, 2 vols., Berlin

Belfiore, E. (1985), 'Pleasure, tragedy and Aristotelian psychology', *The Classical Quarterly*, N.S. 35, 349–61

(1986), 'Wine and catharsis of the emotions in Plato's Laws', *The Classical Quarterly*, N.S. 36, 421–37

Bender, H. (1855), *Die kleinen naturwissenschaftlichen Schriften des Aristoteles*, Stuttgart

Bendz, G. (1943), 'Zu Caelius Aurelianus', *Eranos* 41, 65–76

Bendz, G. and Pape, I. (1990–3), *Caelius Aurelianus. Akute Krankheiten Buch I–III. Chronische Krankheiten Buch I–V*, 2 vols., Berlin

Benes, E. (1971), 'Fachtext, Fachstil und Fachsprache', *Sprache und Gesellschaft* 13, 118–32

(1976), 'Syntaktische Besonderheiten der deutschen wissenschaftlichen Fachsprache', in K.-H.-S. Bausch, W. H. U. Schwewe and H.-R. Spiegel (eds.), *Fachsprachen. Terminologie, Struktur, Normung* (Deutsches Institut für Normung e. V., Normungskunde no. 4), Berlin and Cologne, 88–98

Berry, E. G. (1940), *The History of the Concept of θεία μοῖρα and θεια τύχη down to Plato*, Chicago

Berti, E. (1962), *La filosofia del primo Aristotele*, Padua

Bertier, J. (1972), *Mnésithée et Dieuchès*, Leiden

Bicknell, P. J. (1969), 'Democritus' theory of precognition', *Revue des Etudes Grecques* 82, 318–26

(1970), 'Democritus' parapsychology again', *Revue des Etudes Grecques* 83, 303

(1981), 'Déjà vu, autoscopia and Antipheron. Notes on Aristotle, *De Memoria* 451 a 8–12', *L'Antiquité Classique* 24, 156–9

Bidez, J. and Leboucq, G. (1944), 'Une anatomie antique du cœur humain. Philistion de Locres et le "Timée" de Platon', *Revue des Etudes Grecques* 57, 7–40

Biehl, W. (1898), *Aristoteles. Parva naturalia*, Leipzig

Bien, C. G. (1998), 'Der "Bruch" in Aristoteles' Darstellung des Zeugungsbeitrags von Mann und Frau', *Medizinhistorisches Journal* 33, 3–17

Binswanger, L. (1928), *Wandlungen in der Auffassung und Deutung des Traumes*, Zurich

Birt, T. (1882), *Das antike Buchwesen in seinem Verhältnis zur Literatur*, Berlin

Björck, G. (1946), ' ὄναρ ἰδεῖν. De la perception de rêve chez les anciens', *Eranos* 44, 306–14

Block, I. (1960), 'Aristotle and the physical object', *Philosophy and Phenomenological Research* 21, 93–101

(1961a), 'The order of Aristotle's psychological writings', *American Journal of Philology* 82, 50–77

(1961b), 'Truth and error in Aristotle's theory of sense-perception', *Philosophical Quarterly* 11, 1–9

(1964), 'Three German commentators on the individual senses and the common sense in Aristotle's psychology', *Phronesis* 9, 58–63

(1965), 'On the commonness of the common sensibles', *Australasian Journal of Philosophy* 43, 189–95

(1988), 'Aristotle on the common sense. A reply to Kahn and others', *Ancient Philosophy* 8, 235–50

Blum, R. H. and Blum, E. (1965), *Health and Healing in Rural Greece*, Stanford and London

Bodéüs, R. (1975), 'En marge de la "théologie" aristotélicienne', *Revue Philosophique de Louvain* 78, 5–33

(1981), 'Dieu et la chance à travers les énigmes du Corpus aristotélicien', *L'Antiquité Classique* 50, 45–56

(1986), *Aristote et l'irrationnel en nous* (Cahiers du Département de Philosophie de l'Université de Montréal 86–7), Montréal

(1987), 'Aristote a-t-il fait l'hypothèse de pulsions inconscientes à l'origine du comportement humain?', *Dialogue* 26, 705–14

(1988), 'L'exemple du Dieu dans le discours aristotélicien', *Etudes françaises Montréal* 24, 27–33

(1990), 'La prétendue intuition de Dieu dans le *De Coelo* d'Aristote', *Phronesis* 35, 245–57

(1992), *Aristote et la théologie des vivants immortels*, Paris

(1993), *The Political Dimensions of Aristotle's Ethics*, Albany

Bollack, J. (1965–9), *Empédocle*, 4 vols., Paris

Boncampagni, R. (1972), 'Concezione della malattia e senso dell'individualità nei testi cnidi del Corpus Hippocraticum', *La parola del passato* 145, 209–38

Bonitz, H. (1870), *Index Aristotelicus*, Berlin (2nd edn, 1961)

Bouché-Leclerq, A. (1879–82), *Histoire de la divination dans l'antiquité*, 4 vols., Paris

Bourgey, L. (1953), *Observation et expérience chez les médecins de la Collection hippocratique*, Paris

(1955), *Observation et expérience chez Aristote*, Paris

Bourgey, L. and Jouanna, J. (eds.) (1975), *La Collection hippocratique et son rôle dans l'histoire de la médecine*, Leiden

Bowen, A. C. (ed.) (1991), *Science and Philosophy in Classical Greece*, New York and London

Boyancé, P. (1936), *Le culte des muses chez les philosophes grecs*, Paris

Boylan, M. (1982), 'The digestive and "circulatory" systems in Aristotle's biology', *Journal of the History of Biology* 15, 89–118

(1983), *Method and Practice in Aristotle's Biology*, Washington

Braet, A. (1983), *De klassieke statusleer in modern perspectief*, Groningen

Braet, A. and Berkenbosch, R. (1990), *Academisch debatteren: Theorie en praktijk*, Groningen

Brain, P. (1986), *Galen on Bloodletting*, Cambridge

Bravo García, A. (1985), 'Fisiología y filosofía en Aristóteles. El problema de los sueños', *Cuadernos de Filología del Colegio Universitario de Ciudad Real* 5, 15–65

Brelich, A. (1966), 'The place of dreams in the religious world concept of the Greeks', in G. von Grünebaum and R. Caillois (eds.), *The Dream and Human Societies*, Berkeley and Los Angeles, 293–303

Bremer, D. (1980), 'Aristoteles, Empedokles und die Erkenntnisleistung der Metapher', *Poetica* 12, 350–76

Bremmer, J. N. (1983), *The Early Greek Concept of Soul*, Princeton

Brentano, F. (1867), *Die Psychologie des Aristoteles*, Mainz

Brès, Y. (1968), *La psychologie de Platon*, Paris

Brillante, C. (1986), 'Il sogno nella riflessione dei presocratici', *Materiali e Discussioni per l'Analisi dei Testi Classici* 16, 9–53

(1987), 'La rappresentazione del sogno nella frammento di un *threnos* pindarico', *Quaderni Urbinati di Cultura Classica* 25, 35–51

Brink, K. O. (1932), *Stil und Form der pseudoaristotelischen Magna Moralia*, Berlin

Brock, A. J. (1916), *Galen. On the Natural Faculties*, Cambridge, Mass. and London

Brock, N. van (1961), *Recherches sur le vocabulaire médical du grec ancien: soins et guérison*, Paris

Brothwell, D. and Sandison, A. T. (1967), *Diseases in Antiquity*, Springfield

Brown, C. (1986), 'Seeing sleep: Heraclitus fr. 49 Marcovich (DK 22 B 21)', *American Journal of Philology* 107, 243–5

Bruins, E. M. (1951), 'La chimie du Timée', *Revue de Métaphysique et de Morale* 56, 269–82

Bruun, H. (1997), '*De morbo sacro* and *De aere aquis locis*', *Classica et mediaevalia* 48, 115–48
(1999), 'Sudden death as an apoplectic sign in the Hippocratic Corpus', *Classica et mediaevalia* 50, 5–24
Bryant, J. M. (1986), 'Intellectuals and religion in Ancient Greece; notes on a Weberian theme', *British Journal of Sociology* 37, 269–96
Büchsenschütz, B. (1868), *Traum und Traumdeutung im Altertum*, Wiesbaden
Buck, A. de (1939), *De godsdienstige opvatting van de slaap, inzonderheid in het oude Egypte*, Leiden
Buckley, Th. and Gottlieb, A. (eds.) (1988), *Blood Magic. The Anthropology of Menstruation*, Berkeley, Los Angeles and London
Burckhardt, R. (1904), 'Das koische Tiersystem, eine Vorstufe der zoologischen Systematik des Aristoteles', *Verhandlungen der naturforschenden Gesellschaft in Basel* 15, 377–414
Burguière, P., Gourevitch, D. and Malinas, Y. (1988–2000), *Soranos d'Ephèse. Maladies des femmes*, 4 vols., Paris
Burkert, W. (1977), 'Air-imprints or eidola? Democritus' aetiology of vision', *Illinois Classical Studies* 2, 97–109
Burkert, W. et al. (ed.) (1998), *Fragmentsammlungen philosophischer Texte der Antike – Le raccolte dei frammenti di filosofi antichi*, Göttingen
Burnyeat, M. F. (1970), 'The material and sources of Plato's dream', *Phronesis* 15, 101–22
Bussemaker, U. C. (1854), *Aristoteles. Parva naturalia*, in F. Dübner, U. C. Bussemaker and J. H. E. Heitz, *Aristoteles. Opera omnia graece et latine*, vol. III, Paris
Byl, S. (1968), 'Note sur la place du cœur et la valorisation de la mesotes dans la biologie d'Aristote', *L'Antiquité Classique* 37, 467–76
(1979), 'Quelques idées grecques sur le rêve, d'Homère à Artémidore', *Les Etudes Classiques* 47, 107–22
(1980), *Recherches sur les grands traités biologiques d'Aristote: sources écrites et préjugés*, Brussels
(1998), 'Sommeil et insomnie dans le Corpus Hippocratique', *Revue Belge de Philologie* 76, 31–6
Byl, S. and Szafran, W. (1996), 'La phrénitis dans le Corpus Hippocratique: Etude philologique et médicale', *Vesalius* 2, 98–105
Calabi, F. (1984), 'Gli occhi del sonno', *Materiali e Discussioni per l'Analisi dei Testi Classici* 13, 23–43
Caley, E. R. and Richards, J. F. C. (1956), *Theophrastus. On Stones*, Columbus, Ohio
Cambiano, G. (1980), 'Democrito e i sogni', in F. Romano (ed.), *Democrito e l'atomismo antico. Atti del Convegno internazionale* (Siculorum Gymnasium N. S. 33), Catania, 437–50
(1980), 'Une interprétation "matérialiste" des rêves: du Régime IV', in M. D. Grmek (ed.), *Hippocratica. Actes du troisième colloque international hippocratique*, Paris, 87–96

Cambiano, G. and Repici, L. (1988), 'Aristotele e i sogni', in Guidorizzi (ed.) (1988) 121–36
Campese, S., Manuli, P. and Sissa, G. (1983), *Madre materia. Sociologia e biologia della donna greca*, Turin
Capelle, W. (1925), 'Älteste Spuren der Astrologie bei den Griechen', *Hermes* 60, 373–95
 (1931), 'Straton von Lampsakos', *RE* IV.1, 278–315
Cappelletti, A. J. (1987a), 'La teoria del sueño y los origines de la parapsicología en Aristoteles', *Diálogos* 50, 27–37
 (1987b), *Las teorias del sueño en la filosofía antigua*, Caracas
Capriglione, J. C. (1983), *Prassagora di Cos*, Naples
Casevitz, M. (1982), 'Les mots du rêve en grec ancien', *Ktema* 7, 67–74
Cashdollar, S. (1973), 'Aristotle's account of incidental perception', *Phronesis* 18, 156–75
Castagno, A. M. (1992), 'L'interpretazione origeniana di Mc. 4,10–12: aspetti e problemi della difesa del libero arbitrio', in Perrone (ed.) (1992), 85–104
Castiglioni, A. (1940), 'Aulus Cornelius Celsus as a historian of medicine', *Bulletin of the History of Medicine* 8, 862–6
Chaniotis, A. (1995), 'Illness and cures in the Greek propitiatory inscriptions and dedications of Lydia and Phrygia', in van der Eijk, Horstmanshoff and Schrijvers (eds.) (1995), vol. II, 323–44
Chantraine, P. (1975), 'Remarques sur la langue et le vocabulaire du Corpus hippocratique', in L. Bourgey and J. Jouanna (eds.), *La Collection hippocratique et son rôle dans l'histoire de la médecine*, Leiden, 35–40
Charlton, W. (1970), *Aristotle's Physics I & II*, Oxford
Chroust, A. H. (1974), 'Aristotle's *Protrepticus* versus Aristotle's *On Philosophy*: a controversy over the nature of dreams', *Theta-Pi* 3, 168–78
Clarke, E. (1963a), 'Apoplexy in the Hippocratic writings', *Bulletin of the History of Medicine* 37, 301–14
 (1963b), 'Aristotelian concepts of the form and function of the brain', *Bulletin of the History of Medicine* 37, 1–14
Clarke, E. and Stannard, J. (1963), 'Aristotle on the anatomy of the brain', *Journal of the History of Medicine* 18, 130–48
Clay, D. (1980), 'An Epicurean interpretation of dreams', *American Journal of Philology* 101, 342–65
Codellas, P. S. (1948), 'The hypochondrium syndrome of Diocles of Carystus', in *Festschrift für M. Neuburger*, Vienna, 84–8
Cohen, S. M. (1978), 'Sensations, colors and capabilities in Aristotle', *The New Scholasticism* 52, 558–68
 (1986), 'The credibility of Aristotle's philosophy of mind', in M. Matthen (ed.), *Aristotle Today*, Alberta, 103–21
Coles, A. (1995), 'Biomedical models of reproduction in the fifth century BC and Aristotle's *Generation of Animals*', *Phronesis* 40, 48–88
 (1997), 'Animal and childhood cognition in Aristotle's biology and the scala naturae', in W. Kullmann and S. Föllinger (eds.), *Aristotelische Biologie. Intentionen, Methoden, Ergebnisse*, Stuttgart, 287–324

Collinge, N. E. (1962), 'Medical terms and clinical attitudes in the tragedians', *Bulletin of the Institute of Classical Studies* 9, 43–7
Conrad, L. I. et al. (1995), *The Western Medical Tradition 800 BC to AD 1800*, Cambridge
Cooper, J. (1973), 'The *Magna Moralia* and Aristotle's moral philosophy', *American Journal of Philology* 94, 327–49
Cootjans, G. (1991), *La stomatologie dans le Corpus Aristotélicien* (Académie Royale de Belgique, Mémoires de la Classe des Lettres, 2me série, t. 69. fasc. 3), Brussels
Cordes, P. (1994), *Iatros. Das Bild des Arztes in der griechischen Literatur von Homer bis Aristoteles*, Stuttgart
Corno, D. del (1969), *Graecorum de re onirocritica scriptorum reliquiae*, Milan
 (1982), 'Dreams and their interpretation in Ancient Greece', *Bulletin of the Institute of Classical Studies* 29, 55–62
Corvisier, J. N. (1985), *Santé et société en Grèce ancienne*, Paris
Cosenza, P. (1968), *Sensibilità, percezione, esperienza secondo Aristotele*, Naples
Couloubaritsis, L. (1982), 'Le problème de l'imagination chez Aristote', in *Actes du XVIIIme congrès des sociétés de philosophie de langue française*, Strasbourg, 153–8
 (1990), 'L'art divinatoire et la question de la vérité', in Motte (ed.) (1990) 113–22
Craik, E. (1995), 'Hippokratic Diaita', in J. Wilkins, D. Harvey and M. Dobson (eds.), *Food in Antiquity*, Exeter, 343–50
 (1998), *Hippocrates. On Places in Man*, Oxford
Croce, E. la (1985), 'Etica e metafisica nell' Etica Eudemia di Aristotele', *Elenchos* 6, 19–41
Croissant, J. (1932), *Aristote et les mystères*, Liège and Paris
Cuomo, S. (1998), 'Collecting authorities, constructing authority in Pappus of Alexandria's *Sunagogai*', in Kullmann, Althoff and Asper (eds.) (1998) 219–38
Daiber, H. (1980), *Aetius Arabus*, Wiesbaden
Dambska, J. (1961), 'Le problème des songes dans la philosophie des anciens grecs', *Revue Philosophique de la France et de l'Etranger* 151, 11–24
Dannenfeldt, K. H. (1971), 'Diocles of Carystus', *Dictionary of Scientific Biography* 4, 105–7
 (1986), 'Sleep: theory and practice in the late Renaissance', *Journal of the History of Medicine and Allied Sciences* 41, 415–41
Daremberg, C. (1843), *Hippocrate*, Paris
Dasen, V. (1993), *Dwarfs in Ancient Egypt and Greece*, Oxford
De Bellis, D. (1975), 'Niccolò Leonico Tomeo interprete di Aristotele naturalista', *Physis* 17, 71–93
De Lacy, P. (1978–84), *Galeni De placitis Hippocratis et Platonis* (*CMG* v 4, 1, 2), Berlin
De Meo, C. (1983), *Lingue tecniche del latino*, Bologna
Dean-Jones, L. (1987), 'Morbidity and vitality: interpretations of menstrual blood in Greek science', Stanford (unpublished PhD thesis)

(1989), 'Menstrual bleeding according to the Hippocratics and Aristotle', *Transactions and Proceedings of the American Philological Association* 119, 177–92

(1994), *Women's Bodies in Classical Greek Science*, Oxford

Debru, A. (1982), 'L'épilepsie dans le *De somno* d'Aristote', in G. Sabbah (ed.), *Médecins et médecine dans l'antiquité*, Saint-Etienne, 25–41

(1991) 'Expérience, plausibilité et certitude chez Galien', in J. A. López Férez (ed.), *Galeno: Obra, pensamiento e influencia*, Madrid, 31–40

(1992), 'Les énigmes d'une doxographie latine: le De semine de Vindicianus', paper read at the IVth Coloquio Internacional sobre los textos médicos latinos antiguos, Santiago de Compostela, 17–19 September 1992

(1994) 'L'expérimentation chez Galien', *ANRW* 11. 37.2, 1718–56

(1995), 'Les démonstrations médicales à Rome au temps de Galien', in van der Eijk, Horstmanshoff and Schrijvers (eds.) (1995) vol. 1, 69–82

(1996), 'L'Anonyme de Bruxelles: un témoin latin de l'hippocratisme tardif', in R. Wittern and P. Pellegrin (eds.), *Hippokratische Medizin und antike Philosophie*, Hildesheim, 311–27

(1997), 'Philosophie et pharmacologie: la dynamique des substances leptomeres chez Galien', in A. Debru (ed.), *Galen on Pharmacology. Philosophy, History and Medicine*, Leiden, 85–102

(1999), 'Doctrine et tactique doxographique dans l'Anonyme de Bruxelles: une comparaison avec l'Anonyme de Londres', in van der Eijk (ed.) (1999a) 453–71

(2002), 'La sueur des corps: le *De Sudore* de Théophraste face à la tradition médicale', in W. W. Fortenbaugh and G. Wöhrle (eds.), *On the Opuscula of Theophrastus*, Stuttgart, 163–74

Décarie, V. (1978), *Aristote. Ethique à Eudème*, Paris and Montréal

Decharme, P. (1904), *La critique des traditions religieuses chez les grecs*, Paris

Decharneux, B. (1990), 'Mantique et oracles dans l'œuvre de Philon d'Alexandrie', in Motte (ed.) (1990) 123–33

Deichgräber, K. (1933a), *Die Epidemien und das Corpus Hippocraticum* (Abhandlungen der preussischen Akademie der Wissenschaften, Berlin, Phil.-hist. Klasse, 1933.3), Berlin

(1933b), 'Hymnische Elemente in der philosophischen Prosa der Vorsokratiker', *Philologus* 88, 347–61

(1933c), '*Prophasis*. Eine terminologische Studie', *Quellen und Studien zur Geschichte der Naturwissenschaften und der Medizin* 3, 1–17

(1935), *Hippokrates über Entstehung und Aufbau des menschlichen Körpers*, Περὶ σαρκῶν, mit einem sprachwissenschaftlichen Beitrag von Eduard Schwyzer, Leipzig and Berlin

(1965), *Die griechische Empirikerschule. Sammlung der Fragmente und Darstellung der Lehre*, 2nd edn, Berlin

(1970), *Medicus gratiosus. Untersuchungen zu einem griechischen Arztbild* (Akademie der Wissenschaften und der Literatur Mainz, Abhandlungen der Geistes- und Sozialwissenschaftlichen Klasse, 1970.3), Wiesbaden

(1971), *Die Epidemien und das Corpus Hippocraticum*, 2nd edn, Berlin and New York

Delaney, J., Lupton, M. J. and Toth, E. (1976), *The Curse. A Cultural History of Menstruation*, New York
Delatte, P. (1934), 'Les conceptions de l'enthousiasme chez les philosophes présocratiques', *L'Antiquité Classique* 3, 5–79
Demand, N. (1995), 'Monuments, midwives and gynecology', in van der Eijk, Horstmanshoff and Schrijvers (eds.) (1995) vol. 1, 275–90
Demont, P. (1991), 'Observations sur le champ sémantique du changement dans la Collection hippocratique', in López Férez (1992), 305–18
Demuth, G. (1972), *Ps.-Galenis De dignotione ex insomniis*, Göttingen
Denniston, J. D. (1954), *The Greek Particles*, 2nd edn, Oxford
  (1959), *Greek Prose Style*, Oxford
Derenne, E. (1930), *Les procès d'impiété intentés aux philosophes à Athènes au Vme et au IVme siècles avant J. C.*, Liège and Paris
Desjardins, R. (1980–1), 'The horns of the dilemma. Dreaming and waking vision in the Theaetetus', *Ancient Philosophy* 1, 109–26
Détienne, M. (1958–60), 'Quelques phénomènes psychiques dans la pensée d'Aristote, de Cléarque et d'Héraclide: de la catalepsie à l'immortalité', *La Nouvelle Clio* 10, 123–35
  (1963), *La notion de daimon dans le pythagorisme ancien*, Paris
Deubner, L. (1900), *De incubatione*, Leipzig
Devereux, G. (1976), *Dreams in Greek Tragedy*, Berkeley and Los Angeles
Di Benedetto, V. (1986), *Il medico e la malattia. La scienza di Ippocrate*, Turin
Diano, C. (1970), 'La tyche e il problema dell' accidente', in C. Diano and M. Gentile (eds.), *L'attualità della problematica aristotelica*. Atti del Convegno franco-italiano su Aristotele, Padua, 127–31
Díaz Regañon, J. M. (1976), 'Sueño y ensueño en el Corpus Hippocraticum', *Cuadernos de Investigación Filológica* 2, 19–33
Diels, H. (1879), *Doxographi graeci* (reprinted 1965), Berlin
  (1893a), *Anonymi Londinensis ex Aristotelis Iatricis Menoniis et aliis medicis Eclogae* (Supplementum Aristotelicum III 1), Berlin
  (1893b), 'Über die Excerpte von Menons Iatrika in dem Londoner Papyrus 137', *Hermes* 28, 407–34
  (1893c), 'Über das physikalische System des Straton', *Sitzungsberichte der königlich preussischen Akademie der Wissenschaften Berlin* 1, 101–27
  (1910), 'Über einen neuen Versuch, die Echtheit einiger hippokratischen Schriften nachzuweisen', *Sitzungsberichte der königlich preussischen Akademie der Wissenschaften zu Berlin*, 1140–55
  (1914), 'Corpus Medicorum Graecorum. Bericht', *Sitzungsberichte der königlich preussischen Akademie der Wissenschaften zu Berlin*, 127–30
Diels, H. and Krantz, W. (1961), *Die Fragmente der Vorsokratiker*, 10th edn, Berlin
Diepgen, P. (1912), *Traum und Traumdeutung als medizinisch-naturwissenschaftliches Problem im Mittelalter*, Berlin
  (1937), *Die Frauenheilkunde der alten Welt*, Munich
  (1949), *Geschichte der Medizin*, vol. 1, Berlin

Dierbach, J. H. (1824), *Die Arzneimittel des Hippokrates oder: Versuch einer systematischen Aufzählung der in allen hippokratischen Schriften vorkommenden Medikamente* (reprinted 1967), Hildesheim

Dihle, A. (1998), 'Mündlichkeit und Schriftlichkeit nach dem Aufkommen des Lehrbuches', in Kullmann, Althoff and Asper (eds.) (1998) 265–78

Diller, H. (1933), 'Zur Hippokratesauffassung des Galen', *Hermes* 68, 167–81

(1952), 'Hippokratische Medizin und attische Philosophie', *Hermes* 80, 385–409

(1959), 'Der innere Zusammenhang der hippokratischen Schrift De victu', *Hermes* 87, 39–56

(1970), *Hippokrates. Über die Umwelt*, Berlin

Dirlmeier, F. (1935), 'Theophilia – Philotheia', *Philologus* 90, 57–77 and 176–93

(1956), *Aristoteles. Nikomachische Ethik*, Berlin

(1958), *Aristoteles, Magna Moralia*, Berlin

(1962a), *Aristoteles. Eudemische Ethik*, Berlin

(1962b), *Merkwürdige Zitate in der Eudemischen Ethik* (Sitzungsberichte der Heidelberger Akademie der Wissenschaften, Philosophisch-historische Klasse, 1962.2), Heidelberg

Dittmer, H. L. (1940), *Konstitutionstypen im Corpus Hippocraticum*, Würzburg

Dittmeyer, L. (1907), *Aristotelis De animalibus historia*, Leipzig

Dodds, E. R. (1936), 'Telepathy and clairvoyance in classical antiquity', in *Greek Poetry and Life. Essays Presented to Gilbert Murray*, Oxford, 346–85

(1945), 'Plato and the irrational', *Journal of Hellenic Studies* 65, 16–25 (reprinted in *The Ancient Concept of Progress and Other Essays on Greek Literature and Belief*, Oxford, 1973, 106–25)

(1951), *The Greeks and the Irrational*, Berkeley and Los Angeles

(1971), 'Supernormal phaenomena in classical antiquity', *Proceedings of the Society of Psychical Research* 55, 189–237 (reprinted in *The Ancient Concept of Progress and Other Essays on Greek Literature and Belief*, Oxford, 1973, 156–210)

Dölger, F. J. (1922), *Ichthus. Der heilige Fisch in den antiken Religionen und im Christentum*, vol. II, Münster

Donnay, G. (1983), 'L'âme et le rêve d'Homère à Lucrèce', *Ktema* 8, 5–10

Dönt, E. (1997), *Aristoteles. Kleine naturwissenschaftliche Schriften*, Stuttgart

Dorandi, T. (1993), 'Zwischen Autographie und Diktat: Momente der Textualität in der antiken Welt', in Kullmann and Althoff (eds.) (1993) 71–86

Dover, K. J. (1960), *Greek Word Order*, Cambridge

(1975), 'The freedom of the intellectual in Greek society', *Talanta* 7, 24–54

Drabkin, I. E. (1950), *Caelius Aurelianus on Acute and Chronic Diseases*, Baltimore

Drabkin, M. F. and Drabkin, I. E. (1951), *Caelius Aurelianus, Gynaecia. Fragments of a Latin Version of Soranus' Gynaecia from a Thirteenth Century Manuscript* (Supplements to the Bulletin of the History of Medicine 13), Baltimore

Drossaart Lulofs, H. J. (1943), *Aristotelis De somno et vigilia liber adiectis veteribus translationibus et Theodori Metochitae commentario*, Leiden

(1947), *Aristotelis De insomniis et De divinatione per somnum*, 2 vols., Leiden

(1967), *De ogen van Lynkeus*, Leiden

Dübner F., Bussemaker, U. C. and Heitz, J. H. E. (1848–69), *Aristoteles. Opera omnia graece et latine, cum indice nominum et rerum absolutissimo*, 5 vols., Paris

Dubuisson, M. (1976–7), οἱ ἀμφί τινα, οἱ περί τινα: *L'évolution des sens et des emplois*, Liège

Ducatillon, J. (1969), 'Collection hippocratique. *Du régime*, livre III. Les deux publics', *Revue des Etudes Grecques* 82, 33–42

(1977), *Polémiques dans la Collection hippocratique*, Paris

(1990), 'Le facteur divin dans les maladies d'après le traité hippocratique du Pronostic', in Potter, Maloney and Desautels (eds.) (1990) 61–73

Dulaey, M. (1973), *Le rêve dans la vie et la pensée de Saint Augustin*, Paris

Dulk, W. J. den (1934), *Krasis. Bijdrage tot de Grieksche Lexicographie*, Leiden

Duminil, M.-P. (1983), *Le sang, les vaisseaux, le cœur dans la Collection hippocratique. Physiologie et anatomie*, Paris

(1998), *Hippocrate. Plaies, nature des os, cœur, anatomie*, Paris

Dumortier, J. (1935), *Le vocabulaire médical d'Eschyle et les écrits hippocratiques*, Paris

Dumoulin, B. (1981), *Recherches sur le premier Aristote*, Paris and Irun

Düring, I. (1943), *Aristotle's De Partibus Animalium. Critical and Literary Commentaries*, Göteborg

(1957), *Aristotle in the Ancient Biographical Tradition*, Göteborg

(1966), *Aristoteles. Darstellung und Interpretation seines Denkens*, Heidelberg

(1968), 'Aristoteles', *RE* Suppl. XI, 159–336

Durling, R. J. (1991), 'On *Endeixis* as a scientific term', in F. Kudlien and R. J. Durling (eds.), *Galen on the Method of Healing*, Leiden, 112–13

(1993), *A Lexicon of Medical Terms in Galen*, Leiden

Ebert, Th. (1983), 'Aristotle on what is done in perceiving', *Zeitschrift für philosophische Forschung* 37, 181–98

Edelstein, L. (1931a), 'Antike Diätetik', *Die Antike* 7, 255–70 (reprinted as 'The dietetics of antiquity', in Edelstein (1967a) 303–16)

(1931b), Περὶ ἀέρων *und die Sammlung der hippokratischen Schriften* (*Problemata* 4), Berlin

(1932), 'Die Geschichte der Sektion im Altertum', *Quellen und Studien zur Geschichte der Naturwissenschaften und der Medizin* 3.2, 50–106 (reprinted as 'The history of anatomy in antiquity', in Edelstein (1967a) 247–301)

(1937), 'Greek medicine and its relation to religion and magic', *Bulletin of the History of Medicine* 5, 201–46 (reprinted in Edelstein (1967a) 205–46)

(1940), review of Jaeger (1938a), *American Journal of Philology* 61, 483–9 (reprinted in Edelstein (1967a) 145–52)

(1956), 'The professional ethics of the Greek physician', *Bulletin of the History of Medicine* 30, 391–419 (reprinted in Edelstein (1967a) 319–48)

(1967a), *Ancient Medicine. Selected Papers of Ludwig Edelstein*, edited by O. Temkin and C. L. Temkin, Baltimore

(1967b), 'The Methodists', in Edelstein (1967a) 173–91

Edelstein, E. J. and Edelstein, L. (1945), *Asclepius*, 2 vols., Baltimore (reprinted with a new introduction by G. Ferngren, Baltimore, 1998)

Eemeren, F. van, Grootendorst, R. and Kruijger, T. (1986a), *Drogredenen*, Groningen
(1986b), *The Study of Argumentation*, New York
Effe, B. (1970), *Studien zur Kosmologie und Theologie der Aristotelischen Schrift 'Über die Philosophie'*, Munich
Eger, J.-C. (1966), *Le sommeil et la mort dans la Grèce antique*, Paris
Eichholz, D. E. (1965), *Theophrastus. De lapidibus*, Oxford
Eigler, G., Jechle, T., Merziger, G. and Winter, A. (1990), *Wissen und Textproduzieren*, Tübingen
Eijk, P. J. van der (1991), 'Airs Waters Places and On the Sacred Disease: two different religiosities?', *Hermes* 119, 168–76
(1993a), 'Aristotelian elements in Cicero's *De divinatione*', *Philologus* 137, 223–31
(1993b), 'De fragmenten van Diocles van Carystus. Een verslag van lopend onderzoek', *Gewina* 16, 50–4
(1993c), 'A textual note on Galen, *On the Powers of Foodstuffs* 1 1.3', *The Classical Quarterly* 43, 506–8
(1994), *Aristoteles. De insomniis. De divinatione per somnum* (Aristoteles. Werke in deutscher Übersetzung 14/III), Berlin
(1997), 'Towards a rhetoric of ancient scientific discourse: some formal characteristics of Greek medical and philosophical texts (Hippocratic Corpus, Aristotle)', in E. J. Bakker (ed.), *Grammar as Interpretation. Greek Literature in its Linguistic Contexts*, Leiden, 77–129
(1998), 'Quelques remarques sur la méthode doxographique de Cælius Aurélien', in C. Deroux (ed.), *Maladie et maladies dans les textes latins antiques et médiévaux*, Brussels, 342–53
(ed.) (1999a), *Ancient Histories of Medicine. Essays in Medical Doxography and Historiography in Classical Antiquity* (Studies in Ancient Medicine 20), Leiden
(1999b), 'The Anonymus Parisinus and the doctrines of "the Ancients"', in van der Eijk (ed.) (1999a) 295–331
(1999c), 'Antiquarianism and criticism. Forms and functions of medical doxography in Methodism (Soranus, Caelius Aurelianus)', in van der Eijk (ed.) (1999a), 397–451
(1999d), 'Hippokratische Beiträge zur antiken Biologie', in G. Wöhrle (ed.), *Geschichte der Mathematik und der Naturwissenschaften in der Antike*, vol. 1: *Biologie*, Stuttgart, 50–73
(1999e), 'Historical awareness, historiography and doxography in Graeco-Roman medicine', in van der Eijk (ed.) (1999a) 1–31
(1999f), 'Some methodological issues in collecting the fragments of Diocles of Carystus', in Garzya and Jouanna (eds.) (1999) 125–56
(2000a), *Diocles of Carystus. A Collection of the Fragments with Translation and Commentary*, vol. 1: *Text and Translation* (Studies in Ancient Medicine 22), Leiden
(2000b), 'Aristotle's psycho-physiological account of the soul–body relationship', in J. P. Wright and P. Potter (eds.), *Psyche and Soma. Physicians and*

Metaphysicians on the Mind–Body Problem from Antiquity to Enlightenment, Oxford, 57–77

(2001a), *Diocles of Carystus. A Collection of the Fragments with Translation and Commentary*, vol. 11: *Commentary* (Studies in Ancient Medicine 23), Leiden

(2001b), 'La storiografia delle scienze e la tradizione dossografica', in S. Petruccioli (ed.), *Storia della Scienza*, Rome, vol. 1, 591–601

(2004a), 'Divination, Prognosis, Prophylaxis: the Hippocratic work "On Dreams" (*De victu* 4) and its Near Eastern background', in H. F. J. Horstmanshoff and M. Stol (eds.), *Magic and Rationality in Ancient New Eastern and Graeco-Roman Medicine*, Leiden, 187–218

(2004b), 'Vom Nutzen und Nachteil der Medizinhistorie für das Leben. Form, Gehalt und Funktion der Medizingeschichtsschreibung in der Antike', in T. Rütten (ed.), *Geschichte der Medizingeschichtsschreibung*, Hildesheim (in press)

(2005a), 'Galen's therapeutics', in R. J. Hankinson (ed.), *Cambridge Companion to Galen*, Cambridge, (in press)

(2005b), 'Between the Hippocratics and the Alexandrians: medicine, science and philosophy in fourth century Greece', in R. W. Sharples (ed.), *Proceedings of the Keeling Colloquium on Ancient Philosophy and the Sciences*, Aldershot, (in press)

(2005c), 'The role of medicine in the formation of early Greek philosophical thought', in P. Curd and D. Graham (eds.), *Oxford Guide to Pre-Socratic Philosophy*, Oxford, (in press)

Eijk, P. J. van der, Horstmanshoff, H. F. J. and Schrijvers, P. H. (eds.) (1995), *Ancient Medicine in its Socio-Cultural Context*, 2 vols., Amsterdam

Einarson, B. and Link, G. K. K. (1976–90), *Theophrastus. De causis plantarum*, 3 vols., Cambridge, Mass. and London

Elaut, L. (1952), *Het medisch denken in de oudheid, de middeleeuwen en de renaissance*, Amsterdam

(1960), *Antieke geneeskunde, in teksten van Griekse en Latijnse auteurs vanaf Homerus tot het begin van de Middeleeuwen*, Antwerp and Amsterdam

Elders, L. (1966), *Aristotle's Cosmology. A Commentary on the De caelo*, Assen

(1972), *Aristotle's Theology. A Commentary on book Λ of the Metaphysics*, Assen

Else, G. F. (1957), *Aristotle's Poetics: the Argument*, Cambridge, Mass.

Emonds, H. (1941), *Zweite Auflage im Altertum. Kulturgeschichtliche Studien zur Überlieferung der antiken Literatur*, Leipzig

Empson, J. (2003), 'The psychology of sleep', in T. Wiedemann and K. Dowden (eds.), *Sleep*, Bari, 1–24

Enders, H. (1923), *Schlaf und Traum bei Aristoteles*, Würzburg

Engmann, J. (1976), 'Imagination and truth in Aristotle', *Journal of the History of Philosophy* 14, 259–65

Eucken, R. (1866), *De Aristotelis dicendi ratione. Pars prima. Observationes de particularum usu*, Göttingen

(1868), *Über den Sprachgebrauch des Aristoteles. Beobachtungen über die Präpositionen*, Berlin

(1869), 'Die Etymologie bei Aristoteles', *Neue Jahrbücher* 100, 243–8

Fabricius, C. (1972), *Galens Exzerpte aus den älteren Pharmakologen*, Berlin

Fahr, W. (1969), *Theous nomizein. Zum Problem der Anfänge des Atheismus bei den Griechen*, Hildesheim

Fasbender, H. (1897), *Entwickelungslehre, Geburtshilfe und Gynäkologie in den hippokratischen Schriften*, Stuttgart

Feibleman, J. K. (1958–1959), 'Aristotle's religion', *Hibbert Journal* 57, 126–32

Festugière, A. J. (1945), 'Les "Mémoires pythagoriques" cités par Alexandre Polyhistor', *Revue des Etudes Grecques* 58, 1–65

(1948), *Hippocrate. L'ancienne médecine*, Paris

Fiedler, W. (1978), *Analogiemodelle bei Aristoteles*, Amsterdam

Fischer, J. (1899), *Ad artis veterum onirocriticae historiam symbola*, Jena

Fischer, K.-D. (1998), 'Beiträge zu den pseudosoranischen Quaestiones medicinales', in K.-D. Fischer, D. Nickel and P. Potter (eds.), *Text and Tradition. Studies in Ancient Medicine and its Transmission*, Leiden, 1–54

(1999), 'Bisher unberücksichtigte Handschriftenfunde zur Überlieferung der Werke des Caelius Aurelianus', in Mudry (ed.) (1999) 141–76

Fischer-Homberger, E. (1979), *Krankheit Frau und andere Arbeiten zur Medizingeschichte der Frau*, Bern, Stuttgart and Vienna

Flashar, H. (1956), 'Die medizinischen Grundlagen der Lehre von der Wirkung der Dichtung in der griechischen Poetik', *Hermes* 84, 12–48

(1958), *Der Dialog Ion als Zeugnis platonischer Philosophie*, Berlin

(1962), *Aristoteles. Problemata physica*, Berlin and Darmstadt

(1966), *Melancholie und Melancholiker in den medizinischen Theorien der Antike*, Berlin

(ed.) (1971), *Antike Medizin*, Darmstadt

(1983), 'Aristoteles', in H. Flashar (ed.), *Grundriss der Geschichte der Philosophie. Die Philosophie der Antike*, vol. III, Basel, 175–457

Flashar, H. and Jouanna, J. (eds.) (1997), *Médecine et morale dans l'antiquité*, Vandœuvres and Geneva

Flavion, S. (1950), *La physiologie d'Aristote*, Louvain

Flemming, R. (2000), *Medicine and the Making of Roman Women*, Oxford

Flemming, R. and Hanson, A. (1998), 'Hippocrates *Peri partheniôn* (*Diseases of Young Girls*): text and translation', *Early Science and Medicine* 3, 241–52

Floyd, E. D. (1992), 'Why Parmenides wrote in verse', *Ancient Philosophy* 12, 251–65

Fluck, H.-R. (1980), *Fachsprachen. Einführung und Bibliographie*, Munich

Föllinger, S. (1993), 'Mündlichkeit in der Schriftlichkeit als Ausdruck wissenschaftlicher Methode bei Aristoteles', in Kullmann and Althoff (eds.) (1993) 263–80

(1996), *Differenz und Gleichheit. Das Geschlechterverhältnis in der Sicht griechischer Philosophen des 4. bis 1. Jahrhunderts v. Chr.* (Hermes Einzelschriften 74), Stuttgart

Förster, A. (1932), *Konstruktion und Entstehung der aristotelischen sogenannten Parva naturalia*, Budapest
  (1942), *Aristoteles. De sensu et De memoria*, Budapest
Fortenbaugh, W. W. (1967), 'Recent scholarship on the psychology of Aristotle', *The Classical World* 60, 316–27
  (1970), 'Aristotle's *Rhetoric* on emotions', *Archiv für die Geschichte der Philosophie* 52, 40–70
  (1975), *Aristotle on Emotion*, London
Fortenbaugh, W. W., Huby, P. M., Sharples, R. W. and Gutas, D. (1992), *Theophrastus of Eresos. Sources for his Life, Writings, Thought and Influence*, 2 vols., Leiden
Fortenbaugh, W. W., Sharples, R. W. and Sollenberger, M. (eds.) (2003), *Theophrastus of Eresus on Sweat, On Dizziness and On Fatigue*, Leiden
Fortenbaugh, W. W. and Steinmetz, P. (eds.) (1989), *Cicero's Knowledge of the Peripatos*, New Brunswick and London
Fraenkel, M. (1840), *Dioclis Carystii fragmenta quae supersunt*, Berlin
Fragstein, A. von (1974), *Studien zur Ethik des Aristoteles*, Amsterdam
Frede, M. (1980), 'The original notion of cause', in M. Schofield et al. (eds.), *Doubt and Dogmatism. Studies in Hellenistic Epistemology*, Oxford (reprinted in Frede (1987a) 125–50; references are to the reprint)
  (1983), 'The method of the so-called Methodical school of medicine', in J. Barnes et al. (eds.), *Science and Speculation. Studies in Hellenistic Theory and Practice*, Cambridge, 1–23 (reprinted in Frede (1987a), 261–78; references are to the reprint)
  (1985), 'Introduction' to *Galen, Three Treatises on the Nature of Science*, translated by R. Walzer and M. Frede, with an introduction by M. Frede, Indianapolis, xx–xxxiv
  (1986), 'Philosophy and medicine in antiquity', in A. Donagan et al. (eds.), *Human Nature and Natural Knowledge. Essays Presented to Marjorie Grene on the Occasion of her Seventy-Fifth Birthday*, Dordrecht, 211–32 (reprinted in Frede (1987a) 225–42; references are to the reprint)
  (1987a), *Essays in Ancient Philosophy*, Oxford
  (1987b), 'The ancient Empiricists', in Frede (1987a) 243–60
  (1987c), 'On Galen's epistemology', in V. Nutton (ed.), *Galen: Problems and Prospects*, London (reprinted in Frede (1987a) 279–98; references are to the reprint)
  (1988), 'The Empiricist attitude towards reason and theory', *Apeiron* 21, 79–98
  (1992), 'On Aristotle's conception of the soul', in Nussbaum and Rorty (eds.) (1992) 93–108
  (forthcoming), 'An anti-Aristotelian point of method in three Rationalist doctors'
Frede, M. and Striker, G. (eds.) (1996), *Rationality in Greek Thought*, New York
Fredrich, C. (1899), *Hippokratische Untersuchungen* (Philologische Untersuchungen 15), Berlin
Freeland, C. (1992), 'Aristotle on the sense of touch', in Nussbaum and Rorty (eds.) (1992) 227–48

Frère, J., (1983), 'L'aurore de la science des rêves: Aristote', *Ktema* 8, 27–37
Freud, S. (1900), *Die Traumdeutung*, Leipzig and Vienna
Freudenthal, G. (1995), *Aristotle's Theory of Material Substance: Heat and Pneuma, Form and Soul*, Oxford
Freudenthal, J. (1863), *Über den Begriff des Wortes phantasia bei Aristoteles*, Göttingen
  (1869), 'Zur Kritik und Exegese von Aristoteles' περὶ τῶν κοινῶν σώματος καὶ ψυχῆς ἔργων (Parva naturalia)', *Rheinisches Museum* 24, 81–93 and 392–419
Froschammer, J. (1881), *Über die Prinzipien der aristotelischen Philosophie und die Bedeutung der Phantasie in derselben*, Munich
Fuchs, R. (1903), 'Aus Themisons Werk über die akuten und chronischen Krankheiten', *Rheinisches Museum* 58, 67–114
Fuhrmann, M. (1960), *Das systematische Lehrbuch. Ein Beitrag zur Geschichte der Wissenschaften in der Antike*, Göttingen
Furley, D. and Wilkie, J. S. (1984), *Galen on Respiration and the Arteries*, Princeton
Gallop, D. (1971), 'Dreaming and waking in Plato', in Anton and Kustas (eds.) (1971) 187–201
  (1996), *Aristotle on Sleep and Dreams*, Warminster (revision of 1st edn, Boston, 1990)
García Gual, C. (1984), 'Del melancólico como atrabiliario. Según las antiguas ideas griegas sobre la enfermedad de la melancolia', *Faventia* 6, 41–50
Garcia Novo, E. (1995), 'Structure and style in the Hippocratic treatise *Prorrheticon* 2', in van der Eijk, Horstmanshoff and Schrijvers (eds.) (1995) vol. II, 537–54
Garofalo, I. (1988), *Erasistrati fragmenta*, Pisa
  (1997), *Anonymi medici de morbis acutis et chroniis*, Leiden
Gärtner, H. A. (1983), 'Les rêves de Xerxès et d'Artabane chez Hérodote', *Ktema* 8, 11–18
Garzya, A. (ed.) (1992), *Tradizione e ecdotica dei testi medici tardoantichi e Bizantini* (Atti del Convegno Internazionale, Anacapri, 29–31 ottobre 1990), Napoli,
Garzya, A. and Jouanna, J. (eds.) (1999), *I testi medici greci III. Tradizione e ecdotica*, Naples
Gask, G. E. (1939–40), 'Early medical schools I–III', *Annals of Medical History* 1, 128–57, and 2, 15–21; 383–92
Gatzemeier, M. (1970), *Die Naturphilosophie des Straton von Lampsakos*, Meisenheim am Glan
Gauthier, R. A. and Jolif, J. Y. (1958–9), *Aristote. Ethique à Nicomaque*, 3 vols., Louvain
Gerhard, G. A. (1913), *Ein dogmatischer Arzt aus dem vierten Jahrhundert v. Chr.*, (Sitzungsberichte der Heidelberger Akademie der Wissenschaften, Phil.-hist. Klasse, Nr. 4.13), Heidelberg
Geurts, P. M. M. (1943), 'Εὐθυωρία', *Mnemosyne* II, 108–14
Gigon, O. (1952), 'Die Theologie der Vorsokratiker', in H. J. Rose et al. (eds.), *La notion du divin depuis Homère jusqu'à Platon* (Entretiens sur l'Antiquité Classique 1), Vandœuvres and Geneva, 127–66
  (1959), 'Cicero und Aristoteles', *Hermes* 87, 143–62

(1969), 'Zwei Interpretationen zur Eudemischen Ethik des Aristoteles', *Museum Helveticum* 26, 204–16
(1971), 'Das Prooimion der Eudemischen Ethik', in P. Moraux and D. Harlfinger (eds.), *Untersuchungen zur Eudemischen Ethik*, Berlin, 93–134
(1983), *Aristotelis Opera III: Librorum deperditorum fragmenta*, Berlin
(1985), 'Die Wege zur *aretê* bei Platon und Aristoteles', *Museum Helveticum* 42, 133–50
Gil, L. (1985), 'Procul recedant somnia. Los ensueños eróticos en la antigüedad pagana y cristiana', in J. L. Melena (ed.), *Symbolae Ludovico Mitxelana septuagenario oblatae*, Vitoria, vol. 1, 193–219
Ginouvès, R. (1962), *Balaneutike. Recherches sur le bain dans l'antiquité grecque*, Paris
Ginouvès, R. et al. (eds.) (1994), *L'eau, la santé et la maladie dans le monde grec*. (Bulletin de Correspondance Hellénique, Suppl. 28), Paris
Goltz, D. (1974), *Studien zur altorientalischen und griechischen Heilkunde. Therapie – Arzneibereitung – Rezeptstruktur*, Wiesbaden
Goody, J. (ed.) (1968), *Literacy in Traditional Societies*, Cambridge
Göpferich, S. (1995), *Textsorten in Naturwissenschaft und Technik* (Forum für Fachsprachenforschung 27), Tübingen
Gosling, J. (1993), 'Mad, drunk or asleep? Aristotle's akratic', *Phronesis* 38, 98–104
Gotthelf, A. (ed.) (1985), *Aristotle on Nature and Living Things*, Pittsburgh and Bristol
Gotthelf, A. and Lennox, J. G. (eds.) (1987), *Philosophical Issues in Aristotle's Biology*, Cambridge
Gottschalk, H. B. (1965), 'Strato of Lampsacus, some texts', *Proceedings of the Leeds Philosophical and Literary Society* 11.6, 95–182
(1998), 'Theophrastus and the Peripatos', in J. M. van Ophuijsen and M. van Raalte (eds.), *Theophrastus. Reappraising the Sources*, New Brunswick and London, 281–98
Gould, Th. (1963), 'Aristotle and the irrational', *Arion* 2, 55–74
Gourevitch, D. (1984a), *Le mal d'être femme*, Paris
(1984b), *Le triangle hippocratique dans le monde gréco-romain*, Paris
(1989, 1990), 'L'Anonyme de Londres et la médecine d'Italie du Sud', *History and Philosophy of the Life Sciences* 11, 237–51, and 12, 67–104
(1991), 'La pratique Méthodique: définition de la maladie, indication et traitement', in P. Mudry and J. Pigeaud (eds.) (1991), *Les écoles médicales à Rome*, Geneva, 57–82
Gracia, D. (1978), 'The structure of medical knowledge in Aristotle's philosophy', *Sudhoffs Archiv* 62, 1–36
Graeser, A. (1978), 'On Aristotle's framework of sensibilia', in Lloyd and Owen (eds.) (1978) 69–97
Granger, H. (1990), 'Aristotle and the functionalist debate', *Apeiron* 23, 27–49
Gravel, P. (1982), 'Aristote sur le vin, le sexe, la folie, le génie. Melancolie', *Etudes françaises Montréal* 18, 129–45
Greene, W. C. (1944), *Moira. Fate, Gods and Evil in Greek Thought*, New York and Evanston

Grensemann, H. (1968a), *Der Arzt Polybos als Verfasser hippokratischer Schriften*, (Abhandlungen der Akademie der Wissenschaften und Literatur Mainz, Geistes- und sozialwissenschaftliche Klasse 2), Wiesbaden
  (1968b), *Hippokrates. Über Achtmonatskinder, Über das Siebenmonatskind*, Berlin
  (1968c), *Die hippokratische Schrift Ueber die heilige Krankheit*, Berlin
  (1975), *Knidische Medizin Teil I: Die Testimonien zur ältesten knidischen Lehre und Analysen knidischer Schriften im Corpus Hippocraticum*, Berlin and New York
  (1987), *Knidische Medizin Teil II: Versuch einer weiteren Analyse der Schicht A in den pseudohippokratischen Schriften De natura muliebri und De muliebribus I und II*, Stuttgart
Griffin, M. and Barnes, J. (1989), *Philosophia Togata*, Oxford
Grmek, M. D. (ed.) (1980), *Hippocratica*, Paris
  (1983), *Les maladies à l'aube de la civilisation occidentale*, Paris
  (1989), *Diseases in the Ancient Greek World*, Baltimore and London (English translation of Grmek (1983))
  (ed.) (1993), *Storia del pensiero medico occidentale*, vol. 1: *Antichità e Medioevo*, Bari
Grmek, M. D. and Gourevitch, D. (1985), 'Les expériments pharmacologiques dans l'Antiquité', *Archives internationales d'histoire des sciences* 35, 3–27
Grmek, M. D. and Robert, F. (1977), 'Dialogue d'un médecin et d'un philologue sur quelques passages des Épidémies VII', in R. Joly (ed.), *Corpus Hippocraticum*, Mons, 275–90
Groningen, B. A. van (1958), 'La composition littéraire archaique grecque', *Verhandelingen der Koninklijke Nederlandse Akademie van Wetenschappen*, Afdeling Letterkunde, Nieuwe reeks, Deel 65, no. 2, Amsterdam, 1–394
Grube, G. M. A. and Reeve, C. D. C. (1997), 'Plato: *Republic*', in J. Cooper (ed.), *Plato. Complete Works*, Indiana, 971–1223
Gruner, C. G. (1780–2), *Bibiothek der antiken Ärzte in Übersetzungen und Auszügen*, 2 vols.
Guardasole, A. (1995), 'Per la posizione di Eraclide di Taranto nella storia del pensiero medico', *Koinonia* 19, 63–9
  (1997), *Eraclide di Taranto. Frammenti*, Naples
Guidorizzi, G. (1973), 'L'opusculo di Galeno "De dignotione ex insomniis"', *Bolletino del Comitato per la preparazione dell'Edizione nazionale dei Classici e greci e latini* 21, 81–105
  (1985), 'Sogno, diagnosi, guarigione. Da Asclepio a Ippocrate', in F. Daratta and F. Mariani (eds.), *Mondo classico, percorsi possibili*, Ravenna, 71–81 (reprinted in Guidorizzi (ed.) (1988) 87–102)
  (ed.) (1988), *Il sogno in Grecia*, Bari
  (1989a), 'Ikonographische und literarische Modelle der Traumdeutung in der Spätantike', in A. Pottavicini Bagliarisi and G. Stabile (eds.), *Träume im Mittelalter*, Stuttgart and Zurich, 241–9
  (1989b), 'Tabù alimentari e funzione onirica in Grecia', in O. Longo and P. Scarfie (eds.), *Homo edens*, Verona, 169–76

Guillén, L. F. (1991), 'Hipócrates y el discurso científico', in López Férez (1992) 319–34
Gundert, B. (2000), 'Soma and Psyche in Hippocratic medicine', in J. P. Wright and P. Potter (eds.), *Psyche and Soma. Physicians and Metaphysicians on the Mind–Body Problem from Antiquity to the Enlightenment*, Oxford, 13–36
Guthrie, W. K. C. (1962–81), *A History of Greek Philosophy*, 6 vols., Cambridge
Haberle, J. (1938), *Untersuchungen über den ionischen Prosastil*, Munich
Habrich, C., Marguth, F. and Wolf, J. H. (eds.) (1978), *Medizinische Diagnostik in Geschichte und Gegenwart*, Munich
Hagen, H. (1961), *Die physiologische und psychologische Bedeutung der Leber in der Antike*, Bonn
Hall, R. (1959), 'The special vocabulary of the *Eudemian Ethics*', *The Classical Quarterly* 9, 197–206
Halliday, W. R. (1913), *Greek Divination. A Study of its Methods and Principles*, London
  (1936), 'Some notes on the treatment of disease in Antiquity', in *Greek Poetry and Life. Essays Presented to Gilbert Murray*, Oxford, 277–294
Hamlyn, D. W. (1959), 'Aristotle's account of *aesthesis* in the *De Anima*', *The Classical Quarterly*, N.S. 9, 6–16
  (1963), *Sensation and Perception. A History of the Philosophy of Perception*, London
  (1968a), *Aristotle's De Anima Books II and III*, Oxford
  (1968b), 'Koine aisthesis', *The Monist* 52, 195–209
Hammond, W. A. (1902), *Aristotle's Psychology. A Treatise on the Principles of Life (De Anima and Parva naturalia)*, London and New York
Hankinson, R. J. (1987), 'Evidence, externality and antecedence', *Phronesis* 32, 80–100
  (1991a), *Galen. On the Therapeutic Method*, Oxford
  (1991b), 'Greek medical models of mind', in S. Everson (ed.), *Psychology*, Cambridge, 194–217
  (1995), 'The growth of medical empiricism', in D. Bates (ed.), *Knowledge and the Scholarly Medical Tradition*, Cambridge, 59–83
  (1998a), *Cause and Explanation in Ancient Greek Thought*, Oxford
  (1998b), *Galen. On Antecedent Causes*, Cambridge
  (1998c), 'Magic, religion and science: divine and human in the Hippocratic Corpus', *Apeiron* 31, 1–34
  (1999), 'Hellenistic biological sciences', in D. Furley (ed.), *From Aristotle to Augustine* (Routledge History of Philosophy, vol. 11), London and New York, 320–55
  (2002), 'Doctoring history: ancient medical historiography and Diocles of Carystus' (review of van der Eijk (1999a) and van der Eijk (2000a, 2001a)), *Apeiron* 35, 65–81
Hanse, H. (1939), *'Gott haben' in der Antike und im frühen Christentum*. Berlin.
Hanson, A. E. (1997), 'Fragmentation and the Greek medical writers', in Most (ed.) (1997), 289–314

Hanson, A. E. and M. Green (1994), 'Soranus of Ephesus: Methodicorum princeps', *ANRW* 11.37.2, 968–1075

Hanson, J. S. (1970), 'Dreams and visions in the Graeco-Roman world and in early Christianity', *ANRW* 11.23.2, 1395–427

Hardie, W. F. R. (1964), 'Aristotle's treatment of the relation between the soul and the body', *The Philosophical Quarterly* 14, 53–72

(1976), 'Concepts of consciousness in Aristotle', *Mind* 85, 388–411

Harig, G. (1974), *Bestimmung der Intensität im medizinischen System Galens*, Berlin

(1977), 'Bemerkungen zum Verhältnis der griechischen zur altorientalischen Medizin', in R. Joly (ed.), *Corpus Hippocraticum*, Mons, 77–94

(1980), 'Anfänge der theoretischen Pharmakologie im Corpus Hippocraticum', in Grmek (ed.) (1980) 223–45

(1983), 'Zur Charakterisierung der wissenschaftstheoretischen Aspekte in der Aristotelischen Biologie und Medizin', in J. Irmscher and R. Müller (eds.), *Aristoteles als Wissenschaftstheoretiker*, Berlin, 159–70

Harig, G. and Kollesch, J. (1971), 'Gesellschaftliche Aspekte der antiken Diätetik', *NTM Schriftenreihe zur Geschichte der Naturwissenschaften, Technik und Medizin* 8, 14–23

(1974), 'Diokles von Karystos und die zoologische Systematik', *NTM Schriftenreihe zur Geschichte der Naturwissenschaften, Technik und Medizin* 11, 24–31

Harris, C. (1973), *The Heart and the Vascular System in Ancient Greek Medicine*, Oxford

Hartman, E. (1977), *Substance, Body and Soul*, Princeton

Havelock, E. A. (1982a), *The Literate Revolution in Greece and its Cultural Consequences*, Princeton

(1982b), *Preface to Plato*, Cambridge, Mass.

Hayduck, M. (1897), *Ioannis Philoponi in Aristotelis De anima libros commentaria*, Berlin

Heeg, J. (1911), 'Über ein angebliches Dioklescitat', *Sitzungsberichte der preussischen Akademie der Wissenschaften Berlin*, 911–1007

(ed.) (1915), *Galeni In Hippocratis Prognosticum commentaria III*, in H. Diels (ed.), *Galeni In Hippocratis Prorrheticon commentaria III*; J. Mewaldt (ed.), *Galeni De comate secundum Hippocratem*; J. Heeg (ed.), *Galeni In Hippocratis Prognosticum commentaria III* (*CMG* v 9, 2), Leipzig and Berlin

Heiberg, J. L. (1920), *Naturwissenschaften, Mathematik und Medizin im klassischen Altertum*, 2nd edn, Leipzig and Berlin

Heinaman, R. (1990), 'Aristotle and the mind–body problem', *Phronesis* 35, 83–102

Heinimann, F. (1945), *Nomos und Physis*, Basel

(1955), 'Diokles von Karystos und der prophylaktische Brief an König Antigonos', *Museum Helveticum* 12, 158–72

Hellweg, R. (1985), *Stilistische Untersuchungen zu den Krankengeschichten der Epidemienbücher I und III des Corpus Hippocraticum*, Bonn

Helmreich, G. (ed.) (1923), *Galeni de alimentorum facultatibus* in K. Koch (ed.), *Galeni de sanitate tuenda*; G. Helmreich (ed.), *Galeni de alimentorum facultatibus, De bonis malisque sucis*; C. Kalbfleisch (ed.), *Galeni de victu attenuante*; and O. Hartlich (ed.), *Galeni de ptisana* (*CMG* v 4, 2), Leipzig and Berlin

Herzog, R. (1931), *Die Wunderheilungen von Epidauros* (Philologus Suppl. 22), Berlin
Hett, W. S. (1957), *Aristotle. On the Soul. Parva Naturalia. On Breath*, 2nd edn, Cambridge, Mass. and London
Hey, F. O. (1908), *Der Traumglaube der Antike*, Munich
  (1910), *Die Wurzeln der griechischen Religion in besonderem Zusammenhang mit dem Traumglauben*, Neuburg
Hicken, W. (1958), 'The character and provenance of Socrates' "dream" in the Theaetetus', *Phronesis* 3, 129–49
Hicks, R. D. (1907), *Aristotle. De Anima*, Cambridge
Hirschberg, J. (1982), *The History of Ophthalmology*, vol. 1: *Antiquity*, reprint, Bonn
Hirzel, R. (1895), *Der Dialog*, 2 vols., Leipzig
Hobson, J. A. (1988), *The Dreaming Brain*, New York
Hoessly, F. (2001), *Katharsis. Reinigung als Heilverfahren. Studien zum Ritual der archaischen und klassischen Zeit sowie zum Corpus Hippocraticum* (Hypomnemata 135), Göttingen
Hohenstein, H. (1935), *Der Arzt Mnesitheos aus Athen*, Berlin
Holowchak, M. A. (1996), 'Aristotle on dreaming: what goes on in sleep when the "big fire" goes out?', *Ancient Philosophy* 16, 405–23
  (2001), 'Interpreting dreams for corrective regimen: diagnostic dreams in Greco–Roman medicine', *Journal of the History of Medicine and Allied Sciences* 56, 382–99
Hopfner, T. (1921–4), *Griechisch-ägyptischer Offenbarungszauber*, 2 vols., Leipzig
  (1928), 'Mantike,' *RE* XIV.1, 1258–88
  (1937), 'Traumdeutung', *RE* VI.2, 2233–45
  (1938), *Das Sexualleben der Griechen und Römer*, Prague
Horn, H.-J. (1988), 'Aristote, Traité de l'âme, III, 3 et le concept aristotélicien de la φαντασία', *Les Etudes Philosophiques* 63, 221–34
Horowitz, M. C. (1976), 'Aristotle on women', *Journal of the History of Biology* 9, 183–213
Horstmanshoff, H. F. J. and Stol, M. (eds.) (2004), *Magic and Rationality in Ancient New Eastern and Graeco-Roman Medicine*, Leiden
Hort, A. F. (1916–26), *Theophrastus. Enquiry into Plants*, 2 vols., Cambridge, Mass. and London
Hubert, R. (1999), 'Veille, sommeil et rêve chez Aristote', *Revue de Philosophie Ancienne* 17, 75–111
Huby, P. M. (1973), 'Aristotle, De insomniis 462 a 18', *The Classical Quarterly* 25, 151–2
  (1979), 'The paranormal in the works of Aristotle and his circle', *Apeiron* 13, 53–62
Huffman, C. A. (1993), *Philolaos of Croton. Pythagorean and Presocratic*, Cambridge
Hüffmeier F. (1961), 'Phronesis in den Schriften des Corpus Hippocraticum', *Hermes* 89, 51–84
Hundt, J. (1934), *Der Traumglaube bei Homer*, Greifswald
Hunter, V. (1982), *Past and Process in Herodotus and Thucydides*, Princeton

Hymes, D. (1972), 'Models of the interaction of language and social life', in J. J. Gumperz and D. Hymes (eds.), *Directions in Sociolinguistics. The Ethnography of Communication*, New York, 35–71

Ideler, I. L. (1834), *Aristotelis Meteorologica libri IV*, Leipzig

Ilberg, J. (1910), 'Zur gynäkologischen Ethik der Griechen', *Archiv für Religionswissenschaft* 13, 1–19

Impara, P. (1973), 'θεία μοῖρα e ἐνθουσιασμός in Platone', *Proteus* 4, 41–56

Irmscher, J. and Müller, R. (eds.) (1983), *Aristoteles als Wissenschaftstheoretiker*, Berlin

Iskandar, A. Z. (1976), 'An attempted reconstruction of the late Alexandrian medical curriculum', *Medical History* 20, 235–58

Jackson, H. (1913), 'Eudemian Ethics 8 i, ii (7 xiii, xiv) 1246a 26–1248b 7', *Journal of Philology* 32, 14

Jackson, R. (1988), *Doctors and Diseases in the Roman Empire*, London

Jackson, S. W. (1986), *Melancholia and Depression. From Hippocratic Times to Modern Times*, New Haven and London

Jacques, J.-M. (1997), 'La méthode de Galien pharmacologue dans les traités sur les médicaments composés', in A. Debru (ed.), *Galen on Pharmacology. Philosophy, History and Medicine*, Leiden, 103–29

Jaeger, W. W. (1913), 'Das Pneuma im Lykeion', *Hermes* 48, 29–74

(1923), *Aristoteles. Grundlegung einer Geschichte seiner Entwicklung*, Berlin

(1938a), *Diokles von Karystos. Die griechische Medizin und die Schule des Aristoteles*, Berlin

(1938b), *Vergessene Fragmente des Peripatetikers Diokles von Karystos. Nebst zwei Abhandlungen zur Chronologie der dogmatischen Ärzteschule* (Abhandlungen der preussischen Akademie der Wissenschaften, Phil.–hist. Klasse, 1938.3), Berlin

(1940), 'Diocles. A new pupil of Aristotle', *Philosophical Review* 49, 393–414 (reprinted in Jaeger (1948) 407–25)

(1948), *Aristotle. Fundamentals of the History of his Development*, 2nd edn, Oxford

(1951), 'Diokles von Karystos. Ein neuer Schüler des Aristoteles', *Zeitschrift für philosophische Forschung* 5, 25–46

(1952), 'Diokles von Karystos und Aristoxenos über die Prinzipien', in *Hermeneia. Festschrift für O. Regenbogen*, Heidelberg, 94–103

(1959), *Paideia*, vol. 11, 3rd edn, Berlin

(1980), *The Theology of the Early Greek Philosophers*, reprint Westport (first published Oxford, 1947)

Jakobson, R. (1960), 'Linguistics and poetics', in T. A. Sebeok (ed.), *Style in Language*, Cambridge, Mass., 350–8

Johansen, T. K. (1997), *Aristotle on the Sense-Organs*, Cambridge

(1998), review of van der Eijk (1994), *Journal of Hellenic Studies* 118, 228–9

Johnson, K. (1997), 'Luck and good fortune in the Eudemian Ethics', *Ancient Philosophy* 17, 85–102

Joly, R. (1960), *Recherches sur le traité pseudo-hippocratique Du régime*, Paris

(1969), 'Sur une nouvelle édition de *La nature de l'homme*', *L'Antiquité Classique* 38, 150–7

(1975), 'Le système cnidien des humeurs', in Bourgey and Jouanna (eds.) (1975) 107–28
Joly, R. and Byl, S. (1984), *Hippocrate. Du régime*, Berlin
Jones, W. H. S. (1947), *The Medical Writings of Anonymus Londinensis*, Cambridge
Jones, W. H. S. and Withington, E. T. (1923–31), *Hippocrates*, 4 vols.; vols. I–II (1923), tr. Jones; vol. III (1927), tr. Withington; vol. IV (1931), tr. Jones, Cambridge, Mass. and London
Jordan, D. M. (1986), 'Ancient philosophical protreptic and the problem of persuasive genres', *Rhetorica* 4, 309–33
Jori, A. (1994), 'Les "rêves d'eau" dans le traité du Régime', in R. Ginouvès et al. (eds.), *L'eau, la santé et la maladie dans le monde grec* (Bulletin de Correspondance Hellénique, Suppl. XXVIII), 61–75
(1995), 'Le pepaideumenos et la médecine', in van der Eijk, Horstmanshoff and Schrijvers (eds.) (1995) vol. II, 411–24
Jouanna, J. (1966), 'La théorie de l'intelligence et de l'âme dans le traité hippocratique *Du régime*: ses rapports avec Empédocle et le Timée de Platon', *Revue des Etudes Grecques* 79, 15–19
(1974), *Hippocrate. Pour une archéologie de l'école de Cnide*, Paris
(1975), *Hippocrate. La nature de l'homme*, Berlin
(1982), 'Réalité et théâtralité du rêve: le rêve dans l'Hécube d'Euripide', *Ktema* 7, 43–52
(1983), *Hippocrate. Maladies II*, Paris
(1984), 'Rhétorique et médecine dans la Collection Hippocratique', *Revue des Etudes Grecques* 57, 26–44
(1988a), *Hippocrate. Des vents, de l'art*, Paris
(1988b), 'Ippocrate e il sacro', *Koinonia* 12, 91–113
(1990), *Hippocrate. L'ancienne médecine*, Paris
(1992), *Hippocrate*, Paris
(1996), *Hippocrate. Airs, Eaux, Lieux*, Paris
(1998), 'L'interprétation des rêves et la théorie micro-macrocosmique dans le traité hippocratique *Du régime*: sémiotique et mimesis', in K.-D. Fischer, D. Nickel and P. Potter (eds.), *Text and Tradition*, Leiden, 161–74
(1999), *Hippocrates*, Baltimore (Eng. tr. of Jouanna 1992)
(2003), *Hippocrate. Maladie sacrée*, Paris
Jüthner, J. (1909), *Philostratos. Über Gymnastik*, Leipzig and Berlin (reprinted Amsterdam, 1969)
Kahn, C. (1966), 'Sensation and consciousness in Aristotle's psychology', *Archiv für die Geschichte der Philosophie* 48, 43–81 (reprinted in Barnes, Schofield and Sorabji (eds.) (1979) vol. IV, 1–31)
(1992), 'Aristotle on thinking', in Nussbaum and Rorty (eds.) (1992) 359–80
Kalthoff, P. (1934), *Das Gesundheitswesen bei Aristoteles*, Berlin and Bonn
Kampe, F. F. (1870), *Die Erkenntnisstheorie des Aristoteles*, Leipzig
Kany-Turpin, J. and Pellegrin, P. (1989), 'Cicero and the Aristotelian theory of divination by dreams', in W.W. Fortenbaugh and P. Steinmetz (eds.), *Cicero's Knowledge of the Peripatos*, New Brunswick, 220–45
Kapp, R. O. (1961), *The Presentation of Technical Information*, London

Kassies, W. (1999), 'Gezond leven. Fragment uit de *Hygieina* (Gezondheidsleer) van Diocles van Carystus', *Hermeneus* 71, 72–7

Kauder, E. (1960), *Physikalische Modellvorstellung und physiologische Lehre im Corpus Hippocraticum und bei Aristoteles*, Hamburg

Keil, G. (ed.) (1981), *Fachprosa-studien*, Berlin

Kenner, H. (1939), 'Oneiros', *RE* XVIII.1, 448–59

Kenny, A. J. P. (1967), 'The argument from illusion in Aristotle's Metaphysics', *Mind* 76, 184–97

(1978), *The Aristotelian Ethics*, Oxford

(1992), *Aristotle on the Perfect Life*, Oxford

Kessels, A. H. M. (1969), 'Ancient systems of dream classification', *Mnemosyne* 22, 389–424

(1978), *Studies on the Dream in Greek Literature*, Utrecht

Keuls, E. (1995), 'The Greek medical texts and the sexual ethos of ancient Athens', in van der Eijk, Horstmanshoff and Schrijvers (eds.) (1995) vol. I, 261–73

Kienle, W. von (1961), *Berichte über die Sukzessionen der Philosophen in der hellenistischen und spätantiken Literatur*, Berlin

Kind, F. E. (1927), 'Soranos', *RE* III.A.1, 1113–30

King, H. (1998), *Hippocrates' Woman*, London

King, R. A. H. (2001), *Aristotle on Life and Death*, London

Kinneavy, J. L. (1971), *A Theory of Discourse*, Englewood Cliffs

Klibansky, R., Panofsky, E. and Saxl, F. (1964), *Saturn and Melancholy. Studies in the History of Natural Philosophy, Medicine, Religion and Art*, Edinburgh

(1990), *Saturn und Melancholie. Studien zur Geschichte der Naturphilosophie und Medizin, der Religion und der Kunst*, Frankfurt a.M. (German tr. of (1964) with revisions)

Koelbing, H. M. (1968), 'Zur Sehtheorie im Altertum. Alkmaion und Aristoteles', *Gesnerus* 25, 5–9

Köhnken, A. (1988), 'Der dritte Traum des Xerxes bei Herodot', *Hermes* 116, 24–40

Kollesch, J. (1964), 'Zur Geschichte des medizinischen Lehrbuchs in der Antike', in R. Blaser and H. Buess (eds.), *Aktuelle Probleme aus der Geschichte der Medizin*. Verhandlungen des XIX. internationalen Kongress für Geschichte der Medizin, Basel, 204–8

(1973), *Untersuchungen zu den pseudogalenischen Definitiones medicae*, Berlin

(1974), 'Zur Säftelehre in der Medizin des 4. Jahrhunderts v.u.Z.', in *Acta Congressus Internationalis XXIV Historiae Artis Medicinae*, Budapest, vol. II, 1339–42

(1983), 'Zu Aristoteles' Bewertung von Erfahrung und Theorie in der Medizin und ihren Auswirkung auf die Entwicklung der Heilkunde im Hellenismus', in Irmscher and Müller (eds.) (1983) 179–82

(1985), *Aristoteles. Über die Bewegung der Lebewesen. Über die Fortbewegung der Lebewesen*, Berlin

(1990), 'Vorwort', in Caelius Aurelianus, *Akute Krankheiten I–III. Chronische Krankheiten I–V*, ed. G. Bendz and I. Pape, vol. I, Berlin, 5–6

(1991), 'Darstellungsformen der medizinischen Literatur im 5. und 4. Jh. v. Chr.', *Philologus* 135, 177–83

(1992), 'Zur Mündlichkeit der hippokratischen Schriften', in López Férez (1992) 335–42
(1997), 'Die anatomischen Untersuchungen des Aristoteles und ihr Stellenwert als Forschungsmethode in der Aristotelischen Biologie', in W. Kullmann and S. Föllinger (eds.), *Aristotelische Biologie. Intentionen, Methoden, Ergebnisse* (Philosophie der Antike 6), Stuttgart, 367–73
Kosman, L. (1975), 'Perceiving that we perceive: On the soul 111 2', *The Philosophical Review* 84, 499–519
Krafft, F. (1970), *Dynamische und statische Betrachtungsweisen in der antiken Mechanik*, Wiesbaden
Krug, A. (1985), *Heilkunst und Heilkult*, Munich
Kucharski, P. (1954), 'Sur la théorie des couleurs et des saveurs dans le De sensu aristotélicien', *Revue des Etudes Grecques* 67, 355–90
Kudlien, F. (1963), 'Probleme um Diokles von Karystos', *Sudhoffs Archiv* 47, 456–64 (reprinted in Flashar (ed.) (1971) 192–201)
(1964), 'Herophilos und der Beginn der medizinischen Skepsis', *Gesnerus* 21, 1–13 (reprinted in Flashar (ed.) (1971) 280–95)
(1965), 'Dogmatische Ärzte', *RE* Suppl. x, 179–80
(1967a), *Der Beginn des medizinischen Denkens in der Antike*, Zurich and Stuttgart
(1967b), 'Diokles von Karystos', *Der kleine Pauly* 2, 56–7
(1970), 'Medical education in classical antiquity', in C. D. O'Malley (ed.), *The History of Medical Education*, Berkeley and Los Angeles, 3–37
(1971), *Aretaeus von Kappadozien als medizinischer Schriftsteller* (Abhandlungen der sächsischen Akademie der Wissenschaften zu Leipzig, Philol.-hist. Klasse 63.3), Berlin
(1973), '"Schwärzliche" Organe im frühgriechischen Denken', *Medizinhistorisches Journal* 8, 53–8
(1974), 'Dialektik und Medizin in der Antike', *Medizinhistorisches Journal* 9, 187–200
(1977), 'Das Göttliche und die Natur im hippokratischen Prognostikon', *Hermes* 105, 268–74
(1985), '"Klassen"-Teilung der Ärzte bei Aristoteles', in Wiesner (ed.) (1985) vol. 1, 427–35
(1988), 'Der ärztliche Beruf in Staat und Gesellschaft der Antike', *Jahrbuch des Instituts für Geschichte der Medizin der Robert Bosch Stiftung* 7, 41–73
(1991), 'Endeixis as a scientific term: a) Galen's usage of the word (in medicine and logic)', in F. Kudlien and R. Durling (eds.), *Galen's Method of Healing. Proceedings of the 1982 Galen Symposium*, Leiden, 103–11.
Kühlewein, H. (1894–1902), *Hippocratis opera quae feruntur omnia*, Leipzig
Kühn, C. G. (1820), *De Diocle Carystio*, Leipzig (reprinted in Kühn (1826) 86–127)
(1826), *Opuscula academica medica et philologica*, vol. 11, Leipzig
Kühn, J.-H. (1956), *System- und Methodenprobleme im Corpus Hippocraticum*, Wiesbaden
Kühn, J.-H. and Fleischer, U. (1986–9), *Index Hippocraticus*, 4 vols., Göttingen

Kühner, R. and Gerth, B. (1955), *Ausführliche Grammatik der griechischen Sprache, 2. Teil: Satzlehre*, 2 vols., 4th edn, Hanover
Kullmann, W. (1974), *Wissenschaft und Methode. Interpretationen zur aristotelischen Theorie der Naturwissenschaft*, Berlin and New York
  (1982), 'Aristoteles' Grundgedanken zu Aufbau und Funktion der Körpergewebe', *Sudhoffs Archiv* 66, 209–38
  (1998), 'Zoologische Sammelwerke in der Antike', in Kullmann, Althoff and Asper (eds.) (1998), 121–40
Kullmann, W. and Althoff, J. (eds.) (1993), *Vermittlung und Tradierung von Wissen in der griechischen Literatur*, Tübingen
Kullmann, W., Althoff, J. and Asper, M. (eds.) (1998), *Gattungen wissenschaftlicher Literatur in der Antike*, Tübingen
Kullmann, W. and Reichel, M. (eds.) (1990), *Der Übergang von der Mündlichkeit zur Literatur bei den Griechen*, Tübingen
Labarrière, J. L. (1984), 'Imagination humaine et imagination animale chez Aristote', *Phronesis* 29, 17–49
Lacombe, G. (1931), 'The mediaeval Latin versions of the Parva Naturalia', *The New Scholasticism* 5, 289–314
Lain-Entralgo, P. (1975), 'Quaestiones hippocraticae disputatae tres', in L. Bourgey and J. Jouanna (eds.), *La Collection Hippocratique et son rôle dans l'histoire de la médecine*, Leiden, 315–19
Laks, A. and Louguet, C. (eds.) (2002), *Qu'est-ce que la philosophie présocratique?*, Villeneuve-d'Ascq
Lambert, R. (1966), 'L'observation des ressemblances d'après Aristote', *Laval Théologique et philosophique* 22, 169–85
Lameere, W. (1949), 'Au temps que Franz Cumont s'interrogeait sur Aristote', *L'Antiquité Classique* 18, 279–324
Lanata, G. (1967), *Medicina magica e religione popolare*, Rome
  (1968), 'Linguaggio scientifico e linguaggio poetico. Note al lessico del *de morbo sacro*', *Quaderni urbinati della cultura classica* 5, 22–36
Langholf, V. (1977), *Syntaktische Untersuchungen zu Hippokratestexten. Brachylogische Syntagmen in den individuellen Krankheits-Fallbeschreibungen der hippokratischen Schriftensammlung*, Wiesbaden
  (1980), 'Über die Kompatibilität einiger binärer und quaternärer Theorien im Corpus Hippocraticum', in Grmek (ed.) (1980) 333–46
  (1989a), 'Beobachtungen zur Struktur einiger Traktate des "Corpus Hippocraticum"', *Sudhoffs Archiv* 73, 64–77
  (1989b), 'Frühe Fälle der "Verwendung" von Analogien in der altgriechischen Medizin', *Berichte zur Wissenschaftsgeschichte* 12, 7–18
  (1989c), 'Generalisationen und Aphorismen in den Epidemienbücher', in G. Baader and R. Winau (eds.), *Die Hippokratischen Epidemien. Theorie – Praxis – Tradition*, Stuttgart, 131–43
  (1990), *Medical Theories in Hippocrates. Early Texts and the 'Epidemics'*, Berlin
  (1996), 'Nachrichten bei Platon über die Kommunikation zwischen Ärzten und Patienten', in R. Wittern and P. Pellegrin (eds.), *Hippokratische Medizin und antike Philosophie*, Hildesheim, 113–42

Langslow, D. (1989), 'Latin technical language: synonyms and Greek words in Latin medical terminology', *Transactions of the Philological Society* 87, 33–53
  (1991), 'The development of Latin medical terminology: some working hypotheses', *Proceedings of the Cambridge Philological Society* 37, 106–30
  (1994a), 'Celsus and the makings of a Latin medical terminology', in Sabbah and Mudry (eds.) (1994) 297–318
  (1994b), 'Some historical developments in the terminology and style of Latin medical writings', in M. E. Vázquez Buján (ed.), *Tradición e innovación de la medicina latina de la antigüedad y de la alta edad media*, Santiago de Compostela, 225–40
Lanza, D. (1971), *Aristotele. Brevi Opere di psicologia e fisiologia*, in D. Lanza and M. Vegetti, *Aristotele. Opere biologiche*, Turin
Lara Nava (1992), 'Función literaria del prólogo en los tratados hipocráticos más antiguos', in López Férez (1992), 343–50
Larrain, C. J. (1992), *Galens Kommentar zu Platons Timaios*, Stuttgart
Laskaris, J. (2002), *The Art is Long. On the Sacred Disease and the Scientific Tradition*, Leiden
Lasserre, F. and Mudry, P. (eds.) (1983), *Formes de pensée dans la Collection Hippocratique. Actes du 4me Colloque International Hippocratique*, Geneva
Latacz, J. (1987), 'Funktionen des Traums in der antiken Literatur', in Wagner-Simon and Benedetti (eds.) (1987) 10–31
Latte, K. (1939), 'Orakel', *RE* xviii, 830–66
Laurenti, R. (1987), *Aristotele. I frammenti dei Dialoghi*, 2 vols., Naples
  (1971), *Aristotele. I piccoli trattati naturali*, Bari (reprinted in *Aristotele. Della generazione e della corruzione, Dell'anima, Piccoli trattati di storia naturale*, tr. A. Russo and R. Laurenti, Bari, 1987)
Lausberg, H. (1973), *Handbuch der literarischen Rhetorik*, 2nd edn, Munich
  (1976), *Elemente der literarischen Rhetorik*, 5th edn, Munich
Le Goff, J. (1985), 'Le christianisme et les rêves (ii[e]–viii[e] s.)', in T. Gregory (ed.), *I sogni nel medioevo. Seminario internazionale*, Rome, 171–218
Lee, H. D. P. (1952), *Aristotle. Meteorologica*, Cambridge, Mass.
Leeman, A. (1963), *Orationis Ratio. The Stylistic Theories and Practice of the Roman Orators, Historians and Philosophers*, Amsterdam
Lefebvre, R. (1988), 'Le miroir de l'âme (Aristote, *De insomniis* 459 b 25–460 a 26)', *Les Etudes Philosophiques* 63, 195–206
Lefèvre, Ch. (1972), *Sur l'évolution d'Aristote en psychologie*, Louvain
  (1978), 'Sur le statut de l'âme dans le De Anima et les Parva Naturalia', in Lloyd and Owen (eds.) (1978) 21–68
Leisegang, H. (1919), *Der Heilige Geist. Das Wesen und Werden der mystisch-intuitiven Erkenntnis in der Philosophie und Religion der Griechen*, vol. 1, Berlin
Leitner, H. (1973), *A Bibliography to the Ancient Medical Authors*, Bern, Stuttgart and Vienna
Lengen, R. (2002), *Form und Funktion der aristotelischen Pragmatie*, Stuttgart
Lennox, J. G. (1982), 'Teleology, chance and Aristotle's theory of spontaneous generation', *Journal of the History of Philosophy* 20, 219–38

(1984), 'Aristotle on chance', *Archiv für die Geschichte der Philosophie* 66, 52–60
(2001), *Aristotle. Parts of Animals*, Oxford
Lerza, P. (1986), 'Sogni e incubi dei melancolici. Possibili casi di sindromi narcolettiche nell' antichità?', *Studi Italiani di Filologia Classica* 3, 213–21
Lesky, E. (1951), *Die Zeugungs- und Vererbungslehren der Antike und ihr Nachwirken*, (Abhandlungen der Akademie der Wissenschaften und der Literatur Mainz, Geistes- und Sozialwissenschaftliche Klasse 1950, 19), Wiesbaden
Leumann, M. (1950), *Homerische Wörter*, Basel
Levin, S. R. (1982), 'Aristotle's theory of metaphor', *Philosophy and Rhetoric* 15, 24–46
Lévy, E. (1982), 'Le rêve homérique', *Ktema* 7, 23–42
Liatsi, M. (2002), 'Zur Funktion des Traums in der antiken Medizin (Hippokrates, *De victu* IV)', in J. Althoff, B. Herzhoff and G. Wöhrle (eds.), *Antike Naturwissenschaft und ihre Rezeption*, vol. XII, Trier, 7–21
Lichtenthaeler, C. (1992), 'Zur Kontroverse über das *Theion* des *Prognostikon*', *Rheinisches Museum* 135, 382–3
Liddell, H. G., Scott, R. and Jones, H. S. (1968), *A Greek–English Lexicon*, 4th edn, Oxford
Lieshout, R. G. A. van (1970), 'A dream on a καιρός of history', *Mnemosyne* 23, 225–49
(1974), 'Plato over origine en functie van dromen', *Verhandelingen van het Nederlandse Filologencongres* 33, 152–8
(1980), *Greeks on Dreams*, Utrecht
Lilja, S. (1968), 'On the style of the earliest Greek prose', *Commentationes humanarum litterarum, Soc. Scientiarum Fennica* 41, Helsinki
Lloyd, G. E. R. (1963), 'Who is attacked in *On Ancient Medicine*?', *Phronesis* 8, 108–26 (reprinted in Lloyd (1991) 49–69)
(1964), 'Experiment in early Greek philosophy and medicine', *Proceedings of the Cambridge Philological Society* 10, 50–72
(1968a), *Polarity and Analogy*, Cambridge
(1968b), 'The role of medical and biological analogies in Aristotle's Ethics', *Phronesis* 13, 68–83
(1975a), 'Alcmaeon and the early history of dissection', *Sudhoffs Archiv* 59, 113–47 (reprinted in Lloyd (1991) 164–93)
(1975b), 'The Hippocratic Question', *The Classical Quarterly* 25, 171–92 (reprinted in Lloyd (1991) 194–223)
(1975c), 'Aspects of the interrelations of medicine, magic and philosophy in ancient Greece', *Apeiron* 9, 1–16
(1978), 'The empirical basis of physiology in the *Parva Naturalia*', in Lloyd and Owen (eds.) (1978) 215–40
(1979), *Magic, Reason and Experience*, Cambridge
(1983), *Science, Folklore and Ideology*, Cambridge
(1987a), *The Revolutions of Wisdom*, Berkeley and Los Angeles
(1987b), 'Dogmatism and uncertainty in early Greek speculative thought', in M. Détienne (ed.), *Poikilia. Etudes offertes à J. P. Vernant*, Paris, 297–312

(1991a), *Methods and Problems in Greek Science*, Cambridge
(1991b), 'Galen on Hellenistics and Hippocrateans: contemporary battles and past authorities', in Lloyd (1991a) 398–416
(1992), 'Aspects of the relationship between Aristotle's psychology and his zoology', in Nussbaum and Rorty (eds.) (1992) 147–67
(1996a), *Adversaries and Authorities*, Cambridge
(1996b), *Aristotelian Explorations*, Cambridge
(2002), *The Ambitions of Curiosity*, Cambridge
(2003), *In the Grip of Disease*, Oxford
Lloyd, G. E. R. and Owen, G. E. L. (eds.) (1978), *Aristotle on Mind and the Senses. Proceedings of the 7th Symposium Aristotelicum*, Cambridge
Lokhorst, G. J. (1994), 'Aristotle on reflective awareness', *Logique et Analyse* 37, 129–43
(1996), 'The first theory about hemispheric specialization: fresh light on an old codex', *Journal of the History of Medicine and Allied Sciences* 51, 293–312
Longrigg, J. (1963), 'Philosophy and medicine. Some early interactions', *Harvard Studies in Classical Philology* 67, 147–75
(1975), 'Elementary physics in the Lyceum and Stoa', *Isis* 66, 211–29
(1985), 'A seminal "debate" in the fifth century BC?', in A. Gotthelf (ed.), *Aristotle on Nature and Living Things. Philosophical and Historical Studies Presented to D. M. Balme*, Pittsburgh and Bristol, 277–87
(1993), *Greek Rational Medicine*, London
(1995), 'Medicine and the Lyceum', in van der Eijk, Horstmanshoff and Schrijvers (eds.) (1995) vol. II, 431–45
(1998), *Greek Medicine from the Heroic to the Hellenistic Age*, London
(1999), 'Presocratic philosophy and Hippocratic dietetic therapy', in I. Garofalo et al. (eds.), *Aspetti della terapia nel Corpus Hippocraticum*, Florence, 43–50
Lonie, I. (1981), *The Hippocratic Treatises 'On Generation', 'On the Nature of the Child', 'Diseases IV'*, Berlin and New York
(1983), 'Literacy and the development of Hippocratic medicine', in F. Lasserre and Ph. Mudry (eds.), *Formes de pensée dans la Collection hippocratique* (Actes du 4me Colloque international hippocratique), Geneva, 145–61
López Férez, J. A. (ed.) (1991), *Galeno. Obre, pensamiento e influencia*, Madrid
(ed.) (1992), *Tratados hipocráticos*. Actas del VIIe Colloque international hippocratique, Madrid
Loretto, F. (1956), *Träume und Traumglaube in den Geschichtswerken der Griechen und Römer*, Graz
Louis, P. (1956), *Aristote. Les parties des animaux*, Paris
(1961), *Aristote. De la génération des animaux*, Paris
(1964–9), *Aristote. Histoire des animaux*, 3 vols., Paris
(1982), *Aristote. Météorologiques*, 2 vols., Paris
(1991–4), *Aristote. Problèmes*, 3 vols., Paris
Lowe, M. (1978), 'Aristotle's *De somno* and his theory of causes', *Phronesis* 23, 279–91
(1983), 'Aristotle on kinds of thinking', *Phronesis* 28, 17–30
Lucas, D. W. (1968), *Aristotle: Poetics*, Oxford

Luria, S. (1927), 'Studien zur Geschichte der antiken Traumdeutung', *Bulletin de l'Académie des Sciences de l'URSS*, VIe Série, 441–66 and 1041–72

Lycos, K. (1964), 'Aristotle and Plato on appearing', *Mind* 73, 496–514

Macalister, S. (1990), 'Aristotle on the dream: a twelfth-century romance revival', *Byzantion* 60, 195–212

Majno, G. (1975), *The Healing Hand. Man and Wound in the Ancient World*, Cambridge, Mass.

Maloney, G. (1980), 'L'emploi des particules dans les œuvres d'Hippocrate', *Revue de l'Organisation internationale pour l'étude des langues anciennes par ordinateur* 4, 1–3

Maloney, G. and Maloney, M. (1979), *Distribution des particules selon les œuvres hippocratiques par genres littéraires*, Quebec

Maloney, G., Potter, P. and Frohn, W. (1979), *Répartition des œuvres hippocratiques par genres littéraires*, Quebec

Maloney, G. and Savoie, R. (1982), *Cinq Cents Ans de Bibliographie Hippocratique 1473–1982*, Quebec

Manetti, D. (1985), 'Tematica filosofica e scientifica nel Papiro Fiorentino 115: un probabile frammento di Galeno *In Hippocratis de alimento*', in W. Cavini et al. (eds.), *Studi su papiri greci di logica e medicina*, Florence, 173–213

(1986), 'Note di lettura dell'Anonimo Londinense. Prolegomena ad una nuova edizione', *Zeitschrift für Papyrologie und Epigraphik* 63, 57–74

(1992), 'Hippo Crotoniates 1T', *Corpus dei papiri filosofici greci e latini* 1 1**, Florence, 455–61

(1994), 'Autografi e incompiuti: il caso dell'Anonimo Londinense P. Lit. Lond. 165', *Zeitschrift für Papyrologie und Epigraphik* 100, 47–58

(1999a), ' "Aristotle" and the role of doxography in the Anonymus Londiniensis (PBrLibr Inv. 137)', in van der Eijk (ed.) (1999a) 95–141

(1999b), 'Philolaus 1T', 'Plato 129T', in *Corpus dei papiri filosofici greci e latini* 1 1***, Florence, 16–31; 528–78

Manetti, D. and Roselli, A. (1982), *Ippocrate. Epidemie. Libro sesto*, Florence

(1994), 'Galeno commentatore di Ippocrate', *ANRW* II. 37.2, 1530–635

Mani, N. (1965), *Die historischen Grundlagen der Leberforschung*, vol. 1: *Die Vorstellungen über Anatomie, Physiologie und Pathologie der Leber in der Antike* (Basler Veröffentlichungen zur Geschichte der Medizin und Biologie 9), Basel

Mansfeld, J. (1967), 'Heraclitus on the psychology and physiology of sleep and on rivers', *Mnemosyne* 20, 1–29

(1971), *The Pseudo-Hippocratic Tract Περὶ ἑβδομάδων Ch. 1–11 and Greek Philosophy*, Assen (pp. 164ff. on Diocles)

(1986), *Die Vorsokratiker*, 2 vols., Stuttgart

(1989), 'Chrysippus and the *Placita*', *Phronesis* 34, 311–42

(1990), 'Doxography and dialectic: the *Sitz im Leben* of the "Placita" ', *ANRW* II.36.4, 3056–229

(1993), '*Physikai doxai* e *Problemata physica* da Aristotele a Aezio (ed oltre)', in A. M. Battegazzore (ed.), *Dimonstrazione, argumentazione dialettica e argumentazione retorica nel pensiero antico*, Genova, 311–82

(1994), *Prolegomena*, Leiden

Mansfeld, J. and Runia, D. T. (1996), *Aetiana. The Method and Intellectual Context of an Ancient Doxographer*, vol. 1: *The Sources*, Leiden

Mansion, A. (1946), *Introduction à la Physique aristotélicienne*, Louvain and Paris

(1960), 'Le Dieu d'Aristote et le Dieu des chrétiens', in *La philosophie et ses problèmes, Mélanges offerts à R. Jolivet*, Lyon and Paris, 21–44

Mansion, S. (ed.) (1961), *Aristote et les problèmes de méthode*, Louvain and Paris

Manuli, P. (1977), 'La techne medica nella tradizione encefalocentrica e cardio-emocentrica', in R. Joly (ed.), *Corpus Hippocraticum*. Actes du 2me Colloque international hippocratique, Mons, 182–95

(1980), 'Fisiologia e patologia del femminile negli scritti Ippocratici dell' antica ginecologia greca', in Grmek (ed.) (1980) 393–408

Manuli, P. and Vegetti, M. (1977), *Cuore, sangue, cervello: biologia e antropologia nel pensiero antico*, Milan

Manuwald, B. (1985), 'Die Wurftheorien im Corpus Aristotelicum', in Wiesner (ed.) (1985–7) vol. 1, 151–67

Marelli, C. (1979–1980), 'Il sonno tra biologia e medicina in Grecia antica', *Bollettino dell' Istituto di Filologia Greca* 5, 122–37

(1983), 'Place de la Collection hippocratique dans les théories biologiques du sommeil', in Lasserre and Mudry (eds.) (1983) 331–9

Marenghi, G. (1961), 'Aristotele e la medicina greca', *Rendiconti del Istituto Lombardo*, Classe di Lettere 95, 141–61.

(1966), *Aristotele. Problemi di Medicina*, Milan

Marganne, M.-H. (1981), *Inventaire analytique des papyrus grecs de médecine*, Geneva

Marganne, M.-H. and Mertens, P. (1988), 'Medici et medica', *Proceedings of the XVIIIth International Congress of Papyrology*, Athens, vol. 1, 105–46

Mazzolini, R. G. (1992), 'Müller und Aristoteles', in M. Hagner and B. Wahrig-Schmidt (eds.), *Johannes Müller und die Philosophie*, Berlin, 11–27

McGibbon, D. (1965), 'The religious thought of Democritus', *Hermes* 93, 385–97

McGowen Tress, D. (1999), 'Aristotle against the Hippocratics on sexual generation: a reply to Coles', *Phronesis* 44, 228–41

Meijer, P. A. (1981), 'Philosophers, intellectuals and religion in Hellas', in H. S. Versnel (ed.), *Faith, Hope and Worship* (Studies in Greek and Roman Religion 2), Leiden, 216–31

Mendelsohn, E. (1964), *Heat and Life. The Development of the Theory of Animal Heat*, Cambridge, Mass.

Meslin, M. (1980), 'Significations rituelles et symboliques du miroir', in *Perennitas. Studi in onore di Angelo Brelich*, Rome, 327–42

Mewaldt, J. (ed.) (1914), *Galeni In Hippocratis De natura hominis commentaria III*; G. Helmreich (ed.), *Galeni In Hippocratis De victu acutorum commentaria IV*; and J. Westenberger (ed.), *Galeni De diaeta in Hippocratis in morbis acutis* (*CMG* v 9, 1), Leipzig and Berlin

Michler, M. (1968), *Die alexandrinischen Chirurgen. Eine Sammlung und Auswertung ihrer Fragmente*, Wiesbaden

Mikalson, J. D. (1983), *Athenian Popular Religion*, Chapel Hill and London

Miller, G. L. (1990), 'Literacy and the Hippocratic art: reading, writing and epistemology in ancient Greek medicine', *Journal of the History of Medicine* 45, 11–40

Miller, H. W. (1944), 'Medical terminology in tragedy', *Transactions and Proceedings of the American Philological Association* 75, 156–67

(1945), 'Aristophanes and medical language', *Transactions and Proceedings of the American Philological Association* 76, 74–84

(1948), 'A medical theory of cognition', *Transactions and Proceedings of the American Philological Association* 79, 168–83

(1952), 'Dynamis and physis in *On Ancient Medicine*', *Transactions and Proceedings of the American Philological Association* 83, 184–97

(1953), 'The concept of the divine in *De morbo sacro*', *Transactions and Proceedings of the American Philological Association* 84, 1–15

(1957), 'The flux of the body in Plato's *Timaeus*', *Transactions and Proceedings of the American Philological Association* 88, 103–11

(1960), 'The concept of dynamis in *De victu*', *Transactions and Proceedings of the American Philological Association* 90, 147–64

(1962), 'The aetiology of disease in Plato's *Timaeus*', *Transactions and Proceedings of the American Philological Association* 93, 175–87

Mills, M. J. (1981), 'Eudemian Ethics Θ 2, 1247 a 7–13', *Hermes* 109, 253–6

(1983), 'Aristotle's dichotomy of εὐτυχία', *Hermes* 111, 280–95

Mitropoulos, K. (1961), ''Ιατρικα 'Αριστοτέλους', *Platon* 16, 17–61

Modrak, D. K. W. (1981), 'Koinè aisthèsis and the discrimination of sensible differences in *De Anima* III 2', *Canadian Journal of Philosophy* 11, 405–23

(1986), 'Φαντασία reconsidered', *Archiv für die Geschichte der Philosophie* 68, 47–69

(1987), *Aristotle: the Power of Perception*, Chicago

(1990), 'Aristotle the first cognitivist?', *Apeiron* 23, 65–75

Moog, F. P. (1994), *Die Fragmente des Themison von Laodikeia*, Giessen

Moraux, P. (1951), *Les listes anciennes des ouvrages d'Aristote*, Louvain

(ed.) (1968), *Aristoteles in der neueren Forschung* (Wege der Forschung 61), Darmstadt

(1971), 'Das Fragment VIII 1. Text und Interpretation', in Moraux and Harlfinger (eds.) (1971) 253–84

(1973–2001), *Der Aristotelismus bei den Griechen*, 3 vols., Berlin

Moraux, P. and Harlfinger, D. (eds.) (1971), *Untersuchungen zur Eudemischen Ethik*, Berlin and New York

Morel, G. (1960–1), 'De la notion de principe chez Aristote', *Archives de Philosophie* 23, 487–511 and 24, 497–516

Morel, P. M. (2000), *Aristote. Petits traités d'histoire naturelle. Traduction et présentation*, Paris

(2002a), 'Démocrite dans les Parva naturalia d'Aristote', in A. Laks and C. Louguet (eds.), *Qu'est-ce que la philosophue présocratique?*, Villeneuve-d'Ascq, 449–64

(2002b), 'Les *Parva naturalia* d'Aristote et le mouvement animal', *Revue de Philosophie Ancienne* 20, 61–88

Morsink, J. (1979), 'Was Aristotle's biology sexist?', *Journal of the History of Biology* 12, 83–112

Mortarino, M. (1996), *Galeno. Sulle Facoltà Naturali*, Milan

Most, G. W. (ed.) (1997), *Collecting Fragments – Fragmente sammeln*, Göttingen

Motte, A. (ed.) (1990), *Oracles et mantique en Grèce Ancienne*, Liège (= *Kernos* 3)

Moulinier, L. (1952), *Le pur et l'impur dans la pensée des Grecs d'Homère à Aristote*, Paris

Mudry, P. (1977), 'La place d'Hippocrate dans le De medicina de Celse', in R. Joly (ed.), *Corpus Hippocraticum*, Mons, 345–52

(1982), *La préface du 'De medicina' de Celse*, Lausanne

(1990), 'Médecine et vulgarisation', in *Médecine et communication de l'acte médical à la vulgarisation scientifique* (Cahiers de la Faculté de Médecine de l'Université de Genève 19), 5–31

(1997), 'Ethique et médecine à Rome: la Préface de Scribonius Largus ou l'affirmation d'une singularité', in Flashar and Jouanna (eds.) (1997) 297–322

(1998), 'Caelius Aurelianus ou l'anti-Romain: un aspect particulier du traité des Maladies aiguës et des Maladies chroniques', in C. Deroux, (ed.), *Maladie et maladies dans les textes latins antiques et médiévaux*, Brussels, 313–29

(ed.) (1999), *Le traité des Maladies aiguës et des Maladies chroniques de Caelius Aurelianus: nouvelles approches*, Nantes

Mudry, P. and Pigeaud, J. (eds.) (1991), *Les écoles médicales à Rome*, Geneva

Mugler, Ch. (1964), *Dictionnaire historique de la terminologie optique des Grecs*, Paris

Mugnier, R. (1953), *Aristote. Petits traités d'histoire naturelle*, Paris

Müller, C. W. (1975), *Die Kurzdialoge der Appendix Platonica*, Munich

Müller, J. (1826), *Über die phantastischen Gesichterscheinungen. Mit einer physiologischen Urkunde des Aristoteles über den Traum*, Koblenz

Müri, W. (1947), 'Bemerkungen zur hippokratischen Psychologie', in *Festschrift für E. Tièche*, Bern, 71–85

(1953), 'Melancholie und schwarze Galle', *Museum Helveticum* 10, 21–38

(1986), *Der Arzt im Altertum*, 5th edn, Darmstadt

Natali, C. (1974), *Cosmo e divinità. La struttura logica della teologica aristotelica*, L'Aquila

(ed.) (1981), *La scuola dei filosofi. Scienza ed organizzazione istituzionale della scuola di Aristotele*, L'Aquila

Nestle, W. (1938), 'Hippocratica', *Hermes* 73, 1–16

Neuburger, M. and Pagel, J. (eds.) (1902), *Handbuch der Geschichte der Medizin*, initiated by Th. Puschmann, vol. 1, Jena

Neuhäuser, J. (1878a), *Aristoteles' Lehre von dem sinnlichen Erkenntnissvermögen und seinen Organen*, Leipzig

(1878b), review of Bäumker (1877), *Philosophische Monatshefte* 14, 429–34.

Newhall, S. (1911), *Quid de somniis censuerint quoque modo eis usi sint antiqui quaeritur*, Harvard
Nickel, D. (1979), 'Berufsvorstellungen über weibliche Medizinalpersonen in der Antike', *Klio* 61, 515–18
Nieddu, G. F. (1993), 'Neue Wissensformen, Kommunikationstechniken und schriftliche Ausdrucksformen in Griechenland im sechsten und fünften Jh. v. Chr.: einige Beobachtungen', in Kullmann and Althoff (eds.) (1993) 151–66
Nikitas, A. A. (1968), *Untersuchungen zu den Epidemienbüchern II, IV und VI des Corpus Hippocraticum*, Hamburg
  (1976), *Zur Bedeutung von prophasis in der altgriechischen Literatur. Corpus Hippocraticum*, Wiesbaden
Nilsson, M. P. (1955), *Geschichte der griechischen Religion*, vol. 1, Munich
Nolte, H. J. A. (1940), *Het Godsbegrip bij Aristoteles*, Nijmegen
Norden, E. (1909), *Die antike Kunstprosa*, Leipzig and Berlin
Norelli, N. (1992), 'Marcione e gli gnostici sul libero arbitrio, e la polemica di Origene', in Perrone (ed.) (1992) 1–30
Nörenberg, H. W. (1968), *Das Göttliche und die Natur in der Schrift Über die heilige Krankheit*, Bonn
Nussbaum, M. C. (1978), *Aristotle's De motu animalium*, Princeton
  (1980), review of Hartman (1977), *Journal of Philosophy* 77, 355–65
Nussbaum, M. C. and Rorty, A., (eds.) (1992), *Essays on Aristotle's De Anima*, Oxford
Nutton, V. (1992), 'Healers in the medical market place: towards a social history of Greek and Roman medicine', in A. Wear (ed.), *Medicine in Society*, Cambridge, 15–58
  (1995), 'Medicine in the Greek world, 800–50 BC', 'Roman medicine, 250 BC to AD 200' and 'Medicine in Late Antiquity and the Early Middle Ages', in L. I. Conrad et al. (1995) 11–38, 39–70 and 71–88
  (1997), 'Diokles von Karystos', *Der neue Pauly* 3, 610–13
  (2002), 'Ancient medicine: Asclepius transformed', in C. J. Tuplin and T. E. Rihll (eds.), *Science and Mathematics in Ancient Greek Culture*, Oxford, 242–55
Nuyens, F. (1948), *L'évolution de la psychologie d'Aristote*, Louvain
Oberhelman, S. (1979), 'A survey of dreams in Ancient Greece', *Classical Bulletin* 55, 36–40
  (1983), 'Galen on diagnosis of dreams', *Journal of the History of Medicine* 38, 36–47
  (1987), 'Diagnostic dream in ancient medical theory and practice', *Bulletin of the History of Medicine* 61, 47–60
  (1993), 'Dreams in Graeco-Roman medicine', *ANRW* 11.37.1, 121–56
Oehler, K. (1964), 'Aristotle in Byzantium', *Greek, Roman and Byzantine Studies* 5, 133–46
Ogle, W. (1897), *Aristotle on Youth and Old Age, Life and Death, and Respiration*, London
  (1912), *Aristotle: De partibus animalium*, in W. D. Ross and J. A. Smith (eds.), *The Works of Aristotle Translated into English*, vol. v, Oxford

Önnerfors, A. (1976), 'Traumerzählung und Traumtheorie beim älteren Plinius', *Rheinisches Museum* 119, 352–65
  (1993), 'Das medizinische Latein von Celsus bis Cassius Felix', *ANRW* 11.37.1, 227–392
Orelli, L. (1998), 'Vorsokratiker und hippokratische Medizin', in Burkert et al. (eds.) (1998) 128–45
Osborne, C. (1983), 'Aristotle, *De Anima* 3.2. How do we perceive that we see and hear?', *The Classical Quarterly* 33, 401–11
Oser-Grote, C. (1997), 'Das Auge und der Sehvorgang nach Aristoteles und der hippokratischen Schrift De carnibus', in W. Kullmann and S. Föllinger (eds.), *Aristotelische Biologie. Intentionen, Methoden, Ergebnisse*, Stuttgart, 333–50
  (1998), 'Einführung in das Studium der Medizin. Eisagogische Schriften des Galen in ihrem Verhältnis zum Corpus Hippocraticum', in Kullmann, Althoff and Asper (eds.) (1998) 95–117
  (2004), *Aristoteles und das Corpus Hippocraticum*, Stuttgart
Ostenfeld, E. (1987), *Ancient Greek Psychology and the Modern Mind–Body Problem*, Aarhus
Ostwald, M. and Lynch, P. (1992), 'The growth of schools and the advance of knowledge', *Cambridge Ancient History* vi.2, ch. 13, Cambridge
Otterlo, W. A. A. van (1944), *Untersuchungen über Begriff, Anwendung und Entstehung der griechischen Ringkomposition* (Mededelingen der Nederlandse Akademie van Wetenschappen, Afdeling Letterkunde, Nieuwe reeks, Deel 7, no. 3), Amsterdam
Owen, G. E. L. (1961), 'Τιθέναι τὰ φαινόμενα', in S. Mansion (ed.) (1961) 83–103
Owens, J. (1979), 'The relations of God to the world in the *Metaphysics*', in P. Aubenque (ed.), *Etudes sur la Métaphysique d'Aristote*, Paris, 207–22
  (1982), 'Aristotle on common sensibles and incidental perception', *Phoenix* 36, 215–36
Pachet, P. (1985), 'Le miroir du rêve selon Aristote', in J. Brunschwig (ed.), *Histoire et structure. A la mémoire de Victor Goldschmidt*, Paris, 195–200
Palm, A. (1933), *Studien zur hippokratischen Schrift Περὶ διαίτης*, Tübingen
Parker, R. (1983), *Miasma: Pollution and Purification in Early Greek Religion*, Oxford
Pease, A. S. (1963), *M. Tulli Ciceronis De divinatione libri duo*, Darmstadt (reprint)
Peck, A. L. (1928), 'Pseudo-Hippocrates philosophus; or the development of philosophical and other theories as illustrated by the Hippocratic writings, with special reference to De victu and De prisca medicina', unpublished PhD thesis, Cambridge
  (1937), *Aristotle. Parts of Animals*, London and Cambridge, Mass.
  (1942), *Aristotle. Generation of Animals*, London and Cambridge, Mass.
  (1953), 'The connate pneuma, an essential factor in Aristotle's solutions to the problems of reproduction and sensation', in E. A. Underwood (ed.), *Science, Medicine and History. Essays on the Evolution of Scientific Thought and Medical Practice Written in Honour of Ch. Singer*, vol. 1, Oxford, 111–21
  (1965–70), *Aristotle. Historia animalium, Books I–III* and *Books IV–VI*, 2 vols., London and Cambridge, Mass.

Pellegrin, P. (1988), 'L'imaginaire de la fièvre dans la médecine antique', *History and Philosophy of the Life Sciences* 10, 109–20
Pépin, J. (1964), *Théologie cosmique et théologie chrétienne*, Paris
  (1971), *Idées grecques sur l'homme et sur dieu*, Paris
Pera, M. (1991), 'The role and value of rhetoric in science', in Pera and Shea (eds.) (1991) 29–54
  (1994), *The Discourses of Science*, Chicago
Pera, M. and Shea, W. (eds.) (1991), *Persuading Science: the Art of Scientific Rhetoric*, Canton, Mass.
Perelman, C. and Olbrechts-Tyteca, L. (1983), *Traité de l'argumentation: la nouvelle rhétorique*, 4th edn, Brussels
Perrone, L. (ed.) (1992), *Il cuore indurito del Faraone. Origene e il problema del libero arbitrio*, (Origini. Testi e Studi del CISEC, 3), Bologna
Peters, F. E. (1968), *Aristoteles Arabus. The Oriental Translations and Commentaries on the Aristotelian Corpus*, Leiden
Pfeffer, F. (1976), *Studien zur Mantik in der Philosophie der Antike*, Meisenheim am Glan
Pfister, F. (1959), 'Extase', *Reallexicon für Antike und Christentum* 4, 944–87
Philippe, M. D. (1971), 'Φαντασία in the philosophy of Aristotle', *Thomist* 35, 1–42
Pigeaud, J. (1978), 'Une physiologie de l'inspiration poétique', *Les Etudes Classiques* 46, 23–31
  (1980), 'Quelques aspects du rapport de l'âme et du corps dans le Corpus hippocratique', in M. D. Grmek (ed.) (1980) 417–33
  (1981a), *La maladie de l'âme. Etude sur la relation de l'âme et du corps dans la tradition médico-philosophique antique*, Paris
  (1981b), 'Le rêve érotique dans l'antiquité gréco-romaine: l'oneirogmòs', in J. Pigeaud (ed.), *Rêves, sommeil et insomnie*, Paris 1981 (= *Littérature, Médecine, Société* 3), 10–23
  (1982), 'Pro Caelio Aureliano', in G. Sabbah (ed.), *Médecins et médecine dans l'Antiquité*, Saint-Etienne, 105–18
  (1984), 'Prolégomènes à une histoire de la mélancolie', *Histoire, Economie, Société* 3, 501–10
  (1987), *Folie et cures de la folie chez les médecins de l'antiquité Gréco-romaine. La manie*, Paris
  (1988a), *Aristote. L'homme de génie et la mélancolie*, Paris
  (1988b), 'Le style d'Hippocrate ou l'écriture fondatrice de la médecine', in M. Détienne (ed.), *Les savoirs de l'écriture en Grèce ancienne*, Lille, 305–29
  (1991), 'Les fondements du Méthodisme', in P. Mudry and J. Pigeaud (eds.), *Les écoles médicales à Rome*, Geneva, 7–50
  (1993), 'L'introduction du Méthodisme à Rome', *ANRW* 11.37.1, 565–99
  (1994), 'Caelius Aurélien, Maladies aiguës 1,1, De phrenitide: quelques problèmes philologiques. Remarques en vue d'une édition', in Vázquez Buján (ed.) (1994), 29–44
  (1995), *Aristote. La vérité des songes*, Paris

(1997), 'Les fondements de l'éthique médicale: le cas de Rome', in Flashar and Jouanna (eds.) (1997) 255–96

Pigeaud, A. and Pigeaud, J. (eds.) (2000), *Les textes médicaux latins comme littérature*, Nantes

Pines, S. (1974), 'The Arabic recension of Parva Naturalia and the philosophical doctrine concerning veridical dreams according to al-Risalal al-Manamiyya and other sources', *Israel Oriental Studies* 4, 104–53

Poschenrieder, F. (1882), *Die platonischen Dialoge in ihrem Verhältnis zu den hippokratischen Schriften*, Landshut

(1887), *Die naturwissenschaftlichen Schriften des Aristoteles in ihrem Verhältnis zu den Büchern der hippokratischen Sammlung*, Bamberg

Pötscher, W. (1964), *Theophrastos, Περί εὐσεβείας*, Leiden

(1970), *Strukturprobleme der aristotelischen und theophrastischen Gottesvorstellung*, Leiden

Potter, P. (1980), *Hippokrates. Über die Krankheiten III* (*CMG* I 2,3), Berlin

(1988), *Hippocrates*, vols. V and VI, Cambridge, Mass. and London

(1995), *Hippocrates*, vol. VIII, Cambridge, Mass. and London

Potter, P., Maloney, G. and Desautels, J. (eds.) (1990), *La maladie et les maladies dans la Collection hippocratique*, Quebec

Pradeau, J. F. (1998), 'L'âme et la moelle. Les conditions psychiques et physiologiques de l'anthropologie dans le *Timée* de Platon', *Archives de Philosophie* 61, 489–551

Prantl, K. (1849), *Aristoteles. Über die Farben*, Munich

Preisendanz, K. (1942), 'Oneiropompeia', *RE* XXXV, 440–8

Preiser, G. (1976), *Allgemeine Krankheitsbezeichnungen im Corpus Hippocraticum. Gebrauch von Nousos und Nosema*, Berlin

(1978), 'Diagnosis und diagignoskein. Zum Krankheitserkennen im Corpus Hippocraticum', in Habrich, Marguth and Wolf (eds.) (1978) 91–9

Preus, A. (1968), '*On Dreams* ii 459 b 24–460 a 33, and Aristotle's ὄψις', *Phronesis* 13, 175–82

(1975), *Science and Philosophy in Aristotle's Biological Works*, Hildesheim and New York

(1981), *Aristotle and Michael of Ephesus on the Movement and Progression of Animals*, Hildesheim and New York

(1984), 'Aristotle and Hippocratic gynecology', in J. Irmscher and R. Müller (eds.), *Aristoteles als Wissenschaftstheoretiker*, Berlin, 183–96

Prioreschi, P. (1992), 'Did the Hippocratic physician treat hopeless cases?', *Gesnerus* 49, 341–50

Püschel, E. (1988), *Die Menstruation und ihre Tabus*, Stuttgart and New York

Raalte, M. van (1993), *Theophrastus. Metaphysics*, Leiden

Raible, W. (1993), 'Die Entwicklung ideographischer Elemente bei der Verschriftlichung des Wissens', in Kullmann and Althoff (eds.) (1993) 15–38

Rankin, H. D. (1964), 'Dream/vision as a philosophical modifier in Plato's Republic', *Eranos* 62, 75–83

Rawlings, H. R. (1975), *A Semantic Study of Prophasis to 400 BC*, Wiesbaden

Redard, G. (1953), *Recherches sur χρή, χρῆσθαι*, Paris
Redondo, J. (1992), 'Nivelos retóricos en el Corpus Hippocraticum', in López Férez (1992) 409–20
Rees, D. A. (1971), 'Aristotle's treatment of *phantasia*', in Anton and Kustas (eds.) (1971) 491–505
Regenbogen, O. (1930), 'Eine Forschungsmethode antiker Naturwissenschaft', *Quellen und Studien zur Geschichte der Mathematik*, 1 2, 131–82 (reprinted in O. Regenbogen, *Kleine Schriften*, ed. F. Dirlmeier, Munich, 1961, 141–94)
Renehan, R. (1997), 'On some genitives and a few accusatives in Aristotle: a study in style', *Hermes* 125, 153–68
Renkema, J. (1993), *Discourse Studies. An Introductory Textbook*, Amsterdam and Philadelphia
Repici, L. (1988), *La natura e l'anima. Saggi su Stratone di Lampsaco*, Turin
  (1991), 'Aristotele, gli Stoici e il libro Dei Sogni nel De divinatione di Cicerone', *Metis* 6, 167–209 (also printed in *Atti dell' Accademia delle Scienze di Torino* 125 (1991) 93–126)
  (1995), 'Gli Stoici e la divinazione secondo Cicerone', *Hermes* 123, 175–92
  (2003), *Aristotele. Il sonno e i sogni*, Venice
Revesz, B. (1917), *Geschichte des Seelenbegriffs und der Seelenlokalisation*, Stuttgart
Rist, J. M. (1989), *The Mind of Aristotle: a Study in Philosophical Growth*, Toronto
Rivers, W. H. R. (1894), 'A modification of Aristotle's experiment', *Mind* 3, 583–84
Robert, F. (1976), 'Prophasis', *Revue des Etudes Grecques* 89, 317–42
Robertson, G. C. (1876), 'Sense of doubleness with crossed fingers', *Mind* 1, 145–6
Robinson, D. N. (1989), *Aristotle's Psychology*, New York
Robinson, H. M. (1978), 'Mind and body in Aristotle', *The Classical Quarterly*, N.S. 28, 105–24
  (1983), 'Aristotelian dualism', *Oxford Studies in Ancient Philosophy* 1, 123–44
Robinson, T. M. (1970), *Plato's Psychology*, Toronto
Rodier, G. (1900), *Aristote: Traité de l'âme*, Paris
Roheim, G. (1919), *Der Spiegelzauber*, Leipzig
Röhr, J. (1923), *Der okkulte Kraftbegriff* (Philologus Suppl. 17, no. 1), Berlin
Rolfes, E. (1924), *Aristoteles' kleine naturwissenschaftliche Schriften*, Leipzig
Roscher, W. H. (1913), *Die hippokratische Schrift von der Siebenzahl in ihrer vierfachen Überlieferung zum erstenmal herausgegeben und erläutert*, Paderborn
Rose, V. (1854), *De Aristotelis librorum ordine et auctoritate*, Berlin
  (1863), *Aristoteles pseudepigraphus*, Leipzig
  (1864–70), *Anecdota graeca et graecolatina*, 2 vols., Berlin (reprinted 1963)
  (1867), 'Über eine angebliche Paraphrase des Themistius', *Hermes* 2, 191–213
  (1886), *Aristotelis qui ferebantur librorum fragmenta*, Leipzig
Roselli, A. (1992), *[Aristotele]. De spiritu*, Pisa
  (1996), *Ippocrate. La malattia sacra*, Venice
Rosenmeyer, Th.G. (1986), 'Φαντασία und Einbildungskraft. Zur Vorgeschichte eines Leitbegriffs der europäischen Ästhetik', *Poetica* 18, 197–248
Ross, G. R. T. (1906), *Aristotle. De sensu and De memoria*, Cambridge
Ross, W. D. (1923), *Aristotle*, London

(1924), *Aristotle's Metaphysics*, Oxford
(1936), *Aristotle's Physics*, Oxford
(1949), *Aristotle's Prior and Posterior Analytics*, Oxford
(1955), *Aristotle. Parva Naturalia*, Oxford
(1961), *Aristotle's De Anima*, Oxford
Roth, R. J. (1963), 'The Aristotelian use of phantasia and phantasma', *The New Scholasticism* 37, 491–504
Roussel, P. (1988), 'Le concept de mélancolie chez Aristote', *Revue d'Histoire des Sciences* 41, 299–330
Rousselle, A. (1980), 'Observation féminine et idéologie masculine: le corps de la femme d'après les médecins grecs', *Annales: Economies, Sociétés, Civilisations* 35, 1089–115
Rowe, C. J. (1975), 'A reply to John Cooper on the *Magna Moralia*', *American Journal of Philology* 96, 160–72
  (1992), 'On reading Plato', *Methexis* 5, 53–68
Roy, L. (1981), *Le concept de cholê, la bile, dans le Corpus Hippocratique*, Quebec
Rubinstein, G. (1985), 'The riddle of the Methodist method: understanding a Roman medical sect', unpublished PhD thesis, Cambridge
Rudberg, G. (1911), *Zum sogenannten zehnten Buch der aristotelischen Tiergeschichte*, Uppsala
Runia, D. T. (1999), 'The *placita* ascribed to doctors in Aëtius' doxography on physics', in van der Eijk (ed.) (1999a) 189–250
Rüsche, F. (1930), *Blut, Leben, Seele*, Paderborn
Rütten, T. (1992), *Demokrit. Lachender Philosoph und sanguinischer Melancholiker*, Leiden
Rydbeck, L. (1967), *Fachprosa, vermeintliche Volkssprache und Neues Testament* (Acta Universitatis Upsaliensis: Studia graeca Upsaliensia 5), Uppsala
Ryle, G. (1949), *The Concept of Mind*, London
Sabbah, G. (ed.) (1991), *Le latin médical, La constitution d'un langage scientifique*, Saint-Etienne
Sabbah, G. and Mudry, P. (eds.) (1994), *La médecine de Celse*, Saint-Etienne
Sabbah, G., Corsetti, P.-P. and Fischer, K.-D. (1987), *Bibliographie des textes médicaux latins*, Saint-Etienne
Sager, J. C., Dungworth, D. and McDonald, P. F. (1980), *English Special Languages. Principles and Practice in Science and Technology*, Wiesbaden
Sallares, R. (1991), *The Ecology of the Ancient Greek World*, London
Sallares, R. (2003), *Malaria in Ancient Rome*, Oxford
Sandvoss, E. (1968), 'Asebie und Atheismus im klassischen Zeitalter der griechischen Polis', *Saeculum* 19, 312–29
Santini, C. and Scivoletto, N. (eds.) (1990–2), *Prefazioni, prologhi, proemi di opere tecnico-scientifiche latine*, 2 vols., Rome
  (eds.) (1998), *Prefazioni, prologhi, proemi di opere tecnico-scientifiche latine*, vol. III, Rome
Sarton, G. (1927), *A History of Science*, 2 vols., Baltimore
Sassi, M. M. (1978), *Le teorie della percezione in Democrito*, Florence

Saunders, T. J. (1995), *Aristotle. Politics I and II*, Oxford
Scarborough, J. (1985), *Pharmacy's Ancient Heritage: Theophrastus, Nicander, and Dioscurides*, Lexington
Schell, H. (1873), *Die Einheit des Seelenlebens aus den Prinzipien der Aristotelischen Philosophie entwickelt*, Freiburg
Schenkeveld, D. M. (1997), 'Philosophical prose', in S. E. Porter (ed.), *Handbook of Classical Rhetoric in the Hellenistic Period 330 BC – AD 400*, Leiden, 195–264
Schian, R. (1973), *Untersuchungen über das 'argumentum e consensu omnium'*, Hildesheim and New York
Schiller, J. (1973), 'Aristotle and the concept of awareness in sense perception', *Journal of the History of Philosophy* 13, 283–96
Schmidt, J. (1881), *Die psychologischen Lehren des Aristoteles in seinen kleinen naturwissenschaftlichen Schriften*, Prague
Schmitt, C. B. (1985), 'Aristotle among the physicians', in A. Wear, R. K. French and I. M. Lonie (eds.), *The Medical Renaissance of the Sixteenth Century*, Cambridge, 1–15
Schneble, H. (1987), *Krankheit der ungezählten Namen. Ein Beitrag zur Sozial-, Kultur- und Medizingeschichte der Epilepsie anhand ihrer Benennungen vom Altertum bis zur Gegenwart*, Bern, Stuttgart and Toronto
Schofield, M. (1978), 'Aristotle on the imagination', in Lloyd and Owen (eds.) (1978) 99–140 (reprinted in Barnes, Schofield and Sorabji (eds.), vol. IV (1979) 103–32)
  (1986), 'Cicero for and against divination', *Journal of Roman Studies* 76, 47–64
Schöner, E. (1964), *Das Viererschema in der antiken Humoralpathologie*, Stuttgart
Schrijvers, P. H. (1974), 'Vragen over teksten', *Lampas* 7, 17–30
  (1976), 'La pensée d'Epicure et de Lucrèce sur le sommeil', in J. Bollack and A. Laks (eds.), *Etudes sur l'Epicurisme antique*, Lille, 231–59
  (1977), 'La classification des rêves selon Hérophile', *Mnemosyne* 30, 13–27
  (1980), 'Die Traumtheorie des Lukrez', *Mnemosyne* 33, 128–51
  (1985), *Eine medizinische Erklärung der männlichen Homosexualität aus der Antike*, Amsterdam
Schuhl, P.-M. (1960), 'Platon et la médecine', *Revue des Etudes Grecques* 72, 73–9
Schumacher, J. (1940), *Antike Medizin. Die naturphilosophischen Grundlagen der Medizin in der griechischen Antike*, Berlin
Schumann, H.J. von (1975), *Sexualkunde und Sexualmedizin in der klassischen Antike*, Munich
Schütrumpf, E. (1989), 'Form und Stil aristotelischer Pragmatien', *Philologus* 133, 177–91
Schwyzer, E. (1935), 'Zur Sprache', in K. Deichgräber, *Hippokrates über Entstehung und Aufbau des menschlichen Körpers*, Περὶ σαρκῶν, with a contribution on linguistics by Eduard Schwyzer, Leipzig and Berlin, 62–97
Schwyzer, E. and Debrunner, A. (1950), *Griechische Grammatik*, 2 vols., Munich
Sconocchia, S. and Toneatto, L. (eds.) (1993), *Lingue tecniche del greco e del latino*, Atti del Primo Seminario internazionale sulla letteratura scientifica e tecnica greca e latina, Trieste

Seeskin, K. R. (1975–6), 'Platonism, mysticism, and madness', *The Monist* 59, 575–86

Senn, G. (1933), *Die Entwicklung der biologischen Forschungsmethode in der Antike und ihre grundsätzliche Förderung durch Theophrast von Eresos*, Aarau

Serbat, G. (1995), *Celse. De la médecine, Livres I–II*, Paris

Seyboldt, K. (1984), 'Der Traum in der Bibel', in Wagner-Simon and Benedetti (eds.) (1984) 31–54

Sezgin, F. (1970), *Geschichte des arabischen Schrifttums*, vol. III, Leiden

Sharples, R. (1995), *Theophrastus of Eresus. Sources for his Life, Writings, Thought, and Influence*, Commentary, vol. V: *Sources on Biology*, Leiden

(2001), 'Dicaearchus on the soul and on divination', in W. W. Fortenbaugh and E. Schütrumpf (eds.), *Dicaearchus of Messana. Text, Translation and Discussion*, New Brunswick and London, 143–73

Shields, C. (1988), 'Soul and body in Aristotle', *Oxford Studies in Ancient Philosophy* 6, 103–37

Sieverts, C. W. (1949), *Die Physiologie bei Aristoteles*, Münster

Sigerist, H. E. (1961), *A History of Medicine*, vol. II: *Early Greek, Hindu, and Persian Medicine*, New York

Silverman, A. (1989), 'Color and Color-Perception in Aristotle's De Anima', *Ancient Philosophy* 9, 271–92

Simon, B. (1978), *Mind and Madness in Ancient Greece*, London

Simon, G. (1988), *Le regard, l'être et l'apparence dans l'optique de l'antiquité*, Paris

Singer, Ch. (1927), 'The herbal in Antiquity and its transmission to later ages', *Journal of Hellenic Studies* 47, 1–52

Singer, P. N. (1992), 'Some Hippocratic mind–body problems', in López Férez (ed.) (1992) 131–43

Siniscalco, P. (1984), 'Pagani e cristiani antichi di fonte all' esperienza di sogni e di visioni', in V. Branca, C. Ossola and S. Resnik (eds.), *I linguaggi del sogno*, Florence, 143–62

Sisko, J. (1996), 'Material alteration and cognitive activity in Aristotle's *De Anima*', *Phronesis* 41, 138–57

Sissa, G. (1984), ' "Une virginité sans hymen". Le corps féminin en Grèce ancienne', *Annales* 39, 1119–39

Siwek, P. (1930), *La psychophysique humaine d'après Aristote*, Paris

(1933), *Aristotelis De Anima libri tres graece et latine*, Rome

(1961), 'La clairvoyance parapsychique dans le système d'Aristote', *Sophia* 29, 296–311

(1963), *Aristoteles. Parva Naturalia graece et latine*, Rome

(1969), 'Le Dieu d'Aristote dans les dialogues', *Aquinas* 12, 11–46

Skoda, F. (1988), *Médecine ancienne et métaphore. Le vocabulaire de l'anatomie et de la pathologie en grec ancien*, Paris

Slakey, T. (1961), 'Aristotle on sense-perception', *Philosophical Review* 70, 470–84

Sluiter, I. (1995a), 'The embarrassment of imperfection: Galen's assessment of Hippocrates' linguistic merits', in van der Eijk, Horstmanshoff and Schrijvers (eds.) (1995) vol. II, 519–35

(1995b), 'The poetics of medicine', in J. G. J. Abbenes et al. (eds.), *Greek Literary Theory after Aristotle*, Amsterdam, 192–213
Smith, W. D. (1979), *The Hippocratic Tradition*, Ithaca and London
   (1980), 'The development of classical dietetic theory', in Grmek (ed.) (1980) 439–48
   (1982), 'Erasistratus' dietetic medicine', *Bulletin of the History of Medicine* 56, 398–409
   (1983), 'Analytical and catalogue structure', in F. Lasserre and P. Mudry (eds.), *Formes de pensée dans la Collection hippocratique*, Geneva, 277–84
   (1989), 'Notes on ancient medical historiography', *Bulletin of the History of Medicine* 63, 73–103
   (1990a), *Hippocrates. Pseudepigraphic Writings. Letters, Embassy, Speech from the Altar, Decree* (Studies in Ancient Medicine 2), Leiden
   (1990b), 'Pleuritis in the Hippocratic Corpus, and after', in Potter, Maloney and Desautels (eds.) (1990) 189–207
   (1992), 'Regimen, *krêsis* and the history of dietetics', in López Férez (ed.) (1992) 263–72
   (1994), *Hippocrates*, vol. VII, Cambridge, Mass. and London
Snowden, R. and Christian, B. (eds.) (1983), *Patterns and Perceptions of Menstruation. A World Health Organisation International Collaborative Study*, London
Solmsen, F. (1950), 'Tissues and the soul', *Philosophical Review* 59, 435–68
   (1955), 'Antecedents of Aristotle's psychology and scale of beings', *American Journal of Philology* 76, 148–64
   (1957), 'The vital heat, the inborn pneuma and the *aether*', *Journal of Hellenic Studies* 77, 119–23
   (1960), *Aristotle's System of the Physical World*, Ithaca and New York
   (1961a), 'αἴσθησις in Aristotelian and Epicurean thought', *Mededelingen der Koninklijke Nederlandse Academie van Wetenschappen, Afd. Letterkunde*, Nieuwe reeks 24, 241–62
   (1961b), 'Greek philosophy and the discovery of the nerves', *Museum Helveticum* 18, 151–67 and 169–97
Sorabji, R. R. K. (1971), 'Aristotle on demarcating the five senses', *Philosophical Review* 80, 55–79 (reprinted in Barnes, Schofield and Sorabji (eds.), vol. IV (1979) 76–92)
   (1972a), *Aristotle on Memory*, London
   (1972b), 'Aristotle, mathematics and colour', *The Classical Quarterly*, N.S. 22, 293–308
   (1974), 'Body and soul in Aristotle', *Philosophy* 49, 63–89 (reprinted in Barnes, Schofield and Sorabji (eds.), vol. IV (1979) 42–64)
   (1980), *Necessity, Cause and Blame*, London
   (1992), 'Intentionality and physiological processes: Aristotle's theory of sense perception', in Nussbaum and Rorty (eds.) (1992) 195–225
Souilhé, J. (1930), 'La θεία μοῖρα chez Platon', in *Philosophia Perennis. Mélanges offerts à J. Geyser*, vol. I, Regensburg, 13–25
Souques, A. (1936), *Etapes de la neurologie dans l'Antiquité grecque*, Paris

Spencer, W. G. (1935, 1938), *Celsus. De medicina*, 3 vols., Cambridge, Mass. and London
Spengel, L. (1842), *De Aristotelis libro decimo historiae animalium*, Heidelberg
Spoerri, W. (1996), 'Médecine et formes de connaissance chez Aristote, *Metaphysique* A.1', in R. Wittern and P. Pellegrin (eds.), *Hippokratische Medizin und antike Philosophie*, Hildesheim, 199–202
Sprague, R. K. (1977), 'Aristotle and the metaphysics of sleep', *Revue of Metaphysics* 31, 230–41
　(1985), 'Aristotle on red mirrors (*On Dreams* 11 459 b 24–460 a 23)', *Phronesis* 30, 323–6
Staden, H. von (1975), 'Experiment and experience in Hellenistic medicine', *Bulletin of the Institute of Classical Studies* 22, 178–99
　(1982), 'Hairesis and heresy: the case of the haireseis iatrikai', in B. F. Meyer and E. P. Sanders (eds.), *Self-Definition in the Graeco-Roman World*, London, 76–100, 199–206
　(1989), *Herophilus. The Art of Medicine in Early Alexandria*, Cambridge
　(1990), 'Incurability and hopelessness: the Hippocratic Corpus', in P. Potter, G. Maloney and J. Desautels (eds.), *La maladie et les maladies dans la Collection Hippocratique*, Quebec, 75–112
　(1991), 'Galen as historian. His use of sources on the Herophileans', in López Férez (ed.) (1991) 205–22
　(1992), 'Jaeger's "Skandalon der historischen Vernunft": Diocles, Aristotle, and Theophrastus', in W. M. Calder III (ed.), *Werner Jaeger Reconsidered* (Proceedings of the Second Oldfather Conference, University of Illinois, 26–8 April 1990), Atlanta, 227–65
　(1994a), 'Author and authority: Celsus and the construction of a scientific self', in Vázquez Buján (ed.) (1994) 103–17
　(1994b), '*Media quammodo diuersas inter sententias*: Celsus, the "Rationalists", and Erasistratus', in Sabbah and Mudry (eds.) (1994) 77–101
　(1995a), 'Anatomy as rhetoric: Galen on dissection and persuasion', *Journal of the History of Medicine* 50, 47–66
　(1995b), 'Science as text, science as history: Galen on metaphor', in van der Eijk, Horstmanshoff and Schrijvers (eds.) (1995) vol. 11, 499–518
　(1997), 'Inefficacy, error and failure: Galen on δόκιμα φάρμακα ἄπρακτα', in A. Debru (ed.), *Galen on Pharmacology. Philosophy, History and Medicine*, Leiden, 59–83
　(1999a), 'Caelius Aurelianus and the Hellenistic epoch: Erasistratus, the Empiricists, and Herophilus', in P. Mudry (ed.), *Caelius Aurelianus. Nouvelles Approches*, Nantes, 85–119
　(1999b), 'Celsus as historian?', in van der Eijk (ed.) (1999a) 251–94
　(1999c), 'Rupture and continuity. Hellenistic reflections on the history of medicine', in van der Eijk (ed.) (1999a) 143–87
Stannard, J. (1961), 'Hippocratic pharmacology', *Bulletin of the History of Medicine* 35, 497–518
Steckerl, F. (1958), *The Fragments of Praxagoras and his School*, Leiden

Stein, E. (1990), *Autorbewußtsein in der frühen griechischen Literatur*, Tübingen
Steinhauser, K. (1911), *Der Prodigienglaube und das Prodigienwesen der Griechen*, Ravensburg
Steinschneider, M. (1883–91), 'Die Parva naturalia bei den Arabern', *Zeitschrift der deutschen morgenländischen Gesellschaft* 37, 477–92 and 45, 447–53
   (1893), *Die arabischen Übersetzungen aus dem Griechischen*, Leipzig (reprinted Graz, 1960)
Stevens, P. T. (1936), 'Aristotle and the Koine. Notes on the prepositions', *The Classical Quarterly* 30, 204–17
Sticker, G. (1928–30), 'Fieber und Entzündung bei den Hippokratikern', *Sudhoffs Archiv für die Geschichte der Medizin* 20 (1928) 150–74; 22 (1929) 313–43 and 361–81; 23 (1930) 40–67
Stigen, A. (1961), 'On the alleged primacy of sight in Aristotle', *Symbolae Osloenses* 37, 15–44
Stok, F. (1994), 'Celso e gli Empirici', in Sabbah and Mudry (eds.) (1994) 63–75
Stol, M. (1983), *Zwangerschap en geboorte bij de Babyloniërs en in de Bijbel*, Leiden
   (1993), *Epilepsy in Babylonia*, Groningen
Stratton, G. M. (1917), *Theophrastus and the Greek Physiological Psychology before Aristotle*, London
Strohmaier, G. (1983), 'Al-Farabi über die verschollene Aristoteles-Schrift *Über Gesundheit und Krankheit* und über die Stellung der Medizin im System der Wissenschaften', in Irmscher and Müller (eds.) (1983) 186–9
   (1998), 'Die Fragmente griechischer Autoren in arabischen Quellen', in Burkert (ed.) (1998) 354–74
Strömberg, R. (1944), *Griechische Wortstudien. Untersuchungen zur Benennung von Tieren, Pflanzen, Körperteilen und Krankheiten*, Göteborg
   (1961), *Griechische Sprichwörter. Eine neue Sammlung*, Göteborg
Stuart Messer, W. (1958), *The Dream in Homer and Greek Tragedy*, Columbia
Stückelberger, A. (1994), *Bild und Wort. Das illustrierte Fachbuch in der antiken Naturwissenschaft, Medizin und Technik*, Mainz
   (1998), 'Vom anatomischen Atlas des Aristoteles zum geographischen Atlas des Ptolemaios: Beobachtungen zu wissenschaftlichen Bilddokumentationen', in Kullmann, Althoff and Asper (eds.) (1998) 287–307
Suárez de la Torre, E. (1973), 'El sueño y la fenomenología onírica en Aristóteles', *Cuadernos de Filología Clásica* 5, 279–311
Susemihl, F. (1884), *Aristoteles. Ethica Eudemia*, Leipzig
   (1885), 'Zu den sogenannten *Parva Naturalia* des Aristoteles', *Philologus* 44, 579–82
   (1891–2), *Geschichte der griechischen Litteratur in der Alexandrinerzeit*, 2 vols., Leipzig
Swiggers, P. (1984), 'Cognitive aspects of Aristotle's theory of metaphor', *Glotta* 62, 40–5
Tassinari, P. (1994), 'Il trattato sulle febbri dello ps. Alessandro d'Afrodisia', *ANRW* 11.37.2, 2019–24

Tecusan, M. (2004), *The Fragments of the Methodists*, vol. 1: *Methodism outside Soranus*, Leiden
Tellenbach, H. (1961), *Melancholie*, Heidelberg
Temkin, O. (1933), 'Views on epilepsy in the Hippocratic period', *Bulletin of the History of Medicine* 1, 41–4
  (1935a), 'Celsus *On Medicine* and the ancient medical sects', *Bulletin of the History of Medicine* 3, 249–64
  (1935b), 'Studies on late Alexandrian medicine, 1: Alexandrian commentaries on Galen's *De sectis ad introducendos*', *Bulletin of the History of Medicine* 3, 405–30 (reprinted in O. Temkin, *The Double Face of Janus*, Baltimore and London 1977, 178–97)
  (1936), 'Epilepsy in an anonymous Greek work on acute and chronic diseases', *Bulletin of the History of Medicine* 4, 137–44
  (1956), *Soranus' Gynecology*, Baltimore
  (1971), *The Falling Sickness. A History of Epilepsy from the Greeks to the Beginnings of Modern Neurology*, 2nd edn, Baltimore and London
Theiler, W. (1959), *Aristoteles. Über die Seele*, Berlin
Thesleff, H. (1966), 'Scientific and technical style in early Greek prose', *Arctos* 4, 89–113
Thielscher, P. (1948), 'Die relative Chronologie der erhaltenen Schriften des Aristoteles nach den bestimmten Selbstzitaten', *Philologus* 97, 229–65
Thivel, A. (1965), 'La doctrine des *perissomata* et ses parallèles hippocratiques', *Revue de Philologie* 39, 266–82
  (1975), 'Le "divin" dans la Collection Hippocratique', in Bourgey and Jouanna (eds.) (1975) 57–76
Throm, H. (1932), *Die Thesis*, Paderborn
Tieleman, T. L. (1991), 'Diogenes of Babylon and Stoic embryology: Ps.Plutarch, *Plac.* v 15.4 reconsidered', *Mnemosyne* 44, 106–25
  (1995), 'Galenus over de zetel van het verstand. Medisch experiment en filosofische traditie', *Gewina* 18, 230–42
  (1996), *Galen and Chrysippus on the Soul*, Leiden
  (2001), 'Galen on the seat of the intellect: anatomical experiment and philosophical tradition', in C. J. Tuplin and T. E. Rihll (eds.), *Science and Mathematics in Ancient Greek Culture*, Oxford, 256–73
Tigner, S. S. (1970), 'Plato's philosophical uses of the dream metaphor', *American Journal of Philology* 91, 204–12
Timken-Zinkann, R. F. (1968), 'Black bile. A review of recent attempts to trace the origins of the teachings on melancholia to medical observations', *Medical History* 12, 288–92
Todd, R. B. (1977), 'Galenic medical ideas in the Greek Aristotelian commentators', *Symbolae Osloenses* 52, 117–34
  (1984), 'Philosophy and medicine in John Philoponus' commentary on Aristotle's *De anima*', *Dumbarton Oaks Papers* 38, 103–10
Toohey, P. (1990), 'Some ancient histories of literary melancholia', *Illinois Classical Studies* 15, 143–61

Torraca, L. (1965), 'Diocle di Caristo, il Corpus Hippocraticum ed Aristotele', *Sophia* 33, 105–15
Toulmin, S. (1958), *The Uses of Argument*, Cambridge
Tracy, T. J. (1969), *Physiological Theory and the Doctrine of the Mean in Plato and Aristotle*, The Hague and Paris
  (1983), 'Heart and Soul in Aristotle', in J. Anton and A. Preus (eds.), *Essays in Ancient Greek Philosophy*, vol. 11, Albany, 321–39
Tricot, J. (1951), *Aristote. Parva Naturalia*, Paris
  (1957), *Aristote. Histoire des animaux*, 3 vols., Paris
Ullmann, M. (1970), *Die Medizin im Islam* (Handbuch der Orientalistik, 1. Abt., Ergänzungsband VI/1), Leiden
Ulmer, K. (1953), *Wahrheit, Kunst und Natur bei Aristoteles*, Tübingen
Usener, K. (1990), ' "Schreiben" im Corpus Hippocraticum', in W. Kullmann and M. Reichel (eds.), *Der Übergang von der Mündlichkeit zur Literatur bei den Griechen*, Tübingen, 291–99
Usener, S. (1994), *Isokrates, Platon und ihr Publikum. Hörer und Leser von Literatur im 4. Jh. v. Chr.*, Tübingen
Vallance, J. (1990), *The Lost Theory of Asclepiades of Bithynia*, Oxford
  (1993), 'The medical system of Asclepiades of Bithynia', *ANRW* 11.37.1, 693–727
  (1996), 'Diocles (3)', *Oxford Classical Dictionary*, 470
Vázquez Buján, M. E. (1991), 'Compréhension, traduction, adaptation. De Caelius Aurélianus aux traductions littérales du VIe siècle', in Sabbah (ed.) (1991) 87–97
  (ed.) (1994), *Tradición e Innovación de la Medicina Latina de la Antigüedad y de la Alta Edad Media*, Santiago de Compostela
  (1999), 'La nature textuelle de l'œuvre de Caelius Aurelianus' in P. Mudry (ed.), *Caelius Aurelianus. Nouvelles Approches*, Lausanne, 121–40
Vegetti, M. (1966–9), 'La medicina in Platone, I–IV', *Rivista critica di storia della filosofia* 21 (1966) 3–39; 22 (1967) 251–70; 23 (1968) 251–67; 24 (1969) 3–22
  (1999), 'Tradition and truth. Forms of philosophical-scientific historiography in Galen's *De placitis*', in van der Eijk (ed.) (1999a) 333–58
Vegléris, E. (1982), 'Platon et le rêve de la nuit', *Ktema* 7, 53–65
Verbeke, G. (1945), *L'évolution de la doctrine du pneuma*, Paris and Louvain
  (1961), 'Philosophie et conceptions préphilosophiques chez Aristote', *Revue Philosophique de Louvain* 59, 405–30
  (1978), 'Doctrine du pneuma et entelechisme chez Aristote', in Lloyd and Owen (eds.) (1978) 191–214
  (1985), 'Happiness and chance in Aristotle', in Gotthelf (ed.) (1985) 247–58
Verdenius, W. J. (1952), 'Platons Gottesbegriff', in *La notion du divin depuis Homère jusqu' à Platon* (Entretiens sur l'Antiquité Classique 1), Vandœuvres and Geneva, 241–93
  (1960), 'Traditional and personal elements in Aristotle's religion', *Phronesis* 5, 56–70
  (1962), 'Der Begriff der Mania in Platons *Phaidros*', *Archiv für die Geschichte der Philosophie* 44, 132–50

(1971), 'Human reason and God in the *Eudemian Ethics*', in Moraux and Harlfinger (eds.) (1971) 285–98
(1985), 'The nature of Aristotle's scholarly writings', in Wiesner (ed.) (1985) vol. 1, 12–21
Vernant, J.-P. (ed.) (1974), *Divination et rationalité*, Paris
Versnel, H. S. (1990), *Inconsistencies in Greek and Roman Religion*, vol. 1, Leiden
Vicaire, P. (1970), 'Platon et la divination', *Revue des Etudes Grecques* 83, 333–50
Vidal, M. (1959), 'La theophilia dans la pensée religieuse des Grecs', *Recherches des sciences religieuses* 47, 161–84
Vitrac, B. (1989), *Médecine et philosophie au temps d'Hippocrate*, Saint-Denis
Vlastos, G. (1945, 1946), 'Ethics and physics in Democritus', *Philosophical Review* 54, 578–92 and 55, 53–64
  (1952), 'Theology and philosophy in early Greek thought', *Philosophical Quarterly* 2, 97–123
Vogel, C. (1956), *Zur Entstehung der hippokratischen Viersäftelehre*, Marburg
Volprecht, A. (1895), *Die physiologischen Anschauungen des Aristoteles*, Greifswald
Wachsmuth, C. (1860), *Die Ansichten der Stoiker über Mantik und Dämonen*, Leipzig
Wachsmuth, D. (1975), 'Winddämonen, -kult' *Der kleine Pauly*, 5, 1380–1
Wagenvoort, H. (1946), *Imperium. Studiën over het 'Mana'-begrip in zeden en taal der Romeinen*, Amsterdam and Paris
Wagner, D. (1970), *Das Problem einer theonomen Ethik bei Aristoteles*, Heidelberg
Wagner-Simon, T. and Benedetti, G. (eds.) (1984), *Traum und Träumen. Traumanalysen in Wissenschaft, Religion und Kunst*, Göttingen
Walzer, R. (1929), *Magna moralia und Eudemische Ethik*, Berlin
  (1944), *Galen. On Medical Experience*, Oxford
  (1957), 'Al-Farabi's theory of prophecy and divination', *Journal of Hellenic Studies* 77, 142–8
Walzer, R. and Mingay, J. (eds.) (1991), *Aristotelis Ethica Eudemia*, Oxford
Wardale, W. L. (1940), 'Diocles of Carystus and German popular medicine', *Medium Aevum* 9, 61–78
Waschkies, H.-J. (1993), 'Mündliche, graphische und schriftliche Vermittlung von geometrischem Wissen im Alten Orient und bei den Griechen', in Kullmann and Althoff (eds.) (1993) 39–70
Waszink, J. H. (1941), 'Die sogenannte Fünfteilung der Träume bei Calcidius und ihre Quellen', *Mnemosyne* 9, 65–85
  (1947a), *Quinti Septimi Florentis Tertulliani De anima*, Amsterdam
  (1947b), 'Traces of Aristotle's lost dialogues in Tertullian', *Vigiliae Christianae* 1, 137–49
Waterlow, S. (1982), *Nature, Change and Agency in Aristotle's Physics*, Oxford
Watson, G. (1982), 'Φαντασία in Aristotle's De anima 3.3', *The Classical Quarterly* 32, 100–13
  (1988a), *Phantasia in Classical Thought*, Galway
  (1988b), 'Discovering the imagination: Platonists and Stoics on *phantasia*', in J. Dillon and A. A. Long (eds.), *The Question of Eclecticism. Studies in Later Greek Philosophy*, Berkeley and Los Angeles, 208–33

Webb, P. (1982), 'Bodily structure and psychic faculties in Aristotle's theory of perception', *Hermes* 110, 25–50

Wedin, M. V. (1988), *Mind and Imagination in Aristotle*, London

(1989), 'Aristotle on the mechanics of thought', *Ancient Philosophy* 9, 67–86

(1994), 'Aristotle on the mind's self-motion', in M. L. Gill and J. G. Lennox (eds.), *Self-Motion. From Aristotle to Newton*, Princeton, 81–116

Wehrli, F. (1951a), 'Antike Gedanken über Voraussagung der Zukunft', *Archives suisses des traditions populaires* 66 (also in *Heimat und Humanität, Festschrift für K. Meuli*, 225–32)

(1951b), 'Der Arztvergleich bei Platon', *Museum Helveticum* 8, 177–86

(1951c), 'Ethik und Medizin. Zur Vorgeschichte der aristotelischen Mesonlehre', *Museum Helveticum* 8, 36–62

(1967–9), *Die Schule des Aristoteles. Texte und Kommentare*, 10 vols., 2nd edn, Basel and Stuttgart

Weidauer, K. (1954), *Thukydides und die hippokratischen Schriften*, Heidelberg

Weideger, P. (1976), *Menstruation and Menopause: the Physiology and Psychology, the Myth and the Reality*, New York

Weinreich, O. (1928), 'Zum Zauber des Menstralblutes', *Archiv für Religionswissenschaft* 26, 150–1

Weiss, H. (1942), *Kausalität und Zufall in der Philosophie des Aristoteles*, Basel

Wellmann, M. (1895), *Die pneumatische Schule bis auf Archigenes* (Philologische Untersuchungen 14), Berlin

(1898), 'Das älteste Kräuterbuch der Griechen', in *Festgabe für F. Susemihl. Zur Geschichte griechischer Wissenschaft und Dichtung*, Leipzig, 1–31

(1900), 'Zur Geschichte der Medizin im Altertum', *Hermes* 35, 349–67

(1901), *Die Fragmente der sikelischen Ärzte Akron, Philistion und des Diokles von Karystos* (Fragmentsammlung der griechischen Ärzte, vol 1), Berlin

(1903), 'Diokles von Karystos', *RE* IX, 802–12

(1912), 'Zu Diokles von Karystos', *Hermes* 47, 160

(1913), 'Zu Diokles', *Hermes* 48, 464–8

(1919), 'Eine pythagoreische Urkunde des IV. Jahrhunderts v. Chr.', *Hermes* 54, 225–48

(1922), 'Der Verfasser des Anonymus Londinensis', *Hermes* 57, 396–429

(1924), 'Über Träume', *Sudhoffs Archiv für die Geschichte der Medizin* 16, 70–2

(1931), *Hippokratesglossare*, Berlin

Welsch, W. (1987), *Aisthesis. Grundzüge und Perspektiven der Aristotelischen Sinneslehre*, Stuttgart

Wendland, P. (1902), 'Die Textkonstitution der Aristotelischen Schrift περὶ αἰσθήσεως καὶ αἰσθητῶν', in *Festschrift für Th. Gomperz*, Vienna, 173–84

Wenskus, O. (1982), *Ringkomposition, anaphorisch-rekapitulierende Verbindung und anknüpfende Wiederholung im hippokratischen Corpus*, Frankfurt

(1983), 'Vergleich und Beweis im Corpus Hippocraticum', in Lasserre and Mudry (eds.) (1983) 393–406

Westerink, L.G. (1964), 'Philosophy and medicine in late antiquity', *Janus* 51, 169–77

(1985–94), *Stephani Atheniensi in Hippocratis Aphorismos commentaria* (*CMG* XI 1, 3), 3 vols., Berlin
Wetzel, J. G. (1931), *Quomodo poetae epici et Graeci et Romani somnia descripserunt*, Berlin
Wieland, W. (1962), *Die aristotelische Physik*, Göttingen
Wiersma, W. (1943), 'Die aristotelische Lehre vom Pneuma', *Mnemosyne* 11, 102–7
Wiesner, J. (1978), 'The unity of the treatise *De somno* and the physiological explanation of sleep in Aristotle', in Lloyd and Owen (eds.) (1978) 241–80
  (ed.) (1985–7), *Aristoteles. Werk und Wirkung*, 2 vols., Berlin
  (1985), 'Gedächtnis und Denkobjekte. Beobachtungen zu Mem. 1, 449 b 30–450 a 15', in Wiesner (ed.) (1985–7), vol. 1, 168–90
  (1998), 'Aristoteles über das Wesen der Erinnerung. Eine Analyse von de memoria 2, 451 a 18–b 10', in J. Holzhausen (ed.), *Psuche, Seele, Anima. Karin Alt zum 7. Mai 1998*, Stuttgart, 121–31
Wijsenbeek-Wijler, H. (1976), *Aristotle's Concept of Soul, Sleep and Dreams*, Amsterdam
Wilamowitz-Moellendorf, U. von (1902), *Griechisches Lesebuch*, 2 vols., Berlin
Wili, W. (1955), 'Probleme der aristotelischen Seelenlehre', *Eranos-Jahrbuch* 12, 55–93
Wilkins, J., Harvey, D. and Dobson, M. (eds.) (1995), *Food in Antiquity*, Exeter
Williams, C. J. F. (1982), *Aristotle. De Generatione et Corruptione*, Oxford
Wingate, S. D. (1931), *The Mediaeval Latin Versions of the Aristotelian Scientific Corpus, with Special Reference to the Biological Works*, London
Withington, E. T. (1928), *Hippocrates*, vol. III, Cambridge, Mass. and London
Wittern, R. (1974), *Die hippokratische Schrift De morbis I*, Hildesheim and New York
  (1979), 'Die Unterlassung ärztlicher Hilfeleistung in der griechischen Medizin der klassischen Zeit', *Münchener Medizinische Wochenschrift* 121.21, 731–4
  (1998), 'Gattungen medizinischer Literatur im Corpus Hippocraticum', in Kullmann, Althoff and Asper (eds.) (1998) 17–36
Wöhlers, M. (1999), *Heilige Krankheit. Epilepsie in antiker Medizin, Astrologie und Religion*, Marburg
Wöhrle, G. (1986), 'Zu den Experimenten in den biologischen Schriften des Aristoteles', *Eos* 74, 61–7
  (1990), *Studien zur Theorie der antiken Gesundheitslehre* (Hermes Einzelschriften 56), Stuttgart
  (1992), 'Zur Prosa der milesischen Philosophen', *Würzburger Jahrbücher für die Altertumswissenschaft* 18, 33–47
  (1993a), 'War Parmenides ein schlechter Dichter? Oder: Zur Form der Wissensvermittlung in der frühgriechischen Philosophie', in Kullmann and Althoff (eds.) (1993) 167–80
  (1993b), 'Xenophanes als didaktischer Dichter', *Elenchos* 14, 5–18
  (1995), *Hypnos der Allbezwinger*, Eine Studie zum literarischen Bild des Schlafes in der griechischen Antike, Stuttgart
Woods, M. J. (1982), *Aristotle's Eudemian Ethics. Books I, II and VIII*, Oxford

(1992a), *Aristotle's Eudemian Ethics. Books I, II and VIII*, Oxford (second revised edition of Woods (1982))

(1992b), 'Aristotle on sleep and dreams', *Apeiron* 25, 179–88 (= review of Gallop (1996) [1990])

Woolf, R. (1999), 'The coloration of Aristotelian eye-jelly: a note on *On Dreams* 459B–460A', *Journal of the History of Philosophy* 37, 385–91

Woollam, D. H. M. (1958), 'Concepts of the brain and its functions in classical antiquity', in F. L. N. Poynter (ed.), *The History and Philosophy of Knowledge of the Brain and its Functions*, Springfield, Ill. and Oxford, 5–18

Wright, J. (1920), 'The theory of the pneuma in Aristotle', *New York Medical Journal* 112, 893–900

Yates, F. (1966), *The Art of Memory*, London

Zeller, E. (1879), *Die Philosophie der Griechen, in ihrer geschichtlichen Entwicklung*, part 2, section 2, Leipzig

Zhmud, L. (1997), *Wissenschaft, Philosophie und Religion im frühen Pythagoreismus*, Berlin

Index of passages cited

AESCHINES
3.124   245 n.26

AETIUS
5.9   270 n.46
5.14   270 n.46

ANAXIMANDER
DK A 15   50 n.14
DK A 35   55 n.27
DK A 42   55 n.27
DK B 3   50 n.14

ANAXIMENES
DK A 5   55 n.29
DK A 7   55 n.29

ANONYMUS LONDINIENSIS
IV 13–15   120 n.4
V 37   264 n.22
VI 42   264 n.22

ANONYMUS PARISINUS
3   134

APOLLONIUS
Mirabilia
3   173 n.11

ARISTOPHANES
Aves
724   245 n.26

Vespae
515–17   254 n.58

ARISTOTELES ET CORPUS ARISTOTELICUM
Analytica priora
24 a 20   293 n.61
26 b 23   293 n.62
29 a 7–10   293 n.62

Analytica posteriora
89 b 10ff.   231 n.83
100 a 1ff.   220 n.47
100 a 15ff.   220 n.47

De anima
1.1   209
402 a 5–6   207 n.3
403 a 3-b 16   67 n.90
403 a 8ff.   209 n.11
403 a 8–10   233 n.91
402 a 9   209 n.11; 218 n.44
403 a 16   236 n.100
403 a 25   207 n.5
407 a 32–3   220 n.47
408 b 9   233 n.90
408 b 19–31   224
408 b 24–5   233 n.92
408 b 29   233 n.92
412 a 15   208 n.9
412 a 19–21   207 n.4
412 a 21   208 n.9
412 a 25–6   177 n.23
412 b 5   208 n.9
412 b 12   208 n.9
414 a 22   208 n.9
414 a 26   208 n.9
415 a 26   235
416 a 14   235
2.5   265 n.29
417 a 4–5   207 n.6
2.7   211
420 a 9ff.   207 n.6
421 a 22ff.   212; 226
421 a 23ff.   166
421 a 25   213 n.22
421 b 27–422 a 7   207 n.6
422 b 1   207 n.6
423 a 2ff.   207 n.6
425 b 1   153 n.56
3.2   211 n.17

379

427 b 15	218 n.44	464 a 15	203 n.56
429 a 5–8	224	464 a 15–16	172 n.9
429 a 7–8	176 n.21	464 a 17	203 n.56
3.4–5	217	464 a 19–21	189; 241; 246
3.4–8	209; 233; 237	464 a 20	244
429 a 23–5	130 n.29	464 a 22	234 n.93
429 a 27–8	130 n.29	464 a 24–5	213 n.22
429 a 30-b 6	177 n.22	464 a 24–7	146 n.34; 188
430 a 17–18	176 n.20; 209 n.12	464 a 25	149 n.39
430 a 22–3	176 n.20; 209 n.12	464 a 26	142 n.14
431 a 17	218 n.44	464 a 27	146 n.31
431 b 2	218 n.44	464 a 27–32	188
432 a 3ff.	218 n.44	464 a 32-b 5	188
		464 a 32ff.	143ff.; 146 n.34; 147; 165

De caelo

271 a 33	245 n.27

464 a 33	231 n.83
464 b 1	145 n.28
464 b 1–11	181
464 b 2–3	161 n.78

De divinatione per somnum

462 b 20–2	241; 243	464 b 7	145 n.28; 146 n.31
462 b 24–6	187; 188	464 b 7–16	220 n.49
463 a 3–7	192	464 b 9–10	145; 203 n.55
463 a 3–21	154 n.59	464 b 9–16	171
463 a 3–30	172 n.9	464 b 9ff.	146
463 a 4–5	182; 198; 263 n.16	464 b 10–12	188
463 a 5–7	154 n.58	464 b 16	146 n.31
463 a 7–11	199		
463 a 7–21	197	*De generatione animalium*	
463 a 11–18	187	1–2	265
463 a 19–20	187	1.17–18	35 n.46
463 a 21ff.	174	723 a 29–33	266 n.31
463 a 22–4	187	724 a 4ff.	153
463 a 25	146	725 a 15–16	153
463 b 1–2	172 n.9	725 b 6–18	161 n.74
463 b 1–4	187	727 b 7	270 nn.48–9; 271
463 b 1–11	189; 201	727 b 7–11	272 n.60
463 b 12	187	727 b 9–11	272 n.60
463 b 12–18	189; 204	728 a 10ff.	161 n.74
463 b 12ff.	143f.	729 a 21f.	271 n.53
463 b 14	204; 246; 257	736 a 19	161 n.74
463 b 15	148	736 b 28–9	176 n.20; 209 n.12
463 b 15–18	241	736 b 31ff.	235 n.99
463 b 15–22	220 n.49	737 a 25	235 n.97
463 b 16	146 n.31	737 b 4–7	232 n.86
463 b 16ff.	146 n.31	737 b 28–32	273
463 b 17	150; 161 n.74; 166	738 a 8	153 n.54
463 b 17–22	187	738 a 29	154 n.57
463 b 17ff.	143ff.	739 a 3	273 n.62
463 b 18	146 n.33; 241	739 a 3–5	273 n.64
463 b 22	187	739 a 21	271
463 b 22–3	172 n.9	739 a 28	272 n.59
463 b 22–31	204	739 a 32ff.	272 n.61
464 a 1–4	188	739 a 35	271 n.56
464 a 4	181	739 b 16ff.	271 n.54
464 a 6–19	201	739 b 31–2	232 n.86
464 a 10	203 n.56	743 b 26	222 n.58

744 a 30	228	459 b 7ff.	238 n.39
746 b 16ff.	274 n.67	459 b 10–11	180
746 b 16–25	267 n.36; 269	459 b 11–13	180
746 b 28	270 n.48	459 b 13–18	180
747 a 13ff.	270 n.48	459 b 18–20	180
748 a 21	272 n.59	459 b 20–2	180
749 a 4	223 n.60	459 b 23–460 a 23	180
758 a 30–b 3	93 n.42	460 a 6–7	180 n.24
760 b 27–32	170 n.6	460 a 26–32	180
760 b 27ff.	135	460 b 4–16	181
4	265	460 b 18–19	234 n.96
766 a 15ff.	235 n.97	460 b 21–2	234 n.96
767 a 24	266 n.31	460 b 22–3	181
767 a 25	266 n.31	460 b 26–7	181
767 b 10ff.	235 n.97	460 b 28–461 a 8	182; 197
770 b 10ff.	214 n.26	460 b 29–30	172 n.9
771 b 22–3	270 n.48	461 a 1–3	181
771 b 27ff.	274	461 a 3	183
772 b 30ff.	235 n.97	461 a 6	183
774 a 22	270 n.48	461 a 7	183
775 b 36–7	270	461 a 8–25	220 n.49
776 a 2	273	461 a 8ff.	185
5	210–11	461 a 9ff.	174
5.1	213	461 a 10	256 n.65
778 a 23ff.	213 n.22	461 a 10ff.	145 n.30
779 a 12f.	213 n.22	461 a 11	146 n.33; 147
779 a 13	181	461 a 11–12	181
779 b 22	15	461 a 12	181; 213 n.22
780 b 10	235 n.97	461 a 13	203 n.55
780 b 15ff.	213 n.23	461 a 14ff.	145; 147; 203 n.55
781 a 2	229 n.77	461 a 18–27	181
781 a 21	15	461 a 21–2	181
781 b 12	229 n.77	461 a 22	143ff.; 157 n.66
781 b 20	213 n.24; 222 n.57	461 a 22–3	145; 148 n.36
783 b 29–30	161 n.74	461 a 23–5	221 n.52
786 b 23ff.	211 n.15	461 a 23–4	148
788 a 13	82 n.20	461 a 23–5	161 n.74
788 a 34–b 2	211 n.15	461 a 24	146 n.33
		461 a 25	183; 226 n.71
De generatione et corruptione		461 a 31	183
336 b 27	245 n.27	461 b 3ff.	234 n.96
		461 b 3–7	181
De insomniis		461 b 4	183
458 b 1	179	461 b 11	183 n.26
458 b 5–10	179	461 b 11ff.	226 n.71; 238 n.39
458 b 7	180	461 b 25	234 n.96
458 b 13–15	180	461 b 27	183 n.26
458 b 18–23	180	462 a 1	181
459 a 1–8	179	462 a 2–8	181
459 a 6–8	176	462 a 4	234 n.96
459 a 15	182	462 a 6	234 n.96
459 a 17–18	182	462 a 9–15	185
459 a 21	182	462 a 10–11	181
459 a 23	179	462 a 12	213 n.22
459 a 24	179	462 a 12–15	181

462 a 15–31	184	644 a 17	232 n.86
462 a 19–25	181	644 b 2–3	283 n.13
462 a 25–6	181	645 b 15–28	208 n.8
462 a 29–30	176	645 b 24	232 n.86
462 a 31-b 11	203 n.55	647 b 11–13	142 n.16
		648 a 2ff.	129 n.24; 166; 225; 236 n.105

De interpretatione

16 b 20	220 n.47	648 b 34ff.	161 n.74; 167 n.91
		649 a 24ff.	143 n.21

De iuventute et senectute

3–4	130 n.29	649 a 26	153
468 b 32ff.	129 n.21	649 b 34	153 n.56
469 a 5ff.	222 n.58	650 a 34	153 n.54
469 a 5–7	143	650 b 2	153 n.54
469 b 5–6	222 n.58	650 b 5	153 n.54
469 b 16	211 n.17	650 b 12	153 n.54
		650 b 18ff.	166
		650 b 19ff.	129 n.24; 225; 236 n.105

De longitudine et brevitate vitae

464 b 32ff.	154 n.58; 194 n.42; 263 n.16	650 b 27	161 n.74
466 b 5–9	154 n.57	2.7	129 n.30
		652 b 10ff.	235
		653 a 2	153

De memoria

		653 a 8ff.	194 n.42; 263 n.16
449 b 10	254 n.56	653 a 10	154 n.58
449 b 12	254 n.59	653 a 30	221 n.54
449 b 31–450 a 1	218 n.44	653 b 5	224
450 a 27ff.	38; 228	656 b 5	129 n.24
450 b 1–11	223	660 a 12	226 n.73
450 b 2	213 n.22	3.4	130 n.29
450 b 6	223 n.62	667 a 11ff.	225 n.67; 235 n.98
450 b 8	213 n.22	672 b 16–17	222 n.58
450 b 15ff.	220 n.49	672 b 28ff.	224
451 a 9	213 n.22	672 b 28–33	161 n.74
453 a 10ff.	223	672 b 29	154; 160
453 a 14ff.	141; 145; 228–9; 234	676 b 5f.	168 n.92
453 a 15	149	676 b 11–13	152 n.51
453 a 19ff.	212 n.19	4.2	152
453 a 24	154	676 b 31–2	152; 154
453 a 25	146 n.32; 223 n.61	677 a 10–20	129
453 a 31	223	677 a 16–17	93 n.41
453 b 4	213 n.22; 223 n.62	677 a 16–19	204 n.57
453 b 23–4	160 n.73	677 a 25	152
		677 b 9–10	152 n.51

De motu animalium

		4.10	226 n.72
700 b 18ff.	250 n.41	4.10	227
701 a 27	220 n.47	686 a 7ff.	222 n.59
701 b 17ff.	235 n.99; 236 n.103	686 a 25ff.	221–2
701 b 34	235 n.99	686 a 27ff.	216 n.36
702 a 3ff.	236 n.103	686 a 31	227
703 a 15	235 n.99	686 b 23ff.	224
		686 b 26	162 n.81

De partibus animalium

		686 b 28ff.	225 n.69
1.1	209	687 a 25ff.	227
2.3	153 n.54	687 b 6ff.	216 n.35
640 b 5	193 n.35	692 a 23	161 n.74
641 a 32-b 10	209 n.11	692 b 3ff.	232 n.86

Index of passages cited

De plantis
820 b 5f.   294 n.64

De respiratione
474 b 3   143
474 b 13   211 n.17
480 a 20–3   198 n.50
480 b 22–31   194; 263 n.16
480 b 22ff.   154 n.58; 263

De sensu
436 a 8   209 n.14
436 a 17ff.   154 n.58
436 a 17-b 2   194; 263 n.16
445 a 26   148
6   211 n.17

De somno et vigilia
453 b 11–24   175
453 b 18–20   203 n.55
453 b 22–4   172 n.10; 187; 203 n.55
453 b 23–4   145 n.27; 247 n.30
453 b 26–7   185
454 a 27   176
454 b 5   176
454 b 10   176
454 b 13–14   178
454 b 15ff.   177
454 b 23   186
454 b 26   178; 186
455 a 1–2   177
2   211 n.17
455 a 6   177
455 a 13ff.   176
455 a 23   227 n.74
455 b 3ff.   176
455 b 6   177
455 b 7   177
455 b 14–16   177
455 b 18ff.   176
456 a 5   177
456 a 7ff.   158 n.68
456 a 12   177
456 a 18   178
456 a 25   178
456 a 25–6   186
456 a 25–9   178
456 b 1   178; 222 n.58
456 b 9–16   177
456 b 16   178
456 b 23   178
457 a 2   154 n.57
457 a 3ff.   213 n.22
457 a 4   178
457 a 4–11   133

457 a 10   178
457 a 16   148
457 a 16–17   161 n.74
457 a 18ff.   223 n.62
457 a 20   178
457 a 22ff.   223
457 a 25ff.   142
457 a 26   178; 213 n.22
457 a 29   161 n.74
457 a 29ff.   151
457 a 31   153; 158; 160; 161 n.74; 162
457 a 31–3   143 n.20; 143 n.21
457 b 30   178
458 a 3   153
458 a 10–25   185
458 a 15ff.   178
458 a 25–32   177
458 a 29   176

De spiritu
485 a 28ff.   94 n.42

Ethica Eudemia
1.1   164 n.83; 215 n.30
1214 a 16–24   238; 255 n.60
1215 a 12–20   257 n.66
1219 b 19ff.   244 n.23
1224 b 24   224 n.64
1225 a 25   245 n.28
1229 a 20   161 n.74
1239 a 1–6   243 n.22
1245 b 17   245 n.27
1246 b 10–12   250 n.42
8.2   162 n.81; 238–58
1247 a 2   238
1247 a 4   251
1247 a 7–13   255 n.60
1247 a 13   251
1247 a 23–31   238–40; 256
1247 a 28–9   242 n.19; 243 n.20.22; 244ff.; 256
1247 b 18ff.   240
1247 b 22   232 n.88
1247 b 29–37   251
1247 b 38–1248 a 15   256 n.65
1247 b 39   232 n.88
1248 a 7–8   253 n.50
1248 a 15   243 n.20
1248 a 15–41   247–56
1248 a 22   257
1248 a 25ff.   238–9; 244f.
1248 a 30–1   238
1248 a 32–4   239; 242 n.19; 245
1248 a 34   243 n.20

1248 a 35	242 n.18	1150 b 34	256 n.65
1248 a 38	245	1151 a 1	213 n.22
1248 a 39–40	146 n.31; 148; 241–2; 242 n.18; 244 n.24	1151 a 1–5	146 n.34; 149; 150
		1151 a 20ff.	213 n.22
1248 a 39–41	238–9; 245	1152 a 15	157 n.66; 224 n.64
1248 b 1–2	256 nn.63, 65	1152 a 17ff.	149
1248 b 3–7	238	1152 a 27	151 n.44
1248 b 4	238 n.2; 244; 256f.	1152 a 27–8	150
1249 b 3–23	244	1152 a 29	255 n.60
1249 b 16ff.	244 n.24	7.12–15	150
		1154 a 26	150
Ethica Nicomachea		1154 b 3	150
1094 b 1ff.	262 n.14	1154 b 9ff.	161 n.74
1095 a 18	193 n.38	1154 b 9–11	159 n.71
1095 b 22	193 n.38	1154 b 10	157 n.66; 224 n.64
1097 b 25ff.	214 n.28	1154 b 10–12	152 n.50
1098 a 21ff.	262 n.14	1154 b 11	214 n.27
1098 a 33-b3	93 n.41	1154 b 13	154; 159 n.72
1099 b 10ff.	243 n.21; 257 n.66	1162 a 5	244 n.25
1099 b 17ff.	214 n.29	1175 b 3ff.	224 n.64
1102 a 5 ff.	262 n.14	1177 a 13–17	250
1102 a 18–26	194–5	1177 b 27–31	250
1102 b 2–10	174	1178 b 14	243 n.22
1102 b 3–11	244 n.23	1179 a 21–30	190; 243
2.1	164 n.83	1179 a 23ff.	244 n.25
1103 a 24	215 n.30	1179 a 27–8	250
1114 b 8	232 n.88	10.9	164 n.83
1119 b 10	224 n.64	1179 b 21ff.	145 n.27; 215 n.30; 255 n.60; 257 n.66
4.3	35 n.45		
1127 b 23	193 n.39	1179 b 21–3	239
1128 a 15	193 nn.39–40	1181 a 10ff.	255 n.60
1128 a 31	193 n.39	1181 b 2–6	37 n.51
1138 b 33	283 n.13		
1139 b 19–1140 a 24	193 n.34	*Fragmenta*	
1140 a 1–23	193 n.34; 263 n.15	113–16	264 n.24
1142 b 3–6	231 n.83	123	264 n.24
1143 b 7–9	224 n.66	360	106 n.13
1144 a 24ff.	215 n.32		
1144 b 3	215 n.32	*Historia animalium*	
1144 b 9	215 n.32	487 a 2–4	142 n.16
1144 b 15–16	215 n.31	494 b 17	226 n.73
1144 b 35ff.	215 n.31	511 b 10	153
7	160	511 b 10–15	93 n.42
1145 b 8–14	213 n.22	4.8–10	210
1146 a 16ff.	213 n.22	536 b 27ff.	187; 189
1147 a 13–14	157 n.66; 224 n.64	537 b 13ff.	181; 187
1147 b 6ff.	220	537 b 14ff.	213 n.22
1147 b 7	157 n.66; 224 n.64	7–9	210
1147 b 12	157 n.66	581 b 2	213 n.22
1148 a 30	255 n.60	582 a 15	213 n.22
1150 a 16ff.	152 n.49	582 b 12ff.	272 n.59
1150 b 19	148	586 a 15	273 n.63
1150 b 25	213 n.22	586 a 16	161 n.74
1150 b 25ff.	149	588 a 31ff.	224
1150 b 29ff.	152 n.49	602 b 12–605 b 21	264 n.23

Index of passages cited

10	259–78	637 a 17	273
633 b 12–17	266 n.32	637 a 37	271 n.51
634 a 1	268 n.40	10.6	259
634 a 4–5	267 n.34	637 b 12	271 n.51
634 a 5	267 n.35	637 b 19	271; 271 n.51
634 a 12	267 n.36; 271 n.50	637 b 23–4	259 n.1
634 a 14	267 n.35	637 b 25–32	271 n.55
634 a 21	267 n.36	637 b 29	267 n.36
634 a 26	267 n.35	637 b 30–1	271
634 a 29	267 n.35	637 b 31	271 nn.51–2
634 a 34	267 n.36	638 a 1	271 n.51
634 a 37	267 n.35	638 a 8	271
634 a 39–41	267 n.36	638 a 19f.	273
634 b 7	267 n.36	638 a 20	271
634 b 10–11	267 n.36	638 b 1	273
634 b 12	267 n.35	638 b 15	269 n.44
634 b 29	271 n.51	638 b 30–1	267 n.34
634 b 30ff.	271 n.55		
634 b 31	267 n.36	*Magna moralia*	
634 b 34	273	1185 a 9ff.	244 n.23
634 b 37	271 nn.51–2	1190 a 24	93 n.42
635 a 2–4	267 n.36	1197 a 3	193 n.34; 263 n.15
635 a 7–10	267 n.34	1203 b 1–2	150; 162; 232 n.88
635 a 11	267 n.35	1206 b 28	93 n.42
635 a 12	267 n.35	2.8	240–1
635 a 12–13	267 n.34	1207 a 6–15	240
635 a 17	267 n.35	1207 a 35ff.	240
635 a 21	271 n.51		
635 a 23	267 n.35	*Metaphysica*	
635 a 31–2	266 n.33; 267 n.35	1.1	35 n.45
635 a 36	267 n.36	981 a 7	165 n.86
635 b 2	271 nn.55–6; 272 n.58	981 a 7–12	293 n.63
635 b 15–16	267 n.34	981 a 12	153 n.56
635 b 15–23	272 n.60	981 a 12–b 14	195 n.46
635 b 22ff.	271 n.55	981 b 14–982 a 3	193 n.34
635 b 27	267 n.36	983 a 5–10	245 n.27
635 b 28	269 n.43	993 b 21	262 n.13
635 b 37	271 nn.51–2	1005 b 21	293 n.62
636 a 6	271 n.51; 273	1005 b 28–9	293 n.62
636 a 10ff.	271 n.51	1006 a 6–9	92 n.41
636 a 11–12	271 n.52	1013 a 4ff.	124 n.12
636 a 25	267 n.36	1025 b 25	262 n.13
636 b 3	267 nn.35–6	1044 a 19	153 n.56
636 b 4–5	271 n.51	1059 b 29–39	93 n.42
636 b 6–10	266	1070 a 2–4	93 n.41
636 b 9	266 n.31	1071 b 19	79 n.12
636 b 11–12	267 n.35	1071 b 23	79 n.12
636 b 11–13	259 n.1	1074 b 3	245 n.27
636 b 15–16	271	1074 b 34–5	245 n.27
636 b 15–23	259 n.2	1079 a 25	243 n.22
636 b 37	271 n.51		
637 a 2	272 n.58	*Meteorologica*	
637 a 2–3	271 n.51	357 b 23–4	84 n.22
637 a 8ff.	274	3	211
637 a 15	271 n.51	4	265 n.28

Oeconomica

1344 b 10f.	294 n.64

Physica

196 b 1	243 n.22
199 a 11	296 n.75
199 b 18	296 n.75
199 b 26	296 n.75
215 a 21	296 n.75
246 b 4–5	151 n.46
247 b 1ff.	218
255 b 7	296 n.75
256 a 28–9	93 n.41

Physiognomonica

805 a 1ff.	236 n.100
805 a 3ff.	236 n.102
807 b 12	232 n.88
808 a 37	232 n.88
808 b 10	236 n.101
813 a 29	236 n.101
813 b 7ff.	213 n.22; 228 n.76; 236 n.101

Poetica

1455 a 29ff.	165
1455 a 32	232 nn.87–8; 158 n.70
1459 a 5–7	165; 232 n.87
1459 a 7	232 n.88

Politica

1254 a 2	193 n.34; 263 n.15
1254 b 30	221 n.54
1270 b 40	224
1274 a 28	245 n.56
1282 a 3–4	195 n.46
1287 a 35	37 n.51
1288 b 24	296 n.75
1290 b 22–3	84 n.22
1320 b 7	193 nn.39–40
1325 b 18	193 n.34
1327 b 20ff.	225
1342 a 6	245 n.28
1362 a 32	245 n.27

Problemata physica

1.12	168 n.92
860 a 27	153 n.56
860 b 15	153 n.56
860 b 21ff.	168 n.92
862 a 28	153 n.56
863 a 23	213 n.22
864 a 26–30	294 n.64
864 b 8–11	294 n.64
865 a 1	154 n.57
865 a 6f.	294 n.64
865 a 9–18	294 n.64
3.25a	168 n.92
878 b 16	153
4.30	168 n.92
884 a 23	154 n.57
11.38	168 n.92
14.15	225 n.68
18.1	168 n.92
916 b 7ff.	220 nn.47–8
916 b 16	220 n.48; 224 n.65
18.7	168 n.92
934 a 17	229 n.77
30.1	139ff.; 148; 155ff.; 221 n.55; 243 n.20
953 a 12–15	157
953 a 13	156
953 a 15	156
953 a 16	156
953 a 18	156
953 a 20	157
953 a 27	166
953 a 29	156
953 a 29–31	157; 157 n.65
953 a 30	159
953 a 31	156
953 a 35	158
953 a 38	158
953 b 14–15	146 n.34; 149 n.39
953 b 17	158
953 b 22	158
953 b 23–6	161 n.74
953 b 27–30	161 n.74
953 b 33–954 a 4	161 n.74
954 a 2	161 n.74
954 a 7	142 n.18; 161 n.74
954 a 7–11	143 n.19
954 a 11	158
954 a 13	157; 158; 159
954 a 14	158 n.67
954 a 14–15	160
954 a 14ff.	143 n.21; 150 n.42
954 a 15	151 n.46
954 a 18–20	161 n.74
954 a 20–1	167 n.91
954 a 21	158
954 a 21–2	161 n.74
954 a 22–3	158 n.69; 159
954 a 28–30	158
954 a 29	159
954 a 30	159
954 a 31–8	160
954 a 32	161 n.74; 165; 232 n.88
954 a 33	160
954 a 34	144 n.24
954 a 34–6	161 n.74

954 a 34–8	142 n.16; 158 n.70; 160	1390 b 28	158 n.70; 161 n.74; 232 n.88
954 a 35	224 n.65	1392 b 20	296 n.75
954 a 35–6	161 n.78	1394 a 5	165 n.86
954 b 1	157 n.64; 163	1405 a 8	165
954 b 2	161 n.77	1405 a 8–10	232 n.87
954 b 8	159	1412 a 10	165 n.86
954 b 8ff.	214 n.27	1412 a 12	165; 165 n.87
954 b 8–11	152	1412 a 13	231 n.83
954 b 12	159		
954 b 13	161 n.74	*Topica*	
954 b 24	166	100 b 20ff.	94 n.43
954 b 25	159	108 a 7–14	165 n.86
954 b 26	161 n.77	108 b 7	165 n.86
954 b 26–8	159	108 b 21	165 n.87
954 b 27–8	156	108 b 24	165 n.86
954 b 28–34	166	131 b 5–19	293 n.62
954 b 31	161 n.77	145 a 16	262 n.13
954 b 33	159	151 b 19	231 n.83
954 b 39–40	161 n.74	158 b 1ff.	93 n.41
955 a 40	214 n.27		
955 b 26–7	224 n.66	CAELIUS AURELIANUS	
956 b 39ff.	220 n.47	*De morbis acutis*	
954 a 36	158 n.70	Proem	300 n.7
954 a 39-b 4	156; 157	1.1.9	306
955 a 3	161 n.74	1.1.11	311 n.57
955 a 4	161 n.74	1.1.20	321 n.79
955 a 14	159	1.1.21	316 nn.71, 74
955 a 22–9	161 n.74	1.1.22	315 n.67
955 a 24–5	159 n.72	1.1.23	312 n.58; 315 n.65
955 a 25–8	161 n.74	1.3.34	316 n.74
955 a 29ff.	156	1.3.41	303 n.27
955 a 32–3	158 n.67	1.4.42	300 n.8
955 a 35	158	1.5.47	300 n.8
955 a 36–40	157 n.64	1.8.53–6	119–20; 303 n.24
955 a 36ff.	157	1.8.54	311 n.57
30.5	224 n.66	1.8.55	304 n.34
959 b 29	154 n.57	1.9.58	300 n.8
30.14	168 n.92	1.9.60	300 n.8
		1.11.81	323
Rhetorica		1.11.87	307
2.12–14	213 n.22	1.11.99	300 nn.5, 8
2.12–15	225	1.12.103	303 n.27
2.12–13	152; 159 n.71	1.14.105–16.165	302 n.18
2.15	166	1.14.105	299 n.1
1354 a 7	255 n.60	1.14.113	307 n.47; 308
1355 b 12	117 n.65	1.15.119	307 n.47
1362 b 4	193 n.34	1.15.121	304 n.32; 307 n.41
1362 b 24	231 n.83	1.15.124	307 n.47
1389 a 18–19	152	1.15.127	307 n.47; 324 n.93
1389 a 19ff.	161 n.74	1.15.150	307 n.47
1389 b 29ff.	161 n.74	1.16.155–65	301 n.10
1389 b 29–32	152	1.16.157	322 n.86
1390 b 24	166	1.16.165	322 n.85
1390 b 27	221 n.55	1.17.170	324 n.93
1390 b 27–30	166	2.1–9	303 n.30

2.1.5	319 n.77	3.17.138	307 n.47
2.1.6	302 n.16	3.17.154	314 n.62
2.1.8	300 n.6; 307 n.41; 316 n.71	3.17.159	107
2.3.13	304 n.32; 316 n.74	3.17.172	301 n.10
2.5.23	303 n.25	3.18.177	320
2.6.26	303 n.24	3.19.189	310; 321 n.79
2.6.30	320 n.78	3.19.190	312; 318
2.9.43	324 n.92	3.21.219	306
2.9.46	301 n.13	3.22.220–2	303 n.30
2.9.48	307 n.47	3.22.221	312 n.58; 319
2.10.58	302 n.17		
2.10.61	302 n.17	*De morbis chroniis*	
2.10.64	316	Proem	299 n.1
2.10.65	300 n.6; 311; 315	1.1	303 n.30
2.13.87	106 n.13; 264 n.21; 312	1.1.21ff.	303 n.23
2.14.93	307 n.47	1.1.30	307 n.47
2.19.121	322 n.85	1.1.33	307 nn.47–8
2.20.125	303 n.27	1.1.50	300 n.8; 301 n.10
2.26.142	316 n.70	1.2	303 n.30
2.28.147	300 n.6; 303 nn.24–5; 304 n.34	1.3	303 n.30
		1.3.55	311 n.57
2.29.155	322	1.4.101	307 n.47
2.29.156	322	1.4.105	315 n.66
2.29.160	324 n.93	1.4.129	307 n.41; 324 n.93
2.31.163	300 n.6; 316 n.74	1.4.131–3	135
2.32.172	309	1.4.132	109
2.33.176	320	1.4.135	324 nn.92, 95
2.34.180	307 n.47	1.4.83	306
2.34.183	303 n.24; 327 n.101	1.4.84	307 n.47
2.35.185	303 n.25	1.4.87	324 n.91
2.37.206	323	1.4.97	303 n.23
2.37.217	309; 319	1.5.175	324 n.91
2.38.219	323 n.90	1.5.178	324 nn.93, 95
2.39.225–40.234	302 n.18	1.6	303 n.30
3.1.2	302 n.16	2.1.14	325 n.97
3.1.4–6	313	2.1.16	300 n.3
3.1.5	318 n.76	2.1.32	307 n.47
3.4.45	314 n.62; 324 nn.93–4; 325 n.96	2.1.39	307 nn.47–8
		2.1.55–62	302 n.18
3.4.47	300 n.3; 301 n.10	2.1.60	300 n.4
3.6.62	313 n.59	2.1.60–1	301 n.10
3.6.64–5	314 n.64	2.2.64	323 n.87
3.6.64	312 n.58	2.7.96	301 n.10
3.6.65	317	2.7.109	301 n.13
3.6.66	317; 317 n.75	2.7.112	301 n.10
3.8.87	107	2.9.118	312
3.8.97	322 n.85; 324 nn.91, 93–5	2.10.125	314
3.8.98	301 n.13	2.12.145ff.	303 n.22
3.9.99	313–14	2.12.146	304 n.32; 305 n.40
3.10.101	317	2.12.147	307; 309; 325
3.14.116	323 n.89	2.14.196	312
3.14.117	304 n.34	2.14.202	324
3.15.122	323 n.90	3.1.1–2	321 n.81
3.16.136	303 n.22	3.2.19	307 n.42; 310; 326
3.16.137	323 n.90; 324 nn.91, 93	3.4.65	301 n.13; 307 n.47; 308

Index of passages cited

3.5.71	320	78	90 n.37; 129 n.26
3.8	303 n.30	79	106 n.14
4.1.5	303 n.25	80	90 n.37; 129 n.26
4.8.118	320	85	106 n.14
4.8.119	323	87	90 n.37
4.9	302	92	106 n.14
4.9.134	300 n.4	95	90 n.37
5.1	303 n.30	98	90 n.37
5.2.28	321 n.80	99	106 nn.12, 14; 109 n.17; 135 n.37
5.2.46	324; 324 n.93		
5.2.48	322 n.85	100	106 nn.12, 14; 110 n.18
5.2.51	301 n.10	103	106 n.14
5.10.91–2	309	109	90 n.37; 106 n.14
5.10.103	307 n.41	111a	106 n.14
5.10.105	326 n.99	114	106 n.14
5.11.140	323 n.88	116	106 n.14
		117	90 n.37

CELSUS
De medicina
Prooemium

4	111 n.24
5–11	103–11
47	111 n.26
54	311 n.56
57	306 n.42
59	111 n.26

DEMOSTHENES

24.192	283 n.13

DIOCLES CARYSTIUS
Fragmenta (ed. van der Eijk 2000–1)

3	74 n.1
4	74 n.1
6	37 n.51
16	99 n.57
22	97 n.50
25–8	90 n.37
26	74 n.2
27	74 n.2
28	74 n.2
33	74 n.2
36	74 n.2
49	106 n.14
52	74 n.2; 195 n.45
55a	74 n.3
55b	74 n.3–4
56	25
56b	84 n.23
57	75 n.5
61	24; 195 n.45
63	24
64	24
72	90 n.37; 120 n.4; 120 n.6
73	106 n.14

120	106 n.14
123	106 n.14
125	106 nn.12, 14; 107
128	106 n.14
129	106 n.14
131	106 n.14
132a	106 n.14
136	106 nn.12, 14
139	106 n.14
153	112 n.33
176	75; 76–100
177	25; 84 n.23; 98 n.56
182	117 n.67
183a	112 n.33
185	110 n.19
239a	96
239b	97

DIOGENES APOLLONIATES

DK A 9	55 n.29

DIOGENES LAERTIUS

5.25	154 n.58; 263
5.44	139; 167 n.91
5.62–3	96 n.49

ERASISTRATUS

fr. 117	286 n.23
fr. 156	118 n.70
fr. 176	120 n.5

GALENUS ET CORPUS GALENICUM
De alimentorum facultatibus

1.1.3 (6.454 K.)	280 n.6
1.1.4 (6.455 K.)	282 n.10
1.1.7 (6.457 K.)	280 n.5; 285 n.18; 286 n.20
1.1.7 (6.458 K.)	290 n.47

1.1.7–8 (6.457–8 K.)	281 n.9	2.1 (12.524 K.)	292 n.57
1.1.8 (6.458 K.)	286 n.23	2.1 (12.526 K.)	281 n.7
1.1.9 (6.459 K.)	291 n.49	2.1 (12.529 K.)	281 n.7
1.1.9–10 (6.459 K.)	286 n.24	2.1 (12.532 K.)	281 n.7
1.1.11 (6.460 K.)	295 n.69	3.1 (12.619 K.)	281 n.7
1.1.12–15 (6.460–2 K.)	287 n.25	3.1 (12.620 K.)	284 n.14
1.1.16ff. (6.462ff. K.)	81 n.16	5.1 (12.805ff. K.)	289 n.39
1.1.16–17 (6.462 K.)	287 n.26	5.1 (12.807 K.)	294 n.65
1.1.24–9 (6.467–70 K.)	288 n.36	5.5 (12.884 K.)	283 n.12
1.1.26–8 (6.468–70 K.)	287 n.28	6.1 (12.894 K.)	37 n.53
1.1.27 (6.469 K.)	81 n.17; 98 n.54; 286 n.21	7.2 (13.14ff. K.)	289 n.39
		7.6 (13.107–8 K.)	281 n.7
1.1.30–2 (6.470–1 K.)	287 n.27	8.6 (13.188 K.)	280 n.3
1.1.33 (6.472 K.)	280 n.7; 286 n.21; 294 n.65; 295 n.70	9.1 (13.229 K.)	281 n.7
1.1.34 (6.472 K.)	287 n.31	*De definitionibus medicis*	
1.1.40–1 (6.475–6 K.)	287 n.29	9 (19.351 K.)	117 n.68
1.1.42–3 (6.477 K.)	287 n.30		
1.1.43 (6.478 K.)	281 n.9; 286 nn.21–2	*De diebus decretoriis*	
		2.2 (9.842–3 K.)	281 n.9
1.1.44 (6.478 K.)	290 n.48	2.6 (9.872 K.)	281 n.9
1.1.45 (6.479 K.)	98 n.54; 283 n.13		
1.1.45–6 (6.479 K.)	281 n.9; 286 n.21	*De dignotione pulsuum*	
1.1.46 (6.479 K.)	98 n.54; 283 n.13; 298 n.81	1.7 (8.803 K.)	283 n.11
		2.2 (8.848–52 K.)	281 n.9
1.1.47 (6.480 K.)	37 n.53		
1.12.1 (6.508 K.)	98 n.54; 281 n.9; 285 n.17; 298 n.81	*De experientia medica*	
		1 (pp. 85f. Walzer)	292 n.58
2.59 (6.648 K.)	281 n.9; 285 n.17	13.4–5 (p. 109 Walzer)	99
3.29 (6.723 K.)	280 n.7		
		De locis affectis	
De antidotis		2.8 (8.108 K.)	284 n.13
1.2 (14.12 K.)	280 n.6	3.3 (8.142 K.)	292 n.55
De compositione medicamentorum per genera		*De methodo medendi*	
1.1 (13.366 K.)	292 n.57	1.1 (10.5 K.)	315 n.68
1.4 (13.376 K.)	280 n.6	1.3 (10.30 K.)	315 n.68
1.6 (13.401 K.)	288 n.35	2.5 (10.109 K.)	315 n.68
1.14 (13.426 K.)	281 n.7	2.6 (10.123 K.)	280 n.6
1.16 (13.435–6 K.)	80 n.15	2.7 (10.27 K.)	98 n.54
2.1 (13.463 K.)	292 n.57	3.1 (10.159 K.)	280 n.3
2.5 (13.502 K.)	283 nn.11–12	3.3 (10.181 K.)	281 n.9; 282 n.10; 291 n.52; 292 n.56
3.2 (13.570 K.)	284 n.13		
3.2 (13.594 K.)	292 n.57	3.7 (10.204 K.)	98 n.54; 281 n.9; 292 n.56
4.5 (13.681–2 K.)	281 n.7		
4.5 (13.706f. K.)	280 n.5	3.7 (10.207 K.)	284 n.14; 292 n.55
6.7 (13.886ff. K.)	280 n.5	5.1 (10.306 K.)	280 n.4
6.7 (13.887 K.)	280 n.4	6.4 (10.420 K.)	281 n.7
6.8 (13.891f. K.)	280 n.5	6.5 (10.425 K.)	281 n.7
6.8 (13.892 K.)	292 n.57	13.16 (10.916 K.)	280 n.6
7.4 (13.961 K.)	284 n.13	14.5 (10.962 K.)	280 n.3
De compositione medicamentorum secundum locos		*De naturalibus facultatibus*	
1.7 (12.469 K.)	282 n.10	2.8 (2.124 K.)	80 n.14
2.1 (12.498 K.)	281 n.7		

Index of passages cited

De optima secta
32 (1.192–3 K.)   325 n.98

De placitis Hippocratis et Platonis
7.3.13 (5.604 K.)   293 n.59
9.6.20 (5.767–8 K.)   292 n.56

De sectis ad eos qui introducuntur
2 (1.67 K.)   291 n.53
2 (1.68 K.)   292 n.54
5 (1.75 K.)   281 n.7; 291 n.52; 292 n.58

De sectis
6 (1.79 K.)   303 n.26; 306 n.42; 321 n.82

De semine
1.1 (4.512 K.)   296 n.76

De simplicium medicamentorum temperamentis ac facultatibus
1.1 (11.380 K.)   288 n.36; 296 nn.76, 77
1.1 (11.381 K.)   285 n.19
1.2 (11.382 K.)   288 nn.35, 37
1.2–3 (11.384 K.)   295 n.68
1.3 (11.384 K.)   295 n.69
1.3 (11.385 K.)   280 n.7; 285 n.19; 288 nn.33, 36; 289 n.40
1.4 (11.386 K.)   289 n.41
1.4 (11.388 K.)   280 n.7; 294 n.65
1.11 (11.400 K.).   285 n.19; 287 n.32
1.13 (11.401ff. K.)   280 n.4
1.16 (11.412 K.)   292 n.56
1.18 (11.412 K.)   281 n.7
1.18 (11.413 K.)   289 n.43
1.21 (11.416 K.)   289 n.41
1.21 (11.418 K.)   298 n.80
1.25 (11.424–5 K.)   280 n.4
1.27 (11.428–9 K.)   287 n.28
1.27 (11.429 K.)   281 n.7
1.31 (11.435 K.)   281 n.7; 288 n.35
1.32 (11.437 K.)   289 n.44
1.33 (11.438 K.)   289 n.41
1.34 (11.440ff. K.)   297 n.78
1.34 (11.441 K.)   280 n.7; 286 n.20
1.37 (11.449 K.)   280 n.5
1.40 (11.455f. K.)   288 n.37
1.40 (11.456 K.)   280 n.6; 283 n.12
2.1 (11.459–62 K.)   280 n.5
2.2 (11.462 K.)   280 n.6
2.3 (11.466f. K.)   286 n.20
2.3 (11.467 K.)   288 n.37
2.7 (11.482 K.)   292 n.57
2.7 (11.483 K.)   98 n.54
2.7 (11.483 K.)   282; 283 n.11; 291 n.51
2.9 (11.485 K.)   289 n.41
2.10 (11.485ff. K.)   289 n.42
2.12 (11.490 K.)   281 n.7
2.20 (11.518 K.)   288 n.37
2.21 (11.518 K.)   289 nn.41–2
2.23 (11.523–5 K.)   281 n.7
3.3 (11.545 K.)   288 n.36
3.4 (11.545 K.)   288 n.35
3.6 (11.552 K.)   281 n.9; 288 n.37
3.9 (11.557 K.)   288 n.37
3.12 (11.570 K.).   287 n.27
3.13 (11.572–3 K.)   289 n.41
3.13 (11.573 K.)   281 n.9; 284; 285 n.18; 298 n.81
3.13 (11.573 K.)   98 n.54
3.20 (11.602 f. K.)   295 n.66
4.7 (11.641 K.)   289 n.42
4.7 (11.642 K.)   283 n.12
4.9 (11.650 K.)   288 n.33
4.19 (11.685 K.)   281 n.9; 285 nn.17–18; 298 n.81
4.19 (11.685 K.)   98 n.54
4.23 (11.703 K.)   98 n.54; 281 n.9; 284; 285 n.18; 298 n.81
5.1 (11.705 K.)   80 n.15; 288 nn.33, 36
5.2 (11.712–13 K.)   292 n.56
5.17 (11.760 K.)   288 n.33
5.18 (11.761–4 K.)   288 n.33
6, proem (11.791 K.)   37 n.53; 289 n.42
6.1 (11.800 K.)   98 n.54; 281 n.9; 284 n.16; 285 n.18
6.1 (11.803 K.)   280 n.7
6.1 (11.805 K.)   281 n.7; 298 n.81
7.10 (12.36 K.)   295 n.69
7.10 (12.38 K.)   98 n.54; 281 n.9; 284 n.16; 285 n.18; 298 n.81
7.10 (12.39f. K.)   289 n.42
9.2 (12.192–3 K.)   280 n.3
10.1 (12.246 K.)   281 n.9; 285 n.17
11.1 (12.350 K.)   293 n.59

De temperamentis
1.5 (1.534 K.)   280 n.6
1.9 (1.560 K.)   296 n.73
2.2 (1.590 K.)   296 n.73
3.1 (1.646–7 K.)   296 n.73
3.1 (1.647 K.)   295 n.67; 296 n.74
3.1 (1.651 K.)   295 n.66
3.1 (1.651ff. K.)   287 n.32
3.1 (1.654 K.)   288 n.33
3.1 (1.655 K.)   288 n.36
3.2 (1.655 K.)   80 n.15; 288 n.36
3.3 (1.661ff. K.)   288 n.34
3.3 (1.666 K.)   288 n.35; 296 n.72

Index of passages cited

3.4 (1.670 K.)	288 n.36	*De arte*	
3.4 (1.672 K.)	288 n.35; 296 n.72	6. (6.10 L.)	112 n.27
3.5 (1.684 K.)	288 n.37	8 (6.12–14 L.)	71; 106 n.11; 112 n.27; 115 n.50; 117 n.65
3.5 (1.688 K.)	288 n.38		
3.5 (1.691 K.)	283 n.12; 289 n.39		

In Hippocratis De natura hominis commentaria
1.25–6 (15.25 K.)   264 n.22

De articulis
10 (4.104 L.)   38 n.56

In Hippocratis De victu acutorum commentarium
1.15 (15.444 K.)   283 n.11
1.17 (15.454 K.)   291 n.50

De flatibus
14.1–4 (6.110–12 L.)   132–3

In Hippocratis Prognosticon commentarium
1.30 (18b.93 K.)   281 n.7

De internis affectionibus

1 (7.172 L.)	117 n.66
5 (7.180 L.)	117 n.63
6 (7.182 L.)	115 n.55
9 (7.188 L.)	116 n.58
10 (7.190 L.)	116 n.56
10 (7.192 L.)	116 n.61
12 (7.196 L.)	116 n.56
12 (7.198 L.)	116 n.58
15 (7.204 L.)	112 n.33
17 (7.208 L.)	112 n.33
21 (7.220 L.)	116 n.58
22 (7.220 L.)	115 n.54
24 (7.228 L.)	113 n.38
26 (7. 236 L.)	115 n.52
26 (7.234 L.)	115 n.49
27 (7.238 L.)	115 n.51
29 (7.244 L.)	115 n.55
41 (7.270 L.)	115 n.51
46 (7.280 L.)	117 n.63
47 (7. 284 L.)	115 n.52
50 (7.292 L.)	113 n.37

Quod optimus medicus
1.53–6 K.   123 n.11

Subfiguratio empirica

2 (44.13ff. Deichgräber)	291 n.53
2 (45.18 D.)	292 n.54
4 (50.3 D.)	292 n.54
6–7 (54–65 D.)	291 n.50
6 (59.2 D.)	291 n.50
7 (62.12–13 D.)	291 n.50
7 (62.18ff. D.)	292 n.55
7 (64.22ff. D.)	291 n.52
7 (65.8ff. D.)	292 n.54

HERODOTUS
1.47   245 n.26

HIPPOCRATICUM CORPUS

Aphorismi

1.14 (4.462 L.)	112 n.33
1.20 (4.464 L.)	112 n.33
7.87 (4.608 L.)	113 n.28

De morbis

1.1 (6.140–2 L.)	36 n.49
1.6 (6.150–2 L.)	116 n.56
1.14 (6.164 L.)	112 n.34
2.15 (7.28 L.)	116 n.59
2.29 (7.46 L.)	116 n.59
2.48 (7.72 L.)	115 n.50
2.57 (7.88–90 L.)	115 n.55
2.73 (7.112 L.)	116 n.62
3.1 (7.118 L.)	115 n.55
3.2 (7.120 L.)	115 n.53
3.3 (7.122 L.)	116 n.60
3.5 (7.122 L.)	115 n.55
3.6 (7.124 L.)	115 n.55
3.7 (7.126 L.)	116 n.60
3.10 (7.130 L.)	115 n.55
3.11 (7.132 L.)	115 n.55
3.13 (7.134 L.)	116 n.60
3.14 (7.134–6 L.)	115 n.55
3.15 (7.140 L.)	116

De aere aquis locis

10.12 (2.50 L.)	167 n.91
16 (2.62ff. L.)	225 n.68
22	56; 191–2
22.11–12 (2.80 L.)	56 n.32

De affectionibus

4 (6.212 L.)	112 nn.29–30
9 (6.216 L.)	112 n.29
15 (6.224 L.)	112 n.29
18 (6.226 L.)	112 n.29
20 (6.230 L.)	112 n.33
27 (6.238 L.)	112 n.31
47 (6.256 L.)	101 n.2
55	88
61 (6.270 L.)	101 n.2

Index of passages cited

3.16 (7.150 L.)	114 n.44	5.8 (6.370 L.)	53 n.21
3.17 (7.156 L.)	116 n.60	7	131
		8.1 (6.374 L.)	51
De morbo sacro		8.7 (6.376 L.)	51
1.2 (6.352 L.)	46 n.7; 50; 57	8–9	52
1.3 (6.352 L.)	50 n.15	9.4 (6.378 L.)	51
1.3–4 (6.352 L.)	49 (with n.13)	10	52
1.4 (6.352 L.)	58 n.35; 61 n.39	10.2 (6.378 L.)	54, 55
1.11 (6.354 L.)	61 n.39	10.2ff. (6.378ff. L.)	51
1.12 (6.354 L.)	66	10.4 (6.378 L.)	54 n.24
1.13–14 (6.356 L.)	46 n.7	10.7 (6.380 L.)	54 n.24
1.20 (6.356 L.)	61 n.39	11	52
1.23 (6.358 L.)	47 n.9	11.1 (6.380–2 L.)	51
1.25 (6.358 L.)	47 n.9; 57; 58 n.34; 61	11.3–5	127 n.16
1.25–6 (6.358 L.)	46 n.7	11.5 (6.382 L.)	46 n.7
1.25–31 (6.358–60 L.)	46	11.6 (6.382 L.)	62; 71
1.26 (6.358 L.)	61 n.39	12.2 (6.382 L.)	46 n.7
1.27 (6.358 L.)	61	13	51; 54
1.28 (6.358 L.)	62	13.13 (6.368 L.)	46 n.7; 49; 50 n.15; 54; 58 n.35
1.28 (6.360 L.)	61 n.39		
1.28–30 (6.358–60 L.)	46	14–17	51
1.28ff.	48 n.10	16–17	126
1.29–31 (6.358–60 L.)	55 n.28	16.2 (6.390 L.)	55
1.29	62	17	120 n.4; 124 n.12
1.31 (6.360 L.)	47 n.9; 55 n.26; 57; 58 n.34; 61; 62	17.1–10 (6.392–4 L.)	46 n.7
		18	51
1.32–9 (6.360–2 L.)	58	18.1	54; 58; 59
1.39 (6.362 L.)	65	18.1–2 (6.394 L.)	46 n.7; 50; 54; 70
1.39ff. (6.362ff. L.)	46; 48 n.10; 62; 63	18.2	51; 54; 57; 58; 61; 68 n.56
1.40	66, 67		
1.41 (6.362 L.)	46; 47 n.9; 63, 66	18.3–6 (6.394–6 L.)	60, 61
1.42 (6.362 L.)	46	18.5–6 (6.396 L.)	62 n.42
1.43 (6.362 L.)	47 n.9	18.6 (6.396 L.)	46 n.7
1.43 (6.362–4 L.)	63, 66		
1.44 (6.362 L.)	60	*De natura hominis*	
1.44–5 (6.362 L.)	63, 66 n.52	1 (6.32–4 L.)	36 n.48
1.44–6 (6.362–4 L.)	64–5; 69		
1.45 (6.364 L.)	46; 61; 67	*De natura muliebri*	
1.45–6 (6.364 L.)	46 n.7; 65	1 (7.312 L.)	52 n.19; 56 n.30
1.46 (6.364 L.)	46		
2.1 (6.364 L.)	52	*De septimanis*	
2.1–2 (6.364 L.)	50 n.15; 57	45	198 n.49
2.1–3 (6.364 L.)	50		
2.3 (6.364 L.)	57; 62; 71	*De vetere medicina*	
2.4 (6.364 L.)	62 n.42	1 (1.570 L.)	106 n.10
2.4–5 (6.364 L.)	52; 191	1.1 (1.570 L.)	36 n.48
2.6 (6.366 L.)	50 n.15	1.3 (1.572 L.)	84 n.23
2.6–7 (6.366 L.)	46 n.7	2.1 (1.572 L.)	85 n.26
2.7 (6.366 L.)	47 n.9	2.3 (1.572–4 L.)	91 n.39
3.1	51; 54 n.24	3 (1.574 L.)	113 n.41
3.1 (6.364 L.)	62 n.42	5 (1.580 L.)	113 n.41
3.1 (6.366 L.)	59	7 (1.584 L.)	113 n.41
5	52	7 (1.586 L.)	114 n.47
5.1 (6.368 L.)	50 n.15; 52	11.1 (1.594 L.)	91 n.39
5.1 (6.368ff. L.)	52	12 (1.596 L.)	113 n.40

Index of passages cited

14 (1.600 L.)	117 n.66	3.10 (3.90 L.)	53 n.21
17.1–2 (1.612 L.)	89 n.35	3.16 (3.100 L.)	37
20 (1.620 L.)	106 n.9	3.16 (3.102 L.)	113 n.39
20	91 n.39; 123 n.10; 195 n.44	6.8.7 (5.346 L.)	38
20.2 (1.622 L.)	36 n.48	*Iusiurandum*	102 n.3; 112 n.27
20.3–4 (1.622 L.)	91 n.39		
21.2 (1.624 L.)	91 n.39	*Prognosticon*	
22 (1.626 L.)	113 n.40	1 (2.110 L.)	84 n.25
23.1 (1.634 L.)	91 n.39	1 (2.212 L.)	55 n.30; 71 n.62
		25	56 n.30
De victu			
1.2 (6.470–2 L.)	113 n.42	*Prorrheticon*	
1.35	128; 222 n.57	2.4 (9.20 L.)	38 n.57
1.35–6	230		
1.36	128	HOMER	
2.39	86 n.29; 88	*Odyssey*	
2.40 (6.536 L.)	91	19.560ff.	191
2.40–56	91		
2.42	91	MNESITHEUS	
2.52 (6.556 L.)	91	fr. 11	117 n.68
2.54 (6.556 L.)	91	fr. 22	88
2.56 (6.564 L.)	92		
2.76 (6.620 L.)	117 n.66	PHILOPONUS, JOHANNES	
3.67 (6.592 L.)	113 n.42	*In Arist. De anima I comment.*	
3.69 (6.606 L.)	113 n.42	p. 51,10ff. Hayduck	221 n.53
4.86 (6.640 L.)	169		
4.86–7	128	PLATO	
4.86	199	*Charmides*	
4.87 (6.640–2 L.)	172 n.10; 198 n.49	156 b 3-c 5	195
4.87 (6.642 L.)	71 n.63		
4.89.14 (6.652 L.)	71 n.63	*Ion*	
4.90.7 (6.656 L.)	71 n.63	534 c 7-d 1	245 n.28
4.93.6 (6.662 L.)	71 n.63		
		Leges	
De victu in morbos acutos		686 a	245 n.26
1 (2.224–8 L.)	38		
3 (2.238 L.)	38 n.56	*Phaedo*	
16 (2.254 L.)	38 n.56	96 b	124 n.12
41 (2.310 L.)	114 n.43	96 b 8	220 n.46
44 (2.316–18 L.)	114 n.43	100 e 6-a 1	94 n.42
64 (2.364 L.)	112 n.32		
		Phaedrus	
De victu in morbos acutos (spurium)		244 a–d	254 n.56
4 (2.400 L.)	113 n.35	244 c	67 n.55
8 (2.408 L.)	112 n.33	265 a	156
12 (2.418 L.)	112 n.33	270c–d	24
27 (2.448 L.)	112 n.33		
32 (2.462 L.)	112 n.33	*Respublica*	
56–7 (2.508–10 L.)	113 n.36	379 a–380 c	67 n.55
		380 c 8–9	67 n.55
Epidemiae		403 eff.	118 n.69
1.5 (2.632 L.)	53 n.21	571 cff.	173
1.11 (2.634–6 L.)	101; 117 n.64	573 c 7–9	150 n.41

Timaeus
71 d	245 n.26
89 b 3–4	112 n.33
90 aff.	223 n.63

PLINIUS MAIOR
Naturalis Historia
26.10	74 n.1; 97 n.51

PLUTARCHUS
De defectu oraculorum
437 d–e	146 n.31

PRAXAGORAS
Fragmenta
100	106 n.12
101	106 n.12
102	106 n.12
103	106 n.12
104	106 n.12
105	106 n.12
106	106 n.12
107	106 n.12
108	106 n.12
109	106 n.12
111	106 n.12
112	106 n.12

PRODICUS
DK B 5	53 n.22

SCRIBONIUS LARGUS
Compositiones
praef. 5	101 n.2

SEXTUS EMPIRICUS
Pyrrhoneioi hypotyposeis
1.236ff.	321 n.82

SORANUS
Gynaecia
1.4	305 n.40; 311 n.56
1.12	318 n.76
1.19	318 n.76
1.22	303 n.26
1.29	301 n.11
1.34	307 n.47
1.35	310 n.53
1.36	318 n.76
1.38	307 n.47
1.45	303 n.25; 306 n.42
1.46	322 n.86
1.52	306 n.42; 341 n.63
2.11	307 n.47
2.46	310 n.53
3.17	311 nn.56–7
3.24	301 n.11
3.42	301 n.11
4.1–6	313 n.59
4.35	313 n.59
4.36	313 n.60
4.39	301 n.11

STEPHANUS ATHENIENSIS
Commentaria in Hippocratis Aphorismos
2.33	74 n.4

THEOPHRASTUS
De causis plantarum
2.9.8–9	94 n.42
5.2.5	94 n.42
6.9.4	94 n.42

De igne
35	167 n.91

De lapidibus
5	96 n.48

De pietate
frs. 13–14	66 n.51

Fragmenta
159	93 n.41

Historia plantarum
9	265 n.28

Metaphysica
9 b 1–13	92 n.41

(PSEUDO-?) VINDICIANUS
De semine
2	74 n.1; 96 n.48

General index

abortive 102
Academy, early 92
acoustics 264
actuality (Arist.) 295; first 177, 213
administration of drugs, mode of 288
aetiology 90 n.37; *see also* causal explanation
Aëtius (doxographus) 11
age, of patient 52, 81, 98, 152, 213, 224, 228, 230; *see also* old age, children
Aias 156
air 19, 126, 132, 145; divinity of 55
aitia (cause) 12; *aitios* 54, 59, 132; *see also prophasis*
akrasia 148ff., 220
Alcibiades 166
Alcmaeon of Croton 13, 18, 22, 39; encephalocentric theory of 125, 130
Alexander of Aphrodisias 10, 16, 28
Alexandria 14, 16, 27
alternative medicine 4
analogy 12; medicine used as 264
anaphora 36
anatomy 10, 25; Aristotle on 263; comparative 14; Diocles on 24, 26, 110
Anaxagoras 18, 19, 22; on sterility 17
Anaximander 46, 50 n.14
Anaximenes 19, 55
animals 175, 187, 207, 226; intelligence of 226, 231–2; sexual behaviour of 259
Anonymus Londiniensis 11, 16, 23, 264
Anonymus Parisinus 90 n.37
antecedent cause *see* cause
anthrōpinos 48ff., 52ff., 91
anthropocentrism 259, 262, 268
anthropology, medical 4ff.
antithesis 36, 40
aorta 119, 130
aphoristic style 39
Apollonius the Empiricist 104
apotropaeic ritual 45
Arabic dream theory 171
Aratus 34

archaeology 1, 7
archives 38
area, geographical 81, 98
Aristotle, cardiocentric theory 125; development in his ideas 206–7, 243; on epilepsy 133; on good fortune 238ff.; influence on Galen 293; on the limits of causal explanation 92; medical interests of 10–11, 14ff., 154f., 212, 230, 262ff.; on melancholy 139ff.; on the mind 130, 206ff.; on oral teaching 36, 40; organisation of knowledge 39; relationship to Diocles 24, 95ff.; on relationship between medicine and philosophy 13 ff., 123, 193ff., 263; on sleep and dreams 169ff.; on sterility 17, 259ff.; style of his writings 31, 34; on soul functions 122; theological ideas 69 n.60, 238ff.; on undemonstrables 82
Aristotle, biological works 261; medical works 262ff.; zoological works 206, 231; works: *Dissections* 263; *Eudemian Ethics* 17; *Generation of Animals* 260ff., 264ff., 272ff.; *History of Animals* 15, 175, 259ff.; *Medical Problems* 263; *Nicomachean Ethics* 95, 210, 262; *On Breath* 16; *On Divination in Sleep* 17, 21, 144ff., 156, 170, 186ff., 257f.; *On Dreams* 145ff., 170, 175, 179ff.; *On Health and Disease* 196, 263; *On Remedies* 106, 264; *On Sense Perception* 211, 216; *On Sleep and Waking* 133, 175–7; *On the Soul* 175, 206ff., 209ff., 231, 262; *Parts of Animals* 175; *Parva naturalia* 8, 11, 175, 193, 263, 206ff., 209ff., 231; *Physiognomonica* 236; *Problemata physica* 16, 27, 139ff. 155ff., 231, 263, 265, 270, 273; *Rhetoric* 210
Aristotelian style of reasoning 80, 82, 93
Aristotelianism 14
arteries, as distinct from veins 27
Asclepiades of Bithynia 11, 104, 306f., 310, 319, 321, 326
Asclepius 169; cult of 63
Asia 225
asthmatic complaints 131

396

General index

astronomers 30
atheism 46, 62
Athenaeus of Attalia 13 n.20
Attic dialect 24, 74
audience, of medical/philosophical texts 30, 257–8
authority 6, 30
authorship, multiple 260 n.4
autopsy 130
awakening 220
axioms 279

Babylonian medicine 9 n.17
balance 230; between forces in the body 130
Balme, D. 260–74
bandages, Diocles on 24, 110
Bäumker, C. 234
Bellerophontes 156
bile 152; black 140ff., 159; yellow 140, 153
bio-archaeology 1
biology 206–7
blending (*krasis*) 12
blood 129, 130–1, 132, 135; 166; in Aristotle 140, 153, 176, 185, 218, 220, 225, 230; blood ritual 131; circulation 3 n.3; cognitive role of 26; vessels 142, 178
bloodletting 112–13
body, relation to soul 124ff.; role in mental processes 17, 141–2, 164ff., 207ff., 231, 236; role in sleep 171; studies into 'the body' 8
Boerhaave, H. 3
bones 12
Borysthenes 187
botany, Diocles on 24
brain 20, 28, 119, 126, 129, 131–2, 178, 224, 228; as cause of disease 51, 59; cognitive role of 16, 26
breath 158

Caelius Aurelianus 8, 11, 29, 41, 299ff.; epistemological views 12, 299ff.; *Gynaecia* 301; as a source 107, 119, 135
captatio benevolentiae 40
cardiocentric theory 125
case histories 39
catalogue structure 34–5
catarrhs, Diocles on 110
causal explanation 12, 25, 29, 85, 261; in dietetics 91–2; of disease 90, 115; *see also* aetiology
cause 9 n.17, 45, 59, 132, 175, 188, 259ff., 289; additional 235; antecedent 303, 312ff.; concept of 12–13; in definition 318; of disease 10, 195, 305, 311; and effect 68, 79, 89; of effects of foods and drugs 78ff.; of failure to conceive 271; final 179; four Arist. causes 177, 179; hidden 311; vs. symptom 27

celestial bodies 13, 55
Celsus 10, 303; on early history of medicine 102ff.
central sense faculty 175–6, 183
chance 248–9
change 11; principles of 13
character, affected by physical factors 141, 158, 225
children 178, 181, 218–19, 223
Chinese medicine 5
cholera 310, 318
choleric 52
Christianity 302
chronic disease 116
chronic fatigue syndrome 117
Chrysippus (med.) 104, 110
class distinction between doctors 195 n.46
classification 12
cleansing 46; *see also* purification
Clearchus 27
climate 81, 98, 127, 303
climatic factors 49, 53, 68
clinical practice 13, 18
clystering 113
Cnidian sentences 38
cognition 25, 119ff.
coincidence 188, 201
cold, quality of 12, 19, 89, 143, 220, 225, 228, 230, 236, 315; as cause of disease 51, 55
colour, perception of 180
common, to soul and body 175, 209
common opinions 94 n.43
common sense faculty 170, 175, 221–2, 227
communication of medical ideas 6, 14, 24
communication studies 30
comparative study of medical history 4, 6
compartmentalisation, of medicine 110, 118
competence, claims to 6, 26
complementary medicine 4
concentration, mental 229
conception 271f.
confidentiality 26
conjecture 145, 280
consciousness 120, 127, 171–2
constituents, of nature of foodstuffs 83
constitution, of body 52, 81, 98, 213, 225, 235, 238, 246, 303; types 140ff., 148, 151
contemplation 244 n.24
convalescence 117
cookery 26, 110
cooling 133–4
corpuscular theory 29
Cos 22, 27
cosmology, framework to medicine 18
courage 225
cult, religious 47–8, 67

General index

cultural history of medicine 4, 7; of philosophy 9
curability of disease 50 n.16, 61, 71, 115

daemons 63, 239
daimonios 191; *daimonia phusis* 191, 246–7
data-collection 261
death, causes of 11
definition 12, 29, 232, 279, 315ff.; of dream 184ff.
Defoe, D. 3
deformations 213, 235, 230, 265
Deichgräber, K. 3
deism 69
deliberation 246
Demeter 53 n.22
Democritus 172; 181, 323; anatomical research of 13; on dreams 170; 201ff.; medical interests of 10, 103; on sterility 17
demonstration 315
deontology 4, 5, 101ff.
depression 156; depressive-cold expressions of melancholy 166
Dervenyi papyrus 21
descent 224
description 316
desire, concept of 17, 148
determinism 69
deviations 211, 265
diagnostic character 267
dialect, Attic 24, 74; Ionic 23
dialectics 121, 315; dialectical nature of Aristotle's works 203; presentation 35
dianoia 128, 219, 222ff., 225, 229, 233–4, 236
diaphragm 120, 126
diarrhoea 131
Dicaearchus 27
Diels, H. 3, 33
diet 52, 305, 326
dietetics 5
dietetics 76–100, 104, 123, 279ff.; Diocles on 24; division within 104–5, 110–11, 113ff.; for the treatment of disease 114, 117f.
differentia 316
digestion 133; Diocles on 24, 110
Diller, H. 3
Diocles 5, 7, 8, 23–7, 40, 123, 231 n.81; cardiocentric theory 125; on causal explanation 85ff.; criticised by Caelius Aurelianus 322f.; development of epistemological concepts 12; on epilepsy 134; familiarity with Hippocratic writings 74–5; interest in 'physics' 11; on location of the mind 129; on method of dietetics 74–100; on oral teaching 36; relation to Aristotle and Theophrastus 14, 16, 95ff.; reputation 74; on sterility 17; therapeutic views of 102, 104ff., 117ff.; on the use of experience 99; works: *Affection, Cause, Treatment* 90, 106, 115; *Archidamos* 110 n.19; *On Treatments* 106
Diogenes of Apollonia 48 n.11, 55; on the use of experience 99
Dionysus 53 n.22, 166
diorismos 280ff.
discourse analysis 4, 30–1
discovery, method of 280
disease 218, 224, 228, 236; causes of 11; as distinct from constitution 151, 154, 156; essence of 24; types of 12
disturbance, of vital functions 266
diuretic 78
divination 161 n.78, 169; rational 254ff.
divine, the 57–8, 238; character of disease 45ff.; 48ff., 54ff., 68–70; concern (*theia epimeleia*) 243, 247; dispensation (*theia moira*) 60, 67, 242, 257; intervention 5, 17, 20; movement in the soul 238, 246; principle in man 247, 250; role in healing 5, 62, 71; *see also* gods
division 12; of medicine 104, 110ff.
doctor, duties of 101ff.; gentleness of 26; judgement of 116–17; mentioned by Aristotle 193; professional status of 13; vis-à-vis 'students of nature' 11
doctor–patient relationship 101–2
Dogmatists 12, 25, 28, 77–9, 98–9, 102, 279, 315f., 319, 321ff.
dogs 189
doxography 11, 14, 41, 121, 270, 302 n.18, 321
dreamlessness 181
dreams 8, 11, 17, 128, 143ff., 241; activity of dreaming 216; classification of 190–1; contents of 171; erotic dreams 259, 271; (medical) interpretation of 169, 171; origin of 182–3
drinks 10, 14
dropsy 269 n.44
drugs 10, 14, 62, 282, 288, 294, 326; distinct from foods 99
drugsellers 19
drunkenness 145, 148, 181, 208, 218, 220, 230, 236, 315
dry 19
dualism 128, 172, 198–9
dunamis 12, 295ff.; *see also* power
dwarfs 178, 212, 221ff., 229, 235,

early modern medicine 14
earth 19
earthquakes 13, 19, 61
eclipses 19, 61
ecstasy 156; ecstatic people 212; *ekstatikos* 149
Edelstein, L. 2 n.2, 3
education 208 n.10; medical 7

Egyptian medicine 4, 9 n.17
ejaculation 259, 271f.
elementary qualities, Diocles on 24
elements, four 12, 19; of foodstuffs 83
elite physicians 19
emanatory theory of vision 211
embryo 178; status of 11
embryology 10, 14; Diocles on 24
embryonic development 11
emotion 129, 172, 181, 224, 236
Empedocles 19, 20–1, 33, 34, 156, 165, 231 n.81; haematocentric theory 125; healing activity of 13; medical interests of 10, 103; on sterility 17
empirical method 78, 85; approach to medicine 9 n.17, 123; data 134, 135; evidence 25, 121, 177–8, 282, 286; observation 130, 170; research 10
Empiricists 12, 16, 28–9, 75, 77, 80, 84, 97, 102, 105, 279, 282, 291ff., 321ff., 325
encephalocentric theory 21, 124, 135
Enlightenment 2
enthousiasmos 242 n.19; 251ff.
environment 14, 225
environmental history 1, 7
epilepsy 17, 19, 45–73, 109, 123, 127, 131ff., 156, 191; epileptic seizure 131, 177–8
epilogismos 291
epistemology 12; of medicine 14, 299ff.
Erasistratus 7, 28, 104, 110–11, 118, 326; on *horror vacui* 12; interest in 'physics' 11; on mechanical vs. teleological explanation 12; reception of Aristotelian ideas in 16; on the use of experience 99
error 265; in pharmacology 286
ethics 26; in Aristotle 17; history of medical 4; medical 7; role of nature in 214
ethnography of literature 30
ēthopoion 141, 152, 158, 166
Euclid 31
Eudemus 264
euphuia 145, 165, 227, 232
Euripides, religious beliefs of 46
Europe, Aristotle's views on 225
eutuchia 17
evacuations, Diocles on 110
evidence, medical 26; *see also* empirical method
excretions 53
exercise 113
experience 24, 78, 84–5, 195, 254f., 279ff., 282ff., 321ff.; 'practised' 291; 'qualified' 98, 280ff.; vs. reason 29
experiment 12, 135, 282, 297f.
explanation 9 n.17, 12; *see also* causal explanation
external remedies, Diocles on 110
eyes, rolling of 131

faeces 153
fainting fit 177
falsification 135
fear 156, 236
female, contribution to generation 11; reproductive anatomy 25
fertility 11; fertility test 270 n.48; *see also* infertility *and* sterility
fever 10, 11, 28, 145, 181; Diocles on 24, 110
final cause 204; *see also* cause
fire, element 19, 27, 128, 231
first person, use in scientific literature 40
flesh 226–7; people with hard 166, 213; people with soft 166, 213, 230
fluids, bodily 12, 129, 153
Föllinger, S. 261, 274
fomentations 113
foods 10, 14; Diocles on 24
foodstuffs 282, 288, 294
form–matter distinction 208, 235, 261
fortune, good (*eutuchia*) 17, good 232, 238ff.
Frede, M. 316
Fredrich, C. 86
freedom, intellectual 47–8 n.10
frenzy, Plato on 245

Galen 3, 5, 7, 8, 28–9, 40, 302, 303, 327; on Hipp. writings 21; ideas about distinguished physicians 123; on oral teaching 37; on overlap between medicine and philosophy 13; presentation of Diocles by 97; philosophy of science 12; on reason and experience 279ff.; reception of Aristotelian ideas in 14, 16; relation to Alexander 28; teleology 16; views on the history of medicine 11; works: *On the Method of Healing* 282; *On Mixtures* 287ff.; *On the Powers of Foodstuffs* 76ff., 285; *Thrasybulus* 118
gas 132
gender 213, 287, 303; studies 8
general, vs. particular 10
generalisation 89, 290
generality (*koinotēs*) 303, 325
generation 259ff.
genius 18, 165
genres 32–4
genus 12, 316, 319
Glaucias 104
gnōmē 130
Gnosticism 88
gods 5, 239; in Aristotle 238, 243 n.21, 245, 253ff.; as causes of disease 58, 60, 65, 71; as healers 62, 71; as purifiers of moral errors 65, 71; as senders of dreams 143–4, 189
Gorgianic figures of speech 33, 36

General index

Gourevitch, D. 316
gradualist view on intelligence 222, 231
grammar, ancient 14
Greeks 225
guardian deity 239
gymnastics 26
gynaecology, Diocles on 24, 110

habit 164, 208 n.10, 254f.
haematocentric theory 125, 132
haemorrhage 311, 315, 325
half-sleep 181, 185
hands, human 216, 227; clenching of 131
harm, iatrogenic 101; to do no 26
harmonics 264
Harvey 3
health, causes of 11, 194; regimen in 110, 113ff.; restoration of 114ff.
healthcare system 5, 6
heart 119, 122, 126, 129, 133–5, 177, 228; chambers of 178; cognitive role of 26; left ventricle of 130
heat 158; 218, 236; bodily 129, 273; *see also* hot
Hecataeus 23, 39
Heracles 156
Heracles, Pillars of 187–8; 202
Heraclides of Tarentum 104, 306, 323
Heraclitus 18, 22, 172; on dreams 170
herbs 24
hereditary aspects of disease 131
heritage 213
Hermotimus 173
Herodotus 23, 38–9; on dreams 170
Herophilus 7, 27–8, 104, 110; on causation 12; interest in 'physics' 11; reception of Aristotelian ideas in 16
Hesiod 50 n.14
Hippocrates 3, 5, 7, 10, 21–5, 103; Diocles presented as second to 74; as represented by Galen 327
Hippocratic medicine 20; diversity within 5
Hippocratic writers, on body–soul relationship 124; development of epistemological concepts 12; on melancholy 140, 154–5; on soul functions 122; on status of the medical art 105ff.; therapeutic principles of 26; on therapeutics 110ff.; views on location of mental functions 26–7
Hippocratic writings 2, 13, 19, 34ff., 102; anonymity of 23; diversity within 21ff.; differences with regard to Aristotle 263, 267ff., 269; known to Aristotle 14, 16; similarities with Aristotle 260, 274; works: *Airs Waters Places* 21, 34, 56, 191; *Aphorisms* 75 n.5; *Epidemics* 2, 31–2, 34, 39; *Oath* 2, 5, 21, 26, 101–2; *On Affections* 112; *On Ancient Medicine* 2, 19, 36, 75–6, 86ff., 122, 282; *On the Art of Medicine* 18, 33, 36, 269; *On Breaths* 18, 33, 36, 125, 132f, 134, 269; *On Diseases 1* 36, 115, 125; *On Diseases 2* 115, 125; *On Diseases 3* 115; *On Diseases of Women* 35; *On Fleshes* 9 n.17, 12, 18, 130, 195; *On Generation / On the Nature of the Child/On Diseases 4* 17, 269; *On the Heart* 125, 130; *On Internal Affections* 115; *On the Nature of Man* 9 n.17, 12, 18, 34, 140, 153, 155; *On the Nature of the Woman* 35 *On Places in Man* 18; *On Regimen* 5, 12, 18, 22, 27, 71–2, 75–6, 86ff., 111, 122, 127, 169–70, 172, 175, 191, 195, 198ff., 230–1; *On the Sacred Disease* 2, 5, 9 n.17, 17, 19, 34, 36, 45–73, 123, 131–2, 134, 156, 191; *Pharmakitis* 112
historiography, ancient 14
Homer 50 n.14, 182
homosexuality 302
hopelessness, of cases of disease 57, 71 n.62, 102, 115–16
hot, elementary quality of 12, 19, 89, 225, 228, 230
human, nature of disease 48ff., 51ff., 57–8
humours 9 n.17, 12, 24, 27, 90, 159; theory of 140–1, 153
hupothesis 19, 122
hygiene 14, 24–6
hylomorphism 173, 199
Hymes, D. 32–3

ileus 107
imagination 141, 144ff., 149ff., 223–4; in Aristotle 17, 170, 175, 179, 182
impiety (*asebeia*) 46, 48 n.10, 62–3, 69
impotence 56, 191
imprints 216
impulses (*hormai*) 240, 246
incantations 63, 131
incidental perception 234
incurability 62
Indian medicine 5
indication (*endeixis*) 78, 282, 303; (*tekmērion*) 12, 169
indigestion 315
inference from signs 13, 24, 27, 29; inferential reasoning 279, 282, 315
infertility, female 259ff., 262ff.; male 259, 268
inherited features 11, 265
insects 177
instability 158ff., 161, 166
institutional history of medicine 4
intellectual history 4
intellectuals, religious beliefs of 47, 70
intelligence 55, 120, 166; degrees of 222, 225, 228
intuition 231–2
invisible 84, 309

General index

Ionic dialect 23
irrational 238ff.; nature 240, 246
irrational people 257
irritable people 149, 212

Jaeger, W. 95
John Philoponus 14; medical ideas in 10, 16
judgement 176

katharsis 131
knowledge, nature of medical 28
krasis 12, 151, 157, 159
Kudlien, F. 2 n.2
Kühn, J.-H. 87

laxative 78, 82
left side of the body 52
leptomereia 289, 308
lethargy 123
life, causes of 11
lifestyle, of patient 26, 81, 98, 118, 128, 287
linguistics 1, 7; ancient 14
literacy 31, 37ff.
location of mind 26, 224; of disease in the body 120ff.
locomotion 25
logic 14, 123
longevity 11
looseness, state of 325f.
love 236
luck 106
Lyceum, Diocles and 95–6

madness 165; in relation to genius 18
magic 5, 7–8, 20, 33, 45ff., 63, 131
magicians 20, 57, 65–6
male, contribution to generation 11
man, nature of 11
mania 123, 156
manic-passionate expressions of melancholy 166
market place, medical 7, 33
master craftsman 195
materialism 128, 165 n.89, 236
mathematicians 14, 30
mean 158, 161
mechanical explanation in Aristotle 182ff., 211, 213, 216, 231
mechanics 28, 264
medical examination 266
medical literature on dreams 181, 192
medicalisation 118
medicine, diversity in 5, 18
medieval medicine 14

melancholia 123
melancholics 139ff., 181, 187, 190, 211–12, 229, 241, 253f.
melancholy, Aristotle on 17, 139ff.
Meletius of Sardes 16
memory 8, 11, 17, 128, 175, 216, 223, 228
Meno 264
menstruation 180, 259; menstrual blood 270ff.
mental apprehension 326
mental faculties 126
mental illness 10, 12, 26
metaphor 165, 232
meteorology 14, 24
Methodism 12, 28–9, 119, 299ff.
methodology 12
midwives 269
mind, location of 119ff., 224
mind–body distinction 27, 119ff.
mineralogy 24, 96
mixture 151, 157, 287; *see also krasis*
Mnesitheus 12, 78, 88, 111, 117
moisture 142, 229
mola uteri 259–60, 269–70, 272f.
monstrosities 11
moon 62
moral error 20, 66–7
moral qualification 244
moral values 5, 6
motor signals in the body 129
movement 220, 223; principle of 245
movements, of sense perception 183
mules 11

narcotics 178
narratology 30
natural 233; law 45
natural philosophy 11; 123 *see also phusis and physics*
natural scientist 194
naturalistic theology 45–6, 62, 67
nature 68, 238–9, 257, 296; Aristotle's concept of 212, 214; concept of 12; contrary to 230; of disease 49ff.; of foodstuff 78; formal 235; human 157; material 235; study of 10, 103, 175, 207; theory of, Diocles on 24; *see also phusis*
Near Eastern medicine 4
Nemesius of Emesa 10, 16
nervous system 3, 16, 28
Neuhäuser, J. 234
Nicander 34
Ninos 48 n.10
non-Western medicine 4
nous in Aristotle 122, 130, 176, 222, 233, 243, 258; in sleep 171
number theory 9 n.17

nutrition 177
nutritious 78
nutritive part of soul 235

observable 290–1, 306ff.
observation 10, 12; *see also* empirical method
offspring, multiple 260, 274
old age 10, 11, 224
old people 213
olive oil 24, 110 n.19
optic nerve 125
optics 264
orality 31, 36ff.; oral presentation 35
Oribasius 11
Origen 88
Orphism 171–2

pain 148, 181, 236
palaeopathology 7
palliative care 114
palpitations 131
parallelism 36
paranoia 224
Parmenides 20–1, 34; medical interests of 10
particular 52, 81; vs. general 10
parts, affected 303–4
passages in the body (*poroi*) 128–9, 132
pathology 14, 24, 110
pathos 148, 176
patient 101
perception, in Aristotle 17, 210ff.
Peripatetics 15–16, 27
perittōma 143, 152
peritton, to 18, 157, 161, 163, 165, 167, 221 n.55
phantasia 149ff., 165, 182; thought dependent on 218, 233
pharmacology 14, 29, 104, 111–12, 279ff., 305, 323f.
Philistion 22
Philolaus 10
philosophia, Greek concept of 19
philosophy 106; study of 7, 8ff.; overlap with medicine 10ff.; of mind 206
Philotimus, on the use of experience 99
phlegm 131, 134; in Aristotle 140, 153
phlegmatic 52
phrenes 120
phrenitis 119ff., 123
phronēsis 127, 163, 215, 232
phusa 132
phusiologia 122
phusis 12, 19, 52ff., 57, 73, 81, 82–3, 239, 257; human 141, 144f., 151, 160–1
physics 11, 15, 175
physiology 10, 14, 24, 90

piety 63
Pindar 170
pistis 12
plants 13, 172, 175, 207
Plato 12, 34, 40, 156, 165; on dietetics 118; on dreams 170, 173; medical interests of 10, 11; religious ideas 67, 69 n.60; on wandering uterus 261; works: *Timaeus* 11, 12, 125; *Republic* 21
plausible, the 303
pleasure 148–9, 181, 236
Pleistarchus 77
Pliny the Elder 97
pneuma 129, 132, 145f., 148, 158, 218, 221, 230, 260, 270, 273, 307f.; in Diocles 24, 26, 90; psychic 134
Pneumatists 321
poetry, as medium for communication of knowledge 34
poison 282, 288, 294; Diocles on 24; poisoning by doctors 102
polemical writing 88, 204
pollution (*miasma*) 20, 60, 63, 64
positivism 3, 9 n.17
possession 63, 131
postnatal purgation 52
postulate 19, 84, 106; *see also hupothesis*
potentiality 295
power (*dunamis*) 90; of foodstuffs 77ff., 280
practical science 262, 268
practitioners, medical 6
Praxagoras 23, 27, 104ff., 110; cardiocentric theory 125; on epilepsy 134; *On Treatments* 106; reception of Aristotelian ideas in 16; on the use of experience 99
prayer 5, 71–2
pregnancy 260, 273
prenatal purgation 52
preparation, of foods 287
presentism 3
Presocratic philosophy 19, 62; concept of the divine in 50
prevention of disease 25, 118
principles (*archai*) 11
prognostics 24, 110
progressivism 4
proof (*pistis*) 12
prophasis 12, 49, 51, 52ff., 54, 59, 68, 73, 132
prophecy 232; powers of 144ff., 148, 156; in sleep 172, 186ff., 241, 246
prose writing 34, 38
providence, divine 69
psuchē 127
psychosomatic disease 123
psychology 206–7

pulse 10, 27
punishment, disease as 45
purgation 52
purification 20, 47 n.10, 63, 153; divine 66–7
Pythagoras 13, 20; medical interests of 10, 103
Pythagoreanism 172, 208

qualification 280ff.
qualities, elementary 12, 19; primary and secondary 89–90, 123; of substances 79
question and answer structure 36
quick-witted people 213, 228–9

rapid eye movements 185
ratio 321ff.
Rationalists 25
rationality 9 n. 17, 46, 58, 238, 258; of man 208, 216; of Greek medicine 2, 4, 5, 7, 19
reason, vs. experience 29
reasoning 85, 219, 242, 246, 279ff., 321ff.
reception studies 31
recollection 141, 175, 216, 223, 229, 234
reflection 211
refutation, method of 280
regimen in health, Diocles on 24–5
region 287
relevance, criterion of 306
religion 63, 169; relation to medicine 20–1, 67–8
religious healing 5, 7
religious thought 45
reproduction 10–12, 259ff.
residue 143, 152, 196; *see also perittōma*
respiration 8, 10, 11
rest, state of 219
retrospective diagnosis 3
rhetoric 6, 30–1, 33, 123
right side of the body 52
ring composition 39
ritual 4, 48, 67, 131
Roman medicine 7
rootcutters 19, 110
ruling part of soul 11, 119ff.

sacrifice 71
Scepticism 28, 75, 80, 97, 121, 305; and medicine 13
Schrijvers, P. H. 302
Scythians 56, 191
season 81, 98, 127, 287, 303
sects, medical 12, 28
seed, origin of 11, 12; female 260, 270; male 260, 269, 273

self-control, lack of 148ff.
self-definition, in Greek science 41
sense perception 11, 25, 129, 172, 175, 210, 226; disturbance of 224; principle of in Aristotle 147
Serapion 104
seventh-month children 11
sex differentiation 210
Sextus Empiricus 10, 13, 303
sexual differentiation 261
sexual intercourse 259, 266
sexuality 24, 26, 110
shamanism 173
sharpness of sight 211, 213ff.
shrewdness (*deinotēs*) 215, 232
Sigerist, H. 3
sign (*sēmeion*) 12, 169, 188, 267; of failure to conceive 271; dreams as signs 192ff.
significatio 312, 316
similarity, perception of 144–5, 165
Simplicius 16
skin 230
slavery 214
sleep 11, 128, 142f., 171ff., 175; Aristotle's theory of 8, 133, 175–7, 208, 210, 216, 218, 220, 224, 230; sleepwalking 178; stages of 181, 185
slow-witted people 213, 228
smell 226–7
sobriety 208
social history of medicine 4, 7; of philosophy 9
social position of healers 6, 7
Socrates 24, 156, 165
sophists 18, religious beliefs of 46
Soranus 8, 29, 299ff.
soul 12, 127–8, 262; in Aristotle 170; faculties of 122, 207; part connected with *phusis* 17; parts of 179; principle of movement in 245; relation to body 27, 124ff.; ruling part of 11, 119ff.
sound effects 36
spasm 317
specialisation 13, 118
species 316, 319
speech event 32
sports 26
sprinkling, ritual 66
stability, principles of 13
starting points (*archai*) 82, 92 n.41
sterility 11, 17, 259ff.
Stoicism 11, 27–8, 122, 302
Strato 10, 16, 27
Sudhoff, K. 3
suicide 156
suitability (*epitēdeiotēs*) 216
summetria 266

sun 62; as cause of disease 51, 55
sunesis 127
surgery 104, 305, 326; Diocles on 24, 110; status in the Hippocratic corpus 112
symptomatology 110, 115
systematicity 9 n.17, 24–5

taste 226
teaching 164
technē 18, 195, 215
teeth, grinding of 131
tekmērion 12
teleology 190, 296, 302; teleological explanation 214
Temkin, O. 3, 310
temple medicine 33, 60, 63–4, 66 n.52, 71
temples 63, 67, 71
terminology 39
Tertullian 88
theios 48ff.
Themison 300, 323
Themistius 16
theodicy 69
theology 21, 70, 258, 302
Theophrastus 16, 92ff., 139, 167, 264; medical interests of 10–11, 27; relation to Diocles 24
theoretical nature of medicine 24–5
theoretical reasoning 177, 195
theoretical science 262
Theoris 48 n.10
therapeutics 13, 14, 18, 101ff., 114ff.; Diocles on 24, 26
Thessalus 300
thinking 12, 218; in Aristotle 17, 207ff.; bodily aspects of 207; in sleep 186
Thucydides 3, 46
touch 226–7
toxicology 110
tractatus 31
trance 178
treatment 310, 314; condition in need of 267; different methods of 110ff.; *see also* therapeutics
Tricot, J. 260
triplets 11

twins 11
typological differentiation 212

undemonstrable principles 93 n.41
understanding 127
unguents 180
universals 52, 81
unobservable 306ff., 326f.
upright position 216, 221
uterus 259; wandering 261

Vallance, J. 304
valves of the heart 28
vapours, in the body 133
variations (*diaphorai*) 208ff., 214, 217, 227, 230, 237
vascular system 11–12
vegetables 24, 110
veins, as distinct from arteries 27; people with prominent 142, 213
ventricle, left of the heart 130
vessels, blood 142, 178; *see also* blood
Vindicianus 12; *On the Seed* 110 n.19
virtue 250; natural 215, 232
visual perception 211
viva vox 37
voice 210

waking 208
waste products, bodily 12
water 19, 27, 231; element 128
weather 62
weight, bodily 221f.
Western medicine 4
wet 19
whole, as opposed to parts 24
wind 201–2; as cause of disease 51, 54
wind-pregnancy 259
wine 24, 157, 180
women 215; women studies 8
writing tablet 38

Xenophanes, religious beliefs of 46

young people 213, 221, 228–9
youth 10, 11, 152